Planet of the Toxic Metals

A Reference Book on how chronic Metal Toxicity broke the Human Spirit and our Health and how to fix it

Sacha P. Dobler

This book is dedicated to my daughter Ava Sol

Table of content

Introduction

What is happening to mankind?
We are witnessing an epidemic of chronic diseases, an unprecedented trend to self- destruction, low birth rates, decreasing intelligence and an unraveling de-facto auto- genocide, the first of its kind in human history. Men have less than half the testosterone their grandfathers used to have, a bio- chemical half-castration in 50 years. The same trend is observed for estrogen in women.
How did we get so sick and tired, infertile, angry and stupid? Only within decades?
It turns out within the abundance of toxins and endocrine disrupting chemicals, toxic (heavy) metals or toxic elements play a decisive role in all of these processes.

Are you sick and tired of being sick and tired yet?
A 2019 study referred to by Harvard Social Impact Review revealed that "88% of Americans [adults] are metabolically unhealthy, causing conditions that impact the quality of their lives." [1]
Metabolic health was defined as having optimal waist circumference, glucose, hemoglobin, blood pressure, triglycerides, high-density lipoprotein and no related medication. [2]
66 percent of all adults in the United States use prescription drugs. Three-quarters of those age 50 to 64 use prescription drugs, with an average of 13 prescription drugs in this age group. [3]
"Americans will spend half their lives taking prescription drugs." [4]

Citing the National Survey of Children's Health, the CDC says "In the United States, more **than 40% of school-aged children** and adolescents have at least one chronic health condition." [5]
And 60% of Americans live with at least one chronic disease, like heart disease and stroke, cancer or diabetes. [6]
All of these conditions, on average, can lead to or contribute to early death. When we include chronic mild ailments, close to 100% of all adults are possibly affected.

Did you know that 18 % of deaths of "all causes" in the US are attributed to lead toxicity (according to a 2018 NHANES extension study)? [7]

And these are only the cases attributed to lead, not including the other 40+ toxic metals with potential long-term chronic health effects. Toxic metals can mimic almost every known chronic disease or contribute to it.

One should almost think this would be an important aspect in the discussion of the many health risks in today's general global health crisis: Viruses, bad food, lack of exercise, stress, too much fat, sugar, and so on. Most doctors will tell you every chronic disease you have is either bad luck, bad genes or bad habits or even bad thoughts (psychosomatic), So it's generally your fault.

How is it, almost no one is talking about toxic (heavy) metals? Especially since this is one aspect for which there are established and proven remedies and prevention methods. And if a doctor tells you to have less stress, how are people expected to reduce work related stress in times of a trend to global recession and hyperinflation?

Behavioral problems and the decline of societies

In *Hormonageddon*, we explored the causes and the results of chemically induced hormonal disruption on a societal level. Testosterone levels in men are half of what they were 50 years ago. Which equates to a de-facto chemical half- castration of men. The same trend is observed for estrogen levels in women.

Among the many endocrine disrupting chemicals that contribute to this multigeneration hormonal degradation, toxic metals were mentioned only briefly in the book, a regrettable negligence on my part; which I redeem here. As it turns out, this chronic and ubiquitous metal toxicity is an important contributor to this hormonal degradation, behavior and thus the integrity of societies.

Depression, anxiety and aggression can all be caused or amplified by metal toxicity, and these conditions are not just symptoms of the disintegration of societies and the defeated attitude of people and peoples, but vice versa, the main pathway now turns out to be the following:

Chronic metal- and other toxicity - hormonal disruption and brain damage - psychological illness - societal and economic decline.

How do you expect young men to feal deep satisfaction from hard work and sacrifice when they have less than half the testosterone of the men who built - with their own hands - the infrastructure we

15

are still living of today? It is easy for healthy, high testosterone men to tell others: "just pull yourself up at the bootstraps". Even in wealthy countries in the 1980s, you could still see 65-year-old men in road construction pulling off backbreaking work all day with a pickax in a ditch, right up to the day of their retirement. I remember my schoolfriend's granddad, muscular with his white beard, working with an old-school handheld giant jackhammer, laughing on the construction site. Such a scene seems unconceivable today in the West and elsewhere. The few 65-year-olds still fit to work in heavy construction are machine operators or foremen, not ditch diggers.

Imagine the will power, perseverance and the love of life our ancestors must have had. Only 200 years ago, the average person was mostly starving and freezing, saw half of their children die, they were oppressed by tyrants and they still carried on. In the 1400s, life expectancy at birth was 32 years [8], meanwhile they were building cities and invented the modern world. Fast forward to today and we have a generation of young adults of which half are unable to work or are financially dependent. In Germany, 61 percent of young adults under 24 receive most of their income from their parents or the state. [9]

How do we expect society to function with exponentially increasing numbers of sufferers of mental illness?

"Symptoms of generalized anxiety disorder (GAD) are identical to the most common symptoms of heavy metal toxicity." [10]

Metals as toxic catalysts

Toxic metals are chemical elements that cannot be changed or converted into less toxic substances, and they often remain biologically active in the body for decades after exposure.

Of the thousands of environmental chemicals that we are exposed to these days, many are transformed while generating their deteriorating effect, they are consumed or neutralized in the reaction.

Low levels of bio-transformable toxins, such as organic chemicals, can often be excreted naturally by the body; it is primarily in toxic overload that they cause long-term organ damage and chronic disease.

Things are much different with toxic (heavy) metals: Toxic metals are toxic in all their forms and if untreated, they remain in the body for years to decades; the smallest amounts of them can accumulate and damage the body indefinitely after a certain threshold of accumulation. Theoretically, the same atom of a metal can cause perpetual damage over decades (not to a measurable degree, of course) without being consumed in the chemical reactions; the metal acts as a toxic catalyst.

It is difficult to prevent minimal heavy metal exposure in everyday life. On the plus side, toxic metals can be identified and with some reliability extracted from the body by appropriate chelating agents.

The true costs of metal toxicity

A "global, silent pandemic of neurodevelopmental toxicity" is disabling a generation of children around the world, according to neurology experts Philippe Grandjean and Philip Landrigan in a 2014 report in Lancet Neurology. [11]

The journal *Toxins* notes: "Long-term exposure to environmental toxicants is estimated to account **for 70– 90% of the risks** of acquiring chronic ailments." [12]

A 2018 study published in *The Lancet Public Health* suggests that of the **2.3 million deaths every year in the US, about 412,000 (or 18 %) are attributable to lead exposure**, of which 250,000 are from cardiovascular disease. This concerns only lead, and doesn't include the other 40+ known toxic metals.

"**The population attributable fraction of the concentration of lead in blood for all-cause mortality was 18.0%.**" [13]

So, **400,000 die every year in the US only due to lead, not including the other 40+ toxic elements such as mercury, arsenic and cadmium.**

And when we further consider the synergistic toxic effects of multiple metals - with two or more metals (each within the legal limits) having an exponentially more damaging effect - then we must assume most people alive today are affected to some extent.

But only 100,000 Americans are treated with chelation therapy per year, and only 1,000 by medical doctors. [14]

McFarland M. J. et al, 2022 stated that half of the US population was exposed to adverse **lead** levels in early childhood;

"We estimate that over 170 million Americans alive today were exposed to high-lead levels in early childhood, several million of whom were exposed to five-plus times the current reference level." [15]

How much of a toxic metal is needed to cause continuous damage in the body?

Only 70 µg (70 micrograms or 0.00007 grams) more lead in the blood of a young adult is associated with 2.3 times the odds of major depressive disorder and 4.9 times the odds of panic disorders. [16] 70 micrograms is less than the smallest speck of lead dust that you can see with the naked eye.

In peripubertal U.S. girls, **lead** and **cadmium** are associated with reproductive hormones.

Already 0.00003 grams of lead in the blood of a 10-year-old girl has a measurable negative effect on later fertility.

Here as well, that's less than the smallest speck of dust that you can see with the naked eye. [17]

Now, chelation therapy is recommended by the CDC only for persistent blood lead levels of 45 µg per dL (2.17 µmol per L) or greater. [18]

This ignores the following important facts:

1.) chronic metal poisoning does usually not show up in high blood metal levels. (Conclusive results are provided by a provoked (challenge) urine test after the administration of a chelating agent to extract the metals from the body).

2.) even very low concentrations - well below reference levels – can have detrimental chronic health effects, over longer periods of time.

3.) A combination of 2 or more toxic metals causes synergistic effects and can generate exponentially greater damage than each single metal, but combinations of multiple metals are not subject to regulations or reference levels. See 1.2.2).

"Intellectual impairment in children occurs with blood lead concentrations far **below 10 micrograms per deciliter**."

"Blood lead concentrations, even those below 10 microg per deciliter, are inversely associated with children's IQ scores at three and five years of age, and associated declines in IQ are greater at these concentrations than at higher concentrations." [19]

Endocrine disruption

Historically, heavy metal toxicity targeting the kidney or nervous system has been the focus of most research efforts. "However, accumulating evidence, particularly when studies are performed with low micromolar concentrations, indicates that heavy metals can act as endocrine-disrupting substances through specific, high-affinity pathways." [20]

"Thus far, heavy metals primarily have been described to interact with the estrogen receptor giving rise to the term metalloestrogens." [21]

Recent investigations have yielded the paradoxical observation that heavy metals mimic the biologic activity of steroid hormones, including androgens, estrogens, and glucocorticoids. [22]
"Chronic exposure to **cadmium** - even within the safety values established for cadmium - disrupts the adrenal gland activity." [23]
"**Uranium** mimics estrogen."

Progression of environmental pollution
At the end of the 20th century, emissions of the common heavy metals started to decrease in developed countries: in the UK, emissions of heavy metals fell by over 50% between 1990 and 2001.
This is a positive development on the one hand, but on the other, it must be considered that some toxic metals are being replaced with slightly less toxic metals, sometimes in greater quantities. Newly implemented toxic metals are not discussed publicly, and standard tests for humans and soil include only the known "usual suspects", not exotic metals which are introduced in industrial quantities, as in the case of rare earth metals in electromobility.
As an example of this type of shortsightedness: **lead** in plumbing is being replaced with **antimony** and **bismuth**, both are less toxic, but the long-term toxicity of chronic exposure will take decades to be established, and once antimony will be deemed too harmful, it will take yet more decades to ban it and replace it with another new element. So don't wait for the government to save you.

Prehistoric metal pollution
In case you were wondering about the title of this book: let it be known that there was nothing wrong with the planet per se. We have evolved to be exposed to the natural very low metal concentrations. The problem is the man-made toxic metal pollution from what we have been extracting from the ground.
Prehistoric humans were exposed to small amounts of heavy metals either in nature or by use of fires in huts and cave entrances. But this used to be within the range of neglectable concentrations, which still allows the body to detoxify naturally from the burden.
"In the 20th century, most humans carried concentrations of lead **100 to 1000 times higher than their prehistoric ancestors**, based on analyses of ancient skeletons." [24]
Only under rare conditions, the natural emissions cause harmful concentrations of toxic metals from volcanoes, groundwater etc. Inhabitants near active volcanoes on average have higher levels of several toxic metals.

Actual rates of metal toxicity vs. number of treated cases

In 2009, the Medical Service of Health Insurances in Bavaria, Germany stated:

"In **all persons** in Europe, especially the elderly, heavy metal toxicity from food and inhalation of pollutants must be presumed." [25]

"It is estimated that 8 to 10% of American women have **mercury** levels that would induce neurological disorders in any child they gave birth to, according to both the EPA and National Academy of Science." [26]

When a person only receives half of the ""tolerable lifetime intake" of **cadmium**, they have a 50 % increase of mortality from kidney failure compared with people with low cadmium levels, but the same regulating authorities do not recommend cadmium reducing treatment for the affected groups, but rather discourage it.

According to the *Journal of Patient Safety*, medical errors contribute to more than 400,000 deaths in the U.S. every year, and that estimate only takes hospital patients into account.

"In addition, serious harm seems to be 10- to 20-fold more common than lethal harm." [27]

The CDC says "**no safe blood lead level** in children has been identified." [28]

"The recent findings that no level of lead is considered safe for children have led the Centers for Disease Control and Prevention Advisory Committee on Childhood Lead Poisoning Prevention (ACCLPP) to remove the term "blood lead level of concern." [29]

As it stands now, the CDC's safe level for lead is zero, but at the same time, only children with blood lead levels above the reference value >3.5 µg/dL are considered intoxicated and are evaluated for treatment.

There are 74 million children under 18 in the US (2023).

In a Bangladesh study, 57.5% of the population had skin lesions caused by arsenic poisoning. [30]

In all official statistics on rates of lead toxicity, only cases with high lead levels in the blood are included, not counted are the cases of undiagnosed chronic body burden which do not show up - or only partly - in unprovoked (non-challenge) blood- or urine tests.

And chronic low-level metal toxicity can either mimic any chronic disease or contribute to it.

Infertility

"[...] in **most cases of unexplained subfertility in infertile couples or hypospadias** and/or other idiopathic diseases, a probable factor may be **Cd** reproductive toxicity." [31]
85% of cases with spermiation defects also had high lead (four times higher) and higher nickel levels than controls. [32]

Developmental damage
"Around one-in-three children globally suffer from **lead** poisoning." [33]

"An important tenet is that earlier (developmental) ages of exposure increase the impact of the endocrine-disrupting chemical or heavy metal on the normal development of reproductive organs, which may be permanently affected." [34]
In Taiwan, the mean blood lead concentration of the children with developmental delays is 7.50 µg/dL, which was significantly higher than that of the children with typical development and higher than the suggested threshold concentration of 5 µg/dL. [35]

Intelligence
A Chinese study found that every 1 microgram of **lead** in the blood of children (aged 9 - 11 years) decreased their IQ by 0.1 points.
It was concluded that the reference standard in China of 100 microgram per liter (µg/L) blood **lead** for children above 5 years old should be revised. [36] At about 2 liters of blood for a 10-year-old child, the reference level adds up to 200 microgram of total blood lead.
Thus, even when children have blood lead within the reference levels, it is officially accepted that their IQ is reduced by up to 20 points due to lead contamination.

Everyone born in the US between 1966 and 1975 had childhood levels of lead above the CDC safe levels.
From 1951- 1980, on average, 95,5% of all children had blood lead levels of clinical concern. So, most who were born over these 3 decades are now less intelligent and less healthy than they should have been.
"The average lead-linked loss in cognitive ability since 1950 was 2.6 IQ points per person as of 2015, disproportionately endured by those born between 1951 and 1980." In the latter group the lead-linked deficit is closer to 6 IQ points. [37]
These numbers were based on the CDC's blood lead level of concern of 2021 (>5 µg/dL). Just before the release of the 2022 study, the CDC revised their level of concern (reference value) to

(>3.5 µg/dL) on May 14, 2021 in favor of recommending that the CDC update the reference value to 3.5 µg/dL based on NHANES data.

Based on these values, 16% of US children, every third child globally, and every second adult in the USA are poisoned with **lead**. [38]

In short, things are even much worse than revealed in the above IQ paper.

UNICEF reported that around one in three children globally have lead levels in excess of the 5 µg/dL safe limit. [39]

"Every 1 microgram (µg) of lead in the blood of children (aged 9-11 years) decreased their IQ by 0.1 points." [40]

For a child with 2 liters of blood volume, the new safe level of 3.5 µg/dl would mean a total of 70 µg of lead in the blood, and an accepted reduction in intelligence of 7 IQ points.

Mad hatter syndrome

The classic symptom of chronic **mercury** poisoning, known as erethism [also known as mad hatter syndrome], "is a personality change comprising excessive timidity, diffidence, shyness, loss of self-confidence, anxiety, a desire to remain unobserved and unobtrusive, a pathological fear of ridicule, and an explosive loss of temper when criticized." Does that remind you of any voter demographic in 2024? [41]

"**Lead, cadmium** and **chromium** were significantly raised in newly diagnosed drug free schizophrenic patients compared with controls." Further, **chromium** and **cadmium** were significantly raised in schizophrenic patients on treatment compared with the controls. [42]

Chronic mercury poisoning and erethism has affected light house keepers and hat makers, and still is affecting dentists, goldminers and goldsmiths (see 4.11.).

Cardiovascular disease and lead

Peter Jennich reported: In December 2006, experts from the US NIH came to the conclusion that a connection between **lead** exposure and high blood pressure has been proven in many studies. [43] They established a causal link between lead exposure and high blood pressure, coronary heart disease, peripheral arterial disease and strokes, even with lead exposure that was below the previously considered "safe" limit [translation mine]. [44]

Electromagnetic and metal interactions

22

Radiological interactions enhance the damaging effects of metal toxicity. "Heavy metals and EMFs work synergistically." [45]
A multidirectional effect is observed (or a perfect storm?):
- EMFs increase the toxicity of metals in the body; and vice versa:
- Toxic metals increase the susceptibility to EMFs.
- EMFs can increase the release of metals from metal objects in the body (prosthetics and amalgam).
- EMFs reduce the body's ability to excrete toxic metals.
- Not only the presence of toxic metals can amplify the harmful effects of EMF, but also the lack of essential metals (minerals).
Such interactions may partly explain why people react very differently to wireless radiation, with some being hypersensitive and most people not noticing any effect at all.
For instance, "Co-exposure of metals such as **cadmium** & static magnetic fields (SMF) can aggravate their toxic properties." [46] (See the details in 1.5.).

Multiple metals/ synergistic effects
Robert F. Kennedy Jr. of Children's Health Defense reports:
"Multiple studies have pointed to heavy metals as the leading culprit in the cascade of neurodevelopmental disorders.
Moreover, the effects of heavy metals on cognition and behavior are synergistic: Co-exposure to multiple metals can result in increased neurotoxicity compared to single-metal exposure, in particular during early life." [47]
All throughout the literature on heavy metal toxicity, we find one of the most important treacherous mechanisms of toxic metals: Damage from combinations of several metals in low concentration can not only accumulate, but increase exponentially. The synergistic effects of multiple metals - where the concentration of each metal may be within official limits - are not considered in government regulations (see 1.2.2).
It is a highly problematic fact that those synergistic toxic potentials are not considered in health regulations and guidelines.
Upper limits for toxic metals are given for each single metal, not for the much more dangerous combinations of them.

"In single pollutant models, **arsenic** was significantly associated with reduced birth weight. The effect estimate was doubled when including **cadmium** and phthalate co-exposure." [48]

"The synergistic effect of **lead** and **mercury** is extremely neurotoxic and has been reported to be much worse than the single effects." [49]

"The multi-metal mixtures of **lead, manganese, antimony, tin** and **titanium** are negatively associated with children's IQ, and this when the concentration of each single metal is well within the reference level." [50]

Molecular biologist Ernie Hubbard says: "We now know that heavy metals are additive and synergistic." [51]

Even combinations of non- metals and metal toxins can potentiate the damage generated by the individual toxins.

Fluoride added to public water supplies boosts **lead** absorption by the body (see 7.1.5).

Inversely, deficiencies in essential metals increases the damage caused by toxic metals (see for instance 8.23.4).

Antibiotics
Here as well, a multidirectional interaction of antibiotics and toxic metals is recognized:
- Antibiotics reduce metal excretion from the body.
- Heavy metals (**copper, cobalt, cadmium, zinc** and **lead salts** "enhance the development of antimicrobial resistance in otherwise antimicrobial sensitive strains of bacteria." [52]

"High oral antibiotic usage is concerning because previous rat studies found that **oral antibiotics resulted in a near-total loss of the ability to excrete mercury.** " [53]

In mice with acute **mercury** intoxication, administration of antibiotics reduced the excretion of inorganic **mercury** in the faeces to 26% of that of control mice. [54]

Brain chemistry
"Human exposure to multiple toxic metals results in selective uptake of the metals into locus ceruleus neurons. **Decreased noradrenaline from the locus ceruleus causes multifocal damage to the blood–brain barrier,** allowing toxic metal uptake by astrocytes." [55]

"The human brain and the brains of whales and dolphins (cetaceans) are especially susceptible to a variety of toxic chemicals."

Chelation therapy
Even though the contribution of heavy metals to diet-related cancer deaths is gravely understated, already the official numbers should

raise the question why almost no doctor ever mentions heavy metal chelation in cancer prevention.

Already in the early 1960s," heavy metal detoxification (EDTA chelation therapy) of non-cancer persons has been shown to preemptively **decrease cancer mortality by 90%** in an 18-year controlled clinical study [56] (see 1.13).

Among patients with coronary heart disease and constriction of the coronary arteries, an improvement was determined **in 90 percent of patients after chelation therapy.**

65 patients were originally scheduled for bypass surgery. After chelation treatment, 58 of the bypass candidates improved so well that surgery was no longer necessary (**89.2%!**). [57]

Further, of 207 patients with circulatory heart pain (angina pectoris) who used nitroglycerin as a circulatory drug to control their pain, 189 were able to reduce their drug use after chelation therapy (91.3%!!). Most of them no longer needed nitroglycerin at all. Of 27 patients who were about to have a foot or leg amputation, surgery was avoided in 24 (88.8%). [58]

The American College for Advancement in Medicine says all Americans should know about chelation therapy. They claim "it not only removes toxins but can also remove plaque and calcifications in arteries, capillaries and veins. This implies chelation therapy could prevent the advancement of heart-related events or diseases." [59]

As it stands now, the CDC's safe level for lead is zero, but at the same time, only children with blood lead levels above the reference value >3.5 µg/dL are considered intoxicated and are evaluated for any treatment. but also, the CDC recommends effective chelation therapy only if blood lead levels are persisting at 45 µg/dL or greater. [60]

Regular preemptive chelation

Whoever is aware of the mechanisms at play would do well with regular metal testing and if necessary, professional chelation therapy with the appropriate chelation agents. If a person starts from a theoretical clean slate from conception and birth onward, and is not exposed to excess workplace or environmental heavy metal loads later on, regular testing and if necessary, light and harmless chelation regiments can continuously extract most metals from the bloodstream, before they are deposited in the tissue. From conception onwards means the future mother can be treated with chelation months before conception, never during pregnancy.

The rise and fall of civilizations

"Hard times create strong men, strong men create good times, good times create weak men, and weak men create hard times."

The quote is from a post-apocalyptic novel by the author G. Michael Hopf. [61] Many civilizations have declined in undergoing a process of *'oikophobia'* which has been defined as "the fear or hatred of home or one's own society or civilization."

Most philosophical and political approaches to solve humanity's current problems are futile because they don't pay any heed to chemically induced changes in human behavior, sentiments and persuasions.

In the current era, as most humans now can technically be called epigenetically and endocrinal modified organisms, cynics could justifiably alter Hopf's phrase to:

"People suffering from toxic metals and nanoparticles create hard times!"

Chapter 1
Toxic metals last forever

1.1 Thousands of environmental chemicals

The true cost of pollution

Gilles-Eric Séralini, Professor of Molecular Biology at the University of Caen, said this:

"We need to understand the combined and long-term effects of pollutants in our body. These are probably responsible for 80% of the diseases that will affect human health in the 21st century, in particular, cancers and hormonal diseases. [...] our bodies have become pollutant sponges."

More than 400 pollutants are established in the genes of human fetuses. [62]

Dr. Bryan Stern alleges:

"The list of symptoms related to **mercury** intoxication alone includes virtually any illness known to mankind. Simply put, **mercury** can mimic any illness - or contribute to it." [63]

This encompasses any chronic physical as well as psychological disease.

1.2 Multiple metals

Robert F. Kennedy Jr. of Children's Health Defense reports:

"Multiple studies have pointed to heavy metals as the leading culprit in the cascade of neurodevelopmental disorders.

Moreover, the effects of heavy metals on cognition and behavior are synergistic: Co-exposure to multiple metals can result in increased neurotoxicity compared to single-metal exposure, in particular during early life." [64]

Research indicates, for example, that ADHD and problems such as sleep disturbances are more prevalent in children who live near coal ash (which contains metals such as **lead, mercury** and **arsenic**). [65]

Children with autism have significantly higher blood levels of **arsenic** and **mercury** compared to healthy controls. [66]

And autistic children have higher levels of **mercury, lead** and **aluminum** in their hair compared to matched controls. [67]
"Environmental toxins are causing widespread brain injury and loss of function across a generation of children." [68]
One meta-analysis of nine observational studies showed exposure to **cadmium** is associated to a moderate increased risk of death from all causes. [69]

A "global, silent pandemic of neurodevelopmental toxicity" is disabling a generation of children around the world, according to neurology experts Philippe Grandjean and Philip Landrigan in a 2014 report in Lancet Neurology. [70]
The journal *Toxins* notes: "Long-term exposure to environmental toxicants is estimated to account for 70–90% of the risks of acquiring chronic ailments. Presently, chronic kidney disease and infertility affect a significant proportion of the world population, while research data indicate that exposure to toxic metals may contribute to the looming statistics." [71]

1.2.1 Safe levels are not safe

The Centers for Disease Control and Prevention (CDC) says 'no safe blood lead level in children has been identified." [72]
"The recent findings that no level of lead is considered safe for children have led the Centers for Disease Control and Prevention Advisory Committee on Childhood Lead Poisoning Prevention (ACCLPP) **to remove the term "blood lead level of concern."** [73]
As it stands now, the CDC's safe level for lead is zero, but at the same time, only children with blood lead levels above the reference value >3.5 µg/dL are considered intoxicated and are evaluated for any treatment. But at the same time, the CDC recommends effective chelation therapy only if blood lead levels are persisting at 45 µg/dL or greater. [74]
In a similar vein, when a person only receives half of the ""tolerable lifetime intake" of cadmium, they have a 50 % increase of mortality from kidney failure compared with people with low cadmium levels, but the same regulating authorities do not recommend and even discourage cadmium reducing treatment for the affected groups.

In a 35-year follow-up study in Japan, it was found that a life-time **cadmium** intake of 1 g was associated with a 49% increase in mortality from kidney failure. "Of note, a lifetime cadmium intake of 1 g is half of a "tolerable" lifetime intake guideline of 2 g." [75]

1.2.2 Multiple metals - synergistic effects

All throughout the literature on heavy metal toxicity, we find one of the most important treacherous mechanisms of toxic metals: Damage from combinations of several metals in low concentration can not only accumulate, but increase exponentially. The synergistic effects of multiple metals - where the concentration of each metal may be within official limits – are not considered in official regulations.

For example:

Assume one unit of mercury causes a certain damage (severity 1). One unit of lead causes a certain damage of (severity 1).

But one unit mercury combined with one unit of lead at the same time may cause damage of severity 10.

This mechanism is also well known in animal lethality models. One group of animals is given a LD 10 dose of mercury (Lethal Dose 10, meaning a dose of mercury high enough that 10 percent die. Another group is given LD 10 of lead. if a third group receives LD10 of mercury and LD 10 of lead, the result is not LD 20, but LD 100: all animals die.

Those synergistic toxic potentials are not considered in health regulations and guidelines.
Upper limits for toxic metals are given for each single metal, not for the much more dangerous combinations of them.

"As an example, synergistic effects of multiple metals present at slightly lower concentration than the Australian investigation level can induce phytotoxicity in an ecosystem." [76]

In single pollutant models, **arsenic** was significantly associated with reduced birth weight. The effect estimate was doubled when including **cadmium** and phthalate co-exposure. [77]

"The synergistic effect of **lead** and **mercury** is extremely neurotoxic and has been reported to be much worse than the single effects." [78]

Sri Lankan Agricultural Nephropathy (SAN), a new form of chronic kidney disease among paddy farmers was first reported in 1994 and has now become the most debilitating public health issue in the dry zone of Sri Lanka. Of 19 tested heavy metals, 12 metals and glyphosate levels were greatly increased in SAN patients.

The researchers concluded:
"Although we could not localize a single nephrotoxin as the culprit for SAN, multiple heavy metals and glyphosates may play a role in the pathogenesis." [79]
The multi-metal mixtures of **lead, manganese, antimony, tin** and **titanium** are negatively associated with children's IQ, and this when the concentration of each single metal is well within the reference level. [80] (See also intelligence, 4.17)

A systematic risk characterization related to the long-term dietary exposure of the population to potentially toxic elements showed that the cumulative toxicity was mainly driven by **thallium** and **vanadium**. [81]
Molecular biologist Ernie Hubbard says: "We now know that heavy metals are additive and synergistic. If you get a little thallium, and a little lead, and a little cadmium in your system, you've got one plus one plus one equals five or six, not just three. The reason is that metals and chemicals might each have different effects by themselves, but they "share similar sites of action where they disrupt metabolism." [82]
Metal plus Non-metal pollutants
Even combinations of non- metals and metal toxins can potentiate the damage generated by the individual toxins.
Fluoride added to public water supplies boosts **lead** absorption by the body (see 7.1.5).
Co-exposure with either cadmium or lead with PFAS has a synergistic damaging effect on kidney function. [83]
"The synergistic effects of microplastics (MPs) and heavy metals are becoming major threats to aquatic life and human well-being." [84]

Further, deficiencies in essential metals increases the damage caused by toxic metals (see for instance 8.23.4).

1.3 Toxic metals last forever

In the environment, metals (elements) cannot be broken down and are not biodegradable. Differently from molecular pollutants, as chemical elements, metals can only be transformed into other elements by nuclear reactions.
The safest thing we can do to protect ourselves from toxic metals, is to leave them in the ground. The biological half-life in the body of **lead, mercury** and **arsenic** ranges from 20 to 40 years. A half-life

of 30 years means after 30 years, half of the metal is still in the body; after 60 years, ¼ of the metal is still in the body and so on.
Of the most dangerous toxic substances, the first 3 are the toxic metals **lead, mercury** and **cadmium, arsenic** is ranked 7th (see Table 2). The fourth most toxic substance is the non-metal compound vinyl chloride, a precursor to vinyl plastics. Incidentally, the production of vinyl chloride monomer consumes also 21% of the global mercury production, closing the cycle to toxic metals. Long term exposure to vinyl chloride at a high dose can cause chronic disease, mostly in factory workers. Thus, accumulated damage can cause chronic disease, but extremely small amounts of vinyl chloride do not accumulate over years and decades in the body to cause chronic illness.
Things are much different with toxic heavy metals: the smallest amounts can accumulate and damage the body indefinitely after a certain threshold of accumulation, the same atom of a metal can cause damage over decades.
Metal poisoning may be acute, sub-acute or chronic.
Swaran Flora et al explain: "Usually, acute poisoning is well defined and identifiable, with serious rapid manifestations that may be recovered with immediate medical attention. However, the sub chronic toxicity that may convert to chronic metal toxicities may be ill defined as **general ill health and not identifiable as any classical syndrome**. Moreover, the chronic toxicities may be reversible or irreversible leading to slow development of manifestations like cancer or teratogenic malformations after a latent period." [85]

1.3.1 Metals as toxic catalysts

Biotransfomable chemicals can be excreted naturally by the body, toxic heavy metals only under ideal circumstances.
Of the thousands of environmental chemicals, toxic metals can be relatively easily identified and extracted from the body by appropriate chelating agents. It is difficult to prevent minimal heavy metal exposure in everyday life.
Toxic heavy metals are toxic in all their forms and if untreated, they remain in the body for years to decades to a lifetime, and during this time, they can perpetually damage cells and disrupt every biological function, without being consumed in the chemical reactions, they act as **toxic catalysts**.

1.3.2 Preemptive metal detoxification

Only 100,000 Americans receive some form of chelation each year, while most people have metal levels above the reference values. The 2007 National Health Statistics Report noted an increase of 68%, from 66,000 to 111,000 adults using chelation therapy in the 5 years between 2002 and 2007. [86]

Of these 100,000+ Americans who receive chelation each year, "far fewer than 1 % of these cases are managed by medical toxicologists." [87]

M. Ferrero, 2016: "Chelation therapy is the only procedure able to remove toxic metals from human organs and tissue, aiming to treat damage related to acute and/or chronic intoxication." [88]

The Aetna Clinical Policy Bulletins state:

Chelation therapy with appropriate chelating agents is an established treatment not only for heavy metal (arsenic, cadmium, copper, gold, iron, mercury) poisoning, but also for biliary cirrhosis, **Cooley's anemia (thalassemia major), cystinuria, Wilson's disease, and sickle cell anemia, i.e., secondary hemachromatosis (iron overload from multiple transfusions)."** [89]

For well-informed people, it could be relatively easy to regularly detox from the accumulated heavy metal burden from everyday life via chelation therapy before this becomes harmful.

In *Hormonageddon*, I had pointed out how many bureaucrats defended or covered up the risks to the general public in countless environmental health scandals or accidental public health risks, even though they themselves and their family were exposed to the same toxins:

Lead paint, leaded gasoline, thalidomide causing deformed limbs in babies [90], X-rays directly into the doctor's face, arsenic in newspapers, spraying DDT into children's faces, radioactive bottled water, mercury as treatment for syphilis, radium radioactive watch dials…and so on.

Many who should have known better, small bureaucrats and industrialists, went along even though they were affected themselves. For decades, they had leaded gasoline car exhaust blown in their own and their children's faces, just like everyone else, until the early 2000s.

Today, well-informed people could get tested routinely and undergo regular chelation even for low level metal burden - given, they don't work in high-risk occupations, lead smelting, arsenic industry or other exposure leading to acute heavy metal toxicity. Some private clinics like the Fort Wayne IV Chelation Lounge recommend testing to be performed every 2-3 years to determine heavy metal levels and if needed, chelation with an EDTA I.V. which is complemented with glutathione, vitamin C, magnesium, B vitamins, minerals, and a fiber-rich diet. [91]

And you don't need to be well-connected, either, already reading some of the hundreds of studies going back to the 1960s - such as the 90% cancer reduction by preemptive EDTA chelation - could prompt someone to say: where can I do this? As the TACT study revealed, patients who already had a heart attack and subsequently underwent chelation therapy showed an 18% reduction of vascular events like heart attacks/strokes compared to placebo group. A subgroup of participants that were diabetic had a 39% reduction in risk.

Read the details on preemptive chelation in 1.13.

Now, let's assume someone has a 'good' doctor, who does a routine checkup every year, and performs not only a toxic metal blood test, but also a provoked (challenge) heavy metal urine test, and if indicated, they do a routine protocol, even for low levels of heavy metals, sort of like a routine engine cleaning procedure, and this is called a routine detox treatment.

The key element here is that acute heavy metal burden from recent mild exposure can be removed relatively easily and with almost no side effects, if detected early and treated. But long-term accumulation or heavy burden from years or decades past is difficult and more dangerous to chelate out of the body, as the toxic metals are deposited in bones, fat tissue and the brain. In such cases, unprofessional chelation attempts with pharmaceutical chelation agents can be dangerous and might induce organ damage.

Even naturopathic detoxification methods with chlorella, cilantro and the like can be counterproductive and even dangerous if applied falsely. These agents mostly remobilize metals within the body, actual excretion works only under ideal circumstances.

A person who routinely gets tested and treated for even low amounts of toxic metals will be much less affected by normal, everyday toxic metal exposure over the years, and will not have the accumulated metal burden of the average person.

Plus, if the body is relatively free from toxic metals, it is much more resistant against other (molecular, organic) toxins and pathogens.

The rare side effects in chelation procedures are usually from the toxic metals themselves, when they get temporarily remobilized from long term storage in tissue such as bones and organs, before they are excreted. Even when a pharmaceutical chelator molecule can bind a metal ion securely, the metal ion can still disrupt hormones, neurons and enzymes on its way out.

When talking about chelation in this book, we are primarily talking about "real" pharmaceutical chelating agents such as DMSA, DMPS, EDTA and Prussian Blue. Naturopathic heavy metal detox agents such as chlorella and cilantro are discussed as complementary options.
Today's regulated upper levels for toxic metals are suboptimal and most people (arguably all people) have needless deficits in health and wellbeing due to toxic metal accumulation. Which is particularly true for combinations of multiple metals, as we saw above.

1.4 Definition of toxic metals

According to Mosby et al. 1996, "There are **35 metals that are of concern for us because of residential or occupational exposure, out of which 23** are heavy metals:
Antimony, arsenic, bismuth, cadmium, cerium, *chromium, cobalt, copper*, gallium, gold, *iron*, lead, *manganese*, mercury, nickel, platinum, silver, tellurium, thallium, tin, uranium, vanadium, and *zinc*. [92] Other lists also include osmium, rhodium, ruthenium, iridium, palladium and gadolinium. [93]
Our complete list in Chapter 8 comprises 48 non-essential toxic metals. The elements in the periodic table in Fig. 4 are mostly non-essential metals; in *Italic* are essential elements which are toxic in overdose.
Another non-essential toxic metal is aluminum (it is chemically not classified as a heavy metal).
Gadolinium (as used in MRI contrast agents) and all other rare earth metals as well as all radioactive elements should be added to the list.
As we saw above, not much is known about the long-term health effects of the other rare earth metals other than gadolinium. But since all metals of these high densities for which experimental data exists, are toxic: all rare earth metals and all elements of higher atomic mass than iodine (53) should be treated as toxic until proven otherwise.

"There is no consensus chemical definition of a heavy metal. [94] Recently, it was proposed to replace the term "Heavy Metals" with "Potentially toxic elements (PTEs)". The term 'potentially', however, could lead to a decreased awareness of the toxicity of non-essential metals. All toxic non-essential elements are biologically harmful. Disputes revolve around how much of which metal is how harmful. They have no place in the human body. [95]

In this text, when we refer to heavy metals, we mean primarily non-essential toxic metals, but also essential metals which are toxic in overload (See Fig. 4).

1.5 Electromagnetic and metal interactions

Radiological interactions enhance the damaging effects of metal toxicity.

Theresa Dale, PhD, writes, "We are more susceptible to receive harmful radiation from cell phones, cell towers, etc., due to our level of toxicity in heavy metals." [96]

We can summarize the multidirectional interactions as follows:
- EMFs increase the toxicity of metals in the body and vice versa:
- Toxic metals increase the susceptibility to EMFs.
- EMFs can increase the release of metals from metal objects in the body (prosthetics and amalgam).
- EMFs reduce the body's ability to excrete toxic metals.
- The lack of essential metals (minerals) can amplify the harmful effects of EMF.

"Heavy metal toxicity increases the risk of electromagnetic sensitivity." [97]

"Heavy metals and EMFs work synergistically. A **lead** burden, for example, in the presence of EMF, exacerbates the oxidative damage to plasma proteins as well as the conformational changes in haemoglobin." [98]

"Co-exposure of metals such as **cadmium** & static magnetic fields (SMF) can aggravate their toxic properties, leading, in one study, to increased oxidative damage in rat brain tissue." [99]

A 2018 study showed that EMFs emitted from mobile phones significantly increased the level of **nickel** release from metal prosthetics (orthodontic braces). [100]

Similarly, in 2008, it was found that MRI and microwave radiation emitted from mobile phones significantly release **mercury** from dental amalgam restoration. [101] The findings were confirmed in a later study.[102]

In 2015, Mortazavi and coworkers further corroborated that static magnetic field as well as microwave radiation emitted from mobile phones induced **mercury** to evaporate from amalgam fillings more rapidly. [103]

"**Copper** is highly reactive with strong electrical conductivity. With the large amounts of electrical and magnetic field activity in our environment as a result of electrical grids, telephone poles and wireless, this can result in the creation of excessive free radical activity within the body." [104]

According to research by Dr Yoshiaki Omura, MD, "the more polluted your body is with heavy metals from amalgam fillings, contaminated food and environmental pollutants, the more it acts as a virtual antenna, concentrating radiation, making it far more damaging." [105]

A meta-analysis of 65 studies noted a potential for a synergy of EMF/EMR and toxic metals in autistic children exposed to both. "The children showed a disproportionately increased vulnerability to oxidative stress, impaired neurological adaptability, and increased heavy metal accumulation." [106]

"In these autistic children, heavy metal detoxification was greatly facilitated by the elimination of RF from the treatment environment." [107]

"Another meta-analysis revealed "a synergistic effect exposure occurred primarily when the EMF preceded the exposure to the toxic chemical." [108]

Not only the presence of toxic metals can amplify the harmful effects of EMF, but also the lack of essential metals (minerals).

"It appears that the development of oxidative stress associated with static magnetic field exposure can be ameliorated by **zinc** administration. " [109]

With exposure to EMF at power densities well below current exposure limits, glutathione concentration was found to decrease significantly. [110]

"With increasing RF exposure, the capacity to excrete toxic substances, including metals, may be reduced." [111]

"Metal objects implanted in a human body can cause enhancement of local specific energy absorption rate (SAR) around the objects, although RF exposure guidelines often do not address such situations." [112]

1.6 Toxic metals "hide"

In the important book of Professor Van der Schaar, director of the International Board for Clinical Metal Toxicology, we read: *"it is confirmed that **mercury does not last more than 48 hours in the blood and therefore in the urine**. After that it diffuses in the tissue or is eliminated naturally. Only with chelating products can one find heavy metals in the tissue and make a correct evaluation of mercury poisoning."* [113]

Thus, blood metal levels alone are not conclusive to evaluate chronic lead toxicity. Many studies falsely equate decreased blood metal levels with metal excretion.

One study may show that a certain treatment decreases blood metal concentration. Which is generally a positive sign for the removal of the metal.

However, if blood metal levels are measured, and after a certain treatment - for instance with less effective natural detoxification agents - blood levels are measured to be lower, then that does not necessarily mean that the body's metal content was lowered. It may mean that metals were not chelated, but mobilized and redistributed into organs, bones, fat and the brain.

This has played out to the detriment of metal workers for decades, and still is today. When lead workers show symptoms of lead poisoning and have high blood lead levels, they are put on leave for a few weeks. When they come back, the blood lead levels are lower or normal, the doctor says 'you are ok.' They are not ok, the lead has moved to bones and other tissue, to haunt the patient's health for life or until the metals are removed.

A standard public health screening procedure is described here:
"If a person has a blood lead level of 5 µg/dL (five micrograms per deciliter), they are considered to have an elevated blood lead level. If that happens, healthcare providers will likely confirm the result with a second test anywhere from right away to 1 to 3 months, depending on the initial results. If the test still comes back with high levels, the practitioner will report it to the local health department and go over next steps with the family on what they can do to reduce the blood levels and stop the exposure to lead. In cases of very high lead levels (45 µg/dL or higher), advanced treatment might be needed, especially in kids." [114]

Similarly, urine metal levels are only conclusive when urine is tested after administration of a chelation agent (provoked or challenge urine test), and later retested with the same protocol. A decrease in unprovoked urine levels can also mean the body's ability to excrete metals was further shut down.

In the case of chronic **lead** poisoning, since 95 % of lead is stored in the bones already weeks after absorption, blood tests are not conclusive. Bone lead as an indicator of total body burden can only be measured by L alpha-x-ray fluorescence and lead-induced toxicity can be assessed by erythrocyte protoporphyrin levels. [115]

1.6.1 False diagnoses

The Centers for Medicare & Medicaid Services say: *"There are multiple providers using provoked urine tests to justify chelation therapy - and almost anyone with a provoked urine test will end up with a positive urine screen."* [116]

That is exactly the point, since almost everyone has toxic levels of one or more elements, but regular urine or blood tests will not release all the metals. If unprovoked tests would show significant metal loads in urine, this would mean the natural detoxification mechanisms work sufficiently and the metals would not be retained over decades and thus the problem would solve itself. Even when levels of unprovoked tests are deemed normal in conventional medical practice, in post mortem autopsies, the metals can be measured in diverse organs (see also 1.6.2).

Now, such diagnostic challenges do not only apply to chronic metal burden.

Even in acute poisoning, for instance in the case of the former KGB agent Alexander Litvinenko, who was assassinated in exile in London, the metal thallium was suspected in the first days, but a team of prominent doctors and toxicologists who attempted to save the victims life, could not be sure. On 1 November 2006, Litvinenko was poisoned and suddenly fell ill later that day, he was hospitalized on 3 November. He was initially treated with oral Prussian blue against thallium poisoning. [117] It later turned out, Litvinenko had ingested radioactive polonium-210.

"Dozens of locations were sealed off in one of the biggest health emergencies the capital has ever seen."

The point here being that even in a case of fatal and acute poisoning, the metal toxicity load (non-radioactive metals) is difficult to determine even by leading experts.

This case illustrates that with a suspected toxic metal load, it is reckless to do a simple unprovoked (non-challenge) hair-, blood- or urine- test and then to conclude that a person has no toxic metal load, especially if there is a reasonable suspicion for long-term, chronic toxicity.

Such limitations are an immense danger to public health.

1.6.2 Autopsy results post mortem

Proper testing of a patient with provoked (challenge) urine tests provides relatively reliable values of body metal content. Even bone content can be measured radiologically with some accuracy.

But the exact burden within the brain, bones and organs can only be measured in an autopsy after death.

"Examinations were conducted on deceased workers who had worked in **mercury** mines and had no mercury contact for many years. After their death, mercury levels were found to be elevated in the brain, endocrine glands (e. g. thyroid), pineal gland, kidneys and other organs, suggesting that mercury can remain in the body for longer than previously assumed." (Translation mine). [118]

More recently, in a study of 18 cadavers, Guzzi et al (2006) found **mercury** levels in the **cerebral cortex and pituitary gland** were more than **ten times higher** in subjects with more than 12 occlusal amalgam surfaces than in subjects with three or fewer (for both tissues). **Hg** levels in the blood and occipital cortex, the pituitary and thyroid glands were strongly associated with the subjects' number of dental amalgam surfaces at the time of death. [119]

For the vast majority of affected amalgam carriers, if they die of any disease, their deaths will not be linked to mercury toxicity. Moreover, most likely, no one will ever know of their mercury toxicity.

A further phenomenon reveals how blood tests in the living do not detect actual metal loads. Vast amounts of **cadmium** can be released into the blood from organs after death. The cadmium was not introduced into the body after death.

"The cadmium concentration in the blood collected at autopsy after death was several hundred times as high as the value measured before death." The cadmium had to come from somewhere (brain, other cells and intercellular space).

The residual rates of Cd in the renal cortex in the formalin-fixed organs were only 2.3 % and those in the medulla were only 6.1% of those of the fresh organs. [120]

In forensic autopsies of decease patients who had died of acute illness with no known **lead** exposure, all joint samples showed a highly specific accumulation of **lead** in articular cartilage. [121]

1.7 Toxic metals dispersed to the end of the world

Arsenic in Groundwater

High levels of arsenic have been found in 10 developing countries, including India. In a Bangladesh study, 57.5% of the population had skin lesions caused by arsenic poisoning [122] (see also 8.6.1).

Anthropogenic activities, like the lowering of water table below the organic deposits, accelerate the oxidation process in the natural aquafers. It is hypothesized that in this way, "the origin of arsenic rich groundwater is man-made, which is a recent phenomenon." [123] **So, even though the arsenic itself is present naturally, the mass poisoning is accelerated by land overexploitation, industrialization and overpopulation.**

Toxic metals from industrial sources are dispersed all over the Earth, not only in populated areas, but they fall down on the top of the Himalayans, and in any desert since the Industrial Revolution and they will be there, ready to affect one organism after the other, virtually forever.

"A continuous 500-years trace metal ice core record was established from the Dasuopu glacier (7,200 m altitude, central Himalayas), the highest drilling site on Earth. An early contamination with toxic trace metals, particularly **Cd, Cr, Mo, Ni, Sb,** and **Zn,** emerged at high elevation in the Himalayas at the onset of the European Industrial Revolution (~1780 AD)." [124]

1.7.1 Arctic pollution

Dangerous levels of toxic metals are now found in arctic natives, more or less at the end of the world, arctic fish and other wildlife is contaminated with **mercury** and other metals.

"Arctic indigenous peoples are among the most exposed humans when it comes to foodborne mercury." [125]

Long-range atmospheric transport of mercury, its transformation to more toxic methylmercury compounds, and their bioaccumulation in the aquatic food chain have motivated intensive research on mercury as a pollutant of global concern. [126]

"Today, the rates of hypertension in Inuit adults in Nunavik is associated with their blood mercury levels from fish consumption." [127]

We revisit the interaction of hypertension and toxic metals in Chapter 5.3.1.

Anjali Gopakumar et al estimate:

"Approximately 90% of the present-day **mercury** in Arctic wildlife is of anthropogenic origin. In addition to long-range transported **Hg** that is deposited differently across large spatial scales, there are local sources of Hg in the Arctic, such as the coal mines in Spitsbergen and freshwater runoff from gold and Hg mines in Siberia." [128]

In the Arctic, "remarkably high **cadmium** levels are found in kidney and liver of narwhal (Monodons monoceros) from western Baffin Bay and western Greenland waters. **Mercury** concentrations in muscle of ringed seal and cetaceans frequently exceed 0.5 microgram per gram, especially in older animals." **Cadmium** concentrations in polar bear liver increased from west to east. Other carbon-based toxins such as PCB and DDT are found reaching back to the mid 20th century. [129]

Dastoor et al estimate that 75% of anthropogenic **Hg** deposition in the Arctic is from industrial and ASGM gold mining sources. [130]

Lead pollution from the Australian Broken Hill site – from mining and smelting **lead**, **zinc**, and **silver** - had settled in the snow of the south pole after 1900, causing lead pollution at the time almost as high as at any time since. [131]

1.7.2 Global metal pollution

Travnikov et al compared the global **mercury** emission levels from natural and anthropogenic sources using four models. The proportion of natural emissions and re-emission ranged from 45 to 66% of the total emissions, the rest is from anthropogenic sources. [132]

"Toxic trace metals emitted from mining and metallurgical operations conducted in Western Europe by the Romans (Spain, 200 AD), in South America by the Spaniards (Bolivia, 1570 AD), and in Australia by the colonial population (Broken Hills, 1889 AD) were transported over long ranges and contaminated the atmosphere and the snow in central Greenland and Antarctica with **Pb**, and in South America with **As, Bi, Cu, Mo, Pb,** and **Sb**." [133]

The United Nations Environmental Program (UNEP) estimated anthropogenic **mercury** emissions in 2010 globally at about 1,960 tons per year. [134]

1.7.3 Misleading perspective on the apparent reduction in toxic metal emissions

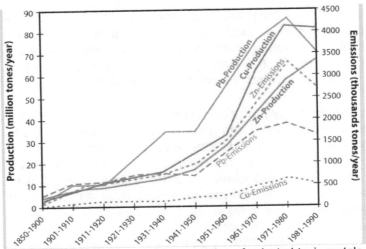

Fig. 1 Global production and consumption of selected toxic metals, 1850–1990. Source: Jaishankar M, Tseten T,et al 2014: Toxicity, mechanism and health effects of some heavy metals. Interdiscip Toxicol. 2014 Jun;7(2):60-72. http://doi.org/10.2478/intox-2014-0009.

1.7.4 Exotic metals vs. the "usual" toxic metals

At the end of the 20th century, emissions of the common toxic metals started to decrease in developed countries: in the UK, emissions of toxic metals fell by over 50% between 1990 and 2001. This is a positive development on the one hand, but on the other, it must be considered that some toxic metals are being replaced with slightly less toxic metals, sometimes in greater quantities. Newly implemented toxic metals are not discussed publicly, and standard tests for humans and soil include only the known "usual suspects", not exotic metals which are introduced in industrial quantities, as in the case of rare earth metals in electronics/ electromobility.

As an example of this type of shortsightedness: **lead** in plumbing is being replaced with **antimony** or **bismuth**, both are less toxic, but the long-term toxicity of chronic exposure will take decades to be established, and once antimony will be deemed too harmful, it will take yet more decades to ban it and replace it with another new element. So don't wait for the government to save you.

For each toxic element, it took decades to centuries after first evidence of public health risks until it was banned.

Further, the metals are accumulated in soil, water, the biosphere, they are toxic forever, which means if the yearly emissions are reduced, then overall environmental contamination still increases.

And as the half-life in the human body for some metals is 20-30 years, people over 50 still carry at least half the lead they absorbed from leaded gasoline before it was banned in the 2000s.

"The presence of harmful environmental [lead] exposure, which disproportionately affects low-and-middle income countries (LMICs), contributes to **>25% of deaths and diseases worldwide** and detrimentally affects child neurodevelopment." [135]

1.8 A global conspiracy?

How could governments and corporations allow this to happen? It rather seems like another case of global stupidity.

When industrialists and politicians forced leaded gasoline upon the world beginning in 1923, every year, millions of tons of bioavailable lead were dispersed into the air everywhere, there was no escaping it. The super wealthy, the 'robber barons' including the owners of Standard Oil - the greatest profiteers of leaded gasoline - lived in unhealthy cities like New York City. Still in the early 2000s, the top dozens of US communities with the highest cancer rates were New York City boroughs and communities in the closer Tristate Area.

And there is no evidence that save and effective lead chelating agents were (secretly) available before 1939 to protect the (accidental) perpetrators of this global lead contamination that began in 1923.

EDTA was first synthesized in 1930, and used for medical purposes only in the 1940s. BAL was developed in 1939 (see 11.1).

When tetra lead ethyl was introduced as a gasoline additive to decrease engine knocking in 1921, the chief chemist Thomas Midgley himself had to go to a medical retreat to recover from lead poisoning, only to come back one week later for a public demonstration to show the world that lead was safe. He even washed his hands in tetra lead ethyl for the reporters (read the full story of leaded gasoline on p. 221).

1.8.1 Experts affected by toxic metals

Let's continue with a tragic example that shows how even highly educated, competent experts are not always aware of the dangers of environmental toxins and particularly toxic metals.

It's the tragic case of a 48-year-old chemistry professor whose research focused on the biologic toxicity of heavy metals. She was admitted to Dartmouth–Hitchcock Medical Center, in Lebanon, New Hampshire, on January 20, 1997.

"An expert in the mechanisms of metal toxicity, Professor Karen Wetterhahn was best known for her research on chromium, but she also conducted significant research on mercury."

"In 1995, Professor Karen Wetterhahn initiated Dartmouth's Toxic Metals Superfund Research Program, an interdisciplinary project exploring the human health effects of metals that are common contaminants in the environment, especially at toxic waste sites." [136]

Let me make it clear that no one is blaming the victim of a fatal accident or of at this point inadequate safety regulations.

The point here is not that she had a chemistry accident in the lab. She was a leading expert in the field, but she couldn't know that dimethyl mercury is vastly more toxic than methyl mercury.

"At that time, it wasn't known that dimethyl mercury could penetrate the rubber gloves and then be absorbed by the skin."

It is super toxic according to the rating in a 1984 clinical toxicology textbook, sited by the EPA. [137]

She knew she had a chemical spill accident on August 14th 1996, with an extremely dangerous substance, and she had taken every precaution to clean up the lab meticulously and made sure she had no direct skin contact.

The Los Angeles Times wrote in 1997:

"At first, friends thought she had caught a stomach bug on her trip to Malaysia. It wasn't until she started bumping into doors that her husband, Leon Webb, began to worry. Karen, always so focused, always so sure of her next step, was suddenly falling down as if she were drunk.

In 15 years together, she had never been sick, never stopped working, never complained. Leon was stunned when she called for a ride home from work.

Over lunch a few days later, Karen confided to her best friend, Cathy Johnson, that she hadn't felt right for some time. Words seemed to be getting stuck in her throat. Her hands tingled. It felt like her whole body was moving in slow motion." [138]

It was not before several months later, in the hospital "she would be tested for everything but heavy metal poisoning."

Even after her dizziness and motor problems led to her almost causing a car crash and her husband had to drive her to work, she didn't go to a doctor, rather, she suspected she 'hadn't slept well'. [139] She had increasing problems of motor control in her hands. Similar deficits were among the key symptoms of the infamous

Minamata Disease, caused by mercury poisoning in Japan in the 1950s to 1970s, and should have sounded an alarm of 'mercury poisoning' with every toxicology student.

When her neurological symptoms began only weeks after the lab accident, but her cognitive capacity was still unaffected, she did not immediately put one and one together (acute and severe mercury poisoning!) and she did not go straight to a metal toxicologist.

"She was admitted to Dartmouth–Hitchcock Medical Center, in Lebanon, New Hampshire, on January 20, 1997, with a five-day history of progressive deterioration in balance, gait, and speech. Beforehand, she had lost 6.8 kg (15 lb) over a period of two months and had experienced several brief episodes of nausea, diarrhea, and abdominal discomfort. " [140]

The doctors were clueless, then she finally told them: "But I work with mercury", she said. "Shouldn't I be tested for the bad stuff?" [141]

"The original body burden of mercury may have been four times the amount at diagnosis, or about 1344 mg, requiring absorption of 0.44 ml (0.1 teaspoon) of liquid dimethylmercury." [142]

From what I learned only from private research, it is clear to me that everyone who has to do with toxic metals in any capacity should know the symptoms of toxicity and react immediately to any related symptoms and get tested for toxic metals routinely.

Metal exposure has a great advantage in that acute metal poisoning can be identified accurately with a single test. Other (organic) toxins are more difficult to diagnose.

People who work in a high-profile chemistry lab have no way of knowing whether another employee spilled something the day before, whether the cleaning lady had dropped a flask, so if they feal slightly unwell, they should have their metal levels checked immediately.

And her husband did not say: you have trouble walking straight, you have trouble talking straight, you can't drive, you have headaches, you work with highly toxic chemicals, maybe you should get checked for exposure to whatever you recently were in contact with.

In summary, after several months of weight loss and episodes of nausea, diarrhea, and abdominal discomfort, it took 5 days of rapid neurological degradation until she finally saw a general practitioner, in the hospital, no specialist came up with the idea that a renowned chemist working with toxic metals could be suffering from toxic metals. After several days in intensive care, she died in June 1997.

Her tragic story led to great improvements in lab safety standards concerning mercury and other compounds.

These are the experts who make official recommendations and together with bureaucrats, they decide what newly introduced toxic metals and other chemicals the public will be exposed to. These are the experts that told the people for a hundred years that leaded gasoline or mercury fillings were safe.

Meanwhile the super wealthy are moving to Paris' inner city which is heavily lead polluted.

1.8.2 Notre-Dame's Fire and lead fall out

In April 2019, the Paris Notre Dame cathedral burnt down.

The same year and the next (during the pandemic), the world's super wealthy were still moving to Paris in droves, mostly to the inner city. This inner city is now contaminated with lead dust from the lead roof. At the beginning of 2022 the BARNES international City Index ranked Paris in the 5th place in the list of the most popular domiciles of the global elites. [143] Here, wealthy or ultra-high net worth (UHNW), means a net worth of 30 million USD or more.

Paris was 1st in the index released in 2020, 7th in 2021, and 5th in 2022 and again number 1 in the 2023 ranking.

"Paris tops the list of the most desirable cities for high-net-worth individuals, followed by Miami and New York." [144]

Meanwhile, the Paris inner city is still contaminated with lead dust, only in trace amounts, but sufficiently to make everyone chronically ill within years. Everybody breathes it in. Apparently, money does not protect from putting oneself in harm's way. Granted, people of 30 million + usually have several homes around the world, they don't spend all their time in their resident city, but that is usually where their children spend most of their time.

"Notre Dame's roof, composed of approximately 450 tons of lead, quickly melted as the fire temperatures exceeded 1,400° F. As the smoke's distinct yellow tinge suggested, the lead vaporized and created a toxic fallout of lead dust that was deposited across Paris."

"Lead oxide is highly soluble in body fluids. The particle size of the metal fumes ranges between 0.1- 0.7 microns [so nanoparticles], which increases the likelihood of inhalation and deposition of the fume directly into the bloodstream." [145]

This finest lead dust is still in every nook and cranny in every pore of architectural structure, in ventilation systems on every wall, it cannot be cleaned up with any efficiency, it is being hurled up by every breeze from gravel parkways and playgrounds. It will take decades for the lead to be dispersed to tolerable levels. And this even after the city took "four months to complete a deep-clean operation of the sidewalks as tourists, residents and merchants walked the streets around the cathedral daily." [146]

According to the New York Times, "the levels of lead dust deposited near the cathedral were up to 1,300 times higher than French safety guidelines."

And already the official safety levels in the environment are inadequate when it concerns chronic, accumulated lead toxicity. As mentioned above, a 2020 US study found that already 30 micrograms of lead (or 0.00003 grams) in the blood of a 10-year-old girl has a statistically measurable negative effect on later fertility. [147] That's less than the smallest speck of dust that you can see with the naked eye.

It is obviously impossible to clean the city so thoroughly that no child ever inhales an invisibly small speck of lead dust, just 3 years after 450 tons of lead rained down.

The CDC, which determines reference levels for the maximum amount of lead in the US, also says 'there is no safe level of lead in the blood of children." [148]

Recall, an NHANES extension study of 2018, published in the Lancet, revealed: "18 % of deaths of all causes in the US are attributed to lead toxicity." [149]

And this is concerning only lead, not including the other 40+ known toxic metals.

"Lead is more commonly detected in the indoor air in houses of children with atopic dermatitis, even with concentrations of airborne lead below the safety levels suggested by health guidelines." [150]

Those international super wealthy who have been flocking to Paris' inner city (especially in the vicinity of Notre Dame) evidently belong to either of two groups:

1. They are just as clueless as the rest of the population when it comes to the long-term effects of accumulated, chronic heavy metal toxicity.

2. Some might be aware of the danger and they don't care because they happen to have a good doctor, are routinely checked with challenge toxic metal tests and routinely undergo preemptive and harmless chelation therapy, before the toxic metal burden can become problematic.

As we'll see in 1.13, already in the 1960s, publicly available studies showed: In patients who had symptoms of lead poisoning, but no sign of cancer, preemptive EDTA chelation therapy showed a 90% reduction in later cancer death. [151]

In Paris, only two families, along with a health association and a trade union, sue authorities for "gross negligence".
"Despite the scale of the fire and knowledge about the risk of pollution and contamination, no precaution in particular was taken by the authorities involved for more than three months after the fire," their legal complaint says, according to AFP news agency. [152]
Unfortunately, 3 months after contamination, 95% of lead has already moved to the bones, only fractions of 0.1 % can be found in the blood, if any.
At least, all workers involved in the Notre Dame restoration are required to wear protective hazardous material suits and respirators and they must regularly take blood tests for lead. Also health authorities 'recommended' lead blood tests for small children and pregnant women. Most residents are not tested at all. [153]
Unfortunately, the recommended blood tests (which are not challenge- or provocation tests) cannot give any meaningful assessment of accumulated toxicity.
The New York Times wrote in September 2019: "The lead created a public health threat that stirred increasing anxiety in Paris throughout the summer." [154]
Half of the drinking water of Paris comes from the rivers Seine and Marne.[155]
Barnes international reports "the high-end real estate market has for decades only concerned certain districts in the west and center of Paris, it now extends to all 20 districts."
Antoine-Marie Preaut, Regional Curator for Historical Monuments, Paris says the smoke traveled east to west, the highest lead concentrations were found on the square in front of the cathedral. [156]

For a bit of trivia, Michelle Obama happened to be on a private cruse on the river Seine passing the Notre Dame as it was burning. [157]

In 2024, Paris is still ranked 5th place in the Barnes City Index, after Dubai, Miami, New York and Madrid. But by now, crime, riots and conflicts between migrant groups are dominating the streets in most districts, with some streets resembling third world cities. So it is unclear whether the ultra-rich are actually living there, or whether they moved their resident address to Paris for other reasons.

1.8.3 Celebrity information deficiency?

American retired professional racing driver Danica Patrick is considered the best female Nascar driver of all times, but also the worst Nascar driver at the peak of her career from 2013- 2017. [158] She tells the story of how she found the source of her health problems and had several metals (including **thallium, cesium, lead** and **mercury**) detected in her body, which she attributed partly to breast implants. She mentions her lead levels were high and as for the source she referred to lead being 'very hereditary', it could have been passed down from her mother in utero. [159]

She is apparently unaware that leaded gasoline is still in use for car racing, where she breathed it in from childhood onwards throughout her career.

Further, she recounts that her mercury levels were "astronomical" (34 times over the reference levels). Famous functional medicine practitioner Marc Hyman told her: "just stop eating sea food for 6 months and you'll be fine."

Apparently, being rich and famous does not ensure getting reasonable health advise when it comes to metal toxicity. Her podcast is called 'pretty Intense', for those who couldn't tell...

The EPA finds even regular motor vehicles contribute to environmental mercury levels. **Mercury** was emitted from fuel (exhausts), lubricants, coolants, brake disks and brake pads. [160]

The reason **lead** is used in race fuels is because it is a great octane booster. [161] **Thallium** is used as an anti-knock additive in some gasoline in areas where high-octane gas is in short supply.

1.8.4 Dentists

Meanwhile, most dentists have no idea they have chronic **mercury** poisoning from being exposed to dental mercury.

Even casually browsing the internet, one can find testimonies of dentists about how they were puzzled finding out their chronic illnesses were related to mercury. With the utmost respect for sufferers of neurological and other chronic diseases: it should be kept in mind, that dentist make important health decisions and recommendations for their clients. If they can't make informed decisions to safe their own health, you can keep your fingers crossed in regards to your health.

One dentist tells the story of her suffering and, luckily her way to recovery, from mercury poisoning after 20 years of dentist practice. She was surprised, when after 6 years of fatigue, eye swellings and gut issues, a blood test revealed high **mercury** levels. Surprised because she herself did not have mercury fillings. [162] A quick search or reading this book would have told her that dentists are at high risk for chronic poisoning with mercury and other metals and they should get tested routinely by a metal toxicologist with provoked (challenge) urine tests. Dentist are disproportionately affected by neurological problems, addiction and suicides. (An in-depth discussion on dentist health and mercury follows in 4.12).

1.9 Lack of Essential Metals

Too many toxic metals, not enough essential metals.
Toxic metals disrupt metal metabolism and homeostasis, they can cause essential metals to not be properly absorbed.
"Many studies in both animals and humans have shown that a deficiency in essential metals such as zinc, calcium or iron can lead to greater absorption and toxicity of **Cd** and **Pb**." [163]

1.9.1 Nutrient deficiency affects almost everyone

According to the US NHANES 2007-2010 report; "94.3% of the US population do not meet the daily requirement for vitamin D, 88.5% for vitamin E, 52.2% for magnesium, 44.1% for calcium, 43.0% for vitamin A, and 38.9% for vitamin C. For the nutrients in which a requirement has not been set, 100% of the population had intakes lower than the Adequate Intake (AI) for potassium, 91.7% for choline, and 66.9% for vitamin K. The prevalence of inadequacies was low for all of the B vitamins and several minerals, including copper, iron, phosphorus, selenium, sodium, and zinc. [164]
Other evaluations find "Over 97% of Americans are potassium deficient: they aren't consuming enough potassium to meet the Institute of Medicine (IOM) daily target of 4.7 grams." [165]
When these percentages are combined, it can be summarized that over 99 % of adults are deficient in uptake of at least one essential mineral or vitamin.
Many people are iodine deficient, therefore governments in many western countries recommend to use table salt fortified with iodine. However, the usual amount of iodine in these salts is very low and basically negligible. Supplementation is often necessary.
The recommended daily value for iodine is 150 microgram/ day for adults. Meanwhile, in most countries, common fortified salt has 15-

25 mg/kg, or micrograms/ gram. So, one gram of fortified salt (a small espresso spoon) covers only 10% of daily iodine needs.

1.9.2 Mineral depletion of soil and food

To make matters worse, the content of essential minerals in soil and in foods has been declining continuously in the last century. Today, even with proper nutrition and healthy intake of fresh natural food, it is increasingly difficult to obtain proper mineral consumption.

The overall long-term comparison of data from 1940 to 2019 shows that the mineral contents of fruits and vegetables remain lower than in 1940. The greatest overall reductions during this 80-year period were Na (52%), Fe (50%) Cu (49%) and Mg (10%). [166]

Looking at 15 different meat items between 1940 and 2002, an analysis found that the iron content had fallen on average by 47%. "The **iron** content of milk had dropped by more than 60%, iron contents of cream and eight different cheeses dropped by more than 50%. Milk appears to have lost 2% of its calcium, and 21% of its magnesium." [167]

Only between 1991 and 2022, the **iron** content of fruit produced in Australia decreased by 55%. [168]

1.9.3 Interactions of Essential and toxic metals

"One reason heavy metals are so toxic is they interrupt the absorption, metabolism, and use of essential minerals, such as **calcium, iron**, and **zinc**."

"Many toxic metals use the same binders or transferors as essential metals.

- **Iron** deficiency leads to an increase in **lead** absorption and cadmium absorption.

- **Iron** and **arsenic** have an antagonistic relationship, meaning that iron competes with arsenic, so if you have sufficient iron, then it mitigates the toxicity of arsenic.

- **Calcium** deficiency increases the intestinal absorption and body retention of **lead**. [169]

- "Sufficiency of essential minerals appears to resist the uptake of toxic metals." [170]

Another example of how toxic metals disrupt metal metabolism, is **lead** toxicity commonly causes **iron** deficiency and anemia, even with proper iron intake.

A lead atom can displace the central iron ion in hemoglobin molecules, and decrease the ability to transport oxygen. When the hemoglobin molecule or the entire red blood cell is replaced, the lead atom is not excreted from the body, but binds to other hemoglobin or other molecules, esp. enzymes, and this can continue for decades or a lifetime.

You have 4 iron ions per hemoglobin, 300,000 hemoglobin per red blood cell and 4 million red blood cells. 4 to the power of 12 integrated iron atoms. **Lead** or **mercury,** for instance, have a half-life in the body of up to 30 years; during their presence, they perpetually displace essential metal ions in important enzymes and render the enzyme useless.

1.9.4 Vitamins and minerals absorption

Vitamin D increases intestinal calcium and phosphate absorption and stimulates the co-absorption of other essential minerals like magnesium, iron, and zinc. "Reciprocally, **lead, cadmium, aluminum**, and **strontium** interfere with normal vitamin D metabolism." [171]

"Inadequate vitamin A in your diet could lead to iron deficiency because vitamin A helps to release stored **iron**. the process of iron absorption is aided by vitamin C, particularly non-haem iron (found in plant foods such as beans and lentils)." [172]

1.10 Non-metal environmental toxins

Other environmental toxins (mostly organic hydro carbons, and especially cyclic hydrocarbons, containing mostly or exclusively C, H, O and N) can be more toxic than metals and some can accumulate in the environment over decades and then be harmful if absorbed by the body. But they are chemically reactive and are usually consumed in the chemical reaction while they are causing their deteriorating effect. The most dangerous of these chemicals are compounds bound to fluorine and chlorine.

The pesticide Glyphosate, for instance, is believed to remain harmful while deposited in the soil for 6 months to a year, and can then still be dangerous to humans and animals. Field studies cited in a report show the half-life of glyphosate in soil ranges between a few days to several months, or even years, depending on soil composition. [173]

Glycine is an essential peptide that is a precursor to the important antioxidant glutathione. Glyphosate mimics glycine, so the body stores glyphosate mistakenly. "Chronic glyphosate- based commercial herbicide (GBH) exposure inhibited glutathione S-transferase (GST), an important detoxifying enzyme." [174]

Glyphosate detoxification can be facilitated with glutathione (preferably IV or suppositories) or oral administration.

"A new study is unearthing the toxic legacy of DDT, finding that the chemical can affect families three generations after the initial exposure." [175] This takes place by epigenetic mechanisms, wherein in utero exposure damages stem cells of the next generation and so on.

And such endocrine disrupting organic chemicals can change a human's physical and psychological constitution for life when they were deployed in utero or childhood or when the dosage was high enough to cause permanent organ damage.

But these non- metal substances such as DDT don't remain chemically active in the body over decades.

1.10.1 Forever chemicals

They behave in similar ways to toxic metals. "The EPA finds no safe level for two toxic 'forever chemicals,' found in many U.S. water systems." More than 96% of Americans have at least one of the per- and polyfluoroalkyl substances (PFAS) in their blood, studies show. [176] in the human body they have a half-life of 4 years, compared to a half-life of 30 years for many toxic metals.

A 2022 study finds "rainwater should be considered unsafe to drink everywhere on Earth (including Antarctica and the Tibetan plateau) due to the levels of "forever chemicals" in the environment". [177]

"They bind to small proteins in our blood," says Megan Romano, an epidemiologist at Dartmouth's Geisel School of Medicine. "And what that means is it's a really excellent delivery system to get to all sorts of places in our body."

Linda Birnbaum, former director of the national toxicology program says: "We know that PFOA and PFOS are predominantly in our liver, our kidney and our blood. We really don't have the data for any of the [thousands of other PFAS] chemicals on where they go in our body." [178]

As of today, there is no effective treatment to remove PFAS from the body.

"PFOA and PFOS stay in the body for many years. It takes nearly four years for the level in the body to go down by half. PFAS leave the body mainly through urine." [179]

A new study shows PFOS (perfluorooctanesulfonic acid, a type of PFAS) is associated with decreased rates of bone mineral density change in adolescents. [180]

Forever chemicals may interfere with bone development in adults as well. [181] And as we saw above, PFAS have synergistic effects with toxic metals.

"The chemicals are associated with low birth weight, high cholesterol, thyroid disease and an increased risk of certain cancers."

Counteractions:

On a positive note, in 2022, scientists claim they have found a method to remove PFAS from water and air. [182]

Researchers found that PFAS can be destroyed using two relatively harmless chemicals: sodium hydroxide or lye, a chemical used to make soap, and dimethyl sulfoxide (DMSO), a chemical approved as a medication for bladder pain syndrome, exposed to low heat (at 115 °C).

The strategy was successful in degrading the chemicals by anywhere from 78% to 100% within a 24-hour period. The method worked on 10 types of common PFAS.

But for body toxicity, prevention and avoidance is the key approach so far. These PFAS chemicals and other 'forever chemicals ' and nanoparticles shall be reserved for a future book. A summery of the present state of research is given in Chapter 9.

As of now, there are no long-term proven, safe protocols to speed up the excretion of these chemicals from the body.

In contrast, we know how to safely chelate toxic metals with 60 years of experience. And the toxic metal load can be measured before and after and thus progress can be monitored. The removal of toxic metals will intermittently even aid the detoxification of other, organic pollutants.

1.11 Rare Earth Elements as a growing hazard in the name of "environmentalism"

Rare earth elements (REE) are a set of seventeen chemical elements in the periodic table, specifically the fifteen lanthanides plus scandium and yttrium.

The lanthanides are found in the 6th period of the periodic table together with some of the most toxic metals known so far (lead, mercury, thallium, tungsten, cesium, polonium, etc.). Lanthanides are very dense metals (very high atomic weight).

"In the last few decades, rare earth metals (REMs) have been extensively used in agriculture to enhance resistance of plants to adverse environments and to improve the quality of crops. [183]

Mainly two REE's are used in electric vehicles [in permanent magnet motors]; neodymium (Nd) and dysprosium (Dy). [184]

Rare earth elements are not even officially discussed in the context of toxic heavy metals, and no standard tests ore reference levels for human exposures are determined, little is known about their health effects. We only know that all similar metals in the lower periods of the periodic table for which data exist, they are all highly toxic. Those elements in the lower half of the periodic table that haven't been studied for health effects should all be banned until proven safe. To politicians who push for more "green" energy at all costs, it seems to be good enough for the time being that workers at electric vehicle factories don't drop dead immediately. The same for firefighters who have to put out the many EV fires and are exposed to rare earth metal fumes.

The average EV uses 1.5kg of rare earth magnets per vehicle. research consultancies believe "the ramp-up of wind turbines and electric vehicles will require very large expansions in rare earth metals production." [185]

Regarding non- rare-earth metals: photovoltaic cells in solar panels contain large amounts of other toxic metal compounds such as **cadmium telluride** (CdTe), a stable crystalline compound formed from cadmium and tellurium. In landfill simulations, 73% of the Cd and 21% of the Te were leached out over the course of 30 days. Several studies have shown that CdTe and CdTe quantum dots are cytotoxic to mammalian cells. [186]

Other panels contain **gallium, arsenic, aluminum, tin, indium, hexavalent chromium, copper** and **selenium**. [187] Acid rain accelerates the leaching of **Zn, Cu, Ni, Ga, Pb, In**, and **Cr** from the damaged panels, contaminating ground water, agricultural and garden soils. [188]

With the global monumental increase in rare earth metal production (mostly for electric cars, wind turbine generators and electronics), we can safely assume we are opening another pandoras box of public health risks in the name of progress.

Imagine a new species of large feline is discovered, the size of a lion. We have known for millennia that all similar large cats are dangerous. Every normal person would stay far away from this new unknown feline, but governments tell you not to worry because they haven't proven that the new cat is indeed dangerous.

REE health effects
Of the rare earth elements, only **gadolinium** is well studied because of its decade- long use in MRI diagnostics and it is known to be extremely toxic without chelation agents or in cases when this chelation fails (see 8.18.).

"REEs are distributed to and accumulated at elevated concentrations in the liver, eyes, bone, spleen, lungs, kidneys, testis, brain, heart and adipose tissue." [189]

"REEs may accumulate in the cerebral cortex by long-term environmental intake of a small amount and cause subclinical damage."

Higher rare earth element levels than in controls were found
- in the maternal serum of pregnant women affected with neural tube defects (NTDs).
- in the blood of sub-Saharan immigrants with anemia and independent of Fe levels.
- in brain-tumor tissues of patients with astrocytoma compared to normal brain tissues. [190]

Exposure of pregnant women to **Cerium** and **Ytterbium** has decreased TSH (Thyroid-stimulating hormone) levels in infants. [191]

-**Cerium** levels in toenails have been associated with an increased risk of acute myocardial infarction. [192]

-**Lanthanum** levels in the serum of women undergoing in vitro fertilization-embryo transfer have been associated with a 230% increase in preclinical spontaneous abortions. [193]

-Both **Lanthanum** and **Cerium** caused adverse effects to wheat plants. [194]

"It has been proven that the lighter lanthanides, as well as **europium** (Eu) accumulate in the microsomal fraction of the liver, in the spleen and other organs rich in reticuloendothelial cells." [195]

-"**Neodymium**-iron-boron magnets [used in wind turbines] are cytotoxic against human oral mucosal fibroblasts." [196]

1.12 Natural sources of toxic metals

The vast part of the heavy metal burden affecting life on earth is man-made, some toxic metals have been present from natural sources, but only sometimes they occur in problematic concentrations. All surviving species have evolved to be adapted to low levels of toxic metals in the environment.

"Flegal & Smith, 1992 estimated that blood **lead** level in a natural, non-contaminated environment amounts to 0.016 µg/dL, i.e. about 600 times lower than the standard adopted for children by the CDC." [197]

"Heavy metals are present in our environment as they formed during the earth's birth. Their increased dispersal is a function of their usefulness during our growing dependence on industrial modification and manipulation of our environment. " [198]

All anthropogenic toxic elements that are now plaguing the biosphere are to a smaller extent also emitted by natural sources, volcanoes, erosion events and dust storms among them.

1.12.1 Volcanic soil fertility and toxic metals

Trace element deposition from a volcano can have advantages for the people living in the vicinity. Beneficial, essential minerals created some of the most fertile soils in the world, near the Vesuvius, in Hawaii, in Java and so on.

"In volcanic regions, pyroclastic materials have formed soils with unique physical, chemical and mineralogical properties, such as low bulk density, large water storage and high phosphate retention." [199]

The British Geological Survey explains: "Volcanic environments can be good locations for farming. Volcanic deposits are enriched in elements such as magnesium and potassium. When volcanic rock and ash weathers, these elements are released, producing extremely fertile soils. Thin layers of ash can act as natural fertilizers, producing increased harvests in years following an eruption." [200]

But an eruption that causes a large **mercury** or **arsenic** deposition can devastate the area and make it uninhabitable for a long time. Even decades after the ashes have settled and the land is again covered in top soil and vegetation, people who resettle may never manage to survive and prosper there. If a volcano does not emit toxic metals, the region is repopulated quickly within years or decades after every eruption, as if nothing ever happened.

"Over 29 million people worldwide live within just 10 km of active volcanoes, and around 800 million people (10 % of the world population) live within 100 km." [201]

A large-scale volcanic eruption produces large amounts of ash and pyroclastic material, which contains not only nutrients (nitrogen,

57

phosphorus, potassium, calcium, sodium, magnesium, etc.) but also toxic elements and metalloids **(arsenic, mercury**, etc.). [202]
Sediments and soils of El Chichón crater lake, Mexico are an important source of heavy metals and toxic elements such as **As** and **Cd.** [203]
Long-lived basaltic volcanic eruptions are a globally important source of environmentally reactive, volatile metal pollutant elements such as **selenium, cadmium** and **lead.** For instance, "the 2018 eruption of Kīlauea, Hawai'i, produced an exceptionally high discharge of metal pollutants." [204]
Volcanic soil and volcanic ash from the Tianchi volcano, a dormant active volcano with a risk of re-eruption, showed **zinc** pollution was high in the study area. [205]
"In the volcanic area *Chengmai County*, a typical volcanic area in Hainan Province, China, "the potential carcinogenic risk of exposure to **Cr, Ni,** and **As** was determined to be unacceptable for residents, with high Cr values far exceeding limits for children."
Aluminum-rich minerals, Fe–Mn oxides, and SOC are the most critical factors affecting heavy metal accumulation in volcanic agricultural soils. [206]

Volcanos health effects
"Volcanic areas have been associated with increased incidence of several diseases, such as fluorosis or even some types of cancer." [207]

"Thyroid cancer incidence is significantly increased in volcanic areas, where relevant non-anthropogenic pollution with heavy metals is present in the environment." [208]
Several site-specific cancers are increased in the region of active Mt. Etna volcano, Sicily, Italy. "Mt. Etna contains a large aquifer providing drinking and irrigation water to most of the Catania province. In the water of this aquifer, the concentrations of boron, iron, **manganese, vanadium** and **radon** (222Ra) are often higher than the maximum admissible concentration." [209]
In this Mt. Etna region, urine concentrations were two-fold or more than two-fold higher for eight metals: **Cd, Hg, Mn, Pd, Tl, U, V,** and **W**. Moreover, the values of **B, Mo, Pd** and **W** were at alarming levels (higher than the 95th percentile of the Italian reference values in more than 20% of the urine specimens from the volcanic area.) [210]

"Thyroid cancer incidence is markedly increased in volcanic areas." [211]

Male residents of O'ahu, Hawaii, older than 65 on average have a **mercury** hair level twice that of the reference level. [212]

"Numerous studies have shown that the inhalation of aerosol particles regardless of source (rural and urban), size range (fine and coarse), and composition is capable of raising blood pressure." The association of volcanic smog (Vog; particle air pollution) and cardiometabolic health let to the term "Hawaiian hypertension." [213] After a 2010 volcanic eruption in Iceland, various long-term negative health effects (skin rash/eczema, back pain, insomnia, PTSD, respiratory symptoms) were recorded in the affected population 3 and more years after the eruption. [214]

1.13 Preemptive chelation therapy/ disease prevention

A long-term observational study showed remarkable cancer prevention by chelation of **lead**. Residents of a small Swiss city of 3000 inhabitants in the 1960s living adjacent to a busy highway who showed symptoms of lead poisoning, but no indication of cancer, were observed.

The **lead** pollution was equivalent to that of any metropolitan area of the world.

Half of them were treated with IV EDTA chelation therapy.

Patients who were treated with calcium-EDTA, previously had symptoms that are commonly associated with lead toxicity, such as hypertension, nervous disorders, headaches, fatigue and gastrointestinal disorders. Depression and substance abuse was also observed with higher frequency. But treated patients had no evidence of cancer at the time of entry into this study.

Within 18 years, only 1.7% (one of 59) **of EDTA treated patients died of cancer, while 17.6 %** (30 of 172) **of untreated controls died of cancer, so mortality from cancer was reduced by 90%.**

"This represents a ten-fold greater incidence of cancer mortality in untreated persons (P=0.002). The two groups were similar in all other respects."

"Death from atherosclerosis and cardiovascular disease was also reduced."

The group of 231 adults was studied beginning in late 1958. Of these 231 people (105 men and 126 women), 31 persons, (17 men and 14 women) died of malignant tumors during the 18-year observation period (1959-1976). This was during the time of leaded gasoline, which was only abolished in the 2000s.

Beginning in 1961, a group of 59 patients with such symptoms was treated with parenteral doses of calcium EDTA. Symptoms improved and urinary delta-amino levulinic acid diminished.
The control group was similar to the treated group in all ways except to the EDTA chelation therapy. [215]
The Faculty of the University of Zurich Medical School reviewed this data.

NOTE: **Observations relate only to long-term prevention of death from malignant disease, if chelation therapy is begun before clinical evidence of cancer occurs**.
"Chelation was administered in relatively young patients who had no evidence of cancer at the time of treatment. The results therefore cannot be applied to patients with an established diagnosis of cancer." [216]

Those who were aware of this publicly available study at the time, when millions of tons of lead were still added to gasoline, would have done well to preemptively undergo EDTA chelation therapy.
Even though the contribution of heavy metals to diet-related cancer deaths is gravely understated in the public discourse, still already the official numbers should raise the question, why doctors don't mention heavy metal chelation in cancer prevention. The German Pharmacist Center (DAZ) claims:
"2 percent of diet-related cancer deaths can be attributed to heavy metals, less than 1 percent to chemical carcinogens, and 8 percent of diet-related deaths are of unknown cause." [translation mine] [217]
"Chelating drugs and chelator metal complexes are used for the prevention, diagnosis and treatment of cancer. Cancer cells and normal cells require essential metal ions such as iron, copper and zinc for growth and proliferation." [218]

1.13.1 Therapeutic results, EDTA trials

A different trial in Denmark yielded comparable results, but in the reduction of cardiovascular disease in patients who were observed for six years after chelation therapy with EDTA:
"Dr. Hancke and Dr. Flytlie, two Danish doctors, conducted a study in 1993 in which they documented the results of 470 patients who were observed for six years after chelation therapy. The results of Hancke and Flytlie were impressive: out of 265 patients with coronary heart disease and constriction of the coronary arteries, an improvement was determined **in 90 percent of patients after**

chelation therapy. 65 patients were originally scheduled for bypass surgery. After chelation treatment, 58 of the bypass candidates improved so well that surgery was no longer necessary **(89.2%!).**

Of 207 patients with circulatory heart pain (angina pectoris) who used nitroglycerin as a circulatory drug to control their pain, 189 were able to reduce their drug use after chelation therapy. **(91.3%!!)** Most of them no longer needed nitroglycerin at all. Of 27 patients who were about to have a foot or leg amputation, surgery was avoided in 24 **(88.8%).** " [219]

Among stable US patients of 50 years and older with previous myocardial Infarction (MI), use of an intravenous chelation regimen with disodium EDTA, compared with placebo, modestly reduced the risk of adverse cardiovascular outcomes, many of which were revascularization procedures. [220]

TACT cardiovascular disease

The TACT study (published in 2013) enrolled 1,708 patients, aged 50 years or older who had experienced a heart attack at least 6 weeks prior. Most of the participants were at high risk for vascular disease. Patients received 30 infusions of a formula containing vitamin/minerals along with disodium EDTA weekly for 30 weeks followed by a maintenance phase every 2-8 weeks for another 10 treatments. The participants were followed for 5 years after the infusions to monitor for progression of vascular disease.

The TACT investigators reported a clinically modest but statistically significant benefit of EDTA chelation therapy for vascular disease; an 18% reduction of vascular events like heart attacks/strokes compared to placebo group. A subgroup of participants that were diabetic had a 39% reduction in risk. "Much better results would have been recorded if the participants had continued the maintenance infusions on a monthly basis, given the ongoing risk factors that the participants had." [221]

1.14 Brain chemistry and metal toxicity

The human brain is one of the main targets of metal toxicity. A study reports on interactions between low dose mixtures of **lead, mercury, arsenic** and **cadmium** and essential metals. In mice, "Exposure to **Pb + Cd** increased brain Pb by 479% in 30 days." Brain copper increased by 221% on Pb + Hg + As + Cd exposure. [222]

Rabbits fed a diet containing increased toxic metals - but still well within the normal range - had higher concentrations of **lead, mercury** and **cadmium** in the brain than in other tissues. [223]

1.14.1 Locus ceruleus

The locus coeruleus is a nucleus in the pons of the brainstem involved with physiological responses to stress or panic. [224]
It is a part of the reticular activating system and the principal site for brain synthesis of **norepinephrine (noradrenaline)**. Norepinephrine may also be released directly into the blood from the adrenal medulla.
Noradrenaline helps you stay focused and alert. Too much can cause anxiety while too little brings on symptoms of depression. [225]
In patients with motor neuron disease (MND) the median percentage of heavy metal-containing locus coeruleus neurons was 9.5%, vs. 0.0% in controls. [226]
Damage to the locus ceruleus has been implicated in the pathogenesis of a number of neurological conditions. Locus ceruleus neurons accumulate toxic metals such as **mercury** selectively.
"In one study, about half of adults had locus ceruleus neurons containing inorganic **mercury**, and elemental analysis found a range of other toxic metals in the locus ceruleus. Locus ceruleus inorganic mercury increased during aging." [227]

It could take only milligrams of mercury or other toxic metals to accumulate in this exact brain region to have detrimental effects in the form of **multiple sclerosis, a disturbed stress response, panic attacks or depression**. A milligram is an invisibly small speck of metal.
As we know, a standard unprovoked blood test will not reveal any amount of this mercury locked in these brain cells, and even a provoked urine test is not likely to release enough mercury from the brain.
Roger Pamphlett et al 2023 explain:
"Human exposure to multiple toxic metals results in selective uptake of the metals into locus ceruleus neurons. **Decreased noradrenaline from the locus ceruleus causes multifocal damage to the blood–brain barrier,** allowing toxic metal uptake by astrocytes." [228]
In tissue doners with multiple sclerosis, individual human locus ceruleus neurons contain varying levels of toxic metals. In contrast,

most toxic metals are absent or at low levels in nearby anterior pons neurons [229] (see also 5.5.4).

"Toxic metals, or alterations in essential trace metals within individual locus ceruleus neurons, could be one factor determining the non-random destruction of locus ceruleus neurons in normal aging and neurodegenerative diseases." [230]

1.14.2 Human and cetacean brains

"The human brain is nearly 60 percent fat." [231]

"The human brain and the brains of whales and dolphins (cetaceans) are especially susceptible to a variety of toxic chemicals."

The high fat content of these brains makes them especially susceptible to long term storage of the same fat-soluble toxic chemicals that accumulate in adipose tissue.

The sulfur amino acids are also highest in these brains, making human and cetacean brains extremely susceptible to neuropsychiatric diseases and criminal behaviors caused by exposures to a variety of toxic chemicals. [232]

Marine mammals are more exposed to **mercury** than any other animals in the world. Reported Hg values in brain of cetaceans (such as whales) surpassed by one or two orders of magnitude those values found in other species such as pinnipeds or polar bears. [233]

1.14.3 Longevity and metals

"Early exposure to heavy metal toxins, such as **lead**, is linked with a 46 percent increase in the mortality rate, according to the CDC in Atlanta. " [234]

In the Hainan Province, China, there was a positive correlation between daily intake of Cu, Se, and Zn from food and water and aging and longevity indices, and a negative correlation between **Pb** intake and these indices. "Compared with water, food is a more important source of trace elements." [235]

"Hechi, China is recognized as a longevity city."

"The longevity index tended to be significantly positively correlated with Silicic acid (**H2SiO3), Ca** and **Fe** in drinking water and significantly negatively correlated with **strontium (Sr)** in soil. [236]

R. Lacatusu et al (1996) reported that soil and vegetables contaminated with **Pb** and **Cd** in Copsa Mica and Baia Mare,

Romania, significantly contributed to decrease human life expectancy (9-10 years) within the affected areas. [237]

Chapter 2
Toxic Metals and 'Hormonageddon'

2.1 Endocrine Disrupting Heavy Metals (EDHMs)

"Heavy metal toxicity is a very common (and overlooked) cause of low hormones and hormone imbalance. Different heavy metals cause different symptoms, ranging from hormone imbalance, fatigue, weight issues, brain fog and headaches." [238]
"There are four main heavy metals that cause hormone imbalance: **mercury, cadmium, lead**, and **arsenic**, they have endocrine disrupting activity." [239]
These are also the four metals with the biggest impact on general human health as listed by the WHO. They are dubbed the "big Four "in this book.
"Metals, as reproductive toxins, may induce hormonal changes affecting other facets of reproductive health such as the menstrual cycle, ovulation and fertility. " [240]

Apart from their common endocrine active properties, several EDCs have been shown to disrupt epigenomic programming. [241]
"Heavy metals that do not act directly on steroid receptors have been shown to alter hormone metabolism via epigenetic alterations." [242]
"Whole blood measurements of toxic metals are associated with genetic variants in metal transporter genes and others." [243]

2.1.1 Cardiovascular disease and testosterone in men

Cardiovascular disease is more prevalent in man, this led to the popular concept that high testosterone is contributing to heart attacks. The opposite is the case.
Toxic metals are a contributor to the epidemic of cardiovascular disease, and low testosterone in turn is associated with more cardiovascular disease.
A study with a follow-up of 11.8 years showed men with lower total testosterone levels (< 241 ng/dL) had a 38% higher risk of CVD. A further confirmation was reported in the larger cohort study: "High

serum testosterone levels (680 ng/dL) predicted a reduced 5-year risk of CV events." [244]

2.2 Pituitary gland disruption

The pituitary gland is also known as the hypophysis.
One of the major causes of *"Hormonageddon"* - and one of the mechanisms that are empirically demonstrated in the book by the same name – is the accumulated disruption of the hypothalamus-pituitary- gonadal axis, an intricate array of hormone- producing and activating glands that determines gonad hormones and thus general-, sexual- and mental health.
Damage to any part of this axis can change a person profoundly.
The first two hormone glands are part of the brain, but they are **not entirely protected by the blood brain barrier**, so toxic metals can easily accumulate there and affect hormone regulation continuously. The gonads are the testis or ovaries.
"**Lead** affects hormones and responsiveness of all levels of the hypothalamic–pituitary–ovarian axis." [245]
"Low levels of pituitary function are associated with depression and suicidal thoughts, and appear to be a major factor in suicide of teenagers and other vulnerable groups. Because of its effect on the pituitary, **mercury** is known to cause frequent urination as well as high blood pressure." [246]
"Lead initially causes some subclinical testicular damage, followed by hypothalamic or pituitary disturbance." [247]

A study analyzing heavy metal concentrations in women with repeated miscarriages, concluded that heavy metals seem to have a negative impact on ovarian as well as on pituitary function. "The heavy metal-induced immunological changes may interfere with the physiological adaptation of the immune system to the state of pregnancy with the result of a miscarriage." [248]
A journal article published by the EPA found "heavy metals can act directly at the level of the pituitary gland to inhibit growth hormone releasing hormone (GRF)." **Zinc, cadmium, nickel,** and **mercury** reduced GRF stimulated growth hormone (GH) release without altering basal GH secretion. [249]
Cadmium affects the hypothalamic activity and pituitary hormone secretion in males. [250] "**Chromium** has a toxic effect on the hypothalamus-pituitary-gonadal axis." [251]

Four areas of the brain are not fully protected by the blood-brain barrier. "These areas include the **posterior pituitary gland, pineal gland, the median eminence of the hypothalamus and the area postrema.**" [252]

Thus, the pituitary gland and the hypothalamus (both instrumental in sex hormone production and regulation) are readily disturbed by the slightest amounts of toxic metals in the blood stream, causing hormonal disruption.

Ultimately, these disturbances may collectively contribute to societal deterioration and the process of "*Hormonageddon*".

The third brain area not protected by the BBB, the **pineal gland**, is instrumental in melatonin regulation and thus circadian rhythms. As toxic metals in the blood can easily enter the pineal gland, it is hardly surprising that insomnia is related to heavy metal toxicity (see p. 174). As we'll see, **mercury** accumulation has been shown in the pineal gland, which participates in circadian function through the secretion of melatonin and serotonin, and toxic metals can cause insomnia. [253]

2.2.1 Adrenal disruption

Environmentally significant metals, viz- **[steel], lead, mercury, cadmium, copper, arsenic** and **nickel** have endocrine/hormonal implications in human and animals, especially concerning the adrenals, thyroid, testis, ovary and pancreas.

"Toxic metals can cause structural and functional changes in the adrenal glands." Exposure to these metals can lead to disturbances in female reproductive performance in exposed subjects. Certain metals can cause injury to the **endocrine pancreas**. [254]

serotonin production
In the central nervous system (CNS), serotonin is almost exclusively produced in neurons originating in the raphe nuclei located in the midline of the brainstem." These serotonin-producing neurons form the largest and most complex efferent system in the human brain." [255]

2.3 Toxic metals and testosterone/ estrogen

"The reproductive health of humans and wild animals has progressively deteriorated in the last 50 years." [256]

"**Cadmium** attenuates [hinders] testosterone synthesis by promoting ferroptosis and blocking autophagosome-lysosome fusion, leading to testicular dysfunction and attenuated testosterone synthesis." [257]

"In children and adolescents (age 6–19 years), blood **cadmium** and **manganese** levels (at low-level environmental metal exposure) were associated with significantly higher serum TT levels in the female adolescents. Additionally, the blood **selenium** levels in male adolescents were related to significantly higher serum TT." Testosterone is a principal sex hormone needed for the normal physiologic processes during all life stages of both sexes. [258]

Testosterone also influences bone mass, muscle strength, mood, and intellectual capacity. [259]

Particularly in males "**testosterone makes strenuous effort feel good**" (work or exercise, etc.). [260]

In females, testosterone is of crucial importance for bone density and is necessary for normal ovarian and sexual function, libido, energy, and cardiovascular and cognitive functions." [261]

Studies have shown a role of the dopaminergic system in heavy metal neurotoxicity. [262]

Heavy metals act as xenoestrogens, mimicking the action of oestrogen in the body and activating cell responses normally mediated by oestrogen.

In particular, **cadmium** mimics estrogen-driven cell proliferation and prolactin secretion from anterior pituitary cells. [263]

In China, it was found that pregnant women with higher blood **lead**, blood **arsenic** or blood **manganese** had higher serum testosterone levels and hemoglobin levels, and testosterone might mediate the effect of **lead** exposure on hemoglobin.

Thus, sex hormones that are generally more prevalent in the opposite sex were increased with toxic metals. [264]

Here we can see one of the 'treacherous' effects of lead toxicity which we have alluded to above. Blood lead hinders the incorporation of the iron atoms in the hemoglobin molecules (hemoglobin accounts for the oxygen transporting property of the red blood cell). If the red blood cells don't function properly, leading to anemia, the body makes more of them, which may be misinterpreted as normal red blood cell counts and it can disguise the root cause of the anemia.

A Serbian study demonstrated the same trend towards more of those sex hormones which are generally more prevalent in the opposite sex, with increasing toxic metals. The researchers at the Clinical Center of Serbia called it a "Puzzling relationship between levels of toxic metals in blood and serum levels of reproductive hormones."

Among the subjects, representative of the general population, males with higher concentrations of the metals **Cd, As, Hg, Cr** and **Ni** in the blood had **higher levels of estradiol and progesterone**. Inversely, females with higher concentration of these metals in the blood had higher levels of testosterone. [265]

"Heavy metals mimic the biologic activity of steroid hormones, including androgens, estrogens, and glucocorticoids."

The metals **Zn(II), Ni(II),** and **Co(II)** in low micromolar concentrations bind the estrogen receptor. The interaction with the estrogen receptor gave rise to the term metalloestrogens." [266]

Further, **uranium** is an estrogen mimic.

Arsenic and hormones

Arsenite may exhibit estrogenic activity. "The altered estrogen signaling may cause over expression of estrogen receptor-alpha, suggesting an epigenetic change was caused by in- utero **As** exposure." [267]

Adult rats that consume drinking water with **arsenite** at 5 mg/kg of body weight per day, 6 days a week for 4 weeks, had reproductive tract abnormalities such as suppression of gonadotrophins and testicular androgen, and germ cell degeneration - all effects similar to those induced by estrogen agonists. [268]

Men with higher environmental **molybdenum** in the blood have significantly less circulating testosterone.

Inversely, men with more **zinc** had higher testosterone levels. [269]

Testosterone levels are correlated with typical male behavioral traits, the propensity for confrontation and heroism. Testes volume showed a moderate positive correlation with testosterone levels [$r(51) = 0.26$, $P = 0.06$]. [270]

If the proverbial "having balls" implies large testicles, then it is based on empirical facts.

2.4 Fertility

2.4.1 Infertility and population decline

In 'Hormonageddon', we elucidated the connection of declining birth rates, infertility, declining male sperm counts, declining male testosterone, declining female estrogen and the lack of interest in having children over the past few decades. We also investigated how the same mechanisms that lower sex hormones and fertility also contribute to the circumstance that most people do not even care about their own genetic extinction anymore. Further, the rate of decline in fertility was massively accelerated since the Covid injections.

A large scale global 2022 meta-analysis by Hagai Levine et al further emphasized the rapid pace towards human extinction, and even though it is all over the news, no one cares:
"This latest meta-analysis includes results from 223 studies." The researchers concluded:
"The new data and analyses confirm our prior findings of an appreciable decline in sperm count between 1973 and 2018 among men from North America, Europe and Australia and support a decline among unselected men from South/Central America, Africa and Asia. This decline has continued, as predicted by our prior analysis, and has become steeper since 2000. This substantial and persistent decline is now recognized as a significant public health concern." [271]

Reproductive health, including fertility, is closely related to behavioral outcomes.
As demonstrated extensively in *Hormonageddon* as well, in societies with below replacement birth rates (societies that are in the actual process of dying out), those individuals with the least desire to have children or with an outright aversion against children, on average have lower fertility in the first place, mostly unknowingly. So, people who don't want children often don't know that they couldn't.
"A substantial proportion of women (35%) who meet the medical criteria of infertility do not view themselves as being infertile."
"Infertility is associated with lower fertility intentions." [272]
Infertility is diagnosed when a couple has regular unprotected intercourse for one year without pregnancy. These conditions are rarely met by people who do not intend to have a baby.

A prospective cohort study showed a history of depression diagnosis was associated with a 4.3-fold increase in the risk of low semen volume in men. [273]

2.4.2 Various metals and infertility

Aluminum chloride (AlCl3), **cadmium** chloride (CdCl2), and **lead** chloride (PbCl4) can cause reduced sperm motility and membrane oxidative damage. [274]

Increased **mercury** levels are associated with infertility or subfertility status. "Further, infertile subjects with unexplained infertility showed higher levels of **mercury** in hair, blood and urine than fertile ones. Mercury exposure induced sperm DNA damage and abnormal sperm morphology and motility." [275]

The toxicity mechanisms of **cadmium, arsenic** and **lead** on reproduction function include oxidative stress, inflammation, apoptosis and endocrine disruption. [276]

The accumulation of **lead, cadmium, arsenic, bismuth**, and other elements, even in low concentrations, induces strong toxic effects on the reproductive tract.

"Characteristic of all heavy metals is that they generate reactive oxygen species (ROS) and induce oxidative stress (OS) in a variety of systems, including the reproductive system." [277]

An overload of **vanadium** (it is disputed as an essential element) is damaging to the reproductive system, affects fertility and it can cause fetuses malformations. [278]

2.4.3 Lead infertility

Chronic **lead** poisoning causes hypogonadism in men. [279]

Epidemiological studies in men (working in a **lead** environment) with blood Pb levels ranging from 10 µg/dl to <40 µg/ dl have shown an increased risk of infertility. [280]

In one study involving 4000 workers with blood **lead** levels higher than 25 µg/dl, it was shown they had significantly decreased insemination potential (childless men or men with a small number of children), compared with the control group. [281]

"Extensive studies presented direct interactions of **lead** with sex hormones and suggest a possible mechanism of lead induced reproductive toxicity at a molecular level." [282]

"Low-to-moderate **lead** exposures may increase the risk for spontaneous abortion at exposures comparable to U.S. general population levels during the 1970s and to many populations worldwide today; these are far lower than exposures encountered in some occupations." [283]

Already the Roman elites used onion and *Sapa* (grape sirup modified with **lead**) for abortions.

*"In both men and women, **lead** has been associated with infertility and damage in serum testosterone. Even In lead smelting workers without clinical symptoms of lead poisoning, a decrease in serum testosterone (T) is observed."* [284]

Studies suggest that **lead** poisoning may lead to a pituitary-hypothalamic defect in LH secretion. [285]

Accumulation of **lead** affects the majority of endocrine glands.

K. Doumouchtsis et al suggest that lead initially causes some subclinical testicular damage, followed by hypothalamic or pituitary disturbance when longer periods of exposure take place. Similarly, **lead** accumulates in granulosa cells of the ovary, causing delays in growth and pubertal development and reduced fertility in females. [286]

In peripubertal U.S. girls, **lead** and **cadmium** are associated with reproductive hormones. At 10 and 11 years of age, higher **lead** was inversely associated with inhibin B, a marker of follicular development, and pubertal delays appeared to be stronger in the context of higher **Cd** concentrations.

Girls with lower **Pb** had significantly higher inhibin B than did girls with moderate Pb (1–4.99 µg/dL). [287]

That's 1 µg of lead per 1 deciliter of blood. For the entire 3 liter of blood) = 30 µg of lead = 0.030 milligram = **0.00003 grams** of lead.

This means: **already 0.030 milligram of lead (30ug or 0.00003 grams) in the blood of a 10-year-old girl has a measurable negative effect on later fertility.**

That's less than the smallest speck of dust that you can see with the naked eye. (For comparison, a tiny grain of salt is about 160 ug or micrograms.)

2.4.4 Lead and gender of offspring

"Lead has been implicated in shifting the sex ratio to fewer boys born and maybe related to low testosterone at the time of conception." Professional drivers exposed to excessive [leaded] petroleum products father fewer sons. [288]

Also workers with higher blood Pb levels had significantly reduced odds of having male offspring. [289]

Accumulation of **lead** affects the majority of the endocrine glands, in particular the hypothalamic-pituitary axis. [290]

72

An analysis of premenopausal women 18– 44 years of age in Buffalo New York demonstrated: higher **lead** levels were associated with higher mean progesterone levels, whereas higher **cadmium** levels were associated with decreased Follicle-Stimulating Hormone (FSH). The researchers observed these associations among healthy, regularly menstruating women at environmentally relevant exposure levels. [291]

Platinum, lead and nickel
Men with spermiation defects have higher estradiol levels and high **platinum** in seminal cells.
85% of cases with spermiation defects **also had high lead (four times higher) and higher nickel levels than controls.** [292]

Lead, copper and infertility
In Saudi Arabian men aged 20-50 years, the heavy metals **copper, lead** and **cadmium** showed a highly significant increase in the serum and blood of infertile men when compared with the concentrations in healthy control men."
Serum **copper** level was negatively correlated with the serum testosterone level among infertile men. [293]
In Nigeria, toxic metals (**lead, cadmium** and **mercury**) in untreated drinking water from hand-dug and borehole wells are associated with lower levels of serum follicle stimulating hormone (FSH), luteinizing hormone (LH), estradiol (E2), and testosterone (T) in men. [294]

Also in Nigeria, it was found that "Endocrine disrupting metals lead to alterations in the gonadal hormone levels in e-waste workers." Levels of TESTO, PROG, LH and FSH; as well as PROL and EST were significantly lower in e-waste workers compared with unexposed participants, due to **chromium, cadmium, arsenic** and **mercury.** [295]
"An excess of the essential trace metals **copper, manganese,** and **molybdenum,** already in low concentrations, has adverse effects on male reproductive function." [296]
"A study on adult male brick kiln workers from Pakistan concluded that increased heavy metal burden in the blood exposes them to the development of general and reproductive health problems due to compromised antioxidant enzyme levels, increased oxidative stress conditions and a disturbed reproductive axis." [297]

2.4.5 Genital malformation

Genital malformation is strongly correlated to in- utero hormone disruption due to phthalates and other organic toxins (as explained in detail in *Hormonageddon)*. GM including hypospadias, cryptorchidism and micropenis now affect over 2.7% of newborn boys. Endocrine disrupting heavy metals can be detected in children with GMF.

"Cryptorchidism is significantly increased by paternal exposure to heavy metals." [298]

Sharma et al established that boys (aged 1- 5) with hypospadias [the opening of the urethra is on the underside of the penis] have significantly higher serum **cadmium** and **lead** levels compared to healthy control boys. [299]

"Similar studies give reason to suppose that in most cases of unexplained subfertility in infertile couples or hypospadias and/or other idiopathic diseases, a probable factor may be **Cd** reproductive toxicity." [300]

In Mexico City, boys who in utero had higher concentrations of **arsenic, cadmium** and **barium,** later had higher testosterone levels in prepuberty. Boys with higher in- utero **aluminum** and peripubertal **barium** concentrations turned out to later have more advanced sexual developmental stage and higher testicular volume at the age of 8 followed by slower pubertal development thereafter. [301]

Meaning, overall, boys with more toxic metal exposure in utero underwent earlier sexual development followed by a slowdown of progression at age 14.

2.4.6 Animal studies fertility

Rams reared near a copper smelter showed reproductive disorders, adversely affecting testicular morphology, sperm production and quality. Greater effects were recorded at closer distances. Higher testicular levels of **Pb, Cd, Cr,** and **Ni** were correlated with higher sperm abnormality. [302]

A similar pattern is observed in the Panda habitat in China (see 14.4.7).

"Fish in bays polluted with **lead** and **cadmium** show disrupted sex hormone levels." The serum levels of sex steroid hormones are sensitive biomarkers for detecting heavy metal pollutants in aquatic environments and their effect on fish reproduction. [303]

A low-dose heavy metal mixture **(lead, cadmium** and **mercury)** induced testicular injury and abnormal sperm morphology in Wistar albino rats. Costus afer and zinc have protective effects. [304]

In female rats, "Subacute oral exposure to **cadmium** may lead to long-term disturbances in the reproductive system."

This includes changes in the plasma levels of steroid hormones and a decrease in estradiol (E2). [305]

2.4.7 Cadmium and fertility

Cadmium also affects the hypothalamic activity and pituitary hormone secretion in males.

The physiological functions controlled by these **pituitary hormones** can be modulated by cadmium. This xenobiotic is associated with deleterious effects on the gonadal function and with changes in the secretory pattern of other pituitary hormones like prolactin, adrenocorticotrophic hormone (ACTH), thyroid-stimulating hormone (TSH) and growth hormone (GH). "The accumulative data indicates the existence of a disruption in the regulatory mechanisms of the **hypothalamic–pituitary axis**." [306]

"Recently, **cadmium** has been shown to act like estrogen in vivo affecting estrogen-responsive tissues such as uterus and mammary glands. Metals that mimic estrogen are called metalloestrogens."

"An important tenet is that earlier (developmental) ages of exposure increase the impact of the endocrine-disrupting chemical or heavy metal on the normal development of reproductive organs, which may be permanently affected." [307]

Already 90 years ago, Alsberg et al reported **cadmium** caused hemorrhaging in testes of rats. [308]

In the 1950's and 1960's, other investigators reported that **Cd** caused hemorrhaging of the testes in a wide variety of species. [309]

"**Cadmium** has been related to impaired semen quality and altered hormonal levels in men. " [310]

"Cd 2+ has been shown to exert significant effects on ovarian and reproductive tract morphology." In addition, **Cd2+** exposure during human pregnancy has been linked to decreased birth weights and premature birth, resulting from maternal exposure to industrial wastes or tobacco smoke. [311]

"The testis is the tissue in which **cadmium** can accumulate in large amounts, with consequent impairment of spermatogenesis and endocrine function." [312]

"In primary ovarian cell cultures from either cycling or pregnant rats or human placental tissue, **cadmium** at concentrations >100 micro Mol suppressed progesterone and testosterone production." [313]

At doses that did not affect most organs, **Cd** caused damage to the testes within 24- 48h. Men with varicocele [mass of varicose veins in the spermatic cord] usually show an increased accumulation of **Cd** in the testicular circulatory system, correlating with the increased percentage of apoptotic germ cells in the seminiferous tubules." [314]

Varicose veins in the scrotum (varicocele) are responsible for >20% of male infertility in the US. Varicocele are associated with decreased sperm fertilizing ability. [315] After vein surgery, NAC supplementation improved male fertility by 22 % compared to surgery without NAC.

2.4.8 Animal studies/ various metals

"Recently, it was demonstrated that heavy metals such as **cadmium, arsenic, mercury, nickel, lead** and **zinc** may exhibit endocrine-disrupting activity in animal experiments." [316]

In rabbit studies, five out of 20 metals tested (**arsenic, cadmium, chromium, mercury** and **vanadium**) reduced sperm motility and curvilinear velocity. **Arsenic, cadmium, mercury and platinum** caused acrosome breakage with formation of various sized microvesicles. The study concluded, all the metal compounds studied, at levels higher than 1 microMol, may reduce sperm kinetic characteristics and probably fertilizing capacity. [317]

2.4.9 Mercury and fertility

"Both organic and inorganic **mercury** compounds highly accumulate not only in the liver and the kidneys but also in major endocrine glands, for example, the hypothalamus, the pituitary gland, the thyroid, the testes, the ovaries and the adrenal cortex." [318]

Animal and in vitro studies have shown that **mercury** can induce abnormalities in sperm morphology and motility. [319]

Choy et al described an association between semen **Hg** concentrations and sperm abnormalities in subfertile males attending an infertility clinic. [320]

In women undergoing in vitro fertilization, higher hair **mercury** concentration was associated with lower oocyte yield and lower follicle number after ovarian stimulation.

"While **mercury** had a deleterious effect, there was a positive effect for zinc and selenium in the ovarian response to gonadotrophin therapy for in vitro fertilization (IVF) treatment." [321]

In *Hormonageddon,* we saw that IVF children have worse health outcomes and lower fertility in later life. The same is true for surrogacy children. A metanalysis showed the medical outcome for the children at age 10 was comparable to previous results for children conceived after fresh IVF and oocyte donation. [322]

serotonin

"The many self-registered symptoms of patients with **mercury** intolerance have revealed many facets in common with those associated with serotonin dysregulation." [323]

2.4.10 Mercury sexual behavior

Hormonageddon covered the sensitive topic of the influence of environmental chemicals on human and animal sexual behavior/ orientation and identity. The substances that have a large immediate impact on sexual development and sex hormones are hydrocarbons, such as polychlorinated hydrocarbons, phthalates, DDT, bisphenols and so on, these accumulate in the environment to some extent, but can decompose over the years.

Toxic metals can act as endocrine disruptors and have similar effects on sexual maturation and behavior in animals as in humans, but in contrast to other (organic) chemicals, toxic metals last forever.

2.5 Animal behavior

Extensive animal studies suggest "wild birds suffer from personality disorders due to the ingestion of heavy metals." [324]

National geography reported: Male birds (ibises) that eat **mercury**-contaminated food show "surprising" homosexual behavior. "These male-male pairs (ibises that ate mercury-contaminated food) did everything that a heterosexual pair would do," said study leader Peter Frederick, a wildlife ecologist at the University of Florida in Gainesville." They built their nest, copulated together, stayed together on a nest for a month, even though there were no eggs— they did the whole nine yards." [325]

Researchers found a strong negative association between methyl **mercury** (MeHg) exposure and the number of breeding Great Egrets, leading to early breeding failure in these birds. [326]

Birds (Parus major, great tit), show variations in personality traits across a metal pollution gradient, where metals, especially **lead** and **cadmium**, are elevated close to a smelter. "At polluted sites, birds of both sexes displayed slower exploration behavior." [327]
These findings were later corroborated on larger scale studies. It was demonstrated that across the year, individuals with high blood **lead** concentrations and high concentrations of multiple metals in the feathers exhibit slower exploration behavior. [328]
Methylmercury exposure also induces sexual dysfunction in male and female drosophila melanogaster (fruit flies). [329]

2.5.1 Thyroid hormones

Autopsy studies in 1975 revealed that the thyroid can retain and accumulate more inorganic **mercury** than the kidneys. [330]
"**Mercury** blocks thyroid hormone production by occupying iodine-binding sites and inhibiting or altering hormone action leading to the impairment of body temperature control, **hypothyroidism, thyroid inflammation and depression.**" [331]
In this way, thyroid disfunction that is connected to iodine insufficiency may also be associated to **mercury** toxicity. Iodine may be present in sufficient quantities, but the mercury blocks thyroid hormone production and function by occupying these iodine-binding sites.
"Thyroid hormone kinetics are affected by a number of metallic compounds." [332]
Thyroid disease associated with cobalt included both thyromegaly and hypothyroidism. [333]

2.5.2 Thyroid goiter

Most goiters are asymptomatic and benign and do not affect the patient's quality of life or longevity.
A study from Iran concluded that toxic metals such as **lead, cadmium** and **chromium** can increase the risk of both hypothyroidism and thyroid cancer." **Mercury** can trigger autoimmune reactions and oxidative damage, which plays a role in the pathogenesis of thyroid cancer, autoimmune thyroiditis, and hypothyroidism. " [334]
Further, **aluminum** can negatively impact the thyroid gland. [335]
Reduced content of essential elements (Mn and Se) and increased content of toxic metals (**Pb, Th, and U**) were found in goiter tissues (GTs) compared with healthy-thyroid tissues (HTTs) [336]

2.5.3 Thyroid cancer

In French Polynesia, an area with a high incidence of thyroid cancer, the risk of this cancer is increased by 30% for each increase in **As** intake of 1 µg/d/kg body weight, despite being within the recommended daily intake indicated by the WHO.

"Thyroid cancer is now the fourth most frequent cancer in women." [337]

Chapter 3
Mechanisms of action

3.1.1 Protein homeostasis disruption

It is surprising to many that humans need so much protein in order to be healthy.

It might seem more plausible when we consider the fact that hunter-gatherer populations in general consume a very high protein diet. But what about in industrialized countries?

Especially since most people do not work in muscle intensive jobs. And why do older people, including retirees, need more protein as they age? People even need more protein when they are critically ill (see below).

Proteins are not directly burned for energy in the way fats and carbohydrates are, they are essential for muscle synthesis and almost every metabolic process. "Under normal circumstances, protein only contributes about 5 to 10 percent of your body's fuel, but certain circumstances can increase protein's role." [338]

In a healthy body, amino acids from used proteins are constantly recycled to build new proteins.

"Proteins participate in virtually every biological process."

"To form these new proteins, amino acids from food and those from protein destruction are placed into a "pool." When an amino acid is required to build another protein, it can be acquired from the additional amino acids that exist within the body." [339]

The continues breaking down of proteins and building of new ones is referred to as protein turnover. "Every day over 250 grams of protein in the body are dismantled and 250 grams of new protein are built." [340]

"General consensus holds that proteins are the prime targets of heavy metal toxicity." [341]

Now, since chronic intoxication with multiple metals is the norm today, the standard recommendation for protein requirements for the average sedentary person must be viewed in the context of how much protein is waisted in protein misfolding and other disruption of protein synthesis. It may turn out that healthy people without toxic metal burden can function and maintain muscle with lower than recommended protein intake.

3.1.2 Metal toxicity and protein excretion

"Some metals can produce reactive radicals which go on to result in depletion of protein sulphhydryls." [342]

Heavy metal ions bind rapidly to albumin, the most abundant protein in plasma.

"Chronic intoxication with heavy metals **(e.g. Cd2+, Hg2+, Pb2+)** induces an increase in urinary flow rate, proteinuria, glycosuria, aminoaciduria and excessive loss of major ions." [343]

(Proteinuria, also called albuminuria, is elevated protein in the urine).

3.2 Toxic metals cause protein misfolding

"Toxic metals disturb native proteins' functions by binding to free thiols or other functional groups, catalyzing the oxidation of amino acid side chains, perturbing protein folding, and/or displacing essential metal ions in enzymes." [344]

Thus, the right proteins may be present in adequate amounts, but cannot be used by the body in their misfolded state.

M. Tamás et al explain:

"*To function, most proteins fold into a strictly defined 3D structure, their native conformation. Misfolded proteins [as can be caused by toxic metals, for instance] are cytotoxic, as they may aggregate and/or interact inappropriately with other cellular components. Numerous neurodegenerative and age-related disorders are associated with protein misfolding and aggregation.*"[345]

"*Heavy metals and metalloids have been shown to inhibit refolding of chemically denatured proteins in vitro, to interfere with protein folding in vivo and to cause the aggregation of nascent (developing) proteins in living cells.*"

"Numerous neurodegenerative and age-related disorders are associated with protein misfolding and aggregation." [346]

Additional studies confirm:

"**Cd2+, Hg2**+ and **Pb2+** proved to inhibit very efficiently the spontaneous refolding of chemically denatured proteins by forming high-affinity multidentate complexes with thiol and other functional groups.

With similar efficacy, the heavy metal ions inhibited the chaperone-assisted refolding of chemically denatured and heat-denatured proteins. Thus, the toxic effects of heavy metal ions may result as well from their interaction with the more readily accessible

functional groups of proteins in nascent and other non-native form. **The toxic scope of heavy metals seems to be substantially larger than assumed so far.**" [347]
These mechanisms of disrupted protein synthesis may cause increased nutritional protein requirement with increasing metal toxicity. Misfolded proteins are cytotoxic, useless and need to be replaced continuously by the body.

In addition:

"Low dietary protein disturbs **cadmium** induced alterations in carbohydrate metabolism, essential trace elements metabolism and offsets the hepatic and renal process of cadmium detoxification. In this way, **protein malnutrition enhances the susceptibility to cadmium intoxication.**" [348]

3.2.1 Required protein intake

"The protein requirement is defined as the lowest level of dietary protein that will balance the losses of nitrogen (N) in persons maintaining energy balance." [349]

For a majority of people worldwide, especially those living in poverty, it would be nearly impossible to acquire the recommended protein intake (for instance, with 3 kg of cooked rice per day, or with 23 chicken eggs or 5 liters of milk per day).

"The Recommended Dietary Allowance (RDA) for protein is a modest 0.8 grams of protein per kilogram of body weight." [350]

For a 70 kg person, that's 56g of protein.

"**People 65 and older need about 50 per cent more protein than younger adults — between about 1 and 1.2 g/kg of protein -** says Heather Keller of the University of Waterloo." [351]

"At age 40- 50, your protein needs increase to about 1–1.2 grams per kilogram" (or 75–90 grams per day for a 75-kilogram person). [352]

Not only do the elderly in general need more protein as they age, but in critically ill geriatric patients throughout the stages of recovery, "It is important to note that protein requirements increase considerably with illness severity." [353]

In order to gain and/or maintain muscle, "most studies suggest that 1.6–2.2 grams per kg of lean mass are sufficient." [354] For a 75 kg person that's between 120g and 165g per day. The higher value would be the equivalent of 5 liters of whole milk or 23 chicken eggs per day.

According to collated national food consumption surveys, the average protein intake of adults in Europe is often at or above the published population reference (PRI) of 0.83 g per kg of body weight per day (between 67 g and 114 g per day for men and between 59 g and 102 g per day for women. [355]

To get the recommended minimum of 75g of protein for a 75 kg person, they would need 780 gram of dry rice or 3 kilos of cooked rice.

3.2.2 Hunter-gatherer protein intake

Large scale analyses by Loren Cordain et al 2000 indicate worldwide hunter-gatherer diets are extremely high in **protein (19– 35% of energy)** and low in carbohydrate (22–40% of energy) by normal Western standards, whereas the fat intake would be comparable or higher (28–58% of energy) than values currently consumed in modern, industrialized societies.

Analyses included 229 hunter-gatherer societies.

"Whenever and wherever it was ecologically possible, hunter-gatherers consumed high amounts (45–65% of energy) from animal food. Most (73%) of the worldwide hunter-gatherer societies derived >56% of energy of their subsistence from animal foods, whereas only 14% of these societies derived >50% of energy of their subsistence from gathered plant foods. This high reliance on animal-based foods coupled with the relatively low carbohydrate content of wild plant foods produces universally characteristic macronutrient consumption ratios in which protein is elevated (19- 35% of energy) at the expense of carbohydrates (22- 40% of energy)." [356]

"Most analyses of hunter-gatherer diets assume caloric intakes of approximately 3000 kcal/day, a surprisingly large figure that exceeds typical contemporary intakes." [357]

Hadza (one of the few remaining "true" H- G groups) men eat and burn about 2,600 calories a day, Hadza women about 1,900 calories a day- the same as adults in the U.S. or Europe.[358]

3.3 Mechanism of action: oxidative stress

The free radical theory of aging arose in 1954, support for this theory has increased progressively since.

The theory postulates that "aging is caused by free radical reactions, i.e., these reactions may be involved in production of the aging changes associated with the environment, disease and the intrinsic aging process." [359]

"The process of oxidative stress via free radicals plays a major part in the development of chronic and degenerative illness such as cancer, autoimmune disorders, aging, cataract, rheumatoid arthritis, cardiovascular and neurodegenerative diseases."

Exogenous ROS/RNS result, for instance, from air and water pollution, cigarette smoke, alcohol and heavy or transition metals (**Cd, Hg, Pb, Fe, As**). [360]

Oxidative stress is also implicated in anxiety (See also 4.7.2)

Chapter 4
Psychiatry and toxic metals

The exponential increase in psychological disorders in recent decades is strongly linked to the progression of *Hormonageddon* in the West and elsewhere. Chronic toxic metal poisoning can cause or exasperate psychological illness.

A National Institute of Health meta-analysis of a total of 415 articles concluded:

"Toxic metal exposure can result in a wide array of common mental health disorders that may mimic many psychiatric diseases and thus lead to psychoactive prescription drug use or other avoidable treatments." [361]

In a paper titled *"Psychotoxicology - the return of the mad hatter,"* the psychiatrist-author alleges that providers of mental health care "have not been attentive to the huge and expanding capacity of neurotoxic substances to induce symptoms of emotional and behavioral dysfunction" and that "patients are being poisoned and rendered psychiatrically disabled as a result of a disregard for occupational and environmental health". [362]

The term 'mad as a hatter', meaning completely crazy, stems from hat makers who often suffered from mental illness as a result of **mercury** exposure [363] (See also mad hatter syndrome 4.10).

A higher concentration of heavy metals in soil is associated with an increased probability of having a mental disorder in the adult population of Spain.

Analysis of data from the Spanish National Health Survey (2011-2012) observed a gradient effect for **Pb, As,** and **Cd.**

"A stronger association of mental disorder with the toxic metals was found in people consuming more than 1 daily serving of vegetables." [364]

"Exposure to **lead** even at levels generally considered safe could result in adverse mental health outcomes." [365]

And **lead** removal from the body has been used in many cases to completely resolve such symptoms.

"**Lead**-exposed workers in foundries, battery plants, or lead smelters are reported to suffer from cognitive and neuromotor deficits, as well as mood disorders such as anxiety, hostility, and depressive states." [366]

According to the U.S. EPA and the Agency for Toxic Substances and Disease Registry, exposure to **mercury, lead** and **arsenic** is known to cause anxiety and/or depression. [367]

"Heavy metal toxicity can disturb the brain chemistry causing depression and anxiety; it can also significantly weaken the immune system." [368]

"Overexposure to **tin** may damage the nervous system and cause psychomotor disturbances including tremor, convulsions, hallucinations, and psychotic behavior. " [369]

4.1 Behavioral disorders, aggression

4.1.1 Various metals and aggression

A study with 299 schoolchildren residing in the heavily polluted Taranto area in Italy revealed: blood **lead** mainly influenced social problems, aggressive behavior, externalizing and total problems. Urinary **arsenic** showed an impact on anxiety and depression, somatic problems, attention problems and rule breaking behavior. "A significant interaction between **lead** and **arsenic** was observed, with a synergistic effect of the two metals increasing the risk of attention problems, aggressive behavior, externalizing problems and total problems." [370]

Excess **copper** can become toxic and trigger symptoms such as hyperactivity and irritability. [371]

Studies show that exposure to **cadmium** is implicated in hyperactivity, increased aggression, impaired social memory processes and altered drinking behavior. [372]

Already in 1983, M. Marlowe et al found increased **lead** and **mercury** levels in emotionally disturbed children. [373]

"Aggression can be caused by internal or external factors, such as exposure to **cadmium**." [374]

A study on 228 adolescents between the ages of 13 and 19 showed a "significant relationship between adolescents' aggression levels and heavy metals. There is an undeniable relationship between the health of adolescents and environmental pollution caused by heavy metals."

Lead, mercury and **manganese** were positively correlated with the tendency to aggression. [375]

4.2 Lead and crime

4.2.1 Lead toxicity and aggression

Lead disrupts neurotransmitter release and neurotransmitter-related systems, particularly those of dopamine. [376]

More precisely, **lead** is known to prohibit the stimulated release of dopamine but to enhance its spontaneous release. [377]

"**Lead** exposure is associated with functional and microstructural changes in the healthy human brain." [378]

"Research has shown that **lead** exposure in children is linked to "a whole raft of complications later in life, among them lower IQ, hyperactivity, behavioral problems and learning disabilities." A significant body of research links **lead** exposure in children to violent crime. [379]

"**Lead** poisoning in our days is also apparent as a relation between hotspots of crime and hotspots of lead exposure. The association between lead and crime appears particularly robust with respect to rates of violent index crime, but less so for rates of property index crime." [380]

"The brain of adults who were exposed to increased **lead** levels during their childhood also shows a decreased volume, especially in the prefrontal cortex." [381]

The prefrontal cortex plays an important role in impulse control and thus deficits are associated to anti-social behavior.

Today, in young adults with even low levels of **lead** exposure, higher blood **lead** levels are associated with increased odds of major depression, panic disorders and other psychological alterations. [382]

As we have seen above "Exposure to lead even at levels generally considered safe could result in adverse mental health outcomes." [383] And lead removal from the body has been used in many cases to completely resolve such symptoms.

Many young children with elevated blood **lead** levels will have iron insufficiency or iron deficiency anemia. Thus, iron deficiency is an important comorbidity of **lead** toxicity; pica behavior has sometimes been associated with iron-deficient status. [384]

(Pica behavior is a tendency or craving to eat substances other than normal food, such as clay, plaster, or ashes, occurring during childhood or pregnancy, or as a symptom of disease).

Not unexpectedly, "Pica behavior is sometimes, but not always, found in conjunction with micronutrient deficiencies", affected people are apparently subconsciously trying to replenish lacking minerals.

"Pica is significantly associated with increased risk for anemia and low hemoglobin (Hb), hematocrit (Hct), and plasma zinc. " [385]

All these conditions are also independently associated with chronic **lead** poisoning.

High **lead** levels have been found to be associated with attention deficit hyperactivity disorder (ADHD), impulsivity and inability to inhibit inappropriate responding. [386]

Recall people born between 1951 and 1980 have average **lead**-linked intelligence deficits of around 6 IQ points. [387]

4.2.2 Manganese and crime

In US-counties where there is no record of environmental pollution from either **lead** or **manganese**, the crime rate is only half of that in counties with pollution of either of the metals according to the government's Toxic Release Inventory.

A group of researchers at Dartmouth College found "the presence of **lead** and **manganese** in a community is directly correlated with the rates of violent crime." [388]

Studies of an area in Australia with much higher levels of violence as well as autopsies of several mass murderers also found high levels of **manganese** to be a common factor. [389]

Manganese is an essential element, but harmful in high doses.

"Studies have found evidence that abnormal metals and trace elements affected by metal exposure appear to be a factor associated with aggressive or violent behavior. [390]

Several studies in the California prison system found those in prison for violent activity had significantly higher levels of hair **manganese.** [391]

"**Manganese** overload is associated with neurobehavioral toxicities including behavioral disinhibition, impulsive errors and attention problems." [392]

4.2.3 Tourette syndrome and tics epidemic of 2021

60 Minutes Australia reported a "global mental health crisis that emerged during the pandemic":

"All over the world, we saw a mysterious explosion in tics in teenage girls." [393]

The epidemic of tics was linked to the emergence of the pandemic.

"Officials at the Centers for Disease Control and Prevention (CDC) observed this concerning trend based on documented emergency department visits by children seeking treatment for tic disorders. [394] But on closer inspection of the timeline, it turns out that the real onset was only at the beginning of 2021, coinciding with the deployment of the c vaccine.

"In 2021 and the beginning of 2022, there were more emergency department visits among adolescents between the ages of 12 and 17 than there were in 2019. For girls in this age group, the proportion of emergency department visits for tic disorders tripled." [395]

"New onset parkinsonism, chorea, and tic-like behaviors have also been reported after COVID-19 vaccination." [396]

The rapid onset of tics in recent years has been linked to the Chinese social media platform *tik tok*. [397]

Obviously, neurologically healthy children are not afflicted with tics only by media consumption alone (social media, video games, TV). Previously, Tourette's syndrome and tics have developed in children from **mercury** poisoning.

"Generally, males suffering from tic disorder are significantly more likely to have received increased organic-**mercury** from Thimerosal-containing hepatitis B vaccines administered within the first month-of-life." [398]

4.3 ADHD / ADD

Attention deficit/hyperactivity disorder (ADHD), which is characterized by inattention, impulsivity, and hyperactivity, is among the most common psychiatric disorders occurring in children. [399]

"ADHD symptoms also include, impulsivity, agitation, irritability and aggressiveness."

According to the statistics on the incidence of autism from the U.S. CDC, one out of 6–8 children suffers from autistic spectrum disorders in the USA. [400]

Polanczyk et al reported a global prevalence of ADHD of 9.5% in a meta-analysis. [401]

4.3.1 Various toxic metals and ADHD

A study by the Norwegian Institute of Public Health found:
"Prenatal exposure to heavy metals such as **cadmium, lead** and **arsen**ic, and increased levels of the mineral **manganese**, were

linked to an increased risk of ADHD and autism spectrum diagnosis in children." [402]

In Korean children, the levels of **lead** and **cadmium** observed in the hair of children diagnosed with ADHD were significantly higher than in the control subjects. [403]

"Even in small amounts, toxic metals are capable of harming neurological development." [404]

In East Asia, ADHD and autism were virtually unknown before 2000. [405] Today, ADHD affects 8.9 % of boys in Hong Kong.

"Seven-year- old children with high blood **mercury** levels (above 29 nmol/L) had a **9.7 times higher risk of having ADHD**." [406]

Also in children aged 6–14 years in Guangzhou, China, ADHD is associated with heavy metal exposure during adolescent development.

The median concentrations of **chromium, manganese, cobalt, nickel, copper, molybdenum, tin, barium,** and **lead** in the urine of ADHD children were significantly higher than those of the control group. [407]

Mercury and ADHD

Prenatal **mercury** exposure, measured through samples of cord blood, is associated with ADHD symptoms in children. [408]

The WHO warns that "effects of **mercury** on the nervous system also include a constellation of effects such as poor school performance, problems with impulse control, and attention deficit." [409]

Copper and ADHD

"One of the major syndromes with which **copper** excess is associated in younger children is attention deficit disorder." [410]

Decreased serum cupper/zinc superoxide dismutase (SOD) is associated with high copper in children with ADHD. [411]

In addition, excess copper blocks the production of serotonin, a mood-balancing neurotransmitter. This triggers emotional, mental, and behavioral problems, from depression and anxiety to paranoia and psychosis. "Copper levels are higher in ADHD children." [412]

Likewise, in children with ADHD in India, hair and urine **copper** levels were increased compared to controls while hair and urine zinc levels were decreased. [413] Copper in adolescent girls is associated with running away, promiscuity and eating disorders (see 8.15).

Cadmium and ADD

Higher cumulative **cadmium** exposure in adults may be related to subtly decreased **attention and perception**. [414] Here again, this association was observed among exposure levels that have been considered to be without adverse effects and these levels are common in U.S. adults.

Antimony and ADHD

"Research on children found that ADHD hyperactivity/impulsivity type (ADHD-H/I) patients demonstrated the highest **antimony** levels and ADHD-I patients demonstrated the highest **cadmium** levels." Further, **cadmium** and **lead** levels were both negatively correlated with Intelligence Quotient. [415]

Recall that **antimony** is contained in PET bottles and increasingly in hundreds of other products and it is marketed as a safe substitution material for lead plumbing.

Lead and ADHD

High hair **lead** levels have been reported to be related to attention-deficit behavior. [416]

A Korean study found: children with blood **lead** levels in the highest quartile (>2.17 hg/ dL) are 1.5 times more likely to be diagnosed with ADHD than children with lower blood lead.

"**Lead** exposure, **even at very low concentrations**, and adverse family environment (e.g., single-parent family) were risk factors for the development of ADHD in children." [417]

These highest quartile blood lead levels are still considered normal by the CDC's and most international government standards.

In school-aged children in the UAE it was found that increased blood concentrations of **lead, manganese** and **zinc** were significantly associated with ADHD. [418]

A study on 270 mother-child pairs in Belgium found that doubling prenatal **lead** exposure (measured in cord blood) was associated with a more than three times higher risk for hyperactivity in boys and girls at age 7- 8. [419]

A study on almost 5,000 US children aged 4-15 found children with the highest blood **lead** levels were over four times as likely to have ADHD as children with the lowest blood lead levels. [420]

Researchers assessing 256 children aged 8-10 concluded, "even low blood **lead** levels (<5 µg/dL) are associated with inattentive and hyperactivity symptoms and learning difficulties in school-aged children". Note again that this is withing the CDC reference level of 2019. [421]

Vanadium ADHD/ chelation therapy

"Vanadium is a trace mineral that in overdose can aggravate bipolar disorder."

A review of 2008 concluded that chelation was an effective treatment for both autism and ADHD. Vitamin C in combination with chelation using EDTA has been used to remove **vanadium** and lessen the symptoms of depression in bipolar patients. [422]

4.4 OCD (obsessive compulsive disorder)

"OCD can arise when a certain amount of **mercury, aluminum,** or **copper** settles close enough to the endocrine glands in the brain or the emotional highway or emotional center of the brain". "The severity of OCD often depends on the amount of toxic heavy metals in the brain." [423]

"There is often a strong correlation to those high in **copper** with other altered minerals and heavy metals that can trigger symptoms of OCD." [424]

Copper toxicity and deranged ceruloplasmin metabolism are strongly implicated in neurological and psychiatric conditions such as OCD and schizophrenia. [425]

A 2008 study found a direct association between elevated ceruloplasmin and OCD. [426]

Iron and OCD

"OCD patients have lower T2 values (suggesting higher **iron** content) in the right globus pallidus (GP) region of the brain, with a trend in the same direction for the left globus pallidus." This effect was driven by patients whose OCD symptoms began from around adolescence to early adulthood. The results suggest a possible relationship between age of OCD onset and **iron** deposition in the basal ganglia. [427]

Vanderbilt University Medical Center investigators have found a 'surprising link' between brain **iron** levels and serotonin, a neurotransmitter involved in neuropsychiatric conditions [including OCD]. Variations in human serotonin transporter protein (SERT) have been linked to many neurobehavioral disorders such as compulsive disorder. [428]

"Low blood levels of the "feel good" hormone serotonin were associated with **iron** accumulation in the dopamine-producing substantia nigra in Parkinson patients."

"Serotonin, a key hormone that stabilizes mood, feelings of well-being, and happiness, is also often lower in the blood of Parkinson's patients and thought to contribute to the high rate of clinical depression among them." [429]

"Either emotional injury or toxic heavy metals such as **mercury, aluminum,** and **copper**, or many times, both causes create the symptoms of OCD in combination with each other." [430]

OCD is commonly treated with SSRIs, substantiating the serotonin connection.

4.5 Autism

In the 1990's, the incidence of autism was estimated to be 1 in every 110 children "but recent studies have shown that this incidence is increasing to 1 in every 88 children." [431]

More recently, an NIH bulletin explained that autism is seen in 1/166 children. Amongst those statistics, it was determined that 1 out of 6 children in the US now have developmental, psychiatric problems. [432]

A systematic review of 44 studies concluded that **mercury** levels are significantly higher in the whole blood, red blood cells, and brains of autistic subjects compared to controls. [433]

In a challenge urine test with DMSA, children with autism had, on average, 3x higher levels of **Hg** excretion than controls. [434]

One study confirmed that children with autistic spectrum disorder had higher levels of **mercury** and **arsenic** in their blood, compared to a control group. [435]

An assessment in 2015 using hair samples from autistic children also found significantly higher levels of **lead, mercury** and **aluminum** than in the control group. [436]

Holmes et al (2003) found that the number of maternal amalgam fillings was significantly associated with the child's hair **Hg** levels in the controls, though not in the autistic children. The major finding of this study was that hair **Hg** levels in autistic children are inversely correlated with severity of autism, suggesting that **autistic children have impaired excretion of Hg.** [437]

The Canadian Lyme disease foundation lists among the **causes of autism:** "metallothionein deficiency, oxidative stress**, childhood vaccinations** which act as triggers to events above through viral persistence in gut and brain, and heavy metal poisoning from additives in vaccines and lastly chronic disseminated Lyme neuroborreliosis disease." [438] (See also Lyme disease in chapter 5.16.7).

4.6 Depression and anxiety

"Depression and anxiety are among the most serious disorders spread-out all over the world."

"A plethora of studies has declared the existence of a relationship between exposure to toxic heavy metals and mood disorders, where the most important are anxiety and depression." [439]

Various studies that have diagnosed patients with depression and panic attacks disorders showed an excess of some metal concentration such as **cadmium, lead,** and **mercury**. [440]

"People in industrialized areas are more affected by mood disorders and are exposed more to heavy metals. " [441]

4.6.1 Depression

The metals most commonly associated with depression are **lead** [442], **mercury** and **cadmium**. [443]

Analyses of datasets of the NHANES of 2017- 2018 "demonstrated blood heavy metals, especially **cadmium, ethyl mercury,** and **mercury** were significantly associated with depression and the prediction of depression was imperative." [444]

"Toxic metals such as **mercury, cadmium, lead** and **tin** affect chemical transmission from one nerve cell to another and they also adversely affect neurotransmitters in the brain causing behavioral and mood changes such as depression." [445]

An earlier investigation of the US National Health and Nutrition Examination Survey on Americans aged 20- 80 years concluded: "The greater the concentration of heavy metals in urine, the higher the prevalence of the developed depressive disorder symptoms." [446]

A study by Fu et al determined heavy metals in combined exposure have a detrimental effect on the risk of depression, which might be attenuated by physical activity. Metals investigated were **cadmium, cobalt, tin, antimony, thallium,** and **mercury.** Urinary **tin** and **antimony** were individually associated with increased odds of depression. [447]

In 2001, the WHO predicted that depression will become "the second most burdensome disease by 2020, with the greatest burden in North America and the United Kingdom." [448]

It turned out they were right on the money, even though they did not forecast the global lockdown of 2020, which massively accelerated the long- developing epidemic of depression and suicide, which was then accelerated after the roll-out of the vaccine programs in 2021.

4.6.2 Cadmium and depression

In male Wister rats, all doses of **cadmium** exposure for 8 weeks provoked depression-like behavior. **Cd** induced an anxiogenic effect in both gender's tests and working memory was affected. [449]
In a nationally representative sample of humans, it was shown that individuals in the highest quartile of blood **cadmium** had higher odds of having depressive symptoms compared to those in the lowest blood cadmium quartile. Smoking status was statistically significantly associated with depressive symptoms. [450]
In a recent Korean study, a doubling of serum **cadmium** was associated with a 21% increase in depression, whereas twofold increases in daily vitamin B1, B3 and vitamin A intake reduced the risk of depression by between 8 and 20 percent. [451]
W. Sciarillo et al suggested that decreasing the amount of **cadmium2+** exposure may be reflected by a reduction in frequency of depression appearance. [452]
"**Cd2+** correlates most often with emotional problems at different age ranges." Prenatal exposure within 281 women have revealed that Cd2+ at means of 0.22 µg/L in umbilical cord blood increase the risk of **emotional problems** to 1.53-fold greater within descending boys at the age of 7– 8 years for every doubling of cord blood Cd2+ concentration. [453]

4.6.1 Depression and mercury

"Mercury has been known to cause several health complications including anxiety and depression." [454]
In a study by Siblerud et al (1994) who compared mood inventories for 25 women with amalgams and 23 women without, it was found that the women with amalgam fillings had higher scores for fatigue, insomnia, anger, depression, and anxiety. [455]
"Amalgam subjects scored as significantly less pleasant, satisfied, happy, secure and steady and had a more difficult time making decisions." [456]
"Acute mercury exposure may give rise to lung damage, whereas chronic poisoning is characterized by neurological and psychological symptoms, such as tremor, changes in personality, restlessness, anxiety, sleep disturbance and depression." [457]
Further observed are irritability, mood swings and nervousness, [458] and loss of self-confidence. [459]

In a group of 50 patients with dental amalgam restoration, 70% had psychiatric disorders including anxiety and depression symptoms, versus 14% in controls. [460]

The many self-registered symptoms of patients with **mercury intolerance** have revealed many facets in common with those associated with serotonin dysregulation. [461]

4.6.2 Lead, depression and anxiety

Persons with blood lead levels in the highest quintile had **2.3 times the odds of major depressive disorder and 4.9 times the odds of panic disorders** as those in the lowest quintile. [462]

A study on middle-aged to elderly men showed that low exposure to **lead** can contribute to depression, anxiety, or other psychiatric issues such as phobic anxiety.

Here again, **bone lead** levels were found to be more decisive than blood lead levels.

Patella (knee cap) bone **lead** was significantly associated with an increased risk of phobic anxiety and the combined outcome measure. Tibia and blood lead had similar associations.

The researchers concluded that cumulative lead exposure, as reflected in **bone lead** levels, could be a risk factor for psychiatric symptoms even at modest levels of exposure. [463]

"After chronic **lead** exposures of 25–50 parts per million (10–19 µg/dL), decreased activities of dopamine and serotonin in certain areas of the brain, especially the nucleus accumbens, were measured." [464]

A 10-year follow-up of 607 metal industry employees showed that **depressive and distress symptoms are predictors of low back pain, neck-shoulder pain**, and other musculoskeletal morbidity. [465]

4.7 Anxiety Disorders

C. Mfem et al 2021 note: "Anxiety is a general term for several disorders that cause nervousness, fear, apprehension and worrying. It is defined as an emotion characterized by feelings of tension, worried thoughts and physical changes like increased blood pressure. Anxiety is not the same as fear, which is a response to a real or perceived immediate threat; it is the expectation of future threat." [466]

"Too many responsibilities or a high-stakes work project trigger a stress response. Anxiety, on the other hand, is more internal. It is how you react to stressors. If you remove those stressors and still feel overwhelmed and distressed, you are likely dealing with anxiety." [467]

4.7.1 Metals and anxiety

In young adults with blood lead levels well within CDC reference levels, persons with blood lead levels in the highest quintile had **2.3 times the odds of major depressive disorder and 4.9 times the odds of panic disorders** as those in the lowest quintile. [468]
Lowest quintile = below 0.7 µg/dL; highest quintile: ≥ 2.11 µg/dL.
You can skip the math, if you like.
At 5 liters of blood for an adult: the lowest quintile= 35 µg in the entire blood volume – the highest q= 105 µg in the entire blood volume. The difference is 70 µg (micrograms) more lead in the blood.

In summary: only **70 µg (0.00007 grams) more lead in the blood of a young adult is associated with 2.3 times the odds of major depressive disorder and 4.9 times the odds of panic disorders. That's less than the smallest speck of lead dust that you can see with the naked eye.**

"Symptoms of Generalized Anxiety Disorder (GAD) are identical to the most common symptoms of heavy metal toxicity."
Patients with GAD have physical anxiety symptoms like tachycardia (abnormally high heart rate) and key psychological symptoms. Restlessness, fatigue, difficulty concentrating, and disturbed sleep are all examples of tachycardia and key psychological symptoms. [469]
"Exposure to heavy metals (**cadmium** chloride in particular) causes severe anxiety disorders." In mice studies, zinc and vitamin E had the capacity to ameliorate anxiety disorder caused by heavy metals. [470]
"Metal mixtures of six metals (**barium, cadmium, chromium, cesium, lead** and **antimony**) are associated with increased anxiety during pregnancy." The authors described the results as a public health concern, as anxiety disorders are highly prevalent and associated with significant co-morbidities, especially during

97

pregnancy when both the mother and developing fetus are susceptible to adverse health outcomes. [471]

"Exposure to heavy metals including **mercury, lead, aluminum and cadmium**, has been found in the cord blood of babies whose mothers were smokers." [472]

"Scores for tension, depression, anger, fatigue and confusion in workers exposed to **aluminum** for more than ten years were significantly higher than those in non-exposed controls." [473]

"**Lead** damages many organs, including the central nervous system, which can lead to provoked anxiety." [474]

In healthy postmenopausal women in Poland, there was a direct relationship between the level of **Pb** and the severity of anxiety. [475]

In open-field tests on rats, "**lead** exposure from the fetal period until adulthood caused anxiety and cognitive impairment.

Permanent exposure to lead caused strong anxiety without locomotor changes."

"These results suggest that the duration of **Pb** exposure is more relevant than the timing of exposure, since the permanent Pb group presented more pronounced effects and a significant increase in the Low Frequency and HF bands and anxiety levels." [476]

4.7.2 Oxidative stress, anxiety and toxic metals

"Heavy metals induce oxidative stress, which may be reversed by chelation therapy." [477]

"The severity of anxiety – but not of depression – is associated with oxidative stress in major depressive disorder." [478]

"All of the data demonstrate that there is a link between oxidative stress and high-anxiety-related behavior. "

"High O2 consumption, modest antioxidant defenses and a lipid-rich constitution make the brain highly vulnerable to redox imbalances. Oxidative damage in the brain causes nervous system impairment. Recently, oxidative stress has also been implicated in depression, anxiety disorders and high anxiety levels." [479]

Oxidative stress has also been reported to be associated with cognitive defects in both human and animal models. [480]

4.8 Anxiety and Hypertension

Multiple cross-sectional studies reveal a positive association between anxiety and hypertension. These associations are bidirectional, with those with hypertension being more likely to have anxiety and those with anxiety being more likely to have hypertension. [481]

We are going to take a closer look at this interaction with the focus on hypertension in 5.3.

The relationship between hypertension and anxiety was confirmed in a systematic review and meta-analysis of 13 epidemiological studies. [482]

To reduce actual stress is not easily done, and everyone knows, when stressed people with hypertension are on an extended vacation, their blood pressure barely drops, if it declines at all. Even when the same patients retire early and dedicate their lives to leisure and well-being, hypertension is usually not resolved.

Even actual retirement has "no clinically significant impact on blood pressure or cholesterol." [483]

By all means, everyone should adopt a healthier lifestyle.

But even those who strictly follow the official government recommended diet to reduce blood pressure called *Dietary Approaches to Stop Hypertension (DASH)*, lower blood pressure only to a slight extent.

Compared with control, DASH lowers BP within a week **without further effect thereafter.** DASH changed SBP/DBP by $-4.36/-1.07$ mm Hg after 1 week. [484]

Study participants lowered their BP from an average SBP from 135 mm Hg to 131 Hg. That is a reduction of 3 % by drastically changing their diet.

At the same time, it is well accepted that blood pressure will simply rise and rise over time, unless the patient is medicated.

In adults in Hong Kong, hypertension was associated with anxiety but not depression." [485]

In summary: Toxic metals generate antioxidant stress and can propagate hypertension.

Toxic metals can cause or enhance psychological conditions such as anxiety. Anxiety is determined as a psychological reaction or expectation of stress. In practice, reduction of actual stress only leads to a slight reduction of hypertension, if the underlying causes, such as metal toxicity, are not addressed.

4.9 Suicide and toxic metals

According to a 1977 review, "in severe cases of chronic **mercury** poisoning, depression may reach suicidal proportions." [486]

In a study of occupational exposure of former **mercury** miners, Kobal Grum et al (2006) reported that miners at the Idrija mercury mine in Slovenia have a historically high rate of suicide – 40 of 1589 miners (2,5 %) in 1950 -1995. Miners who had retired (for 1 year or longer) "tended to be more introverted and sincere, more depressive, more rigid in expressing their emotions and are likely to have more negative self-concepts than controls." [487]

In autopsies of deceased people, it turned out those who died of suicide had on average 3 times higher **mercury** contents in brain, liver and thyroid than non-suicide cases. [488]

Workers with toxic metal exposure at the Paducah gaseous diffusion plant from 1952 to 2003 had an increased suicide risk. Within exposure likelihood categories, several suicide SMRs were typically elevated for several metals. **Beryllium** exposure likelihood was associated with an increased hazard ratio (HR).

Uranium urine concentration was associated with an elevated suicide risk. [489]

"Decades of **mercury** exposure has been linked to the high youth suicide rates in an Indigenous community in Canada." 40% of indigenous adolescents in the region have attempted suicide. Grassy Narrows was the site of mercury dumping for nearly a decade after 1963, when a paper company released more than 20,000lb of mercury into the Wabigoon and English river systems. [490]

Additionally, **low zinc** levels are found in patients who have attempted suicide. [491] Zinc is depleted from the body by various toxic, non- essential metals.

Independently of toxic metals, in the new age of medicine of 2022: "a rising number of suicide attempts among young children worries North West physicians and poison centers." [492]

4.10 "Mad Hatter Syndrome" and mercury

Historically, hatters or hat-makers commonly exhibited slurred speech, tremors, irritability, shyness, depression, and other neurological symptoms; hence the expression "mad as a hatter." The symptoms were associated with chronic occupational exposure to mercury. Hatters toiled in poorly ventilated rooms, using hot solutions of mercuric nitrate to shape wool felt hats. [493]

Even low-level mercury exposure affects mood:

The classic symptom of chronic mercury poisoning, known as **erethism**, is a personality change comprising **excessive timidity,**

diffidence, shyness, loss of self-confidence, anxiety, a desire to remain unobserved and unobtrusive, a pathological fear of ridicule, and an explosive loss of temper when criticized. [494]
The term `erethism' was first coined by Pearson in 1805.
"Erethism is also known as erethismus mercurialis, the said mad hatter disease or mad hatter syndrome, it is a neurological disorder which affects the whole central nervous system, as well as a symptom complex." [495]

4.11 What do light house keepers, hat makers, dentists and goldminers have in common?

In the 19th century, also lighthouse keepers had a high frequency of madness and suicide. For a hundred years, lighthouses were often considered haunted, possessing the souls of the keepers or pushing them to go insane and commit murder. [496] This is reflected in numerous horror stories and thrillers. Before the 1800s, lighthouses were rather associated with tales of enchantment and romanticism.
"In order to turn the light and the Fresnel lens accurately, a zero-friction bearing of the day floated the light and the lens on a circular track of liquid mercury, the mercury evaporated and fumes were inhaled constantly." [497] Since the late 1800s, the large Fresnel lens was floated on 200 kg of mercury in a ring-shaped tray, the lamp was stationary in the center. [498]
Keepers breathed and touched the mercury on their daily cleaning rounds. [499]
According to Michaela Walter of the University of Calgary:
"Keepers were not aware of the many dangers of mercury and did not wear protective gear in those days. Another prevailing factor was the amount of time they spent in the area where the lens and lighting system was kept. Keepers routinely cleaned and maintained the lens and mercury bath, lit and cleaned the lamp, as well as reset the gears every three hours to allow the light to rotate." [500] When dust, dirt or other impurities built up in the mercury, part of the light house keeper's job was to strain the mercury through a fine cloth. Thus, "mercury fumes were making light house keepers mad as hatters." [501]
One of the most infamous light house keepers was Victoriano Álvarez, the last man on Clipperton island, an outpost abandoned by the Mexicans. Álvarez had lived secluded in his decommissioned lighthouse. After the remaining men died at sea

in 1917, Álvarez, now the only male survivor together with 15 women and children, came out of his lighthouse and started raping, enslaving and murdering women over months, until the last 3 surviving women managed to kill him. [502]

Naturally, human simplicity led to the conclusion that it was the loneliness that drove lighthouse keepers crazy and caused psychoses and aggression. No such symptoms were observed in guards of fire watch towers in the US, in solitary monks or in lonely shepherds over millennia.

4.12 Dentists

Dentists and their assistants are continuously exposed to **mercury** from amalgam fillings, even if the dentist practice itself does not use **mercury**; old remnants of amalgam can be covered by newer ceramic or composite fillings and are occasionally drilled into. "Dentists have been shown to have a higher urine **mercury** level, and a higher mercury body burden than the general population." [503]

Toxic metals other than mercury used in dentistry work include: "**nickel, aluminum, cadmium, chromium, titanium**, and unhealthy resin fillings with **aluminum**, hormones, and fluoride." [504]

"The use of **beryllium** (one of the most toxic metals) in the dental industry creates additional occupational exposure risks." [505]

"An Israeli case series study demonstrated that dental technicians are exposed to **beryllium** and various other occupational dusts and chemicals and are at high risk of developing chronic beryllium disease and other lung diseases." [506]

Dental assistants were found to have a relative risk of 2.0 (double the risk) for having five or more cognitive symptoms with a frequency of "often" or greater, relative to controls. [507]

A representative sample of 600 dentists showed dentists purchased significantly more illness-specific prescribed medications than controls, for the following disease categories: neuropsychological, neurological, respiratory, and cardiovascular. [508]

"Dentists, particularly male dentists, have significantly higher blood pressure than controls. " [509]

A 2019 review revealed a significant occurrence of neurological and sensory symptoms in dental workers occupationally exposed to chronic, low levels of metallic **Hg**.

"Some studies have reported a high prevalence of memory disturbance among dentists and dental personnel compared with the general population."

"Dental personnel reported more often neurobehavioural problems, reduced psychomotor speed, reduced cognitive flexibility, attention deficits, as well as memory loss, fatigue and sleep problems." [510]

Further, "dental personnel more often develop uncharacterized symptoms like fatigue, weakness and anorexia than unexposed people." [511]

A similar trend was shown for neurobehavioral effects, like idiopathic disturbances in cognitive skills, affective reactions, and motor functions. [512]

Studies show that dental health personnel who are occupationally exposed to **Hg** appear to suffer not only a higher body burden of Hg but also a higher total illness burden than is found in the general population. [513]

Insomnia and other sleep disorders have been reported among dental assistants exposed to **mercury**. [514]

4.12.1 Substance abuse and suicide in dentists

According to Dr. James Roberts, dentists have higher alcoholism rates than medical doctors. Roberts attributes this to mercury poisoning.

"Some dentists use specific drug groups to deal with stressors and pain. These include alcohol, opiates, benzodiazepine, illicit drugs and nitrous oxide. According to data, alcohol is the drug of choice for 37% of dentists with substance abuse problems, while 31% use opioids, 10% consume street drugs, and 5% abuse nitrous oxide." [515]

Curtis (2011) reported that "while 10 -12 percent of the general American population become addicted to **alcohol or drugs** at some point during their lives, the prevalence for dentists and physicians is probably 12-19 percent. "[516]

"In 1983, Christen quoted figures indicating that 12,000 dentists in the USA had a drinking problem." [517]

In a ten-year prospective cohort study, Arnetz et al (1987) found "an elevated standardized mortality ratio (SMR) for suicide in male dentists compared to other male academics." [518]

Throughout academia, it is broadly denied that dentists have high rates of drug- and alcohol- abuse and higher suicide rates. However, there is a disproportionate abundance of literature

103

concerning mental health and alcoholism of dentists, proclaiming that dentist work is extremely stressful and poorly rewarded and dentists are "stigmatized". Dentists are said to suffer from work-related stressors such as:

"A high patient load; lack of sufficient control, especially over resources for effective service delivery, especially in community-based dentistry; lack of recognition and appropriate reward; lack of social support; quality of working life; occupational hazards, ocular problems, eye injuries, latex allergy and musculoskeletal pain." [519]

According to a search of 'mental health' within the BDJ archives, there are 662 results, the first of which is dated 24 January, 1987, where Cooper, Watts and Kelly wrote 'Job satisfaction, mental health, and job stressors among general dental practitioners in the UK'. [520] The paper reads:

*"This study assesses the levels of job satisfaction and mental health among a sample of 484 general dental practitioners. It was found that about one-third of the sample were job dissatisfied. In addition, **male dentists showed significantly higher mean scores on four sub-scales of the mental health index (free-floating anxiety, phobic anxiety, depression and hysterical anxiety)** than the normal population; while female dentists had higher scores on only two sub-scales (free-floating anxiety and hysterical anxiety). Type A coronary-prone behaviour was also higher for male in contrast to female dentists."* [521]

"Dentists have been described as 'melancholic perfectionists' frustrated because they are often unable to achieve the ambitious goals within the stringent timetables set up by themselves or, purportedly by others. The mechanical minutiae and constant dealing with a nervous public inevitably cause feelings of frustration, resentment, and inferiority." [522]

All these symptoms and personal grievances are consistent with chronic mercury poisoning. For one of the best paid white-collar professions, this sounds like "*Mad hatter syndrome.*" The physical complaints are also consistent with mercury "ocular problems, eye injuries, latex allergy and musculoskeletal pain. "

When was the last time you heard an entire profession (say fast food workers) complain about 'latex allergy' and 'lack of social support'?

Why aren't brain surgeons - whose job performance is usually a matter of life or death - complaining about "*constant dealing with a nervous public.*"

In the US, a general dentist makes $167,160 a year for their "poorly rewarded" work. [523] In Switzerland, it's between 65 and 200,000 Euro per year, [524] including parttime work.

Compare all of these problems to the minute number of articles written on the stressful occupations of oil rig workers, underpaid EM nurses and garbage collectors. How many dentists look at a delivery driver and think: "He has got the good life, poor me, I'm so stigmatized and poorly rewarded."

Since the above psychological symptoms can be enhanced by low level chronic mercury poisoning, it is likely that the chronic mercury exposure is the decisive factor here. Anecdotally, you might be able to spot a 'mad hatter dentist'. I have met two of them, overly shy dentists with temper tantrums and anger issues, unexpected traits for a high education profession, in which patience, composure and a calm, steady hand are absolute requirements.

Medical doctors

"The rate of substance abuse disorders in medical doctors and dentists is estimated to 10% to 15%, more than double that of the general population." [525]

In the general population of people 26 and older, SUD affects 6.7%. [526]

"One medical doctor commits suicide in the U.S. every day -- the highest suicide rate of any profession. And the number of doctor suicides - 28 to 40 per 100,000 - is more than twice that of the general population, new research shows. "The rate in the general population is 12.3 per 100,000. [527]

In India, while an average person lives up to 72 years, a doctor is expected to live up to 59 years. The study conducted in Maharashtra found that the majority of them die due to cardiovascular diseases and early malignancy. [528]

4.13 Gold workers mercury

Goldsmiths often suffer from Mad Hatter Syndrome as well.

The burning process of amalgamated gold is a significant source of **Hg** exposure to goldsmiths.

"Gold workers in Pakistan had 20 times higher **mercury** levels in their Red Blood cells as well as plasma than controls.

Urine mercury levels were 61 times higher. All workers participating in this study were suffering from physical and mental diseases." [529]

In manual, artisanal gold mining – which produces 10 percent of the world's gold - 3 kg of mercury is used to produce 1 kilo of gold. [530] But only milligrams of mercury remain in the finished gold, which is then evaporated by soldering in jewelry making. Wearing the finished jewelry is unlikely to cause any mercury toxicity effects, reactions to nickel in jewelry, called nickel contact allergy, are more common.

Gold jewelry sold in the west has been tested to contain up to 5 ppm of mercury and 1 ppm of arsenic. [531]

Today, western jewelers work primarily with bulk gold from big industrial refineries which contains less mercury (most refineries are in Switzerland). But, when old jewelry is repaired or amended, the gold smith might solder old gold that can be 100 % artisanal, with a high mercury content. Whatever the purity of the gold is (e.g., 99%) the remainder can be expected to be mostly mercury.

So, in artisanal jewelry gold, the mercury comes either from the mining process, or from traditional fire- gilding, a thin gold coating of objects made of other metals.

Not only **mercury**, but also **lead** exposure is related to health problems in metal artisan workplaces and high-risk household contacts.

In Thimphu, Bhutan, blood **lead levels are elevated in** 38.4% **and mercury levels** are elevated in 51.9% of the workers.

"In traditional goldsmith work, mercury is mixed with gold to form an amalgam, which is then applied to metal objects and sublimed by fire to obtain a rich metallic glow and durable golden appearance (burnished gold)." [532]

During this fire- gilding process, the mercury is mostly evaporated and released in the air of the workshop, to be directly inhaled by the goldsmith, depending on safety ventilation.

Gold miners

During the 1800s California Gold Rush, based on estimates by researchers, it is possible that 10 to 13 million pounds (5,000-6,000 tons) of mercury were discharged into the environment. "A significant portion of this mercury has migrated downstream to the Sacramento Delta and San Francisco Bay." [533]

Today, the mercury that was left behind creates problems for human health and the environment in much of the state.

"California's mining sediments may continue to release mercury into waterways over at least the next 10,000 years." [534]

"Mercury is everywhere in the waterways and ecosystems of the Sierra Nevada. Liquid mercury can be seen on the bottom of streams." [535]

During the California Gold Rush, mercury was distilled from cinnabar rocks (orange or pink rock, often found on the surface). Most of the mercury used for the gold rush was mined from the Coast Range between Los Angeles and Eureka. For the gold mining, sediments of entire hill slopes were washed down with pressure hoses, the sand panned and filtered, the black sand was then mixed with mercury to isolate the gold. The mercury was then evaporated and dispersed in the environment. Today, In the state of California, there are 74 lakes listed as impaired from mercury pollution by the State Water Resources Control Board.

"During the present gold rush, Brazil is first in the world in gold production (with 90% coming from informal mining or garimpos)." At least 2000 tons of mercury have been released to the environment in the present gold rush. [536]

Artisanal gold mining is now thought responsible for over half the global stream flux of Hg, followed by the burning of coal. [537]

The region of Diwalwal, dominated by Mt. Diwata, is a gold rush area on Mindanao (Philippines) where approximately 15,000 people live. Of the population, 0 % of the controls, 38% of the people living downstream, 27% from Mt. Diwata - non-occupational exposed -and 71.6% of the workers were classified as **Hg** intoxicated. [538]

In 2003, workers suffering from **mercury** poisoning in this region were treated with chelation therapy with oral DMPS. Already after 14 days most of the patients reported a marked improvement of the complaints and increase mercury excretion was measured. [539]

Other toxic metals are detrimental to gold miners:

In the Zamfara gold mining disaster where hundreds of children were killed by **lead** poisoning, treatment with oral DMSA (Succimer) reduced lead-related childhood mortality from 65% reported in the literature to 1.5%. **Lead** was also present in the gold-containing ore and was spread in dust in high concentrations. [540]

4.13.1 Metal implants and bizarre effects

People with dental fillings or crowns of different metals on opposing teeth sometimes experience specific pain due to the effects of a galvanic cell in the mouth (for instance a mercury filling on a bottom tooth and a gold filling on the opposite upper tooth, see 8.20).

There have been many cases of people with **mercury**, and even **gold** fillings, picking up (receiving) radio stations in their mouth – even before cell phones were invented. [541]

According to Robert Hunsucker of the University of Alaska Fairbanks, "a receiver is so simple that anything from a phone to a person's mouth can act as one" [even without metal implants]. [542]

"There have been reports that go back to nearly a century of people claiming to pick up radio signals through their teeth."

These examples are mostly anecdotal, however. And they involve solid metal fragments or objects in the body, rather than chronic metal poisoning with dissolved metal compounds.

"One notable case of a seemingly sane person picking up radio signals through their fillings (in this case temporary **lead** fillings) is actress Lucile Ball from the famous 1950s TV show "I Love Lucy". [543]

During WWII, she heard what sounded like morse code when driving through Coldwater Canyon. When it happened again a week later, she told MGM security. She stated that the FBI located the source of the signals, an underground Japanese radio station. [544]

American Radio ARCHIVES report: "if you have fillings in your teeth, you may be able to hear faint radio signals – but don't expect to be able to listen to your favorite station clearly! The metal in your fillings will cause interference, making the signal sound fuzzy and difficult to understand." [545]

Other reports exist of radio broadcasts being received even through shrapnel fragments embedded in the skull of a Vietnam veteran. [546]

It is obvious that most people who experience such interference and claim to 'hear faint voices or music in their head' are diagnosed with insanity and medicated or institutionalized.

Underlying metal toxicity does indeed often go along with mental disorders and mental disorders can produced such voices with no external influence, which leaves a challenging task for psychological assessors. If the sounds are distinct enough to identify text, it would be possible for an examiner to find the causing radio program. Few of those who actually heard real radio signals are as lucky as Lucile Ball, and are able to explain their case and have the cause investigated and proven to be real.

4.14 Substance abuse/ addiction

There is a bi-directional relationship between substance abuse and heavy metal toxicity.

1.) Many pharmaceutical as well as illicit drugs contain toxic metals in harmful doses, which cause the usual health degradation as listed above. "Prevalent sources for heavy metals are alcohol, cigarettes, E-cigarettes, opium, opioids, cocaine and so on."

2.) Metals from any source can contribute to the addiction behavior of the consumer and heavy metal removal has been used to resolve addiction. The symptoms of metal toxicity often lead to an urge to self-medicate and to a decreased capacity of impulse control, propagating the vicious circle. Addiction is not just a weakness or character flaw. Rather, toxicity can cause weakness, hormonal disruption and lack of impulse control.

Further, alcohol consumption may increase the absorption of toxic metals in the body (see below).

Animal models demonstrated cocaine addiction is not only a matter of the addictiveness of cocaine, but it can be influenced by developmental metal toxicity. Rats have no knowledge or awareness of the long-term consequences of cocaine and no social stigma concerning drugs, so it could be assumed they consume as much of it as is available, but they don't. When we observe the average person who enjoys moderate alcohol consumption, we might get the impression that if it wasn't for conscious knowledge of the consequences of alcohol, then we would all be alcoholics. Or if it wasn't for the observation of how cocaine users usually end up, everyone would do it. But it turns out even substance addiction is influenced by developmental and adult toxin burden, including toxic metal burden.

Developmental exposure to **cadmium** alters responsiveness to cocaine in the rat. Cocaine sensitization was attenuated (reduced) in animals perinatally exposed to cadmium. [547]

In adult rats, those animals exposed to **lead** during early development self-administered cocaine at significantly greater rates at a low dose of the drug, even after the blood **lead** levels had returned to normal. [548]

Douglas C. Jones and Gary W. Miller found in humans, "Heavy metals, including **lead, manganese,** and **cadmium** have differential effects on dopaminergic activity. All three metals have been shown to disrupt the behavioral response to drugs of abuse and may contribute to the addiction process." [549]

Persons with dental **amalgams** are 2.5-times more likely smokers than persons without amalgams. This is probably because "**mercury** decreases dopamine, serotonin, norepinephrine, and acetylcholine in the brain, and nicotine has just the opposite effect on these neurotransmitters." [550]

Among Chinese smokers, metal ions in cerebrospinal fluid, including **zinc** and **lead**, were found to have a significant correlation with nicotine dependence (PSQI) scores in the general group (see also 14.4.3). [551]

Alcoholism:

Workplace **beryllium** exposure is linked to susceptibility to alcoholism and suicide risk. [552]

Natural Health Group claims: "**Beryllium** is linked to **alcoholism** or alcohol addiction, basically beryllium finds its way to the pleasure center of the brain and steals the seats normally used by important amino acids, this prevents normal pleasure chemicals from working properly causing depression, alcohol addiction results from attempting to activate the pleasure center but only getting a limited response thanks to beryllium toxicity." [553]

"Disulfiram (Antabuse) is a chelating agent used as a therapy for contact dermatitis for metals such as **nickel** and **cobalt**, but its main use is as supportive therapy for alcohol addiction." [554]

There are further indications of a bidirectional relationship of chronic metal toxicity and alcoholism.

Brzóska et al, 2000 conclude that even short-term ethanol consumption in conditions of exposure to **cadmium** can increase this heavy metal body burden and lead to more serious disturbances in metabolism of important elements such as zinc and copper. [555]

In Eastern Poland, the serum concentration of **cadmium** was significantly higher in patients with advanced alcoholic liver cirrhosis compared to the control group. [556]

Inversely, "Experimental evidence suggests that ethanol could enhance the absorption of metals in the body and alcoholics may be more susceptible to metal intoxication." [557]

Dopamine and drugs

"Exposure to low-levels of heavy metals [**lead** and **mercury**] can increase the risk for altered dopamine (DA) neurotransmission/ turnover following the use of psychostimulants (cocaine and methamphetamine), resulting in an exaggerated response or increased risk for toxicity." [558]

On a positive note: "magnesium reduces the intensity of addiction to opiates and psychostimulants (cocaine, amphetamine, nicotine, and others). "It also decreases the auto-administration of cocaine and the relapse into cocaine and amphetamine intake, as well as reducing the experimental addiction to morphine, cocaine and other substances in animals." [559]

"Zinc dietary supplementation in patients treated with opioids for cancer-related chronic pain should be considered, due to the high incidence of zinc deficiency also well-documented in opioid consumers." [560]

4.15 Additional psychological disorders

4.15.1 Mania

Analysis of toxic trace metals in mentally ill patients showed that **cadmium** was raised in depressives.

Lead was increased in depressives and schizophrenics. Serum zinc was reduced in all mental patients. [561]

Vanadium is associated with manic- depressive psychosis. Raised levels of vanadium have been reported in plasma of patients with mania and depression. Raised vanadium hair levels were reported in mania patients. [562]

4.15.2 Schizophrenia and toxic metals

A higher concentration of **lead** and **chromium** is significantly associated with schizophrenia. [563]

Modabbernia et al 2016 found higher early-life **Pb2+** exposure among patients with schizophrenia in adulthood than among controls. Moreover, they found a negative correlation between Pb2+ levels and adult IQ." [564]

Iron and **selenium** levels were significantly reduced in newly diagnosed and medicated-schizophrenic patients compared with non- schizophrenic controls. **Pb, Cd** and **Cr** were significantly raised in newly diagnosed drug free schizophrenic patients compared with controls. Further, **Cr** and **Cd** were significantly raised in schizophrenic patients on treatment compared with the controls. [565]

In China, the concentrations of **antimony** and **uranium** were significantly higher in schizophrenia cases than in controls. [566]

4.16 Cognitive deficits/ intelligence

Studies have found that heavy metals such as **mercury, cadmium, lead** and **tin** affect chemical synaptic transmission in the brain and the peripheral and central nervous system. [567]

Methyl mercury is a potent cytotoxic agent, prenatal exposure results in widespread cortical and cerebellar alterations characterized by reduced myelination and loss of neurons. [568]

Cadmium levels are negatively correlated with the Full Scale Intelligence Quotient. **Lead** levels were negatively correlated with most indices of the Wechsler Intelligence Scale for Children -Fourth Edition (WISC-IV). [569]

Metals (**Cu, Co, Al,** and **Pb**) can negatively affect children's cognitive flexibility by disturbing the gut microbiota. [570]

Lead and intelligence

Epidemiologists believe "over 50% of all U.S. children have had their learning ability or mental state significantly adversely affected by prenatal and/or postnatal exposure to toxics substances." [571]

Numerous studies have demonstrated that **lead** exposure has a negative effect on the central nervous system with regard to cognitive function, e.g., reaction time, pattern comparison, vocabulary, memory, and intelligence. " [572]

Since 1990, "more than 6,000 studies have all shown that exposure to low levels of **lead** early in life has been linked to effects on IQ, learning, memory, and behavior." [573]

"Blood **lead** concentrations, even those below 10 microg per deciliter, are inversely associated with children's IQ scores at three and five years of age, and associated declines in IQ are greater at these concentrations than at higher concentrations." [574]

A Chinese study found that every 1 microgram of **lead** in the blood of children (aged 9 - 11 years) decreased their IQ by 0.1 points. It was concluded that the reference standard in China of 100 microgram per liter (µg/L) blood **lead** for children above 5 years old should be revised. [575] At about 2 liters of blood for a 10-year-old child, the reference level adds up to 200 microgram of total blood lead.

Thus, even if children have blood lead within the reference levels, it is officially accepted that their IQ is reduced by up to 20 points only due to lead contamination.

In corroboration of this, a meta-analysis of 8 case-control studies demonstrated "that the concentration and duration of **lead** exposure have a large effect on mental function in children.

For children who were exposed to lead high enough to result in lead levels slightly exceeding the reference level for more than 4.5 years, the **reduction in intelligence was 22.5 IQ scores**. [576]

Further, **titanium** and **antimony** levels have a synergistic relationship, with a decline in children's IQ score in China.

In addition, the multi-metal mixtures of **lead, manganese, antimony, tin** and **titanium** were negatively associated with children's IQ. [577]

4.17 Infant/ child development

Body size, height

Prenatal low- dose **mercury** exposure significantly reduces growth in children from birth to age 9. The height gain deficit was not seen at birth. Also prenatal exposure to airborne polycyclic aromatic hydrocarbons (PAH) showed a significant negative association with height growth from 0 to 9 years (more than 1.1cm). [578]

"**Lead** can result in a higher risk of stunted growth." [579]

In a Chinese study, exposure to **arsenic** impaired children's physical development in height. [580] The effect was amplified with metal mixtures.

Exposure to **Cd** and **As** reduced children's weight, height, and growth velocity at age 5. [581]

Further effects

Exposure to metal mixtures [Hg, Al, V] in early pregnancy, both individually and as a mixture, was associated with the risk of hypertensive disorders in pregnancy. [582]

In Nigeria, maternal blood **aluminum** was strongly inversely correlated with body weight (r=-0.61) and birth length (r=-0.61).

Toxic metals were associated with altered anthropometric parameters at birth. "Anthropometric parameters at birth are important indicators of child vulnerability to the risk of childhood illness, and consequently, the chance of survival and risk of diseases later in life." [583]

"Considering all the confounding factors, mothers with dental **amalgam** have about double the risk of perinatal death (child death weeks or immediately before and after birth) of their babies compared to mothers without amalgam." [584]

In Japan, **cadmium** levels were found to be significantly associated with early preterm birth. [585]

In northern Sweden, the erythrocyte concentrations of **cadmium** and **mercury** in pregnancy were inversely associated with the infants' birth weight and birth length. Further, the women's urinary **Cd** concentrations were positively associated with thyroid hormone levels in pregnancy. [586]

Prenatal heavy metal exposure with **Hg, Cd, As** and **thallium** measured in cord blood concentrations were associated with delayed neonatal development (NBNA) in Shanghai, China.

Levels of **arsenic** considered safe by authorities were found to be 'not safe' for the newborns' development. [587]

A study in the Republic of Congo - published in the Lancet - found that fathers having mining-related jobs (**copper** and **cobalt** exposure) had a 5.5 times higher probability of having neonates with visible birth defects. [588]

Cobalt production has been increasing exponentially in recent years for electric vehicle manufacturing.

Children who had higher heavy metal loads in utero at 17 weeks of gestation, turned out at 3 years of age to have lower scores in standard children's ability tests and more childhood illnesses.

"Many similar studies measuring child hair levels of the toxic metals **aluminum, arsenic, cadmium, lead** and **mercury** have found that these toxic metals have significant effects on learning ability and cognitive performance, explaining as much as 20 % of cognitive differences among randomly tested children who have low levels of exposure." [589]

A systematic review on heavy metals and neurodevelopment of children in low and middle-income countries concluded:

"94 % of all available studies on postnatal **lead** and all studies on postnatal **manganese** show a negative association with metal exposure and neurodevelopment. **Lead** and **manganese** appear to consistently have a detrimental effect on the neurodevelopment of children." [590]

"The fetus has been found to get significant exposure to toxic substances through maternal blood and across the placenta, with fetal levels of toxic metals often being higher than that of maternal blood." Likewise, infants have been found to get significant exposure to toxins, such as **mercury**, that their mother is exposed to, through breast-feeding. [591]

Even low-level exposure to toxic metals **(As, Cd, Hg,** and **Pb)** in infancy is associated with delayed growth, lower post-birth weight gain and head circumference, but longer duration of breastfeeding and iron deficiency (with or without anemia). [592]

Brain volume

MRI scans showed childhood **lead** exposure was associated with brain volume loss in adulthood. "Individuals with higher blood lead levels as children had less gray matter in some brain areas. The main brain region affected was the prefrontal cortex, which is responsible for executive function, behavioral regulation, and fine motor control." [593]

The prefrontal cortex is instrumental in impulse control (see also the association of **lead** and crime 4.2).

4.17.1 Lead and childhood development

Children with a blood **lead** level of 70µg/dl have been either severely compromised cognitively or seriously mentally handicapped. "At lower doses, a blood **lead** level of 15µg/dl, Sciarillo and colleagues have observed in 4 to 5 year-old children an increased incidence of a range of behavioral troubles including depression." [594]

Babies born to mothers with higher bone-**lead** burden have a decreased birth weight. Researchers concluded **that lead can mobilize from bone into plasma without detectable changes in whole blood lead**. [595]

Maternal bone **lead** is also an independent risk factor for fetal neurotoxicity. "Higher maternal trabecular bone **lead** levels constitute an independent risk factor for impaired mental development in infants at 24 months of age." [596]

The increase risk of adverse maternal, infant, or childhood health outcomes due to **lead** exposure during pregnancy may be caused by the interference with hypothalamic-pituitary-adrenal-axis function. Concurrent blood **Pb** levels were associated with cortisol awakening response in these pregnant women. [597]

A 1993 study found significantly abnormal levels of trace minerals and toxic metals in the head hair of children (mostly **lead**) with learning and behavior disorders. [598]

Lead and neurodevelopment

Nigg et al, 2008, confirmed that even low blood **lead** levels are associated with clinically diagnosed attention-deficit/hyperactivity disorder and mediated by weak cognitive control. [599]

"Today, approximately 8- 15% of Taiwanese children with physical, mental, communication, social, behavioral, or emotional developmental delays require special health assessment and care." [600]

"The toxic metals lead and mercury inhibit the mesenchymal stem cell metabolism. In fact, MSCs are more sensitive to these metals than differentiated cells such as lung fibroblasts and HUVEC." [601]

During prenatal development, the human brain is more vulnerable to xenobiotics than the brain of an adult. Indeed, the placenta does not provide an effective protection against environmental contaminants, [602] and the blood-brain barrier is not formed until 6 months after birth. [603]

"Already very low **lead** exposure is detrimental to children's neurodevelopment." [604]

Wodtke et al found that sustained exposure to disadvantaged neighborhoods reduces vocabulary skills during early childhood and that this effect operates through a causal mechanism involving **lead** contamination. [605]

4.17.2 Various metals and neurodevelopment

There is compelling evidence that heavy metals not only adversely affect neurodevelopment but also increase the risk of autism spectrum disorders (ASD). [606]

In a systematic review, "Most of the studies reported a relationship between exposure to metals during perinatal and early childhood periods and increased risk for autism. "Moreover, the effects resulting from co-exposure to multiple metals should not be underestimated." [607]

Cerebral palsy (CP) is the most common motor disability in childhood. Elevated levels of **copper** and **manganese** measured in maternal blood during the second trimester could be related to increased risk of CP in children. [608]

A blood **cadmium** concentration higher than 1.0 µg/L was found to have a 2-fold greater association with developmental delays in comparison with a blood cadmium concentration of 0.6 µg/L. [609]

Higher blood **cadmium** concentration also showed a significant positive association with developmental delays. [610]

Some studies have reported that postnatal **cadmium** exposure is associated with the development of learning disabilities in children and cognitive deficits in boys. [611]

4.17.3 Dyslexia

A study of dyslexic children with normal IQs found the dyslexic group had a **cadmium** hair level average 25 times that of the control group. [612]

In China, children with higher **silver** levels had a higher risk of dyslexia, while **selenium** was negatively associated with dyslexia. [613]

Hair from dyslexic children also showed significantly higher concentrations of **magnesium, aluminum, cadmium** and **copper** than did hair from control subjects. [614]

Lead was positively associated with Chinese dyslexia in a multiple-metal exposure model. [615]

As for puberty, "through an analysis of national big data, a study found evidence that Korean girls showed a younger age at menarche in response to higher blood **lead** and **mercury** concentrations." [616]

4.17.4 Increased heavy metal load with increasing age of pregnancy

With increasing metal toxicity in the environment, the fact that women are having children at increasingly later ages (if they have children at all), also means a higher accumulated heavy metal load to be transferred to the child.

"Prenatal exposure to heavy metals can cause impaired cognitive development even at very low concentrations." [617]

The toxic trace elements **mercury, lead, cadmium** and **antimony** are transferred over the placenta to the fetus and secreted into the breastmilk. "In a group of healthy Norwegian never-pregnant women, age contributed to **Hg** and **Sb** levels, but diet and life style factors were stronger determinants of whole blood **Hg, Pb, Cd** and serum **Sb** levels." [618]

4.18 Down Syndrome

"It is well established in research that people with Down Syndrome (Trisomy 21) have elevated levels of heavy metals compared to the typical population." [619]

Most research on this connection is focused on the mechanism by which Down Syndrome increases the absorption of toxic metals.

However, research shows that children in India with DS had elevated concentrations of **arsenic**, while their parents had toxic levels of **arsenic**.

"Parents' exposure to **arsenic** greatly increases the possibility of a fetus developing the extra chromosome that causes this incurable disease." [620] So here as well, the relationship between cause and effect is not fully established.

"All people with DS suffer from cognitive decline and develop Alzheimer's disease (AD) by the age of 40." [621]

Children with Down's Syndrome, 1-2 years old, have elevated hair mineral and trace element contents.

"Hair levels of **magnesium, phosphorus, iodine, chromium, silicon, zinc** and **lead** in Down's syndrome patients all exceeded the control values (by between 28 and 57%)." [622]

"Also **mercury** levels have been found to be significantly elevated in Down Syndrome children." Further, down syndrome children have higher levels of DNA damage. [623]

"Mutations can result in the enhanced absorption of **aluminum** across the gastrointestinal tract in individuals with Down's syndrome." [624]

This increased gastrointestinal absorption of **aluminum** observed in people with Down Syndrome is also associated with the progression of Alzheimer's Disease.

"People with DS have a permeable blood brain barrier,
and a deficit of glutathione and selenium compared to the typical population, and are at high risk of developing brain damage following **mercury** exposure." [625]

Chapter 5
Physical diseases and heavy metals

5.1.1 "Death by Doctors"

The grave health ramifications of even low levels of toxic metals are generally disregarded by medical institutions and governments. Most chronic illnesses can either be solely caused or accelerated by toxic metals, and metal toxicity can mimic many chronic illnesses.

According to their own reports, the said medical industry kills millions of people annually by prescription drugs and false treatments (see below). All of these drugs are primarily used to alleviate the symptoms and they may cure an acute illness but they are not designed to treat the cause of a chronic illness.

According to a Johns Hopkins study, "Over **250,000 people** in the U.S. die each year because of medical errors, making it the third leading cause of death in this country behind heart disease and cancer." [626]

But according to the Journal of Patient Safety, medical errors contribute to more than 400,000 deaths in the U.S. every year, and that estimate only takes hospital patients into account.

"In addition, serious harm seems to be 10- to 20-fold more common than lethal harm." [627]

The updated estimate was developed from modern studies published from 2008 to 2011.

The official number of patients who are "killed by doctors' prescriptions" doubled in only 10 years (for instance in the UK between 1996 and 2006, according to the NHS). [628] The German federal agency of medical products estimates "1,400 cases of death annually due to prescription drugs in Germany alone." 'Die Welt' writes: "The number of unrecorded cases is enormous: official estimates already claim 90 percent of cases are unreported." [translation mine] [629] Not included here are casualties of false diagnosis and unnecessary treatments, which may cause new symptoms as side effects, as describe in the package insert, and these are then countered with yet more prescription drugs with more side effects.

5.2 Cardio-vascular disease and toxic metals

Analysis of the data of 42,749 male participants showed the correlation between 15 heavy metals and coronary heart disease (CHD) ranges from − 0.238 to 0.910 (the latter is a very strong, positive association). There was also a significant positive correlation between total **arsenic, monomethylarsonic acid**, and **thallium** in urine and CHD (all P < 0.05). [630]

"**Lead, cadmium, antimony, cobalt**, and **tungsten** have been associated with cardiovascular disease." [631]

Experts warn of cardiovascular risk from heavy metal pollution, even at low doses: "Exposure to **arsenic, lead, cadmium** and **copper** is associated with an increased risk of cardiovascular disease and coronary heart disease." [632]

In December 2006, the US National Institutes of Health published a comprehensive systematic review of the scientific research results on the subject of "lead exposure and cardiovascular disease". [633] Peter Jennrich reported: "The experts came to the conclusion that a connection between **lead** exposure and high blood pressure has been proven not just in a few studies, but in many studies. They say there is enough evidence to establish a causal link between **lead** exposure and high blood pressure, an increased incidence of coronary heart disease, peripheral arterial disease and strokes. These cardiac and vascular events occur even with lead exposure that was below the previously considered "safe" limit of 5 ug/dl lead in the blood" [Translation mine]. [634]

The Department of Epidemiology and Welch Center for Prevention, Baltimore, USA states: "**Mercury** levels are increased in heart attack patients." [635]

Johns Hopkins Bloomberg School of Public Health confirms: "**Mercury** is directly associated with the risk of heart attack." [636]

Barregard et al 2021 found blood **cadmium** in the highest quartile was associated with coronary artery calcium score (CACS) in a general population sample with low to moderate cadmium exposure. "Atherosclerosis is an important mechanism underlying the associations between **cadmium** and incident cardiovascular disease." [637]

Higher blood **cadmium** levels were also associated with increased incidence of heart failure in a cohort with comparatively low exposure to cadmium. [638]

Frustachi et al have shown a very strong correlation between cardiomyopathy (heart disease) and heavy metal accumulation in the coronary arteries and heart muscle. "The role of heavy metal detoxification in the prevention and/or treatment of cancer and heart disease is paramount for optimum healing or prevention." [639]

As we saw above, a 2018 study published in The Lancet Public Health found that of the 2.3 million deaths every year in the US, about 412,000 (or 18%) are attributable to **lead** exposure, of which 250,000 are from cardiovascular disease. [640]
"Studies have reported statistically significant associations between cardiovascular disease (CVD) and exposure to **As, Cd, Hg,** and **Pb."** Additionally, imbalanced levels of Zn, Cu, Cr, Co, Mg, Se, Ni and W are associated with an increased CVD risk. [641]
In 49 patients with acquired, severe, calcified aortic valve stenosis with indicated heart surgery, the aortic valves contained significantly higher concentrations of **Ba**, Ca, Co, Cr, Mg, P, **Pb**, Se, **tin**, **strontium** and zinc than the control group. [642]

Now, since unprovoked (non-challenge) blood tests are inconclusive for chronic metal toxicity, as the metals are not in the blood, then where are they? For instance, with patients of idiopathic dilated cardiomyopathy?
Myocardial and muscular biopsy samples of 13 (alive) patients, all without past or current exposure to trace elements, revealed:
"A large increase of trace element concentration **(>10,000 times for mercury and antimony)** has been observed in myocardial but not in muscular samples in all patients with idiopathic dilated cardiomyopathy (IDCM)."
In patients with IDCM, the mean concentration of **mercury** was 22,000 times, **antimony** 12,000 times, **gold** 11 times and **chromium** 13 times higher than in control subjects. [643]
Thus, whenever a cardiomyopathy patient is told by their doctor that antimony from PET bottles is harmless, they can ask the doctor where he thinks they accumulated their antimony from, in concentrations 12,000 times higher than normal.

In one study, "the highest hair **Al, As,** and **Pb** levels were observed in obese CHD patients, significantly exceeding the respective values in other groups. " [644]

5.2.1 Atrial fibrillation (AFib, irregular heart beat)

"Workplace exposure to metals or pesticides is associated with an increased likelihood of coronary heart disease and atrial fibrillation." [645]

Metal exposure was associated with a four-fold increase in risk for atrial fibrillation. [646] Inversely, selenium deficiency is associated with new-onset AFib. [647]

Paroxysmal atrial fibrillation "may be related to the additive toxic effects induced by the combination of multiple exposures to heavy metals [i.e., elemental metallic **mercury, arsenic** and **lead**]." [648]

Untreated AFib can raise your risk for problems like a heart attack, stroke, and heart failure. [649] AFib shortens life expectancy after diagnosis by about 2 years. [650]

CVD/ cholesterol - Cause and effect

An NHANES analysis found "Increasing blood **Pb, Hg,** and **Cd** levels were associated with significantly increased odds of high total cholesterol after adjusting for age, sex, and socioeconomic status."

People with the highest level of **Hg** were almost twice as likely to have high total cholesterol levels, compared to the average.

"Elevated cholesterol has a significant relationship with incremental levels of heavy metals." [651]

Serum copper and zinc levels were found to be high in individuals with high LDL-C levels in Iran. [652]

"HDL helps rid your body of excess cholesterol so it's less likely to end up in your arteries. LDL is called "bad cholesterol."

Calcification or plaque in heart and vessels contains cholesterol and calcium.

Excess cholesterol from the diet is often cited as a cause of heart disease, so decreased intake of cholesterol and calcium or cholesterol blockers are prescribed. However, when plaque is produced as a cause of metal toxicity, oxidative stress on the vessel intima and the following arthrosclerosis, then calcium or cholesterol restriction has little benefits; on the contrary, lack of calcium can damage the heart muscle and disrupt heart rhythm, lack of cholesterol is detrimental to the brain.

Dilated cardiomyopathy

In a mining area in the Democratic Republic of Congo, urinary toxic metals (**arsenic, copper** and **chromium** were strongly associated with dilated cardiomyopathy in the miners as well as the general population. [653]

5.2.2 Cerebral small vessel disease

Small vessel disease accounts for up to 25% of all ischemic strokes. [654]

Small blood vessels are highly vulnerable to heavy metals, as they are directly exposed to the blood circulatory system.

"Heavy metals (**As, Cd, Pb, Hg,** and **Cu**) in small vessels are strongly associated with the development as well as the progression of cerebral small vessel disease (CSVD). Chelation therapy may be an effective strategy to reduce the toxic metal load and the associated complications." [655]

"Serum and urine **cadmium** concentrations are positively associated with the risk of ischemic stroke." [656]

5.2.3 Chelation Therapy in CVD

The average mortality for coronary artery bypass grafting (CABG) surgery is 4% to 10%. [657] "In fact, CABG has **no overall effect on improving survival**." According to one study published in the New England Journal of Medicine, "as compared with medical therapy, coronary artery bypass surgery appears neither to prolong life nor to prevent myocardial infarction in patients who have mild angina or who are asymptomatic after infarction in the five-year period after coronary angiography." [658]

For chelation therapy for CVD prevention and treatment see also 1.13.

The hitherto largest systematic review of published studies was conducted to examine the effect of repeated EDTA on clinical outcomes in adults with cardiovascular disease (CVD).

Of 24 selected studies, 17 studies suggested improved outcomes, "Repeated EDTA for CVD treatment may provide more benefit to patients with diabetes and severe peripheral arterial disease." [659]

5.2.4 Atherosclerosis and hypertension

Dr. Houston urges "**mercury** toxicity should be evaluated in any patient with hypertension, coronary heart disease, cerebral vascular disease, cerebrovascular accident, or other vascular disease." [660]

Scientists at the University of California showed that **lead** can cause the production of free radicals und cause damage to the intima of the blood vessels. [661]

"The clinical consequences of **mercury** toxicity include hypertension, coronary heart disease, myocardial infarction, cardiac arrhythmias, reduced heart rate variability, increased carotid intima-media thickness and carotid artery obstruction, cerebrovascular accident, generalized atherosclerosis and renal dysfunction, insufficiency, and proteinuria." [662]

"In general, a higher heart rate variability (HRV) is considered better as it indicates a more adaptable and resilient autonomic nervous system, which can respond effectively to different stressors." [663]

Carotid atherosclerosis

"Among men aged 42-60 years, high hair **mercury** content was one of the strongest predictors of the 4-year increase in the mean common carotid intima-media thickness (IMT)." [664]

Environmental exposure to low levels of toxic metals can raise the risk for developing clogged arteries of in necks, hearts and legs, according to a study on auto workers in Zaragoza, Spain.

Titanium, arsenic, cadmium and potentially **antimony** are atherosclerosis risk factors. [665]

Metal levels were correlated to a buildup of plaque in the arteries of the workers necks, hearts and legs. [666]

EDTA chelation has been used to improve arteriosclerosis, even when the positive effect was not individually linked to a reduction of toxic metals in the arteries (see below).

5.3 Hypertension

"Hypertension, one of the most common diseases worldwide, is estimated to affect one quarter of all adults, and has been identified as the leading cause of mortality and the third cause of disability-adjusted life years worldwide." [667]

According to the WHO, the number of cases has doubled since 1990. [668]

The U.S. CDC estimates that about one out of every three American adults have hypertension. [669]

Hypertension-related disease burden is a major challenge globally [670], with an estimated 1.56 billion adults in all regions of the world expected to be affected by hypertension by 2025. [671]

5.3.1 Metals and hypertension

The risk of hypertension over 10 years was highly correlated to **mercury** exposure in a group of chemical factory workers. [672]
Meanwhile in remote Nunavik, Canada, in Inuit adults, blood **mercury** level was correlated with higher systolic and diastolic blood pressure and pulse pressure. [673]
"**Mercury, cadmium** and other heavy metals inactivate catechol-o-methyltransferase (COMT), which increases serum and urinary epinephrine (adrenalin), norepinephrine, and dopamine. This effect will increase blood pressure and may be a clinical clue to heavy metal toxicity." [674]
In several Asian countries, urinary **lead** concentrations at low levels of exposure/intake are positively associated with both systolic and diastolic blood pressure.
Inversely, urinary **selenium** concentrations were associated with lower blood pressure. [675]
"In a study of 47,595 US women, it was found that living with higher residential exposure to **arsenic, lead, chromium, cobalt,** and **manganese** was related to higher risk of hypertension, whereas living in areas with higher **selenium** was inversely related to the risk of hypertension. [676]
Joint exposure with five metals (**cadmium, copper, magnesium, molybdenum** and **zinc** at low concentrations) was found to be positively related to the risk of hypertension. [677]
Further, in middle-aged women of all ethnic backgrounds, urinary heavy metal concentrations (**arsenic, mercury, lead** and **cadmium**) were associated with diastolic blood pressure. [678]
A nationwide study among adults in South Korea revealed:
Higher blood concentrations of **Pb, Hg,** or **Cd** were positively associated with increasing levels of blood pressure and the prevalence of hypertension. "Co-exposure to these three metals collectively increases the risk of hypertension." [679]
Exposure to metal mixtures is even related to blood pressure among 5 - 7-year- old children. Associations were observed for **selenium, molybdenum, tin** and **mercury, chromium** and **copper**. [680]

5.4 Poverty and hypertension

Factors generally attributed to blood pressure include stress, lack of exercise, overeating, too much salt, alcohol, fat and sugar, and thus many still regard it as a result of over-indulgence, a disease of wealthy countries or a civilization illness. But the prevalence of hypertension throughout the world shows that other factors - such as environmental toxins/ heavy metals - are just as important.

As we'll see below, lifestyle changes have a limited effect in lowering blood pressure. Even strictly following the official government diet plan lowers blood pressure on average by only 3 %.

Among the countries with the highest rates of hypertension are wealthy as well as poor countries. Among women with the highest hypertension rates, Jamaica is ranked 6th, with a rate of 48% of the population; Haiti – the poorest country in the western hemisphere - is in 7th place (48%).

The top countries with the largest increases in hypertension prevalence in the last 30 years are among the poorest countries, whereas the top countries with the largest decline in hypertension prevalence are wealthy, western countries. [681]

According to conventional medicine, hypertension cannot be cured: "Hypertension is a chronic disease. It can be controlled with medication, but it cannot be cured. Therefore, patients need to continue with the treatment and lifestyle modifications as advised by their doctor, and attend regular medical follow up, usually for life." [682]

"If left untreated, high blood pressure shortens life considerably: For example, if a 35-year-old man with a persistent blood pressure of 150/100 mmHg remains untreated, his life expectancy decreases by 16.5 years from an average of 76.5 years to 60 years." (Translation mine). [683]

150/100 mmHg is categorized hypertension stage 2 out of 3.
Hypertension stage 1 is   130-139/80-89 mmHg
Hypertension stage 2 is   140/90 mmHg or more
Hypertensive crisis is higher than 180/120 or higher

So, in the view of academic medicine, high blood pressure is not curable, it can only be alleviated for some time with medication and premature death can be delayed. And with lifestyle adjustments and stress avoidance, mild high blood pressure can be slightly lowered.

Those patients who go on an extended vacation of several months know they do rarely lower their blood pressure.

Even actual retirement has on average "no clinically significant impact on blood pressure or cholesterol," not even after 3 years. [684]

Whatever you do in terms of lifestyle adjustments, most doctors will always tell you: you need to do better, not enough exercise causes hypertension, if you do exercise and nothing changes, then it must be too much exercise. Too much meat, if you say you don't eat much meat anyways, then it must be not enough meat. Plus, you need to relax and have more positive thoughts. It's always your fault, bad habits, bad genes, bad luck.

This view of incurability is reminiscent of similar absolute dogma in conventional medicine: the general assertion that cancer can only be cured with very invasive interventions such as chemo, radiation or surgery, and if anyone cures cancer with prescription-free or alternative means, then they didn't have cancer in the first place, and the diagnosis was false (which should raise the question how many people die each year of the side effects of chemotherapy who also didn't have cancer in the first place?)
On the other hand, the difference here is obviously that people with high blood pressure don't have a false diagnosis, they know for a fact they have high blood pressure. So it is true, that if the root cause is not treated, their blood pressure usually increases and lowers life expectancy. But if 'alternative" medicine does not evaluate the heavy metal load as a possible cause and if detected, the metals are not addressed with effective (pharmaceutical) chelation agents, then mainstream medicine will usually be right about the end outcome and hypertension keeps worsening.

5.4.1 Mercury - mechanism of action on blood pressure

"Because of its effect on the pituitary, **mercury** is known to cause frequent urination as well as high blood pressure." [685]
Already low **mercury** concentration, below the reference values, produces vasoconstriction, decreases nitric oxide (NO) bioavailability and increases oxidative stress in rat conductance artery.
"Acute low concentration mercury exposure, occurring time to time, could induce vascular injury due to endothelial oxidative stress, contributing to increase peripheral resistance, being a high-risk factor for public health." [686]

Anxiety and hypertension
As we saw in 4.8, multiple cross-sectional studies reveal a positive association between anxiety and hypertension. [687]
Hypertension is often connected to kidney dysfunction (see 5.10.1).

127

5.4.2 Chelation in cardio-vascular disease

"Chelation therapy will generally lower raised blood pressure. Blood pressure lowering medication can frequently be diminished or even discontinued." [688]

A study by L.T. Chappell concluded: "EDTA chelation therapy should be more commonly used in the treatment of vascular disease." [689]

Already in the 1950s, Clarke et al tested the effect of EDTA in a group of patients with severe angina, and found remarkable symptomatic and/or electrocardiographic improvement after repeated EDTA infusions in 17 out of 20 patients. [690]

Dr. Garry Gordon found in the treatment of hunnerts of patients in 50-plus years of medical practice: "Chelation therapy [with EDTA] does not predictably by itself decrease plaque." [691] "However, improved blood flow happens in over 80% of patients." [692]

Mg-EDTA chelation therapy improves pulse wave velocity (PWV) and lowers arterial stiffness. "These improvements demonstrate that atherosclerosis is a dynamic and (partially) reversible process." [693]

Hypertension in children with **mercury** poisoning has been resolved by chelation therapy. "In children with severe hypertension and elevated catecholamines, the physician should consider **mercury** intoxication as well as pheochromocytoma." [694]

5.4.3 Varicose veins

"Physicians have used EDTA chelation therapy to treat varicose veins in a very effective manner for more than forty years. It is also a good alternative treatment for people affected by varicose veins." [695]

"EDTA reduces dark pigmentation associated with varicose veins." [696]

"Rectal varices are only found in people with high blood pressure in the veins that lead to the liver. Hemorrhoids develop from increased pressure in the lower rectum." [697]

5.5 Neurological/ neurodegenerative disorders

5.5.1 Alzheimer's Disease/ Dementia

"High **aluminum** levels have been found to be related to encephalopathies and dementia. " [698]

"There is a strong association between accidental metal exposure and various neurodegenerative disorders, including Alzheimer's disease (AD)." [699]

"Researchers have found proof of a correlation between Alzheimer disease and **mercury** exposure. Studies have shown that deceased patients who suffered from neurodegenerative diseases have higher levels of **Hg** in their nerve tissue than healthy people." [700]

"Adult human epidemiologic studies have consistently shown **lead, cadmium,** and **manganese** are associated with impaired cognitive function and cognitive decline."

Results of trials suggest **manganese** chelation therapy as a possible strategy for the intervention of AD pathogenesis. [701]

Compared to controls, circulatory levels of **aluminum, mercury, and cadmium** are significantly higher in AD patients. [702]

Alzheimer's and aluminum

"Aluminum is exponentially accumulated in the body with ageing." [703]

Aluminum has been associated with Alzheimer's disease. [704]

"Even low levels of aluminum can lead to behavioral and morphological changes associated with Alzheimer's disease and age-related neurodegeneration." [705]

Aluminum is linked to processes in the cell that eventually lead to premature cell death. [706]

In US women, cause of "death by neurological disease" has increased 663 % (almost 7-fold!) in the last 20 years. [707]

Researchers estimate degenerative brain diseases affect more than 50 million people worldwide (moving toward 1 % of the population). [708]

"Epidemiological and clinical studies have shown a strong correlation between aberrant metal exposure and a number of neurological diseases." [709]

A. Fulgenzi et al found that toxic-metal burden plays an important role in the etiology of neurodegenerative diseases (ND).

"The presence of toxic metals such as **lead, cadmium, cesium, and aluminum** was always significantly more elevated in ND patients than in healthy controls." For instance, in 379 patients with neurodegenerative or other chronic diseases, levels of 20 out of 21 tested metals (all tested metals but thorium) were much higher than in healthy controls. [710]

"**Al** levels were significantly higher in neurodegenerative diseases (ND) patients than in healthy subjects. " [711]

In Mosul, Iraq, there was a significant increase in patients with Alzheimer's, epilepsy and migraine in levels of **lead, nickel** and **chromium** compared with the control group, as well as a significant increase in the level of **copper** for Alzheimer's and epilepsy patients when compared with the control group. [712]

"Administration of low doses of **copper** ion can induce epileptic seizures in animals. [713]

"Cerebral and cerebellar calcification was described in adults with raised serum **lead** levels and known exposure to lead for 30 or more years. Calcification patterns were found in the subcortical area, basal ganglia, vermis, and cerebellum." [714]

5.5.2 Lead neuropathy

"Patients with **lead** neuropathy present with weakness that primarily involves the wrist and finger extensors, but which could also spread to involve other muscles." [715]

"Diagnosis of **lead** neuropathy is important because it is potentially reversible and also because its early detection and treatment may prevent other systemic complications. " [716]

Lead encephalopathy is characterized by sleeplessness and restlessness.

"People who have been exposed to **lead** for a long time may suffer from memory deterioration, prolonged reaction time and **reduced ability to understand**. Individuals with average blood lead levels under 3 µmol/l may show signs of peripheral nerve symptoms with reduced nerve conduction velocity and reduced dermal sensibility." [717]

5.5.3 Peripheral neuropathy (nerve impairment)

"Exposure to several metals has been shown to cause peripheral neuropathy and may be discovered on laboratory testing of a 24-hour urine sample." [718]

"In cases of **lead**-induced peripheral neuropathy, chelation therapy should be used." [719]

"Common causes of environmentally induced peripheral neuropathy include: exposure to **lead, mercury, arsenic** and **thallium.**" [720]

Koszewicz et al found co-exposure to many heavy metals (in low doses) results in explicit impairment of peripheral nerves. "The lesion is more pronounced within small fibers and is predominantly connected with greater impairment of temperature-dependent pain thresholds." [721]

Obvious changes in psychological status, neuromotor speed and accuracy were observed in workers exposed to **aluminum** for long periods. [722]

5.5.4 MS / multiple sclerosis

"A meta-analysis including 16 studies with 1650 participants showed that patients with MS had significantly higher levels of circulatory **As** and **Cd** compared to the controls." [723]

An observational study of 20,000 participants found that **mercury** dental amalgams may increase the risk of multiple sclerosis. [724]

Mercury or **silver** from the environment can contribute to the loss of nerve function.

"Heavy metals were found in motor neurons and also in a special class of nerve cells called interneurons, which relay electrical signals between different types of nerve cells." [725]

A study of archived tissue from deceased autopsied brains of people with and without MS showed that combinations of **iron, silver, lead, aluminum, mercury, nickel** and **bismuth** were present more often in the locus ceruleus of MS patients than of controls. "The metals were located predominantly in white matter tracts." [726]

As we saw in 1.14.1, metal toxicants in locus ceruleus neurons **weaken the blood–brain barrier**.

5.5.5 Parkinson's

A study of 20,000 people revealed a 57% increased risk of Parkinson's disease in those who had amalgam (**mercury**) fillings. [727]

Johns Hopkins medicine confirms "Heavy metals such as **iron, mercury, manganese, copper,** and **lead** have been linked to PD and contribute to its progression. In addition, the interactions

131

among the components of a metal mixture may result in synergistic toxicity." [728]

"The typical manifestation of **manganese** overexposure is parkinsonism, which may be difficult to differentiate from the more common idiopathic Parkinson's disease." [729]

High-dose **manganese** exposure is linked to certain occupations, such as welding. [730]

Other studies also showed an association between PD and an exposure to **aluminum, bismuth, thallium,** and **zinc**. [731]

"One of the hallmark features of PD brains is the increased accumulation of **iron** in the substantia nigra (SN), with a smaller accumulation of iron in the red nuclei, globus pallidus, and cortex of PD patients." [732]

"In recent clinical trials, **iron** chelation therapy has been shown to open the way to a treatment of Parkinson's disease, which potentially slows the disease progression." [733]

5.5.6 ALS

"Exposure to heavy metals has been associated with the pathogenesis of ALS for over 150 years, when heavy metals were detected in the tissues of patients with motor neuron diseases (MND)."

"Among the various possible causes that can favor the development of the disease, heavy metals cannot be excluded." [734]

"The observed associations suggest that **cadmium, lead,** and **zinc** may play a role in ALS etiology. Cadmium and lead possibly act as intermediates on the pathway from smoking to ALS." [735]

"Exposure to heavy metals (including **lead, mercury** and **selenium**) increase odds ratios of developing ALS." [736]

In the study by Fulgenzi et al 2020, ALS patients were gravely intoxicated with **lead, cadmium, cesium** and **aluminum** as compared to controls.

"Metal uptake is dysregulated during childhood in individuals eventually diagnosed with ALS." Metal levels of **chromium, manganese, nickel** or **zinc** were between 1.5 and 2.6 times higher in cases than in controls and different ages between birth and the age of 8.

"Co-exposure to 11 elements indicated that childhood metal dysregulation was associated with ALS." [737]

In a case report, a 49-years- old ALS patient with increased **mercury** was fully restored after 3 years of DMPS treatment. [738]

"High levels of metallothionein, a sign of exposure to heavy metals, have been found in brain tissue of deceased ALS patients." [739]

'Lead and mercury have been indicated most often [in ALS], but manganese and selenium have also been posited because of increased occupational exposure or increase in tissue levels in ALS patients." [740]

"Heavy metals are present in many spinal interneurons, and in a few α-motoneurons, in a large proportion of older people. Damage to inhibitory interneurons from toxic metals in later life could result in excitotoxic injury to motoneurons and may underlie motoneuron injury or loss in conditions such as ALS/MND, multiple sclerosis, sarcopenia and calf fasciculations." [741]

5.5.7 Guillain-Barré syndrome

Genchi et al found Guillain-Barré resembles the ascending paralysis of **thallium** poisoning in both time course and distribution. However, the prominence of sensory involvement in thallium poisoning distinguishes it from Guillain-Barré. [742]

Chronic or acute exposure to **mercury** has been reported to cause Guillain–Barre syndrome in isolated cases. [743]

Acute toxic neuropathy mimicking Guillain Barre syndrome has been induced by **arsenic** poisoning from ayurvedic drugs. [744]

Further, **mercury** from skin lightening cream and hair dyes has caused membranous nephropathy and Guillain–Barre syndrome. [745]

5.5.8 Epilepsy

"Neurological symptoms associated with **lead** overexposure include an impaired ability to coordinate voluntary movements (ataxia), brain damage (encephalopathy), seizures, convulsions, swelling of the optic nerve (papilledema), and/or impaired consciousness." [746]

Lead poisoning has been reported to cause persistent seizures, requiring ventilator support when BLL exceeds 244 µg/dl. [747]

"**Lead** and **mercury** are the heavy metals that are most likely to cause seizures, whether the child is on the autism spectrum or not, as they are very harmful and powerful. The contributing factor to Kanner's syndrome is the very presence of **arsenic, cadmium, lead, mercury, aluminum,** or **nickel** in the blood of the child." [748]

In pregnant women in South Korea, **Pb** in the first trimester of pregnancy and **Cd** in the third trimester of pregnancy were associated with the incidence of epilepsy in the infant. [749]

5.5.9 Muscle spasms/ motor control/ tremors

Mercury, manganese, thallium and **tin** are all associated with tremor and motor control issues (See each individual paragraph of metals and their symptoms).

Exposure to heavy metals can trigger dystonia (jerky movements, muscle spasms).

Acquired neuromyotonia syndrome is a rare form of peripheral nerve hyperexcitability syndrome, characterized by spontaneous and continuous muscle contractions. "In rare cases, it is a neurological clinical manifestation in patients with **mercury** poisoning." [750]

5.5.10 Restless leg syndrome

Among the elderly in North West Wales, subjects with restless leg syndrome (RLS) had a significantly higher number of amalgam dental fillings. [751]

We saw that RLS was described in **mercury** workers already in the 1700s.

Serum **copper, magnesium, selenium**, and **calcium** concentrations have been found to be significantly higher in restless legs syndrome patients than in controls. [752]

"**Iron deficiency** is an important comorbidity of **lead** toxicity. Iron deficiency anemia has been associated with restless legs syndrome. " [753]

"Cerebrospinal fluid (CSF) ferritin levels are reduced in restless legs syndrome, a condition caused by **low brain iron** levels that are treated with iron supplements." [754]

Restless leg syndrome is a common complication in patients with end-stage renal disease (ESRD). Elementary heavy metals, such as **copper**, predicted the incidence of uremic RLS. [755]

5.5.11 Treatment of neurodegenerative diseases

"The chelating agent EDTA - previously used to treat cardiovascular diseases - is known to be useful for the treatment of neurodegenerative diseases." [756]

"Treatment with EDTA chelation therapy removes toxic-metal burden and improves patients' symptoms of neurodegenerative diseases." [757]

5.5.12 Migraines/ chronic headaches

According to Dr. Lawrence Wilson, "High **copper** levels are probably the most common biochemical causes of migraine headaches." [758]

"When the health effects of **mercury** were investigated by O. Donma et al, the most frequently observed symptom was cephalalgia [headache or any type of pain affecting the head, face, or neck]." Continuous exposure to **lead** was concomitant with the appearance of symptoms such as headache. [759]

In 2015 Turkey's Yuzuncu Yil University found that migraine patients had significantly higher blood levels of the toxic heavy metals **cadmium, iron, lead** and **manganese**, 2 to 4 times the average amount found in the control group. [760]

In Mosul City, Iraq, male migraine patients had significantly increased levels of **lead, nickel** and **chromium** than controls. [761]

Around 65% of patients with cluster headaches are smokers or have a history of smoking. "However, smoking cessation does not seem to alter the clinical course of the disorder. " [762] Which supports the findings that the main chronic toxicity driver in smokers is accumulated metal toxicity and recall toxic metals last "forever".

"Both zinc and magnesium deficiencies are more common in patients with headaches than in headache free patients." [763] **Cadmium** displaces zinc and increases zinc deficiencies.

Inversely, treatment with magnesium (Mg) oxide did lead to a significant reduction in headache days in children.

Zinc supplementation has shown promise in research studies as a treatment for migraines. [764]

5.6 Anemia (lack of healthy red blood cells)

"Exposure to heavy metals must be considered in the differential diagnosis of many types of anemia. The heavy metals most commonly associated with hematologic toxicity are **arsenic** and its derivative arsine, **copper, gold, lead,** and **zinc**." [765]

Mount Sinai institute lists among metals that "can cause anemia": **arsenic, chromium/chromates, platinum salts, nickel compounds, copper, lead** and **cis-platinum**. [766]

"High **lead** levels (≥ 10 µg/dl) were significantly associated with anemia, decreased iron absorption and hematological parameters and low ferritin." [767]

See also retained bullet fragments and metal poisoning (14.3.).

"Serum **lead** concentration is high in iron deficiency anemia (IDA) adults subjects versus healthy individuals. In addition, iron deficiency may increase susceptibility to **lead** poisoning." [768]

Cadmium induces anemia through interdependent progress of hemolysis, body iron accumulation, and insufficient erythropoietin production in rats. [769]

In Chinese women, **Pb** and **Ni** were significantly negatively associated with hemoglobin (Hgb). Pb and Ni were significantly negatively associated with mean corpuscular volume (MCV) and mean corpuscular hemoglobin concentration (MCHC) in males and females. Female hemogram parameters were more susceptible to heavy metal poisoning such as **Pb, Ni** and **Cr**. [770]

5.7 Respiratory disorders

"Exposure to **cadmium** may lead to emphysema. Bronchial asthma may be caused by complex **platinum** salts, **nickel**, **chromium** or **cobalt**, presumably on the basis of allergic sensitization." [771]

"Many studies have reported an association between heavy metal exposure and asthma." [772]

Elevated levels of **Cd** in cord blood were associated with a greater risk of asthma and food allergy. [773]

In Taichung City, combined exposure to **Pb with As, Cd,** and **Hg** during early and late gestational weeks was associated with the incidence of pediatric asthma. [774]

Exposure to **cadmium, cobalt, lead**, and **manganese** has been associated with decreased pulmonary function in adults (e.g., decreased *forced expiratory volume in one second* (FEV1). [775]

"The fumes or gaseous forms of several metals, e.g. **cadmium, manganese, mercury, nickel carbonyl** ($NI(CO)4$, **zinc chloride** ($ZnCl2$), **vanadium pentoxide** ($V2O5$), may lead to acute chemical pneumonitis and pulmonary oedema or to acute tracheobronchitis." [776]

5.7.1 COPD (chronic obstructive pulmonary disease

A large-scale study of US NHANES data from 1999 through 2019 found that increased blood **cadmium** and blood **lead**

136

concentrations were independently associated with increased all-cause mortality in COPD patients. [777]

Kim et al found a high concentration of **copper** may increase COPD risk in males in the general US population. [778]

Serum **mercury** levels are associated with post-bronchodilator FEV1 and with Obstructive Lung Disorder (OLD) prevalence. [779]

5.7.2 Inflammation

"Even very low levels of chronic **mercury** exposure promote endothelial dysfunction as a result of increased inflammation, oxidative stress, reduced oxidative defense, reduction in nitric oxide (NO) bioavailability, which increases the risk of cardio vascular disease and CVA (cerebrovascular accidents)." [780]

"Oxidative stress caused by reactive oxygen species (ROS) is a well-known mechanism of heavy metal-induced damage." [781]

(See also the *free radical theory of aging* 3.3.).

5.8 Gastrointestinal illnesses

Cd exposure induces a significant alteration of intestinal bacterial populations. Cd exposure in the intestinal wall induces inflammatory response and cell damage including disruption of tight junctions, ultimately leading to increased gut permeability. [782]

"Exposure to **cadmium** causes profound toxic effects on microbiota of mice intestinal tract." The probiotics including Lactobacillus and Bifidobacterium were notably inhibited and the gut barrier was impaired. [783]

The gut is an important target tissue of **mercury** toxicity. "Both **IHg** and **MeHg** were found to cause intestinal microbial disorders, abnormal metabolites production, tight junction damage, and immune responses in the gut." [784]

Exposure to contaminants including metals is associated with an increase in gut permeability, leading to 'leaky gut syndrome."

"Chelating agents as well as gut microbes reduce intestinal absorption of metals by forming complexes, thereby making them less permeable." [785]

"Exposure to inorganic **arsenic** can lead to gut microbe perturbations and hepatocellular carcinoma." [786]

5.9 Cancer

"Almost all heavy metals are serious toxicants as carcinogens."
Arsenic, cadmium, chromium and **nickel** are classified as group 1 carcinogens by the International Agency for Research on Cancer. "Analyzed data showed that above-mentioned metallic substances induce oxidative stress, DNA damage, and cell death processes, resulting in increased risk of cancer and cancer-related diseases." [787]

Exposure to **cadmium** has been associated with carcinogenesis in multiple tissues including breast, esophagus, stomach, intestines, prostate, lungs and testes. [788]
Cadmium revealed moderate to high-risk scores for prostate, renal, bladder, breast, pancreatic, and endometrial cancers. [789]
"Arsenic increases the risk of basal cell carcinoma and other cancers." [790]
High concentrations of **As** and **Fe** in the soil of Golestan province, Iran was determined to be a high stomach cancer risk factor. [791]
The genotoxic metal **mercury** is found in normal pancreatic cells in more people with, than without, pancreatic cancer. Hg concentrations were up to 4 times higher in patients as compared to controls. [792]
"Metal composition of pancreatic juice was distinctive in patients with pancreatic cancer relative to those without such a cancer. The metal concentrations that were found to have the strongest association with pancreatic cancer were **chromium, selenium** and **molybdenum.**" [793]
In a study performed on **lead** exposed workers, a positive correlation was observed between exposure to **lead** and increased risk of carcinogenesis in lung tissue and a marginal positive correlation for malignant growth in brain, larynx and bladder tissues. [794]
"High blood **lead** levels increase the risk of colorectal cancer."
"**Aluminum** and **cadmium** long-term exposure induces [cancerous] cellular survival and proliferation." [795]
Manganese and **cadmium** are positively associated with nasopharyngeal carcinoma (NPC) risk. [796]

5.9.1 Lymphoma (Hodgkin's/ Non- Hodgkin's disease)

"On the average, **Ni, Cr, Cu** and **Cd** revealed significantly higher contents in the blood and scalp hair of [Lymphoma] patients than the controls. **Cr** as well as other chemicals had a direct carcinogenic effect on Hodgkin's disease." [797]

Deubler et al observed a significant positive association between high erythrocyte **lead** concentration and risk of lymphoid malignancies overall. [798]

Preliminary data suggest being a metal worker is a significant risk factor for nodal marginal zone lymphoma. [799]

Retrospective analysis of various specimens from a patient who had died from Hodgkin's lymphoma showed intracellular heavy metal nanoparticles within lymph node, bone marrow, and liver samples. The debris consisted of stainless steel, **chromium, nickel** and **gold** compounds. [800]

People with extensive tattoos often show metal deposits in lymph nodes (see 14.4.4).

5.9.2 Brain tumors

"Prolonged exposure to heavy metals such as **lead, nickel, arsenic** and **cadmium** is strongly correlated with an increased likelihood of malignancy, specifically for brain tumors." [801]

Arslan et al. reported higher concentrations of **Cd, Fe, Mg, Mn, Pb** and **Zn** in the serum of patients with malignant gliomas compared to those of healthy subjects. [802]

"**Lead** and **cadmium** was detected in significantly higher concentrations in glioma patients, suggesting these two metals combined may produce excessively toxic effects." [803]

Patients with malignant brain tumors had 2.1 times more **lead** and 2.3 times more **silver** in the cortical spinal fluid than controls. [804]

A. Stojsavljević et al found the most noticeable change in metal homeostasis in malignant brain tumors (MBT) patients was the elevated **uranium** content, indicating its considerable role as a major cerebral discriminator of the presence/absence of MBTs. "The **uranium/selenium** ratio could be considered as an appropriate blood marker in diagnostic MBT evaluation." [805]

When brain tumor tissue was tested for toxic metals, "all of the 47 tested elements were detected in the brain tumor tissue, and 22 were detected in > 80% of samples; this implies that these elements can cross the blood-brain barrier." [806]

"Underground mining of e.g. **uranium** or **iron** is associated with a high incidence of lung cancer, as a result of exposure to **radon**. At least some forms of **arsenic, chromium** and **nickel** are well established lung carcinogens in humans. [807]

5.9.3 Breast cancer

Analyses found that **aluminum** was significantly higher in the breast tissue of breast cancer patients versus healthy women in the control group. [808]

A German research team analyzed breast cancer tissue and found "a highly significant accumulation of **iron, nickel, chromium, zinc, cadmium, mercury** and **lead** in the cancer samples when compared to the control group."

They concluded that gradual accumulation of transition metals in the breast tissue may be closely related to the malignant growth process and explain the anti-tumor effects of current therapies with high doses of vitamin C and substituted phenols. **Zinc** levels were 5 times higher, **mercury** 3 times higher and **cadmium** 2.5 times higher in cancer cases. [809]

Cadmium was markedly increased in the urine of patients with breast cancer compared with the control population (approximately 2-fold). **Cr** and **As** were also increased in the urine of patients with BC. [810]

"Studies demonstrated that **aluminum** in the form of aluminum chloride or aluminum chlorhydrate can interfere with the function of oestrogen receptors of MCF7 human breast cancer cells." [811]

Another analysis found that **aluminum** was significantly higher in the breast tissue of breast cancer patients versus healthy women in the control group. "Aluminum can lead to iron dysregulation, and there was a distinct correlation between increased aluminum and higher ferritin (the protein that stores iron) in the breast cancer patients." [812]

Specific commercial products containing **aluminum** salts include certain antacids and antiperspirant deodorants.

"**Aluminum** exposure has been strongly correlated with carcinogenesis in the breast tissue." [813]

It is believed that aluminum from deodorants is transported to the breast tissue via lymph nodes in the armpits.

Mice subjected to **AlCl3**, the same aluminum salt used in antiperspirant deodorants, displayed malignant growth of mammary gland epithelial cells. [814]

This same result was observed in studies performed on samples of human breast cells. [815]

"**Aluminum** appears to directly affect the secretion of protein from dispersed parathyroid cells. " [816]

Kidney cancer

A study has determined a strong correlation between **lead** exposure and the development of kidney cancer. [817]

Other studies determined a strong positive association between metal exposure and mortality rates of cancers including kidney cancer. [818]

Bladder cancer:

"A significantly higher concentration of **As, Mn,** and **Pb** was noted in the blood and urine of carcinoma urinary bladder (CAUB) patients compared to controls." [819]

In Iran, environmental **cobalt** was shown to be associated with higher rates of colon cancer in men. [820]

Treatment

The most effective use of metal chelation in the context of cancer is in prevention, evidence for cancer treatment after the fact is scarce.

"**Copper** chelation using the metal chelator TPEN, selectively kills colon cancer cells through redox cycling and generation of reactive oxygen species." [821]

5.10 Kidney disease

Each nephron in the kidney contains a filter (glomerulus) that has a network of tiny blood vessels called capillaries. "When blood flows into a glomerulus of a healthy kidney, tiny molecules - water, essential minerals and nutrients and wastes - pass through the capillary walls. Large molecules, such as many proteins and red blood cells, do not. " [822]

"The kidney is a target organ in heavy metal toxicity for its capacity to filter, reabsorb and concentrate divalent ions."

Meaning, the structure is made to reabsorb the 'good', essential heavy metals, so they can be recycled, the kidneys also reabsorb the toxic metals which have similar physical properties. Some essential metals are located just next to toxic metals in the periodic table.

"Heavy metals in plasma exist either in an ionized form, which is toxic and leads to acute toxicity or a bound, inert form when metals are conjugated with metallothionein and are then delivered to the liver, possibly causing chronic kidney damage." [823]

"Studies in animals and humans primarily demonstrate a clear association between exposure to the metals **cadmium, lead, arsenic** and **mercury** [the "Big Four"] and the presence of chronic renal damage."
"The kidney is the main organ affected by chronic **cadmium** exposure and toxicity. Continued and heavy **Cd** exposure can progress to the clinical renal Fanconi syndrome, and ultimately to renal failure." [824]

"In older adults, urine **arsenic** and **vanadium** were significantly associated with chronic kidney disease in single metal models and made major contributions to kidney function among mixtures." [825]
In a Bangladesh study, chronic kidney damage patients exhibited significantly higher levels of **Pb, Cd** and **Cr** levels in their urine samples than controls. The serum levels of **Cu** were also much higher in CKD patients. [826]
"Sri Lankan Agricultural Nephropathy (SAN), a new form of chronic kidney disease, has now become the most debilitating public health issue in the dry zone of Sri Lanka." [827] And it is associated with multiple heavy metal exposure, of course.
In a systematic review, Satarug et al 2017 dubbed the synergism between kidney **cadmium** toxicity, diabetes and high blood pressure: "The Perfect Storm". [828]
"The most common metals implicated in kidney toxicity are **arsenic, barium, cadmium, cobalt, copper, lead, lithium, mercury** and **platinum**." [829]
Lewis et al found an increase in the mortality rate in kidney disease in men, but not in women, due to exposure to high concentrations of **As**. [830]
Blood **cadmium** levels were correlated with chronic kidney disease, especially in adults with hypertension or diabetes. [831]
Not only do toxic metals damage the kidneys, but excessive excretion of essential minerals can be an indication for renal dysfunction.
"Early indication of renal dysfunction can be gleaned from urinary wasting of essential elements such as **magnesium, calcium, potassium** and **sodium** in an unprovoked [urine test] specimen. "

142

5.10.1 Kidney disease and hypertension

Kidney disease and hypertension often go hand in hand, the exact cause and effect relationship is very complex and not yet fully established. Both conditions can occur individually and both conditions are enhanced by or can be individually cause by toxic metals.

The NHS says "*High blood pressure can constrict and narrow the blood vessels, which eventually damages and weakens them throughout the body, including in the kidneys. The narrowing reduces blood flow. High blood pressure is the second leading cause of kidney failure in the United States after diabetes.*" [832]

But vice versa, it is accepted that restricted renal vessels can increase blood pressure to ensure circulation.

"*Hypertension (HTN) is ubiquitous in the renal failure patient. It has long been thought that renal disease interferes with salt excretion, leading to volume overload and consequent hypertension. This theory gives prominence to the kidney in long-term regulation of blood pressure. It is assumed that the excess salt and water retention increases the blood flow to the tissues, which sets in motion the phenomenon of autoregulation. The tissue arterioles vasoconstrict to decrease the excessive blood flow. The resulting vasoconstriction raises the peripheral vascular resistance, which is the cardinal most consistent findings in HTN (whether essential or renal in origin).*" [833]

The Cleveland Clinic says:

"Renal hypertension happens when the arteries that transport blood to your kidneys get smaller. Complications of renal hypertension include heart attack, aneurysm and stroke." [834]

The association of hypertension and toxic metals is discussed in 5.3.

5.10.2 Gout

Gout manifests as a buildup of uric acid in the blood, often caused by decreased uric acid excretion by the kidney.

Blood heavy metal mixtures are associated with an increased prevalence of hyperuricemia and gout, with the greatest effect coming from **lead**. [835]

"The findings of a study suggest that chronic low-level environmental **lead** exposure may interfere with urate excretion of chronic renal insufficiency (CRI) patients."

"Importantly, the inhibition of urate excretion can be markedly improved by **lead** chelating therapies" (with a weekly intravenous infusion of 1 g of calcium disodium EDTA for four weeks). [836]

The results of a different study demonstrated a significant dose-dependent relationship between **mercury** exposure from dental amalgams and kidney integrity biomarkers such as glutathione-S-transferases (GST)-α (suggestive of kidney damage at the level of proximal tubules (PTs). [837]

"Even low blood **lead** levels, in the range currently considered acceptable are associated with increased prevalence of gout and hyperuricemia." After adjustment for confounders, the highest quartile of blood lead levels was associated with a 3.6-fold higher risk for gout and a 1.9-fold higher risk for hyperuricemia compared with the lowest quartile. [838]

E. Krishnan says "It's not clear why low-level **lead** would boost gout risk." The theory is that even small amounts of lead can hinder the kidneys' ability to excrete uric acid. [839]

"Higher levels of **mercury** and **lead** are both associated with gout, serum uric acid [SUA] and hyperuricemia." [840]

Cadmium intake is positively associated with hyperuricemia (elevated uric acid level in the blood) among Chinese adults. "There is an increasing body of evidence that suggests hyperuricemia increases the risk of gout." [841]

Further, **cadmium** exposure had a positive association with serum uric acid levels in the nationally representative Korean population. [842]

Already the ancient Roman elites suffered from gout, evidently due to their high **lead** consumption in wines and sweets (see 14.5.1).

5.10.3 Metals, kidney, gout and porphyria

The body **lead** stores (BLS) of patients with both chronic renal insufficiency (CRI) and gout are higher than those of patients with CRI only (see below). [843]

In a cohort of patients diagnosed with neurological disorders (NDs), **Hg** body-burden was associated with brain dysfunction.

"Patients with neurological disorders and more severe brain dysfunction had significant increases in the mean urinary concentration of uroporphyrins (uP)."

A significant positive correlation between **Hg** body-burden associated porphyrins and increased brain dysfunction was observed. [844]

Porphyria is a group of liver disorders in which substances called porphyrins build up in the body, negatively affecting the skin or nervous system. [845]

"The presence or elevation of various urinary porphyrin species can flag a potentially toxic condition. Metals and other toxic chemicals with prooxidant reactivity can inactivate porphyrinogenic enzymes, deplete glutathione and other antioxidants, and increase oxidant stress, all of which lead to damage to membranes, enzymes, and other proteins in cells." [846]

Urinary porphyrins are oxidized metabolites of heme biosynthesis. Specific urine porphyrin profiles are associated with high-level exposure to **mercury, arsenic** and **lead**. [847]

Lead poisoning can mimic acute porphyria

Tsai et al concluded "**Lead** poisoning can be easily misdiagnosed as acute porphyria and nonspecific abdominal pain." [848]

The American Association for Clinical Chemistry says:

"Heavy-metal poisoning is another cause of increased urinary porphyrins. **Lead**, and to a lesser extent, **mercury** and **arsenic** toxicity mimic acute porphyria attacks and can trigger porphyria investigations." [849]

"These metals can lead to false positive urine porphyrin tests. [850]

"Studies proved the disturbance of iron-reducing activity by moderate **lead** exposure. Gene carriers of porphyrias are considered to be a high-risk group to chemical pollutants." [851]

"Ferritin positively associates with serum urate and an interventional study suggests that **iron** has a role in triggering gout flares." [852]

"Urinary porphyrin profiles are used as biomarkers of trace metal exposure and toxicity in rats during prolonged exposure to methyl **mercury**." [853]

5.10.4 Chelation in cases of kidney insufficiency

Kidney insufficiency is generally considered a counterindication for vigorous chelation protocols with EDTA or DMSA/ DMPS, which excrete metals mainly via kidney. However, with low- doses and slower chelation protocols with constant monitoring of kidney function, kidney health is often improved or restored by chelation: Sears 2013 elaborates: "A concern with chelation therapy is that renal insufficiency may be a contraindication for therapy. The opposite appears to be the case." In patients with chronic renal insufficiency with elevated body burden of **lead** and without diabetes, three months of CaNa2EDTA weekly infusions resulted in slowing or reversing degeneration in the chelation group. [854]

Renal dysfunction may alter **Pb** chelatability with CaNa2EDTA, bone-blood **Pb** reequilibration, PbEDTA distribution, or PbEDTA excretion. [855]

Already in 1986, a study in creatinine clearance found improvement in renal function following EDTA chelation and multi-vitamin-trace mineral therapy.

"Subjects with chronic degenerative disorders and with renal damage were treated with infusions that included EDTA, vitamins, mineral and oral supplements. Following 20 infusions, creatinine clearance significantly improved." [856]

A **lead** poisoned adult (blood lead level 384 micrograms/dL) with a specific urinary porphyrin profile of elevated porphyrins, was fully restored after 2 5-day courses of DMSA. [857]

"Short-term **lead**-chelation therapy has been used to improve renal function and slowed the progression of renal insufficiency in lead workers." [858]

A meta-analysis of available randomized controlled trials - published by the NIH - showed that calcium disodium EDTA chelation therapy can effectively delay the progression of chronic kidney disease in patients with measurable body **lead** burdens. [859]

"For more than a decade, Ja-Liang Lin and colleagues have published randomized placebo-controlled clinical trials reporting that treatment with calcium disodium EDTA slows chronic kidney disease progression (caused by environmental **lead** exposure)." [860]

In a rat model, acute renal failure was induced by 60 minutes ischemia (inadequate blood supply). "EDTA treatment was able to protect rat kidneys from ischemic damage possibly through the stimulation of nitric oxide (NO) production." [861]

So here, EDTA administration improved renal function after a mechanical kidney injury, where toxic metals were not evaluated.

"Chelation with another chelating agent, DMSA, improved renal function and was efficacious in treating nephropathy and hypertension, induced in animals by long-term exposure to low-levels of **lead**." [862]

5.11 Liver disorders

Johns Hopkins Medicine reported:

People with higher levels of **cadmium** in their urine appear to be nearly **3.5 times more likely to die of liver disease than those with lower levels.** "The cadmium-liver disease link disproportionately affects men." [863]

The global prevalence of non-alcoholic fatty liver disease (NAFLD) is between 25.2% and 29.8%. [864]

In the overweight population, the global prevalence of NAFLD is 70%. [865]

Heavy metal exposure showed an association with liver damage among the general adult population in Korea. [866]

Blood **lead** levels are associated with non-alcoholic fatty liver disease in the Yangtze River Delta region of China in the context of rapid urbanization, especially in women. [867]

In the Korean adult population, **cadmium, mercury** and **lead** all demonstrated positive correlations with liver enzymes and NAFLD indices. "Key molecular pathways implicated in the pathogenesis include activated oxidative stress, altered lipid metabolism, and increased cytokines and inflammatory response." [868]

In another nationwide Korean study on the same metals (**lead, mercury** and **cadmium**) it was demonstrated that a higher blood **Hg** level was associated with hepatic steatosis in men and women. And a higher blood **Cd** level was associated with hepatic fibrosis in women. [869]

In Taiwanese men, the prevalence of moderate to severe fatty liver disease is 26.5%. "The presence of soil heavy metals **[arsenic, mercury, cadmium, chromium, copper, nickel, lead** and **zinc]** is a significant risk factor for fatty liver disease in men. Lean men with a BMI <24 kg/m2 are the most susceptible to soil heavy metals." [870]

"Chronic exposure to **lead** causes lead to accumulate mainly in the liver." In vivo studies have shown that lead toxicity is related to alterations in the inflammatory response. [871]

Arsenic and liver

Frediani et al demonstrated a positive association between urinary **arsenic** exposure and the risk of NAFLD among U.S. adolescents and adults, that is highest among Mexican Americans and among those obese, regardless of race/ethnicity. [872]

Lead is also one of several heavy metals observed in statistically higher concentrations in gallstones. [873]

5.11.1 Prostate disorders

"Four heavy metals (**As, Zn, Mn, and Sb**) are significantly and positively associated with prostate cancer risk." [874]

Croatian and Serbian cohorts showed significantly higher blood **Hg** levels and significantly lower serum SH levels in prostate cancer patients than in controls. [875]

"The repercussions triggered by heavy metals on the prostate include hormonal imbalance and oxidative damage, leading to morphological alterations." [876]

5.12 Muscular health

Handgrip strength is a commonly used marker of muscle strength. Grip strength was strongly correlated with total muscle strength, with correlation coefficients between 0.736 and 0.890.

"Weaker grip strength has been associated with an increased risk of cardiovascular disease, cognitive decline and mortality, both in middle-aged and older adults." [877]

Poor muscular strength has been shown to be associated with increased morbidity and mortality in diverse samples of middle-aged and elderly people. [878] Sarcopenia is the age-related progressive loss of muscle mass and strength.

Data from the Korea National Health and Nutritional Examination Surveys demonstrated that "high levels of blood **lead, mercury** and **cadmium** increase the prevalence of sarcopenia in both genders of elderly populations." [879]

Elderly Koreans with higher **cadmium** levels not only had weaker handgrip strength but also more depression. [880]

Children and adolescents with higher heavy metal exposure (**cobalt, molybdenum, lead, antimony, strontium, thallium** and **cesium,** measured in urine) have significantly lower muscle strength. "Higher heavy metal exposure and the exposure levels of a mixture of metals in urine are inversely related to handgrip strength." [881]

Also in US adults, **cadmium** exposure is associated with reduced grip strength. [882]

Levels of **Co, Cd, Cr** and **Hg** in muscles are correlated with decreased muscle fibers' diameter." [883]

By the way, hand grip strength is a common marker for overall muscle strength, because it is easy to measure also in elderly people without endangering the subjects. Obviously, one cannot test the general population's muscular fitness by assessing a maximum dead-lift exercise. This does not mean that grip training in particular promotes overall health and longevity - as has been suggested by fitness trainers - but full body muscle training can do so. And people who are generally healthy have better muscle health even without training.

5.13 Skeletal health

Bone health is a predictor of longevity.
Patients over 90 years of age had an overall low prevalence of fractures and relative preservation of bone health. "The low percentage of osteoporosis and fractures likely reduced the morbidity and mortality in this population, potentially contributing to their overall longevity." [884]
Bone health is also associated with mental health.
"Evidence exists that mental health disorders (i.e., depressive disorders, anxiety disorders and PTSD) and osteoporosis have a bidirectional relationship." says Dr. Traci Speed of Johns Hopkins University School of Medicine. [885]
"Of the key elements that seek the hydroxyapatite of bone, two have been identified as the agents responsible for most of the toxicological pathologies. They are **lead** and **aluminum**, with **lead** being identified as the most dangerous to skeletal metabolism at the present time." [886]
"Metals such as **cadmium, arsenic, mercury, chromium** and **aluminum** are toxic to bone cells even at low concentrations." [887]
In postmenopausal women (aged 53–64 years), bone mineral density (BMD) is negatively correlated with **cadmium** levels in the urine. [888]
And **cadmium** levels were negatively correlated with **Zn** levels in the intervertebral discs of patients with degenerative changes. [889]
"Heavy metals can incur disordered bone homeostasis, leading to the development of degenerative bone diseases, including osteoporosis, osteoarthritis, and degenerative disk disease."
Cadmium is the best-characterized heavy metal involved in bone homeostasis disorder and osteoporosis." [890]

5.13.1 Chronic back pain

"8 percent of all adults experience persistent or chronic back pain, and as a result are limited in certain everyday activities. Back pain is the sixth most costly condition in the United States. " [891]

"Chronic **mercury** poisoning can mimic the low back pain form of spondyloarthritis." [892]

Spondyloarthropathy (SPA) is a family of chronic inflammatory diseases affecting the spinal structure and joints. Comparison of metals data indicated that **Cd, Co, Cr, Cu, Fe,** and **Mn** levels were significantly higher in SPA patients, whereas **Ca, Mg,** and **Zn** contents were substantially higher in healthy subjects. [893]

Spondyloarthritis is frequently characterized by a dull ache felt deep in the lower back, or buttocks. It is associated with inflammation of the sacroiliac (SI) joints, which are the joints linking the lowest part of the spine to the pelvis.

As we have seen above, in metal industry employees, depressive and distress symptoms are predictors of low back pain, neck-shoulder pain, and other musculoskeletal morbidity.

"Musculoskeletal disorders were considered as predating the development in depressive and distress symptoms." [894]

"With increasing age, the concentrations of **chromium, cobalt,** and **thallium** in bone decreases significantly, while the concentration of **cadmium** in bone markedly increases."

As bone density decreases with age, toxic metals that were stored in the bones, can be redistributed into soft tissue.

"There is a close correlation between the concentration of **cobalt** in bone and the presence of osteopenia." [895]

"Occupational exposers to heavy metals such as **cadmium, lead** and **mercury** cause extensive health deteriorations, such as asthma and back pains." [896]

Long-term high **cadmium** exposure may cause skeletal damage, which was first reported from Japan, where the itai-itai (ouch-ouch) disease (a combination of osteomalacia and osteoporosis), was discovered in the 1950s. "The exposure was caused by **cadmium**-contaminated water used for irrigation of local rice fields. A few studies outside Japan have reported similar findings." [897]

Itai-itai disease manifests as severe back pain, especially in the lumbar region, as well as bone and muscle pain, demineralization of the skeleton and a characteristic duck-like gait. [898]

5.13.2 Osteoarthritis

Osteoarthritis is often associated with toxic metals in different ways, one because sufferers of advanced joint degradation receive artificial joint replacements which may release toxic metals (**chromium, cobalt**, etc.) But metal toxicity is also strongly associated to the initial cartilage damage in the first place.

Rheumatic arthritis patients in Pakistan had significantly higher blood levels of **Pb, Cd, Cr,** and **Ni** than healthy controls. [899]

Osteoarthritis (OA) is the gradual loss of articular cartilage. **Cadmium** (e.g., from tobacco smoke) 'has been identified as a major OA risk factor.' [900]

Lead and **cadmium** promote the prevalence of osteoarthritis (OA) in the population of the United States as demonstrated by analysis of the NHANES 2011- 2020 datasets. [901]

In a study with 12,584 U.S. adults, **Cd, Co,** and **Cs** were identified to be positively associated with osteoarthritis (OA) risk.

"**Cd, Co, Cs, Pb** and **Tl** were positively associated with biological aging markers, while all biological aging markers had significant associations with OA risk."

Cadmium and **lead** are cumulative bone-toxicants and contribute to musculoskeletal disease. [902]

Knee- and hip osteoarthritis is ranked as the 11th highest cause of global disability and the 38th highest cause of disability-adjusted life years (DALYs).

95% of all knee replacements are performed for osteoarthritis. [903]

Lead toxicity involves alterations on calcitropic hormones' homeostasis, which increase the risk of skeletal disorders. [904]

"High blood **cadmium** levels were related to increased risk of disease symptoms onset in inflammatory arthritis patients."

"These changes partly explain why **cadmium** exposure and a high cadmium body burden may raise the risk of IA and of disease symptoms exacerbation." [905]

Patients with osteoarthritis of the spine/ spinal degenerative disease had the following parameters as compared to controls:
- lower median concentration of **Mg** in the serum
- higher median concentration of **Cd** in the blood
- Significantly lower molar ratios of Ca to **Cd** and **Pb** as well as Mg to **Pb** and **Cd**. [906]

In osteoarthritis, we see a similar helplessness by the medical community as in other chronic diseases such as hypertension. If you have osteoarthritis, doctors might tell you it's because you don't do enough exercise, if you tell them you exercise every day, then it must be because of too much exercise. Or it's because you consume too little calcium. if you have arteriosclerosis, then you consume too much calcium.

5.13.3 Osteoporosis

Heavy metal exposure is a risk factor for osteoporosis.
"A significant association is observed between blood heavy metals (**lead** and **cadmium**) levels and low bone mineral density (BMD)."[907]

A systematic review and meta-analysis of 14 studies confirms:
"Exposure to **cadmium** and **lead** is associated with an increased risk of osteopenia or osteoporosis in adults."[908]
"Among middle-aged and elderly adults, there was a significant positive relationship between **cadmium** levels and a higher prevalence of osteoporosis." Inversely, higher selenium level led to a lower prevalence of osteoporosis and exerted a protective effect.[909]

"Low-level exposure to **cadmium** during a lifetime also increases the risk of osteoporosis and fractures of the lumbar spine in the elderly."[910]
"**Cobalt** induces alterations in serum parameters associated with bone metabolism in male adult rats." The results of a study suggest that cobalt can induce bone resorption in adult rats and, therefore, behave as an osteoporotic agent.[911]

Osteoporosis and lead
Blood **lead** levels are associated with an increased risk of falls and osteoporotic fractures.[912]
Exposure to **lead** is associated with increased risk for fracture in premenopausal women, according to study results published in the Journal *Bone*.[913]
"**Lead** exposure inhibits fracture healing and is associated with increased chondrogenesis, delay in cartilage mineralization, and a decrease in osteoprogenitor frequency."[914]
Campbell et al found a significant inverse association between **lead** exposure and bone mineral density in the US population, but only among white subjects.[915]
In a Nigerian study, 62% of welders had elevated blood pressure and high blood **lead** levels. The measured significant relationship between serum lead levels and low back pain and knee pain was attributed to lead's effect on the musculoskeletal system.[916]

In Korean adults, the risk for osteopenia or osteoporosis significantly increased with an increasing blood **lead** or **cadmium** level. The highest quartile group in blood **lead** had a 1.47 times higher risk of osteopenia or osteoporosis. With higher blood **cadmium**, the risk for osteopenia or osteoporosis increased 2.1 times. [917]

Now, here is a common practice failure of general practitioners and even some bone specialists. X-rays of healthy bones look solid white; osteoporosis bones appear gray and less dense. Bones laden with **lead** are also more brittle, but appear solid white in the X-ray as well, on closer inspection mostly near the joints, characterized as lead bands or lead lines. "The minimum blood levels at which 'lead bands' are seen is much lower than previously described." [918] But an average doctor just sees "bones white, therefore 'bones good'.

5.13.4 Rickets in children or osteomalacia in adults

Factory children during the Industrial Revolution often had rickets and osteomalacia or soft bones. This is generally believed to have been caused by lack of sun light in the factories and smog cities and thus vitamin D deficiency. Lack of sunlight is obviously a contributor, but can only partly explain the phenomenon.

Today as well, **lead** poisoning in children induces rickets.

"A meta-analysis found that compared with healthy controls, the body **lead** levels in rickets children were significantly higher than controls." [919]

"**Cd** exposure induced nephrotoxicity through impaired vitamin D metabolism in the kidney, leading to subsequent impairment of bone metabolism and bone fragility." [920]

"During the Industrial Revolution in England, families streamed to urban areas, the lack of sunlight was severe."

"Rickets appeared in epidemic form in temperate zones where the pollution from factories blocked the sun's rays." [921]

What was not considered here, is that the factories emitted vast amounts of toxic metals, the pollution did not just block sunlight, but caused chronic metal poisoning, affecting especially the children working in these factories or playing nearby.

The Smithsonian reported that many children in ancient Rome suffered from vitamin D deficiency.

"New research suggests rickets was common long before the Industrial Revolution, when pollution blocked out sunlight."

The Roman physician Soranus noted that infants in Rome suffered from bone deformities more often than infants in Greece.
The rate of rickets in children was found to be 5.7 percent." [922]
Unfortunately, the archeologists in charge of this investigation did not bother to examine these ancient bones for **lead** poisoning, which is a common denominator for people with bone deformities in Roman, Victorian and present times. See an extended discussion on **lead** poisoning in ancient Rome in Chapter 14.5.

5.13.5 Cartilage, ligaments and tendons

In forensic autopsies of decease patients who had died of acute illness with no known **lead** exposure, all joint samples showed a highly specific accumulation of **lead** in the tidemark (the transition zone between calcified and non-calcified articular cartilage). [923]
"Cartilage and bone are target tissues for toxic materials such as **lead** and **cadmium**." [924]
"**Mercury** is taken up selectively by cells involved in joint, bone, and connective tissue disorders." These cells are predominantly affected in rheumatoid arthritis and osteoarthritis. [925]
Preliminary study results imply that "subjects with occupational **lead** exposure have smaller Achilles tendons than healthy subjects." Chronic **lead** exposure may affect the tendons due to reduction of collagen synthesis. [926]

5.13.6 Tooth decay and periodontitis

Periodontitis (bacteria induced inflammation of tooth supporting tissue or advanced gingivitis).
Several studies have reported an increased risk of periodontitis due to excessive exposure to individual metals. For example, a cross-sectional study of 4716 participants demonstrated associations between **cadmium**, **lead** and periodontitis.[927] Metal mixtures increased the effect.
Increased **lead** levels on root surfaces of periodontally diseased teeth in smokers explained the increased clinical attachment loss (CAL) and periodontal destruction in these cases compared to non-smokers. Further, **arsenic** and **cadmium** were raised in periodontitis teeth. [928]
Mixed metal exposures were significantly associated with periodontitis, **Cd, Pb, Tl** and **Ba** had the greatest effect. [929]
Mercury exposure was independently associated with periodontitis in Korea (odds ratio = 3.17). [930]

Exposure to **uranium** has been found to inhibit periodontal bone formation in rats. [931]

The results of a Polish study indicated that impacted mandibular teeth and the surrounding mandibular bones reflected the exposure of people to **cadmium** and **lead** in the environment. [932]

Periodontal patients had a fivefold increase in the concentration of **Cu**, a threefold-elevated level of **Mn** and a twofold increase in the concentration of **Mg** in the oral fluid compared to controls. [933]

"**Lead** poisoning increases the risk of tooth decay by weakening tooth enamel development." [934]

"Both primary and permanent teeth (due to their similar structure) are reliable bioindicators of environmental exposure to heavy metals [such as **Sn, Sr, Al, Sb, Hg, Zn, Pb** and **Cr**]." [935]

"Heavy metals in human teeth dentine are a bio-indicator of metal exposure and environmental pollution." [936]

Results from the Veterans Affairs Normative Aging Study showed: "Men in the highest tertile of bone **lead** had approximately three times the odds of having experienced an elevated degree of tooth loss as those in the lowest tertile." [937]

Military personnel, firearm instructors and police officers often have **lead** toxicity from firearm training. When firing a gun, minute quantities of abrasion dust are released when a bullet leaves the barrel, the dust is inhaled at shooting ranges.

Leaded ammunition is being phased out for police use, it is mostly substituted with **antimony** and **bismuth**, both are also toxic, but less so than lead (see also 14.3).

5.14 Autoimmune diseases

"Heavy metals are capable of altering the immune response; they have been implicated in influencing autoimmunity. In fact, they are usually inhibitory to immune cell proliferation and activation." [938]

"Heavy metals such as **mercury, silver** and **lead** are associated with autoimmunity." [939] Further metals that "provoke immune reactions include **gold, platinum, beryllium, chromium**, and **nickel**." [940]

"**Mercury**- containing compounds can profoundly affect the immune system at concentrations well below those that damage the central nervous system." [941]

"**Aluminum** accumulation is associated with autoimmune ASIA syndrome, cause by vaccines, where it is used as an adjuvant to enhance a desired immune response." [942]

The **silver** content of dental amalgam can contribute to autoimmune disease, more so than the **mercury** content (see also 8.38).

"In genetically susceptible strains of experimental animals, **mercury** and **silver** can induce autoimmune responses." [943]

"Preliminary data suggest that dental amalgam and dental **nickel** alloys can adversely affect the quantity of T-lymphocytes. Human T-lymphocytes can recognize specific antigens, execute effector functions, and regulate the type and intensity of virtually all cellular and humoral immune responses." [944]

"Heavy metals can manipulate the immune system into mounting an inappropriate immune response. " [945]

5.14.1 Lymphatic system disorders

Pyroptosis is a form of inflammasome-triggered programmed cell death in response to a variety of stimulators, including the environmental cytotoxic pollutant **cadmium**.

"**Cd** exposure causes pyroptosis not only in vascular endothelial cells, but also in lymphatic endothelial cells. Cd treatment significantly decreased the viability of human dermal lymphatic endothelial cells (HDLECs)." [946]

Cadmium induces apoptosis of pig lymph nodes [947]

Arsenic causes lymphadenopathy as a side effect.[948]

"Lymph nodes are an essential part of the body's immune system. Due to their function, they come into contact with toxins [such as metals], which can cause them to swell." [949]

5.15 Obesity and toxic metals

Some toxic metals have been associated with overweight and obesity, others with underweight and anorexia. [950]

"**Arsenic** and **tin** are the toxic elements most often associated with obesity. Some heavy metals accumulate in the body and are stored in various tissues, including the adipose tissue." [951]

5.15.1 Weight loss and mental health

Metal toxicity can be one of the reasons why some people feel worse when they lose weight quickly, they can have metals transferred from the fat tissues to organs and the brain, and thus suffer from increased symptoms of heavy metal toxicity when dieting, including mental health problems such as anxiety and depression. Many people on a diet report feeling like a 'part of their soul is being taken away from them'.

"Some describe losing excess body fat as being easier than dealing with the aftermath when it comes to dramatic weight loss. Others feel that along with the weight lost, so too is their ability to 'be happy' or feel content." [952]

A 2014 study "casts doubt on the common belief that weight loss success leads to psychological benefits such as reduced levels of depression."

"Weight loss over four years in initially healthy overweight/obese older adults was associated with no psychological benefit." [953]

According to a PLOS report, "the results of a study showed a positive correlation between physical health and weight loss, but a **negative correlation between mental health and weight loss**."

"Losing weight won't necessarily make you happy," the researchers said. [954]

5.15.2 Calories, standard of living vs obesity

Calorie intake and expenditure are not solely representative of BMI, thus it is neither sensible nor helpful to carelessly blame people for being overweight or underweight. "A poor diet cannot fully explain the prevalence of obesity. Other environmental factors (e.g., heavy metals) have been reported to be associated with obesity." [955]

"Even physical activity has shown an inconsistent negative association with BMI." [956]

In 1971, the average population BMI for adults aged 20 years and older was 25.7. By 2020, the mean BMI increased to 30.0. During this period, obesity increased by 20%. [957]

It is self-evident that people who exercise regularly are on average leaner and healthier. But also, for people who happen to be lean and healthy, it is easier and more satisfying to exercise regularly, so they tend to exercise more. For fit people, exercise is fun, for obese and chronically ill people, it can be torture. Likewise, strength training can increase testosterone in men, inversely: "testosterone reduces feelings of stress and anxiety, lessens pain, and **makes strenuous effort feel good**" (work, exercise, etc.). [958]

In this way, it's easy for healthy, lean people to tell obese people: 'just work out and you feel good.'

In the same way, it is easy for healthy, high testosterone men to tell others: "just pull yourself up at the bootstraps and work hard and work out regularly."

Here again, cause and effect are not clearly distinguished. For morbidly obese people with chronic endocrine disfunction, oxidative stress, mitochondrial damage and adrenal fatigue (whether cause by metal toxicity or other factors), they sometimes don't need to drastically overeat to maintain their weight. The various chronic conditions may cause them to gain weight and the urge to overeat can be increased by these imbalances.

Just like different types of addictions, morbid obesity is not solely the result of weakness or a character flaw.

Many doctors and fitness coaches insist: ' It's simple: when you eat more calories than you burn, you gain fat, when you eat less than you burn, you lose fat." Most people over 40 know from experience: it's not that simple; a young adult can usually eat a lot without gaining weight, as they get older, they eat less, even start working out and still gain weight.

Having said that, of course people are mostly responsible for their weight problems. Everyone with or without any chronic disease should be encouraged to eat well and exercise at a reasonable capacity. And no one should be encouraged to indulge in unhealthy habits by telling them they can't change their body anyways.

On a societal scale, there is an obvious general trend towards wealthy countries having more food energy intake and higher obesity. However, calory- intake and availability are not absolute predictors of obesity.

The findings of a study involving hunter-gatherers by Pontzer et al "seem to contradict popular beliefs that weight management is simply a matter of balancing what we eat with enough purposeful physical activity."

"The similarity in [total energy expenditure (TEE)] among Hadza hunter-gatherers and Westerners suggests that even dramatic differences in lifestyle may have a negligible effect on TEE." [959]

Studies among the Hadza, traditional farmers in Guatemala, the Gambia and Bolivia, as well as rural farmers in Nigeria showed their energy expenditures were broadly similar to those of city dwellers.

Similarly, primates, kangaroos, sheep and pandas living in zoos expend the same number of calories each day as those in the wild, despite obvious differences in physical activity. [960]

BMI vs. food energy intake by country
Some people are literally malnourished while being overweight or obese. Calorie quality is just as important as quantity. High fructose sugars and seed oils are some of the obesity risk factors, aside from toxins such as metals.

Haiti, the poorest nation in the western hemisphere (ranked 162 of 188 in GNI (PPP, per capita globally), has a higher rate of obesity (22.7%) than most western European countries. In Switzerland, one of the richest nations worldwide, the rate of obesity is 19.5%. The population of Haiti is genetically mostly of West African descent. In West Africa today, obesity rates are among the lowest in the world, so genetics are not the major factor. Wealthy Japan has an obesity rate of 4.8 %. [961]

While obesity rates can also reflect inequality within a country, body mass index (BMI) is more meaningful for the relationship between food intake and body weight.

Papua New Guinea, one of the poorest countries in the world, has a higher BMI than France or Denmark. Belgium is number 3 in food energy intake, but below the world average in BMI.

You can find many such apparent inconsistencies when comparing the list of BMI by country [962] with the list of food energy intake by country. [963]

'Arabian obesity' and arsenic:
Even the types of food staples don't give a clear picture. For instance, Middle Eastern countries, Saudi Arabia, Qatar etc. have some of the highest obesity rates in the world, rice is one of the important staple crops, imported from South East Asia, where obesity rates are low.

"Among different age groups the main source of **arsenic** exposure is grains and grain-based food products, particularly rice and rice-based dietary products."

"The source of carbohydrates through rice is one of the leading causes of human **arsenic** exposure. The Gulf population consumes primarily rice and ready-to-eat cereals as a large proportion of their meals." [964]

In Saudi Arabia, other nutritional markers were found highly relevant: People with low consumption of omega-3 showed a 5.7

times increased risk of higher body mass index and a 20.5 times increased risk of higher waist circumference. [965]

The inconsistencies in the relationship between obesity and living standards are similar to those between hypertension and living standards (see 5.4.).

5.15.3 Various metals and obesity

"Heavy metals (**Cd, Pb**, and **Hg**) were inversely associated with abdominal and peripheral obesity risks."

Further, heavy metals might counteract the beneficial effect of healthy dietary patterns on obesity. [966]

"Some heavy metals (e.g., **arsenic, cadmium, lead** and **mercury**) have been associated with obesity and obesity comorbidities among U.S. adults." The results of a 2003-2014 study showed that cumulative exposure to heavy metals as mixtures is associated with obesity and is related to chronic conditions such as hypertension and type-2 diabetes mellitus (T2DM). [967]

In a prospective cohort of US children, it was demonstrated that among children born to mothers with overweight or obesity (OWO), low-level in-utero co-exposure to **mercury, lead,** and **cadmium** increased the risk of childhood OWO. "The risk was mitigated by adequate maternal selenium and folate levels." [968]

The Arkansas Rural Community Health Study with 270 randomly selected women showed significant positive associations in postmenopausal women with obesity for both **arsenic** and **cadmium** concentrations, at concentrations well below governmental and industrial standards for acute toxicity.

"The rate at which individuals gain weight is affected by metal concentrations and may play a role in the rapid increase in weight in postmenopausal women." [969]

"Epidemiological studies demonstrated an association between heavy metal exposure and the incidence of obesity and metabolic syndrome." [970]

"Exposure to environmental pollutants may play a significant role in the development of obesity because of their role as endocrine disruptors, raising the concept of **"obesogens"**. [971]

The EPA refers to analysis of adipose tissue of random subjects in southern Spain that showed: "**Nickel, lead, tin,** and **titanium** were detected in 100% of adipose tissue samples, and **arsenic** in 51% of them. "**Ni** was the metal showing the highest median concentration (0.56 µg/g), followed by **Ti, Pb, Sn** and **As**. [972]

Known chemical **obesogens** include different organic chemicals and metallic compounds "Exposure to markers of **mercury, cadmium, lead** and **arsenic** as well as metal mixtures were found to be correlated with anthropometric and metabolic parameters in obesity and metabolic syndrome. **However, the only metal considered a classic obesogen is tin (Sn),** particularly its organic compounds." [973]

H.N Duc et al identified associations of serum **cadmium, lead,** and **mercury** with obesity in individuals ≥50 years of age with comorbidities. In a study with 6434 subjects, serum **Hg** levels were associated with obesity and abdominal obesity as well as with body mass index (BMI) and waist circumference (WC).

"The overall effect of the mixture of all 3 metals was significantly associated with all the above parameters." [974]

"Among the general adult population of Korea, both **Pb** and **Hg** exposure was associated with an increased risk of obesity." In addition, both **Hg** and **Cd** exposure was associated with increased odds of nonalcoholic fatty liver disease.

The metal levels were 1.5 to 2 times the levels of those in the people of the lowest quartile of obesity. [975]

In adults living along the Yangtze River, China, researchers measured a positive association between **molybdenum** exposure and waist circumference /obesity. [976]

"**Cu, Ni** and **Pb** were positively associated with 4 different anthropometric indices, incl. body roundness index (BRI), conicity index (CI), body adiposity index (BAI) and abdominal volume index (AVI)." [977]

In people living in southern Taiwan, several heavy metals - **lead, nickel, arsenic** and **copper** - were positively correlated with metabolic syndrome (MetS).

5.15.4 Arsenic in obesity and diabetes

"There is a positive association between salivary **arsenic** concentration and obesity in a pilot study of women living in rural communities in the United States." [978]

"A recent study found that obese individuals are at higher risk of developing Type 2 diabetes, when exposed to inorganic **arsenic** (iAs)." [979]

"In those parts of the world with the most elevated levels of environmental **arsenic** in drinking water, there is a proposed relationship to type 2 diabetes, as arsenic may cause insulin resistance and impaired pancreatic-cell functions including insulin synthesis and secretion." [980] A bidirectional relationship is evident: "Several epidemiologic studies have shown that the risks of **arsenic**-caused disease are markedly higher in obese individuals, highlighting obesity as an important susceptibility factor." [981]

Arsenic and obesity have both been linked to inflammation, oxidative stress, adipokine expression, and insulin resistance, and these pathologic processes are thought to play a role in the diseases caused by each." [982]

"**Arsenic** exerts negative effects on the white adipose tissue by decreasing adipogenesis and enhancing lipolysis. " [983]

"Obesity and excess weight in early adulthood is also associated with high risks of **arsenic**-related cancer in later life." [984]

Cadmium and obesity

"It has been shown that "BMI values correlated significantly with hair **cadmium** levels in women as well as **lead** and **tin** levels in men." [985]

"**Cadmium** exposure was reported to upregulate pro-inflammatory markers and downregulate anti-inflammatory markers." **Cd** plays an adverse role on adipose tissues (AT) structure, function, and secretion patterns of adipokines. [986]

Cadmium exposure results in a significant increase in free fatty acids and serum glucose level. "Fat cells exposed to this Cd^{2+} significantly decreased dose-dependent cell viability."

A lower concentration of zinc and a higher concentration of **copper** in the blood can further increase the risk of obesity. [987]

Mercury obesity

High total blood **mercury** levels were found to be associated with significantly increased visceral adipose tissue mass in Korean adults. "Those in the highest tertile of blood mercury had a higher body mass index (BMI), waist circumference (WC), and visceral adipose tissue (VAT); had higher levels of blood pressure, fasting glucose, and insulin resistance." [988]

Lead obesity

"**Lead** effectively accumulates in human adipose tissue." [989]

Blood **lead** levels were positively associated with BMI in Chinese women. BLLs in Chinese adults were twice as high as in the US population. "China's lead-acid battery industry is the world's largest in terms of production and consumption, using over 67% of China's total lead production." [990]

5.15.5 Thyroid and obesity

"Hypothyroidism (thyroid under-function) is usually associated with a modest weight gain, decreased thermogenesis and metabolic rate, whereas hyperthyroidism is related with weight loss despite increased appetite and elevated metabolic rate." [991]
So, the latter are people who are never cold, can eat a lot and don't gain weight, but are low in energy.
"Endocrine disruption in the adrenal and thyroid glands can mean weight gain and problems managing blood sugar. " [992]
Among the causes of obesity are also "damage to the hypothalamus and abdominal-medial hypothalamic nuclei." [993]
(See also thyroid dysfunction and toxic metals in Chapter 2.5.1).

5.15.6 Obesity and other Endocrine Disrupting Chemicals (not restricted to metals)

"There are between fifteen and twenty chemicals that have been shown to cause weight gain, mostly from developmental exposure," says Jerry Heindel, who leads the extramural research program in obesity at the National Institute of Environmental Health Sciences (NIEHS)."
"Most known or suspected *obesogens* are endocrine disruptors." [994]

"Environmental pollutants contribute to the rising prevalence of the obesity epidemic." An expanding body of scientific evidence from animal and epidemiological studies has begun to provide links between exposure to EDCs and obesity. [995]

5.15.7 Diabetes

"Human and laboratory studies indicate the role of **cadmium** in diabetes." [996]
"It was shown that patients with gestational diabetes mellitus in Beijing, China had significantly higher levels of **endocrine-disrupting heavy metals (EDHMs) mercury** and **tin** than the control group." [997]
The results from multi-pollutant models among Chinese elderly all indicated that metal mixtures were positively associated with the risk of diabetes, and **zinc** and **thallium** were the major contributors to the combined effect. [998]
Another Chinese study identified increased odds of Type 2 Diabetes with **arsenic** exposure, which is significantly increased in individuals with excess BMI. [999]

In type 2 diabetes mellitus patients with foot ulcers, **lead, barium, cobalt, cesium** and **selenium** levels were increase compared with control subjects. [1000]

5.15.8 Anorexia (loss of appetite and underweight)

"In toddlers, anorexia is the earliest symptom of **lead** poisoning." [1001]

"Acute **lead** overexposure may cause children to be less playful, clumsier, irritable, and sluggish (lethargic). In some cases, symptoms include vomiting, abdominal pain, **lack of appetite (anorexia)** and constipation." [1002]

Workers and/ or patients exposed to **mercury** may lose approximately 10- 15 kg in body weight. [1003]

"When **mercury** and other heavy metals interfere with neurotransmitters in certain parts of the brain, bulimia or anorexia can develop." [1004]

Cobalt and **cesium** are negatively associated with body mass index and waste circumference. [1005]

"Cobalt, a metal used in making jet engines, may cause nausea, vomiting and **lack of appetite (anorexia)**." [1006]

"The clinical manifestations of **zinc deficiency** and anorexia nervosa are remarkably similar."

Zinc therapy enhances the rate of recovery in anorexia nervosa patients by increasing weight gain and improving their levels of anxiety and depression. [1007]

"In female patients admitted to the hospital with a diagnosis of anorexia nervosa, plasma **zinc** and **copper** levels were significantly reduced, whereas zinc and copper content of hair was found to be in the normal range," indicating exaggerated zinc and copper excretion. [1008]

"Chronic **Tl** (thallium) poisoning, characterized by symptoms such as anorexia and headaches, can result from prolonged exposure to low levels of Tl." [1009]

5.16 Parasites/ pathogens/ infections

Analyses of the NHANES have reported associations between the following conditions and metal toxicities:
- Chronic HBV infections are associated with blood **mercury** levels in women of child-bearing age. [1010]

- Higher blood **cadmium** levels are reported among HIV-infected individuals.
- Elevated blood **lead** levels are associated with an increased risk of herpes simplex virus type 2 infections. [1011]

5.16.1 Chronic infection

NHANES data showed elevated blood **lead** and **cadmium** levels are associated with chronic infections (with seropositivity for Helicobacter pylori, Toxoplasma gondii, and Hepatitis B virus (HBV)). [1012]

Dr. Bryan Stern is one of the leading holistic practitioners in the U.S. with over 35 years of experience. "The discovery of the PCR test (polymerase chain reaction), which identifies microorganisms by their DNA structure, has led to the understanding that virtually all illnesses are caused by or contributed to by a chronic infection." Recall: "The list of symptoms related to **mercury** intoxication alone includes virtually any illness known to mankind. Simply put, **mercury** can mimic any illness - or contribute to it." [1013]

5.16.2 Parasites

In animal studies, high heavy metal toxicity is consistent with higher parasite load. Parasites, over long times of infestation, have much higher metal concentrations than the surrounding host tissue.

As in Lyme disease, so in similar parasite infestations, the exact relationship between cause and effect is not settled:

Whether it is primarily the metals that foster the proliferation of the parasite and metal contaminated organisms are more susceptible, or whether the main process is the parasites absorbing metals from the host. It is established that in animals, parasites can protect the host from toxic metal overload (see below).

Not only the parasites that remain in the host for prolonged times, but also material that is constantly excreted from the host body - such as pin worms, eggs or fragments of tapeworm bodies - contain high levels of toxic metals. Thus, for the duration of the infestation, metals are constantly excreted. Many studies show the parasites thrive in metal toxic hosts, while the host keeps lowering the body metal burden, unless the host is continuously reabsorbing new metals. It is proposed here that also in humans, some parasites have a limited potential symbiotic relationship with the host. In ideal cases, the damage of the actual infection could be less detrimental than the long-term effects of the metal toxicity.

However the exact cause and effect relationship may turn out to be, as metals are closely associated with parasites, what is certain, is this: no non- essential toxic metals at all are better than any amount of toxic metals.

Tapeworms

Nature magazine reported: parasites suck toxins from sharks Intestinal worms collect heavy metals from the sea.

"The worms could be saving the sharks from metal poisoning - at least for now." The tapeworms had 278 to 455 times higher metal **[lead and cadmium]** concentrations than the sharks themselves, the researchers report in *Parasitology*. [1014]

Red foxes in Croatia without **Echinococcus** multilocuralis (Dwarf fox tapeworm) had twice as much toxic metal burden of **cadmium** and **lead** compared to infected foxes. "The researcher summarized that this could support the hypothesis that tapeworms are able to absorb toxic heavy metals from the host body into their tissues." [1015]

Likewise, liver samples of cow and sheep collected from slaughterhouses in Erbil and Koya cities revealed: Cow liver parasitized with Echinococcus parasite had lower levels of toxic metals. **Cadmium** levels in infected cows were 6 times lower than in the uninfected cows. **Cadmium** levels in parasitized sheep liver were 8 times lower than in uninfected sheep; whereas the **lead** level was 14 times lower than in uninfected sheep. [1016]

Echinococcus multilocuralis (fox tapeworm) infection in humans, causing the live disease alveolar echinococcosis (AE), is considered to be ultimately fatal unless early surgical intervention can remove the parasite cyst. [1017]

It is assumed the parasite destroys the liver over the course of 10-20 years. Many dog owners are infected from their own pet. Dog owners are between 4 and 13 times more likely to contract alveolar echinococcosis than non- dog owners. [1018]

Fish

The accumulation of **Hg** in fish is "related to the possible parasitic infestation of fish. Fish intestinal nematodes accumulate heavy metals at high concentration. " [1019]

"In some fish species in the Mediterranean Sea, **mercury** accumulation was greater with higher rates of Anisakis parasites." [1020]

Alternatively, "the presence of the parasite in fish is considered an important factor for **Hg** accumulation." [1021]

166

"It has been proposed that even if parasites do not accumulate organic pollutants, they are able to alter the uptake of chemicals of their hosts, including metals." [1022]

In the intestinal parasite helminth Pomphorhynchus laevis and its host fish species Barbus barbus in the Danube River, ten out of twenty metals analyzed were found at higher concentrations in the acanthocephalan than in different tissues (muscle, intestine, liver and kidney) of the host barbel itself, 'indicating that there is competition for metals between the parasites and the host.' [1023]

A study by Hassan et al concluded that the infection of marine fish with Cestoda parasites showed a much higher bioaccumulation capacity of some heavy metals (**As, Fe, Zn, Pb, Cu, Cd**) than the fish organs, "therefore, it might act as a biological indicator for heavy metal pollution." [1024]

In catfish in the Nile Delta in Egypt, the total prevalence of parasitic infection is associated with uptake of metals. [1025]

Rodents

"Intestinal *Helminths* in Urban Rats have a high heavy metal bioabsorption capacity." [1026]

Lead inhibits the intracellular killing of *leishmania* parasites and of extracellular *cytolysis* of the target cells in mice in vitro. [1027]

In Nigeria, highly significant positive correlations were observed between heavy metal concentrations in organ tissues of the African Giant Rat and cestode parasite [a tapeworm]. [1028]

Bacteriological and parasitological studies in Poland detected a correlation between the concentrations of **lead** and **chromium** and the presence of the eggs of helminths (ATT), as well as between the concentration of **zinc** and the presence of Salmonella bacteria in municipal sewage sludge. [1029]

5.16.3 Bacteria / Metals and Antibiotic Resistance

A multidirectional interaction of antibiotics and toxic metals is recognized:

- antibiotics reduce metal excretion from the body.
- Heavy metals (**copper, cobalt, cadmium, zinc** and **lead salts**) "enhance the development of antimicrobial resistance in otherwise antimicrobial sensitive strains of bacteria." [1030]

Various pathogens - antibiotic resistance

Omura and Beckman, 1995 found "antibiotics used to treat various infections often were ineffective in the presence of abnormal

167

localized deposits of heavy metals like **Hg** and **Pb,** which were often observed to co-exist with Chlamydia trachomatis, Herpes Simplex Types I & II, Cytomegalovirus (CMV), and other micro-organisms."
Therefore, the research team hypothesized that the infectious micro-organisms mentioned above somehow **utilize the Hg or Pb to protect themselves from what would otherwise be effective antibiotics**, and/or that heavy metal deposits in some way make antibiotics ineffective. [1031]
Heavy metals including **lead** and **cadmium** "are increasingly of concern with respect to the propagation of antibiotic-resistance."
An NHANES analysis showed that general population levels of blood **Pb** are associated with differences in nasal carriage of Staphylococcus aureus. [1032]
"If highly toxic metals such as **mercury, cadmium, copper** and **zinc** reach the environment and accumulate to critical concentrations, they can trigger co-selection of antibiotic resistance. Furthermore, co-selection mechanisms for these heavy metals and clinically as well as veterinary relevant antibiotics have been described." [1033]
"Heavy metal exposure creates antibiotic resistant bacteria (ARB)."
Pb exposure is associated with increased colonization by antibiotic resistant bacteria, and resistant Gram-negative bacilli (RGNB) are particularly resistant to Pb. 34% of participants tested positive for ARB, they had on average 6 % more urinary lead than those who tested negative. [1034]

5.16.4 Toxoplasmosis

Toxoplasmosis is an infection caused by a single-celled parasite called *Toxoplasma gondii*.
"In humans in different age groups, an association was determined between blood **lead** and *Toxoplasma gondii* seropositivity. " [1035]
Children with above median blood **lead** levels and positive for IgG anti-T. gondii showed a 5.51-fold increase in the chance of displaying disobedient behavior. "The results suggest that T. gondii infection may be contributing to the high indices of behavioral changes." [1036]

5.16.5 Virus infections

"Metal ion chelators have achieved widespread success in the development of antiviral drugs." Heavy metal (**lead, cobalt,**

168

cadmium, manganese, iron and **copper**) concentrations are significantly higher in the blood of Hepatitis C Virus (HCV) patients as compared to normal persons. "Chelation therapy with monoisoamyl DMSA (MiADMSA) led to a significant excretion of heavy metals in the urine. This chelation therapy will be helpful to reverse the HCV related health problems." [1037]

Covid
"Whole blood **iron**, age, and sex were determined to be independent factors associated with COVID-19 disease severity, while **chromium, cadmium**, and the comorbidity of cardiovascular disease were determined to be independent factors associated with mortality." [1038]
Zinc deficiency was associated with Covid severity (see also 5.17.3: Covid and taste and smell).

Candida/ Fungal infections
Dr. Melina Roberts explains: "Heavy metals have a symbiotic relationship with candida. Heavy metals bind to candida as a protective mechanism to bring heavy metals out of circulation. Therefore, if you are struggling with fungal overgrowths, the root cause may be heavy metal toxicity." [1039]

5.16.6 Parasites/ pathogens - Treatment/ Chelation

"**Nickel** chelation therapy with Dimethylglyoxime (DMG) has been applied as an approach to combat multi-drug resistant enteric pathogens."
"DMG inhibited activity of two Ni-containing enzymes, Salmonella hydrogenase and Klebsiella urease. **Oral delivery** of nontoxic levels of DMG to mice previously inoculated with S. Typhimurium led to a 50% survival rate, while 100% of infected mice in the non-DMG control group succumbed to salmonellosis." [1040]

A Giannakopoulou et al 2018 found: "Metal-chelating inhibitors of viral and parasitic metalloproteins constitute attractive, promising and safe therapeutic agents for the treatment of serious infectious diseases." [1041]

An EU patent has been filed for "Uses of metal ion chelating compositions for the treatment or prophylaxis of parasitic infestations such as nematodes and other parasitic organisms, including protozoan species in human and non-human animals." [1042]

"**Iron** chelation (with DFP or EDTA) is able to potentiate the antibacterial activity of conventional antibiotics by destroying bacterial biofilms." This combination is recommended as a promising strategy for the treatment of chronic device infections with biofilm producing coagulase-negative staphylococci (CNS)." The addition of the **iron** chelator DFP amplified the antibacterial activity of conventional antibiotics against S. epidermidis. [1043]

Iron chelation has been successfully used to treat malaria.

"Compared with placebo, treatment with the chelator desferrioxamine B was associated with an almost 10-fold enhancement of the rate of parasite clearance.

No drug toxicity was detected. "Iron chelation may provide a new strategy to be developed for the treatment of malaria." [1044]

5.16.7 Lyme disease

Dr. Jay Davidson says: "Parasites absorb heavy metals."

"From what we understand research- wise, Lyme disease, which is technically a bacteria or spirochete, has been shown to live inside of certain nematodes, which is essentially a type of parasite like a roundworm. So, parasites can actually house Lyme disease, bacteria, or viruses." [1045]

"Studies continuously fail to find the spirochete pathogens in most cases of either symptomatic cases or in cases with confirmed antibody test. "

In 1983, of 36 Lyme patients in Long Island and Westchester County, New York, who had signs and symptoms suggestive of Lyme disease, spirochetes could be isolated from the blood of only 2 patients. [1046]

"Lyme bacteria can hide inside parasitic worms, causing chronic brain diseases." Board-certified pathologist Alan B. MacDonald, MD, found two Borrelia pathogens, including B. burgdorferi - the causative agent of Lyme disease - thriving inside parasitic nematode worms, worm eggs or larvae in the brain tissue of nineteen deceased patients. [1047]

Like the other parasites listed above, in many host species, nematode worms (roundworms) have much higher concentrations of toxic metals than the hosts. "Anguillicola crassus, a nematode, was observed to harbour **lead** concentrations while parasitizing the fish Anguilla anguilla." [1048]

If nematodes thrive in toxic metal- infested hosts, and Borrelia can hide in nematodes and Borrelia are protected by metal induced biofilms, this would (partly) explain how metal chelation has been successfully used to treat Lyme disease.

"Although many Lyme patients have had success with long-term antibiotics, Lee Cowden, MD, integrative medical researcher and physician, believes many patients being treated with antibiotics recover completely for months or years only to suffer a recurrence." [1049]

On this note, we also recall that antibiotic use shuts down the body's ability to excrete **mercury**.

In 2014: experts called Lyme disease "the fastest-spreading vector-borne illness in the US".

"**Lead, mercury, cadmium**, and other toxic metals fuel inflammation and suppress immune function." [1050]

5.16.8 Metal toxicity and Lyme Disease

"Most pathogen infections initiate a classical defense response of the immune system based on chelation of **iron**." Borrelia has circumvented this strategy by using **manganese** as the main 'survival' metal.

"Borrelia uses **zinc and manganese** for proliferation and to protect itself against oxidative pressure." [1051]

In one study, patients with chronic Post Treatment Lyme disease Syndrome (PTLDS) showed high levels of **mercury** and **lead** in urine after a DMSA challenge. More than 84% of the patients had evidence of exposure to heavy metals, including **mercury, lead**, **arsenic, cadmium** and **aluminum**. [1052]

The Lyme spirochete B. burgdorferi does not require iron, but "has the capacity to accumulate remarkably high levels of **manganese**. This high manganese is necessary to activate the SodA superoxide dismutase (SOD) essential for virulence."

"B. burgdorferi has uniquely evolved without a cellular requirement for iron, and the organism accumulates high levels of **manganese** compared with other more iron-philic organisms, such as E. coli and S. cerevisiae." [1053]

"Because immune dysfunction and inflammation are associated with chronic diseases, it is crucial to know if someone has elevated levels of heavy metals in conditions like chronic Lyme disease." [1054]

"The symptoms of heavy metal poisoning are similar to those of Lyme disease. Toxic metals interfere with other medical treatments, even those for Lyme disease. Not only does the buildup of heavy metals interfere with metabolic functions, but it also provides a barrier that protects Lyme bacteria." [1055]

"Certain heavy metals, in particular **mercury,** greatly impair the immune system's ability to get to the bacteria." [1056]

"As a powerful immuno-suppressant, **mercury** poisoning is particularly troublesome for persons with cancer or Lyme disease." [1057]

"Manganese, iron, copper, and **zinc** are the most prevalent transition metals in the Lyme disease spirochete Borrelia burgdorferi." [1058]

In particular, a **manganese**- rich environment supports superoxide dismutase activity in Borrelia burgdorferi. [1059]

Dr. W. Lee Cowden, MD, from the University of Texas Medical School states:

"As people becomes sicker [with LD], their levels of toxicity increased; this has been accompanied by an increase in heavy metal poisoning." [1060]

SeAY wellness claims: "For people suffering from Lyme disease, heavy metals are the rate-limiting step in their ability to get better." [1061]

Lyme distribution patterns

Regional analysis revealed that Lyme disease risk appeared in **urbanizing areas rather than urbanized and rural areas.** "These results suggested that rapidly urbanizing areas may become LD hotspots."

"Geographical detector analysis further proved that urban expansion is the dominant factor for LD cases increase." [1062]

If urbanizing areas (or suburbs) are more affected than urban areas, how many people living in suburbs and urbanizing areas are regularly wading through high grass in comparison to rural residents of mostly farmland?

The distribution pattern of infection strongly indicates that the monocausal theory of a tick bite is lacking. Even though rural areas are generally more affected than urban, the question should be how city dwellers who are rarely in nature should ever get a tick bite, from a tick that was on a deer before and then on a rodent recently.

"Deer are important sources of blood for ticks and are important to tick survival. However, deer are not infected with Lyme disease bacteria and do not infect ticks." [1063]

Ticks are small, spider-like arachnids but they are not spiders.

For a tick to be able to suck blood from a host and survive, it must be undisturbed, but most humans notice ticks on them or their

172

children immediately and kill them. Or at the latest they notice them when they are pumped full of blood. How many people leave a tick on their body for 48 hours unnoticed?

The CDC says: "In most cases, a tick must be attached for 36 to 48 hours or more before the Lyme disease bacterium can be transmitted. If you remove a tick quickly (within 24 hours), you can greatly reduce your chances of getting Lyme disease." [1064]

It should be added that the CDC doesn't site any scientific study - only other statements by their institutes - to support their explanations of transmission patterns.

Thus, even though ticks can live for weeks without food, ticks living off humans only and over several feeding cycles, is an unlikely and unproven scenario. The accepted wisdom is still the following:

"Ticks can bite people, but it is very rare that you will 'catch' one directly from your pet. You would be most likely to pick one up when walking through long grass." [1065]

"During colder weather, from November to April, Lyme disease diagnoses occurred more often in urban than rural areas." [1066]

"Ticks and Lyme disease are a threat for cities, too. An examination of black-legged ticks in New York City raises concerns about Lyme disease spreading in urban communities." [1067]

These distribution patterns and the symptoms suggest that metal toxicity of the human host is an important and underappreciated factor in Lyme disease. Reduction of metal toxicity may play a role in prevention and treatment.

5.16.9 Kryptopyrroluria (KPU) and heavy metals.

"KPU is usually a genetic condition whereby the body cannot easily absorb vitamin B6 and zinc, excreting too much in the urine. In 1964, however, Thompson and King reported that aside from acute and inherited conditions, there are milder constitutional forms caused by heavy metal contamination or chemical toxicity." [1068]

Dr. Klinghardt has found a high correlation between patients with chronic Lyme disease and those with kryptopyrroluria (KPU). "Klinghardt has found the incidence of KPU in Lyme disease to be 80% or higher; in patients with heavy metal toxicity (**lead, mercury, aluminum, cadmium**, and others) over 75%; and in children with autism over 80%." [1069]

5.16.10 Adrenal insufficiency

"Cancer patients often have low adrenalin levels." [1070]

173

"Auto-immunity is the most common cause of primary adrenal insufficiency in adults and genetic defects, especially enzyme defects, is the most common cause in children." [1071]

"Mercury in the human adrenal medulla could contribute to increased plasma noradrenaline in aging." [1072]

"The heavy metal substances that are accumulated in the adrenal gland will make the adrenal gland produce fewer hormones and cause adrenal fatigue, which will quickly degenerate the body and cause high stress." [1073]

"The many self-registered symptoms of patients with **mercury** intolerance have revealed many facets in common with those associated with serotonin dysregulation." [1074]

5.17 Insomnia

"Sleep wake disorders are identified as one of the predominant molecular mechanisms involved in the pathophysiology of sleep disorders induced by heavy metals (**cadmium, lead,** and **mercury**)." [1075]

Already in 1761 Venice, Joannes Antonius Scopoli identified sleep disorders as a "prominent sign of **mercury** toxicity, in addition to tremor, respiratory difficulties, personality changes, difficulty eating, dream disturbances and what today would be termed restless leg syndrome." [1076]

A study by Spiegel, 1999 claims that 9 hours of sleep for adults was the norm before 1910, while the average adult in 1999 got 7.5 hours of sleep on average. [1077]

"Various heavy metals are known to contribute to insomnia, for instance **lead, nickel** and **arsenic.**" [1078]

Lead exposure in early childhood is associated with increased risk for sleep problems and excessive daytime sleepiness in later childhood, according to research from the University of Pennsylvania. [1079]

Among e-waste workers in Thailand, high urinary **mercury** levels were associated with high rates of insomnia (46.8%), muscle atrophy, weakness, and headaches. [1080]

The NIH lists insomnia and depression as two of the symptoms of **manganese** toxicity. "Other metals implicated in sleep pattern disruption and sleeplessness are, **mercury, aluminum, lead, copper** and **zinc.**" [1081]

"Circadian disruption is observed in patients with Parkinson's disease (PD), Alzheimer's disease (AD) and Huntington's disease

174

(HD), all neurodegenerative diseases that - in addition to a genetic component - are thought to be influenced by metal exposures." [1082] Metals implicated in neurodegenerative diseases and sleep disruption include essential metals in overload (**manganese, copper,** and **zinc**) or non-essential metals (such as **lead, mercury,** and **aluminum**). "**Manganese** toxicity is mediated by dopamine so it is possible that Mn-dopamine interactions have an adverse effect on the sleep-wake cycle." [1083]

Workers exposed to **mercury** are often affected by insomnia.

"Adaptive efficiency indicated that in all out of 15 studied subjects, the adaptive solutions were frustrating and led to psychic suffering and/or environmental conflict confirming the severity of the involvement in inorganic **mercury** poisoning." [1084]

Insomnia and other sleep disorders have been reported subsequent to **mercury** exposure in workers in fluorescent light bulb plants (mercury). [1085]

Further, "Low levels of **arsenic** exposure were observed to be associated with sleep disturbance in **copper** smelter workers." [1086] **Arsenic** and other toxic metals are associated with a variety of sleep disorders. According to data from the U.S. NHNES, 2005 - 2006: "Higher levels of urinary **arsenic** were associated with waking up at night. Higher levels of other toxic metals were associated with leg cramps while sleeping."

The tested metals were **barium, cadmium, cobalt, cesium, molybdenum, lead, antimony, thallium, tungsten, uranium** and **arsenic.** [1087]

"Low vitamin D levels can also play an important role in time to fall asleep at bedtime." [1088]

"Duration of sleep correlates with the ratio of **zinc** to **copper** in adult women, suggesting that a balance between these two metals is important for sleep-wake regulation." [1089]

The findings were corroborated for men in a different study.[1090]

"Cortisol levels rise dramatically first thing in the morning and decline throughout the day. High levels of stress can result in daytime cortisol production, disrupting this pattern." [1091]

Braun et al found concurrent blood **lead** levels were associated with Cortisol Awakening Response in pregnant women from Mexico City and this might explain adverse health outcomes associated with **lead**.[1092]

We saw above (2.2) that **mercury** and other metal accumulation has been shown in the pineal gland, which participates in circadian function through the secretion of melatonin and serotonin. [1093]

Recall the pineal gland is one of the 4 parts of the human brain that is not protected by the blood brain barrier and can thus easily be affected by toxic metals in the blood stream.

5.17.1 Insomnia and liver

Sleep disturbance is a common feature of chronic liver disease (CLD) with impact on health-related quality of life; 60–80% of patients with CLD report subjective poor sleep. [1094]

"People with poor nighttime sleep and prolonged daytime napping have the highest risk for developing fatty liver disease," says Dr. Yan Liu. [1095]

"The risk of nonalcoholic fatty liver disease (NAFLD) is significantly higher in patients with insomnia and daytime sleepiness." [1096]

Recall that fatty liver disease is strongly related to **chronic metal toxicity** (see also 5.11).

The Times Of India suggests: "Waking up between 1 am and 4 am could signal a risk for non-alcoholic fatty liver disease. " [1097]

If you go to a practitioner of Traditional Chinese Medicine in China, and you tell them you regularly wake up at 3 in the morning for no apparent reason, they probably say "liver". By the way, Dr. Klinghardt claims: "Traditional Chinese Medicine practiced in the West is Traditional Chinese Medicine minus the chlorella." In Traditional Chinese Medicine in China, chlorella (a natural metal chelator) is administered proficiently.

"In East Asia, chlorella algae are also added to rice, tea, and pancakes. Chlorella has been used for thousands of years by Traditional Chinese Medicine practitioners." [1098]

Insomnia, metal toxicity and anxiety

Carol Gillette explains: "Toxins also disturb the naturally occurring processes within the neurology and the body in general. **Mercury** debilitates the ability of serotonin to convert into melatonin, resulting in sleepless states. **Mercury** toxicity also debilitates the ability of norepinephrine to convert to epinephrine (also known as adrenaline). This results in a build-up of norepinephrine. Elevated **norepinephrine means anxiety**, as norepinephrine is a chemical marker for anxious states." [1099]

"Smoking is a significant risk factor of insomnia." [1100]

Of the more than 600 chemicals in tobacco, the toxic heavy metals are the ingredients that can contribute to the increased rates of insomnia of smokers.

5.17.2 Chronic fatigue syndrome

Studies have shown that delayed-type hypersensitivities (type 4 allergy) to **nickel** and **mercury** are more frequent in patients with chronic fatigue syndrome (CFS) as compared to healthy controls. [1101]

In 2001, **nickel** allergy was found in a majority of women with chronic fatigue syndrome and muscle pain. "Furthermore, improvement in CFS symptoms following removal of dental amalgams has been reported." [1102]

5.17.3 Taste and smell

Cadmium, chromium, arsenic and **nickel** compounds are specifically associated with olfactory (smell) impairment.
"The olfactory bulb tends to accumulate certain metals (e.g., **Al, Bi, Cu, Mn, Zn**) with greater avidity than other regions of the brain." [1103]

"Early signs of chronic **tin** poisoning include loss of smell." [1104]
"Uptake and transport in the olfactory neurons may be an important means by which some heavy metals gain access to the brain." [1105]
"Among adults between 40- 80, those with higher **cadmium** exposure have higher rates of taste and smell dysfunction." [1106]
"In clinical studies, **cadmium** and **nickel** compounds have been specifically associated with olfactory impairment." [1107]

During the Covid pandemic, loss of taste and smell was strongly correlated with **zinc deficiency**. "Zinc deficient COVID-19 patients had a more prolonged hospital stay." [1108]
J. S. Al-Awfi (2020) stated one of the symptoms in COVID-19 patients - loss of taste - has been associated with zinc deficiency. It is undetermined whether the virus is causative or those patients had zinc deficiency pre COVID-19.
"Approximately 57.4% of COVID-19 patients have low zinc serum levels which may indicate an advantage to administer zinc therapeutically to those patients." [1109]

5.17.4 Erectile dysfunction

In a 2022 study, participants with ED were found to have higher blood **cadmium, mercury** and higher urinary **lead** and **cadmium** levels. It was concluded that "heavy metal exposure is closely correlated with the development of ED, and a high blood **cadmium** level is an independent risk factor of ED." [1110]

177

Further, **cobalt** and **antimony** were positively associated with ED. [1111]

ED patients were shown to have significantly lower dietary intake of trace metals **(Mg, Zn, Cu,** and **Se).** "Increasing dietary intake of these trace metals within the upper limit is beneficial in reducing the prevalence of ED." [1112]

5.18 Skin disorders

Collateral damage from skin disorders:
"The skin is a sensitive organ and the largest organ of the body. Small, non- cancerous skin irregularities are usually not life threatening, but they can have a profound effect on the wellbeing of people, not just in cases of vanity." Studies have demonstrated "a strong correlation between skin diseases and anxiety." [1113]
In the field now known as *psychodermatology*, psychologists are getting more involved in helping dermatology patients.
Dr. Gorbatenko-Roth describes three types of psychodermatology disorders:
-Skin problems affected by stress or other emotional states.
-Psychological problems caused by disfiguring skin disorders.
-Psychiatric disorders that manifest themselves via the skin, such as delusional parasitosis." [1114]
There are deeper archaic reasons that skin and hair disorders cause social anxiety and exclusion: they can give a rough superficial impression of a person's health, chronic illness or malnourishment and may subconsciously deter potential sexual partners or social contacts. Whenever times were hard, people with severe skin lesions and marks in the face were generally avoided 'like the plague'. Skin diseases are, on average, less fatal than diseases of most inner organs. But they often correlate with or are outwards symptoms of such organ diseases.
"The skin frequently serves as a marker for underlying internal disease. The type of lesion typically relates to a specific disease or type of disease." [1115] "There is an extensive correlation between vitiligo and other organ-specific or generalized autoimmune disorders. Vitiligo is now recognized as more than just a skin disease, what a dermatologist observes as a white spot of skin is just the "tip of the iceberg" of the condition." [1116]
Chronic toxic metal poisoning can cause or proliferate chronic skin disorders. And chronic toxic metal poisoning can in itself lead to psychological stress, anxiety and low self-esteem. A recent study
178

found that adults with active or severe atopic dermatitis had "an increased risk of all-cause death and certain causes of death, such as infectious and respiratory diseases. " [1117]

M. Oaten et al present a model of the system of disease avoidance and stigmatization, which includes an emotional component, whereby visible disease cues directly activate disgust and contamination, motivating avoidance. The authors argue that "stigmatization of many different groups may result either directly or indirectly from an evolved predisposition to avoid diseased conspecifics". [1118]

"The results of a study support the theory that humans have an evolved predisposition to avoid individuals with disease signs, which is mediated by the emotion of disgust. This implicit avoidance occurs even when they know explicitly that such signs result from a noncontagious condition." [1119]

Repeated experiments showed for instance: strangers in public keep a greater distance to people with a false disfigurement/ mark (such as a port wine stain) in the face than they did to a person without a mark. [1120] No wishful thinking about our own unbiased personality can trick our archaic instincts.

88% of patients with atopic dermatitis, psoriasis, skin cancers, alopecia, acne or chronic urticaria considered their skin disorders to be embarrassing in their personal lives and at work. 14.5% of participants felt they were rejected by others because of their skin condition, 19.2% felt they were looked at with disgust.[1121] And they aren't all wrong.

"Some studies suggest that psoriasis shortens the lifespan of patients by 4 years and maybe up to 10 years." [1122]

Lead and skin

Chronic occupational exposure to **lead** leads to significant mucocutaneous changes in lead factory workers. In one study, all tested subjects had elevated blood **lead** levels; the mean level was 74.15 µg/dL.

The most frequently observed signs were gingival brown pigmentation in 83.6%, gingivitis in 82.8% and **lead** line in 49.3% of patients. "Even in normal-appearing skin, the level of hydration and elasticity decreased in **lead**-intoxicated patients. " [1123]

Arsenic and skin

As we already learned, more than half the population of Bangladesh has skin lesions due to chronic **arsenic** poisoning (see 8.6.1).

A systematic review of epidemiologic studies showed

exposure to **arsenic** was associated with an increased risk of keratinocyte carcinoma (in the epidermis). Further, **cadmium** and **chromium** are toxic and carcinogenic. [1124]

"Chronic **arsenic** toxicity can cause hardened patches of skin (hyperkeratosis), unusual darkening of certain areas of the skin (hyperpigmentation), and a scale- like inflammation of the skin (exfoliative dermatitis)." [1125]

An Argentinian community had a very high incidence of skin lesions up to 1969. When the **arsenic** concentration in the drinking water was lowered by a factor of 7 by 1971, the incidence of skin lesion dropped by a factor of 17 in the same year. [1126]

5.18.1 Dermatitis

A systematic review in cement industry areas found:

"**Chromium, nickel, cobalt, zinc, cadmium** and **mercury** may play an important role in human skin disease."

"Of these metals, **chromium, cobalt** and **nickel** are almost certainly present in every case of dermatitis and eczema." Elements such as **cadmium, lead** and **mercury** usually are found in chronic skin disease (psoriasis and skin cancer) on a biologic test." [1127]

Serum levels of heavy metals (**lead, mercury** and **cadmium**) are significantly associated with atopic dermatitis (see below).

The results of a study on prenatal heavy metal exposures found that **lead** exposure in late pregnancy increases the risk of atopic dermatitis (AD) in 6-month-old boys. [1128]

In children aged between 4 and 13 years, "**lead** was more commonly detected in the indoor air in houses of children with atopic dermatitis, even with concentrations of airborne lead below the safety levels suggested by health guidelines." [1129]

A Taiwan cohort study found that prenatal exposure to inorganic **arsenic** and coexposure to inorganic **arsenic** and **cadmium** was associated with a higher risk of atopic dermatitis in young children. [1130]

Eczema

In patients with eczema and miscellaneous skin conditions in Hong Kong, **lead** levels have significant correlations with disease severity. [1131]

Elevated levels of **manganese** in maternal serum are associated with eczema. [1132]

Hyperpigmentation

"Heavy metals produce increased pigmentation in part from deposition of metal particles and in part from an increase in epidermal melanin production." [1133]

5.18.2 Vitiligo (loss of pigments)

In a case-control study, vitiligo patients had significantly higher concentrations of **lead** than healthy controls. "Vitiligo patients also had significantly lower values of **selenium /mercury** ratios than healthy controls." [1134]

Vitiligo patients on average had a 20 to 50% lower content of copper, manganese, selenium and zinc in hair analysis, but an increase in the toxic elements **lead** and **cadmium**. [1135]

Serum **zinc** level was highly significantly decreased in Sudanese vitiligo patients. [1136]

5.18.3 Psoriasis

"The results of a study showed that the mean values of **Cd, Cr, Ni** and **Pb** were significantly higher in scalp hair, blood and urine samples of mild and severe psoriasis patients as compared to referents." [1137]

A nationally representative sample confirmed psoriasis patients had significantly higher blood **cadmium**. "Psoriasis is common and affects approximately 2– 3% of the white population. Environmental exposure to **cadmium** may compromise immunity." [1138]

"Furthermore, metabolic syndrome, smoking and obesity are known to be more prevalent in psoriasis patients." [1139]

Multiple epidemiologic studies have consistently demonstrated higher prevalence of metabolic syndrome in patients with psoriasis. [1140]

Acne

"In the Nigerian population, acne sufferers have significantly higher blood **Cd** and **Pb**." [1141]

The New York Times says: "Heavy metals also convert the skin's oils into a waxy, gland-blocking substance, resulting in acne, blackheads, stretched-out pores, redness and irritation." [1142]

"Heavy metal dermatoses are a heterogeneous group of skin diseases related either to direct contact with or systemic absorption of heavy metals (mostly **mercury, nickel** or **arsenic**)." [1143]

Among adolescence in Moscow, the results obtained in a study indicate at least two mechanisms of the formation of acne vulgaris in adolescents. The first is associated with a violation of the regulation of sex hormones, and the second with the dermatotoxicity of anthropogenic ecotoxicants. "Adolescents with predominantly intoxicating etiology were characterized by low concentrations of selenium and zinc, high **mercury** and **lead** in hair samples, as well as an increase in the number of micronuclei in the buccal epithelium." [1144]

It is plausible that acne in puberty is a process of radically excreting toxic metals from sensitive tissues such as the brain and hormone glandes, before the body is fully developed. As acne is often concentrated in the face, this may also deter potential sexual partners during a process of excessive metal excretion.

Contact dermatitis

"It is currently estimated that around 20% of the global population exhibits allergic sensitivity to at least one metal (Schultzel et al. 2020)."

The allergens **nickel**, **cobalt** and **palladium** are among the most prevalent sensitizers. "Exposure to **Co** may lead to metal allergy." [1145]

Nickel contact allergy often affects people who have high chronic nickel toxicity in the first place. any further contact to nickel objects can trigger dermatitis skin reactions locally or in an unspecific distribution. "Allergic nickel dermatitis may be localized to the nickel exposure site, be more widespread, or present as hand eczema." The widespread type makes it more difficult to identify the condition and the triggering metal. Touching nickel containing coins, cookware, keys, doorhandles or jewelry - all common occurrences - may cause constant non-specific skin reactions anywhere; these are not likely to be identified as cause by nickel.

Allergic contact dermatitis can even occur with an inert metal such as **gold**. [1146]

5.18.4 Alopecia, hair loss

"The presence of **thallium, arsenic, mercury, selenium, cadmium, bismuth, lithium** and **copper** should be taken into account when dermatologists are considering toxic metals as a potential cause of alopecia areata in humans." [1147]

In acute **thallium** poisoning, alopecia typically occurs within 2 to 3 weeks of exposure. [1148] In fact, "alopecia is a feature that should lead to suspicion of **thallium** toxicity." [1149]

"**Thallium, arsenic, selenium** and **mercury** are the most common cause of metals-related alopecia areata in men and women." [1150]

"In alopecia areata patients, serum Zn and Mn levels were significantly lower whereas **Cd, Fe**, **Mg, Pb, Co** and **Cu** levels were significantly higher compared to those of the control group." [1151]

A systematic review confirmed agents with the strongest evidence of association to alopecia include **thallium, mercury, selenium** and **colchicine** (Colchicine is used to prevent gout attacks). [1152]

"Men with male pattern baldness have a 32 percent increased risk of developing coronary artery disease and a 40 percent increased risk of developing aggressive prostate cancer." [1153]

Both of these conditions are also independently associated with toxic metal burden.

5.19 Allergies

"Allergy and autoimmunity are caused by an abnormal immune response and have the same clinical outcomes, including local and systemic inflammation resembling autoimmune/inflammatory syndrome induced by adjuvants (ASIA)." [1154]

"In the general population of Korean adults, serum levels of heavy metals (**lead, mercury** and **cadmium**) were significantly associated with asthma, atopic dermatitis, allergic rhinitis, allergic multimorbidity, and airflow obstruction." [1155]

"It has been found that **mercury, nickel, cadmium, lead, aluminum** and **arsenic** can exert immunotoxic effects through epigenetic mechanisms." [1156]

"New research links another health issue to inadvertently ingesting low doses of **cadmium**: high activation of the antibodies that cause an allergic response." [1157]

Heavy metals from heavy traffic exposure have been associated with increases in the incidence and prevalence of childhood asthma and wheeze as well as allergic sensitization, bronchial hyperresponsiveness and respiratory symptoms in children. [1158]

"A gluten-free diet is recommended for people with celiac disease. In 2015, one-quarter of Americans reported eating gluten-free, a 67 percent increase in only two years, from 2013." This number alone should be a sign of highest alarm, either because everyone suddenly contracted the same allergy or everyone suddenly believes they must not eat what they always ate.

People who reported eating gluten-free had higher concentrations of **arsenic** in their urine (almost twice as high), and **mercury** in their blood (70 percent higher), than those who did not. [1159]

Here once again, there are different possible cause-and-effect pathways. Unlikely: gluten free foods contain higher levels of arsenic and mercury. More probable: the metals contribute to celiac disease.

Lactose intolerance

"Lactic acid bacteria (LAB) biosorption may aid the detoxification of people exposed to heavy metals."

Of 103 tested bacteria strains, all showed **Cd (II)** biosorption.

The tested bacteria were isolates from various foods, including Lactobacillus strains, unidentified LAB derived from yogurt, Weissella, strains of Pediococcus, Streptococcus, Enterococcus and 18 strains of unidentified bacteria. [1160]

Seyed Jalil Masoumi et al revealed that probiotic yogurt fortified with Lactobacillus acidophilus and Bifidobacterium sp for 7 days could safely and effectively decrease **lactose intolerance** symptoms and improve hydrogen breath test outcomes (HBT). These probiotics were recommended as a treatment of choice in lactose intolerance patients. [1161]

5.19.1 Fibromyalgia syndrome

Patients with fibromyalgia syndrome (FMS) have significantly elevated blood levels of **lead** and **cadmium**, whereas serum levels of calcium and magnesium is significantly reduced in FMS patients. [1162]

In female FM patients, reduction of metal exposure was achieved by replacement of dental metal restorations and by the avoidance of known sources of metal exposure. "All FM patients tested positive to at least one of the metals tested. The most frequent reactions were to **nickel,** followed by **inorganic mercury, cadmium** and **lead.**" After 5 years, objective examination showed that half of the patients no longer fulfilled the FM diagnosis, 20% had improved and the remaining 30% still had FM. All patients reported subjective health improvement. [1163]

5.20 Decreased body temperature, metabolic rate

Over the past 157 years, mean body temperature in US men and women has been decreasing continuously. "After adjusting for cofactors - body temperature decreased monotonically by 0.03°C per birth decade. A similar decline within the Union Army cohort as between cohorts, makes measurement error an unlikely explanation." [1164]

This substantive and continuing shift in body temperature is a marker for the metabolic rate. "The body temperature is not just a good measure of the metabolic rate, it's an exact measure." [1165] And the metabolic rate is a good measure for general health, however, high body temperature can also be caused by hyperthyroidism.

Even in the Bolivian Amazon, average human body temperature is getting cooler. "A new study finds the average body temperature among Bolivia's Tsimane people dropped by nearly a full degree in just 16 years." [1166]

"Chills or a low body temperature are among symptoms of heavy metal poisoning." [1167]

Lead and **cadmium** induce hypothermia in mice. [1168]

In another trial with 11 metals on mice, **Hg, Cd**, and **Ni** had the greatest effect in lowering body temperature. "The hypothermia and hypometabolism test may prove to be a sensitive and rapid test for the evaluation of toxicity of environmental contaminants." [1169]

Nickel and **cadmium** cause large reductions in body temperature when injected at a T of 20 and 30 degrees C. [1170]

"Central administration of **lead** or **cadmium** to mice produced a marked decrease in body temperature (1.9°C for **lead** and 2.8°C for **cadmium**)." [1171]

5.21 Eyes/ ocular disorders

"Heavy metal toxicity has been linked to the development of neurodegenerative diseases and various ocular pathologies." [1172]

"**Lead** and **cadmium** are toxic heavy metals that accumulate in the retinal pigment epithelium and choroid, ciliary body and the retina of humans." [1173]

Mercury was found to be significantly associated with dry eye disease in Korean women. [1174]

Cobalt is neurotoxic and can cause optic neuropathy and retinopathy. [1175]

Lead, mercury, cadmium, aluminum, and other xenobiotic metals are implicated in structural and physiological damage in the mammalian eye. **"Thallium** shows an affinity for melanin (in skin and eyes). " [1176]
"Case series of **mercury** exposed workers showed that acute exposure to mercury vapor had a hazardous effect on the visual system." [1177]
Systemic **silver** toxicity can lead to loss of night vision. [1178]

Cataract
Cataract is a major cause of visual dysfunction and the leading cause of blindness. "Elevated levels of **cadmium** and **lead** have been found in the lenses of cataract patients."
"Cumulative **cadmium** exposure may be an important under-recognized risk factor for cataract." [1179]
"Heavy metals are deposited in the tissues of the eyes, damaging them and accelerating cataract."
"Correlations of analyzed chemical elements (**Cd, Pb** and **Hg**) are important in the development of cataracts." [1180]
"**Cadmium** exposure can also cause conjunctivitis and damage the cornea."
One hundred patients suffering from **organomercury** poisoning who were hospitalized in the Medical City, University of Baghdad, were examined ophthalmologically in the period between March and December 1972, and were reviewed again 10 months later. Most of the patients who suffered visual disturbance had a blood **mercury** level above 100 ng/ml at the time of onset of symptoms. No visual disturbance could be detected in patients who had a blood mercury level of less than 500 ng/ml early in March 1972, 2-3 weeks after the onset of symptoms. [1181]
A study by the University of Sydney examined the eyes from tissue donors (after death) and concluded **lead, nickel, iron, cadmium, mercury,** and other metals could be found in the retina, while **iron, mercury, nickel,** and **aluminum** were found in the head of the optic nerve." [1182] The retina and the optic nerve are technically extensions of the brain.

5.22 Hearing

In a systematic literature review, all of the 49 relevant studies supported that "exposure to **cadmium** and mixtures of heavy metals induce auditory dysfunction." [1183]

In adolescents 12- 19 years old, a blood **lead** level greater than or equal to 2 µg/dL compared with less than 1 µg/dL was associated with double the odds of high-frequency hearing loss. Individuals with higher quartile urinary **cadmium** levels had significantly higher odds of low-frequency hearing loss.

"Blood **lead** levels well below the current recommended action level are associated with substantially increased odds of high-frequency hearing loss." [1184]

Chapter 6
Spurious correlations between mining (coal and metals/ minerals) and drug overdose/ despair

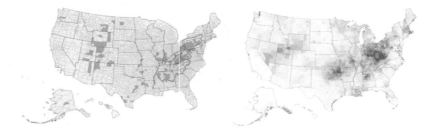

Fig. 2 Active coal mining vs death from despair. Left: Active coal mining in the US. The map shows US counties with active coal mines. The line plots show the evolution of coal mines and coal mining jobs in Appalachia and the rest of the US from 2001 to 2016. Data and Image Egli, Florian et al (2022). Backlash to fossil fuel phase-outs: the case of coal mining in US presidential elections. Environmental Research Letters. 17. http://doi.org/10.1088/1748-9326/ac82fe. Right: Deaths by Despair, including Murder, Suicide, and Drugs; Image: BuzzFeed News These Maps Show Where "Deaths Of Despair" Are Most Likely, Including Murder, Suicide, And Drugs"; Caroline Kee; March 22, 2018, https://www.buzzfeednews.com/article/carolinekee/maps-despair-deaths-drugs-alcohol-homicide-suicide

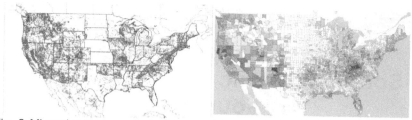

Fig. 3 Mineral resources and mines vs drug overdose. Left: Interactive map of mineral resources and mines across the United States. The U.S. Geological Survey (USGS) Mineral Resources Data System https://www.americangeosciences.org/critical-issues/maps/mineral-resources-data-system-map-viewer Right: drug overdoses, 1999: Age-adjusted death rates for drug poisoning per 100,000 population by county and year https://data.cdc.gov/NCHS/NCHS-Drug-Poisoning-Mortality-by-County-United-Sta/pbkm-d27e/about_data?category=NCHS&view_name=NCHS-Drug-Poisoning-Mortality-County-Trends-United

Chapter 7
Sources of toxic metals (prevalent sources)

Measures to avoid toxic metals from such sources or a healthy lifestyle are no guarantee for lower metal burden. Only proper metal testing reveals the actual metal burden. For unconventional, less prevalent sources see Chapter 14.

Table 1 shows the most dangerous elements according to the Substance Priority List (a function of toxicity and prevalence in the environment). Compare with the complete list of top 10 toxic substances in Table 2.

Element	Anthropogenic and natural sources	Ranking Substance Priority List
Mercury (Hg)	Is passed from mother to baby, Vaccinations, Dental Amalgams or 'Silver Fillings', contraception pills and contact lens solution	1
Lead (Pb)	Drinking water, fossettes, old lead paint.	2
Cadmium (Cd)	Cosmetics, air pollution, fossil fuel combustion, fertilizers, smoking	3
Arsenic (As)	Drinking water, food, pesticides	7
Beryllium (Be)	Industry,	43
Cobalt (Co)	Industry, welding	51
Nickel (Ni)	Jewelry	57
Zinc (Zn)		74
Uranium (U)		99

Table 1 The most relevant toxic metals (according to the Substance Priority List) and some of their main sources

7.1 Sources of toxic metals (common sources)

7.1.1 Industry

7.1.2 Coal mining

Coal and biomass combustion release various pollutants into the atmosphere, including soot particles, sulfur dioxide, and carbon dioxide. An important component of these emissions is the fine fraction of soot (fly ash), which is enriched in trace metals. Coal fly ash is characterized by **Ba, Bi, Co, Cr, Cs, Mo, Ni**, and, particularly, **As, Cd, Ga, Pb, Sb, Ti** and **Zn**. the emission factors of which are significant. [1185]

Today, coal mining is one of the main sources of poisoning with **mercury, lead** and other metals.

Psychological distress levels among Australian coal miners were significantly higher in comparison with a community sample of employed Australians. [1186]

Potentially toxic metals (PTMs) from coal mining posed a significant health risk to children 0- 6 years, particularly revealed by blood lead levels. [1187]

7.1.3 Appalachia mining

In the US Appalachia region, mining companies literally blow the tops off mountains to reach thin seams of coal. They then dump millions of tons of rubble into the streams and valleys below the mining sites.

Toxic heavy metals such as **cadmium, selenium,** and **arsenic** leach into local water supplies, poisoning drinking water.

"Cancer rates are twice as high for people who live near mountaintop-removal sites, and the risk of heart defects in babies born to mothers who lived near these sites while pregnant is 181 percent higher than for babies in non-mining areas."
[1188] See also spurious correlation (Chapter 6).

Indiana University researcher Michael Hendryx calls this mining a public health disaster, with more than a thousand extra deaths each year in areas of Appalachia where mountaintop removal (MTR) operations take place. [1189]

Here again, the majority of deaths from diseases caused by long-term, chronic metal poisoning will not be correctly identified as such but rather attributed to unknown causes.

7.1.4 Geological sources

Both volcanoes and forest fires send **mercury** into the atmosphere. However, as seen at the beginning, human activities are responsible for much of the **mercury** that is released into the environment. "The burning of coal, oil and wood as fuel can cause mercury to become airborne, as can burning waste that contains mercury. "[1190]

Some sources claim human **mercury** emissions are 2- 9 times greater than natural emissions.

"Estimates of anthropogenic contributions to the atmospheric **Hg** budget vary between 3,000 and 11,500 tons/ yr and are substantial compared to our natural Hg flux estimate." [1191]

Twenty-five percent of total worldwide emissions come from fossil fuel combustion. In the United States, 26 percent (64.7 tons/year) of atmospheric mercury emissions come from medical waste incineration, such as cremation." [1192]

Living downwind from a waste incinerator plant is a mercury hazard. So is living downwind from a crematory even in countries like Germany or Switzerland, some of the few countries where crematories have air filters, but they don't remove mercury from amalgam from the exhausts. [1193]

7.1.5 Drinking water

Recently, people in the US have heard a lot about Flint Michigan and the **lead** poisoning of children due to drinking water contamination. Meanwhile, all over the world, drinking water is shown to contain harmful levels of toxic metals.

In 2010 Sawan, et al reported in *Toxicology*: Fluoride added to public water supplies boosts **lead** absorption in lab animals' bones, teeth and blood. [1194]

Fluoride added to our water is actually fluorosilicic acid. "Technically classified as hazardous waste, this acid is an unsafe byproduct of fertilizer manufacturing and phosphate mining.

Excess fluoride increases absorption of lead and other heavy metals." [1195]

7.1.6 Food

"In the general non-smoking and non-occupationally exposed population, **food** is the most important source of heavy metals in the human body (e.g., **Cd, Hg,** and **Pb**)." [1196]

Metals are present in most foods at different concentrations as plant crops can absorb them from polluted soil or water and spread them through the food chain. [1197]

In 2012, the US FDA found **arsenic** in almost all of the 193 brands of rice, rice baby foods, and rice cereals it tested. [1198]

Consumption of 100 g/day of liver Sarpa salpa (a fish belonging to the Sparidae family, common on the coasts of the Canary Islands which is normally available in local markets) may pose a serious health risk due to the intake of **cadmium**. 100 g/day is responsible for 572% of the tolerable weekly cadmium intake for adults and 117% of the tolerable daily intake of **lead** for adults. [1199] The Canary Islands have no heavy industry to speak of.

"In a recent study, molecular biologist Ernie Hubbard found that kale - along with cabbage, broccoli, cauliflower, and collard greens - is a hyper-accumulator of heavy metals like **thallium** and **cesium**. What's more, traces **of nickel, lead, cadmium, aluminum,** and **arsenic** are also common in greens, and this contamination affected both organic and standard produce samples." [1200]

Of 11 tested common vegetables, watercress, radish, turnip and green cabbage have the highest **thallium** levels. [1201]

Elevated concentrations of **thallium** have been found in French vegetables (particularly in green cabbage) and up to 40 mg/kg in rape seed (Brassica napus L.) [1202]

"A value of 0.25 mg/kg (fresh mass) has been proposed for human foods." So, the **thallium** content was 160 times higher than the safe levels.

The German Federal institute of Risk Assessments determined a maximum **thallium** intake of 10 microgram per day. [1203]

Testing by *Consumer Reports* found: of the 28 dark **chocolate** bars tested in 2022, 23 had heavy metal (**lead** and **cadmium**) levels above 100% of the maximum allowable dose. In the 46 products tested in 2023, they found detectable levels in every product.

Perugina premium dark chocolate had 539% of the maximum allowed dose of **lead**. [1204]

Pesticides in foods

As if glyphosate in soil, water and food wouldn't be bad enough, glyphosate-based herbicides are shown to also contain heavy metals such as **arsenic,** which is the component that accumulates and lasts forever. [1205]

Okra vegetable crop was grown on a soil irrigated with treated wastewater in the western region of Saudi Arabia during 2010 and 2011. The concentrations of **nickel** in the edible portions were above the safe limit in 90% of the samples, **Pb** in 28%, **Cd** in 83% and **Cr** in 63% of the samples. [1206]

Marine predator fish at the end of the food chain (tuna and cod) are known to have high levels of **mercury** even in remote arctic waters, but also fresh water fish are contaminated. In the Iranian Kor River, industrial activities have polluted the river and the maximum concentrations of **Cd, Pb,** and **Hg** are higher than the permissible levels for human consumption. [1207]

A study in northern Thailand compared heavy-metal contamination in the eggs, blood, feed, soil, and drinking water on chicken farms, duck farms, and free-grazing duck farms in an area less than 25 km to an area farther than 25 km distance from a gold mine. The following parameters were significantly increased in the area nearer to the gold mine.

- **Hg, Pb,** and **Mn** concentrations in the eggs of free-grazing ducks
- blood **Hg** concentration in free-grazing ducks
- **Pb** concentration in the blood of farm ducks
- concentration of **Cd** in drinking water on chicken farms. [1208]

Baby Food

In 2021, the U.S. Government released a shocking report on toxic metals in baby food with the title: Baby foods are tainted with dangerous levels of **arsenic, lead, cadmium,** and **mercury**. (This includes many of the leading baby food brands). [1209]

CNN reported: "Making baby food at home with store-bought produce isn't going to reduce the amount of toxic heavy metals in the food your baby eats, according to a new report." [1210]

"The FDA failed to warn consumers of the risk." [1211]

A report released by *Consumer Reports* stated that organic foods are no safer than conventional baby and toddler foods when it comes to heavy metals. Among the metals found in some of the

194

more popular baby food products are **arsenic, cadmium** and lead. [1212]

7.2 Air pollution - Multiple chemical sensitivity

"There is an explicit correlation between exposure to air pollutants and high levels of toxic metals in the body with consequent development of diseases." [1213]

In the context of air pollution, we must of course refer to the leaded gasoline disaster that went on for a century and the aftermath is still plaguing humanity and the rest of the biosphere (see 8.23.2).

Heavy metals other than lead that are associated with traffic include "**nickel**, which is also added to gasoline and is contained in engine parts, **zinc**, and **cadmium** from tires, lubricating oils, and galvanized parts such as fuel tanks." [1214]

7.2.1 Occupational sources

Various industrial occupations lead to high toxic metal exposure, as above-mentioned mining operations, electronics, foundries,

The welding fume generated during the welding process possesses at least 13 metals, including **manganese, beryllium, cadmium, chromium, cobalt, copper, iron, lead, mercury, molybdenum, nickel, zinc, antimony**, and **vanadium**. Welders are known to be at risk, particularly to manganese. These metals are increased in the blood of professional welders by factors of 2-5 compared to controls. [1215]

7.3 Pharmaceutical drugs and heavy metals

"Over-the-counter antacids are the most important source for human **aluminum** exposure from a quantitative point of view." (See also aluminum in 8.5).

Among 39 samples of randomly tested pharmaceuticals available in the United Arab Emirates, all exhibited a positive response for **lead, cadmium** and **nickel** except three products whose Ni levels were below quantification levels.

"Three products showed higher levels of lead than oral permitted daily exposure levels." [1216]

Active pharmaceutical ingredients (API)

Process steps involving transition metal catalysts are now commonplace in API manufacture, presenting the real possibility for traces of these metals to remain in the API after purification. Common metals used in this way include **chromium, copper, nickel, palladium, rhodium, platinum** and others. Historically, the most likely culprits for trace metals in drug products were **arsenic, cadmium, lead** and **mercury**, all of which are much more likely to enter the manufacturing chain from natural sources. [1217]

Painkiller drugs contain high levels of toxic metals.
Of 30 Nigerian locally manufactured painkiller drugs, 83 % of the samples contain **arsenic**, 80 % contain **cadmium**, 36 % contain **chromium** while 33 % contain **mercury.**
63.33 %) of the painkiller drugs contain **nickel, arsenic** and **cadmium**, while 100 % of the drugs contained **nickel**. 76.67 % of the drug samples contain **lead**. [1218]

During the Covid pandemic, metallic taste in the mouth was reported. "This can also be due to a COVID antiviral treatment with Nirmatrelvir and Ritonavir, which is currently on sale as Paxlovid." [1219]

7.3.1 Antidepressants

Lithium drugs are commonly used in the management of bipolar disease. "Long-term lithium treatment is relatively frequently associated with different endocrine complications." [1220]

"More than 160 million antidepressant prescriptions are written annually, despite the fact that a recent meta-analysis shows they are no more effective than placebo to treat mild to moderate depression, the most common condition for which they are prescribed." [1221]

7.3.2 Cosmetics

Many cosmetic products contain toxic metals, **aluminum** in deodorants, **cadmium** in makeup, aluminum in deodorants and so on.
EDTA is contained in small quantities in some cosmetic products (CaNa2 EDTA is a standard metal chelator). Ironically, this can theoretically remove (chelate) some of the toxic metals from cosmetic products or from other sources. In small quantities, it is mostly absorbed locally, which may indeed rejuvenate a skin area.

So, it may actually counteract some of the harmful effects of said metals in the same products. This might be a rare case of a somewhat valid promise by beauty products.

A CIR Expert Panel concluded in 1998 that EDTA, **Calcium Disodium EDTA (CaNa2 EDTA),** is safe as used in cosmetic formulations. [1222]

But we can't have that, can we? So this is then called out by health bureaucrats as potentially harmful, even though EDTA is poorly absorbed by the skin (Dermal application of radiolabeled CaNa2EDTA to human skin showed that 0.001% was found in the urine and none was found in the blood). [1223]

So, people who use cosmetics and body care products, are either exposed to toxic metals that are absorbed and accumulated, or low dose chelators that can actually unwittingly remove different heavy metals from different sources from the body. Or it's a little bit of both.

The same applies for contact lens solutions. Many products contain mercury or EDTA or both.

Hygiene products: Apart from aluminum in deodorants, tampons contained 16 different metals. "Tampon use is a source of exposure to metals in menstruating people" [until recently known as women]. [1224]

7.3.3 Prosthetic joints

The most common traditional metals used for THA are **stainless steels, titanium** alloys (Ti6Al4V) and – mainly - **cobalt-chromium-molybdenum** alloys. [1225]

Stainless steel is an alloy of iron that contains at least 11% **chromium**.

Dental implants

"When dental implants are in good conditions, wearers have serum concentrations of **cobalt, chromium, molybdenum, titanium** and **vanadium**, which are around 5 times higher than in people without implants. if implants show significant wear, the serum levels are 5 to 10 times higher than in people without dental implants." [1226]

"**Nickel** is used in most silver-colored cast metals for crowns, usually partially covered by porcelain. These alloys typically contain 75 percent nickel and 2 percent **beryllium. Nickel** is the most carcinogenic metal known, and many women are allergic to it. Many orthodontic brackets are about 10 percent nickel." [1227]

7.3.4 Drug withdrawal

"Heavy metal toxicity disrupts benzodiazepine withdrawal and worsens withdrawal symptoms." [1228]

Chapter 8
The Toxic Metals of Concern and their Treatment

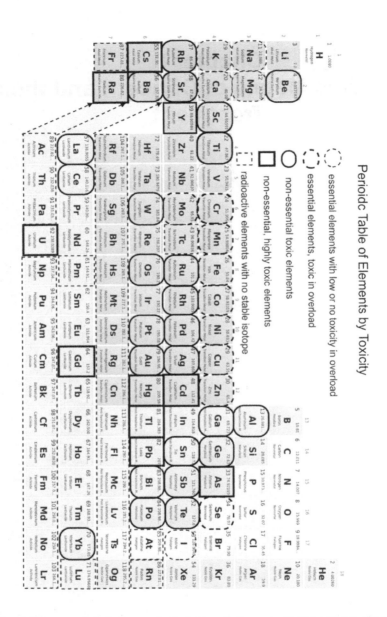

Fig. 4 Heavy metals in the periodic table of elements (these are the elements of the greatest interest for biology and human health. Bold circles: highly toxic heavy metals (non-essential); Thin lined circles: toxic heavy metals (non-essential); Dotted line circles: essential (heavy) metals (in overdose toxic) Dotted square lines: all isotopes of these elements are radioactive

Aluminum is a toxic, non-essential metal, but not a heavy metal in the technical sense.

Arsenic is a metalloid, but due to its high toxicity and ubiquitous use, it is usually counted as a heavy metal in the lteratre.

Nickel (Ni) has also been suggested to be an essential mineral, important for cellular growth, but toxic in overdose. [1229]

Vanadium is officially regarded as non-essential. [1230] (Evidence for it being essential is detailed below).

In the 5th period, molybdenum (Mo) with the atomic number 42 out of 118, is the last essential metal in the periodic table (not including the essential, non-metal Iodine, of course).

A fun question: is that why 42 is 'the answer to life, the universe and everything'...? [1231]

In the 6th and 7th period, every element is non-essential and most are toxic.

The following are radioactive elements without a stable isotope: all elements of the 7th period (including all actinides) plus Pm, Tc, Po, At, Rn. [1232]

There is no place in the human body for any element of the 6th and 7th period or denser than iodine (atomic number 53).

In my humble opinion, for a restart of civilization we will have to seriously think about whether we should put every metal denser than molybdenum back into the ground, with the possible exception for restricted use of tungsten, silver and gold.

8.1 Essential metals

Based on current knowledge it is ascertained today that metals such as **P, Na, K, Mg, Ca, Fe, Mn, Co, Cu, I, Zn, Se** and **Mo** are essential elements for life and our body must have appropriate amounts of them. [1233]

Sodium (Na) and phosphorus (P) are important essential elements of which deficiency is rare and thus supplementation is also rarely considered.

Disputed essential elements are V, Li, B, Ni, Sr. they are demonstrated to have some biological roles, but no cases of actual deficiency in these elements were proven, so supplementation is generally not recommended (8.50).

Needless to say, essential elements also include the non-metal elements C, O, H and N, the basic elements of life.

In the Substance Priority List provided by the Agency for Toxic Substances and Disease Registry (ATSDR) the three most relevant toxic substances are toxic metals (Table 2.). Cadmium is ranked 7th. These four comprise the "Big Four" of toxic metals.

"The listing algorithm prioritizes substances based on frequency of occurrence at NPL sites, toxicity, and potential for human exposure to the substances found at NPL sites.

This priority list is not a list of "most toxic" substances, but rather a prioritization of substances based on a combination of their frequency, toxicity, and potential for human exposure at NPL site."
[1234]

2019 Rank	Substance Name	Total Points
1	ARSENIC	1676
2	LEAD	1531
3	MERCURY	1458
4	VINYL CHLORIDE	1356
5	POLYCHLORINATED BIPHENYLS	1345
6	BENZENE	1327
7	CADMIUM	1318
8	BENZO(A)PYRENE	1307
9	POLYCYCLIC AROMATIC HYDROCARBONS	1278
10	BENZO(B)FLUORANTHENE	1253

Table 2 The most relevant toxic substances. In the Substance Priority List provided by the Agency for Toxic Substances and Disease Registry (ATSDR). table from ATSDR's Substance Priority List; What is the Substance Priority List (SPL)? https://www.atsdr.cdc.gov/spl/index.html

8.2 Essential metals that are toxic in overload

See list below for toxicity and treatment of each element.
Cobalt (Co)
Chromium (Cr)
Copper (Cu)
Iron (Fe)
Manganese (Mn)
Molybdenum (Mo)
Selenium (Se)
Zinc (Zn)

8.3 Toxic, non-essential and essential metals (alphabetical order)

non-essential elements have no beneficial biological role in the body. Any amount of them is too much, useless and potentially harmful.

One single atom of these metals can theoretically weaken the organism over decades (not to a measurable degree, of course).

In the following paragraph, the beforementioned 4 elements are the most relevant for public health: **lead, mercury, arsenic** and **cadmium** (dubbed 'the big four' in this text).

Thallium is the most toxic non-radioactive element, but less prevalent in the environment. Due to its unique physical properties, it is often overlooked in the diagnosis and treatment of toxic metals, even by clinical toxicologists.

These five metals are given extended treatment in the list below.

Again, all elements lower than iodine in the periodic table (greater atomic number) are non-essential and most of them are toxic, they have no place in the human body.

8.4 Antimony (Sb)

With all the negative press about lead, in recent years, many lead applications were replaced with antimony, which is also toxic, but a little less so than lead, at least for most uses. It's much like replacing mercury in vaccines with aluminum.

Antimony is a naturally occurring, silvery-white, hard, brittle metal. It is also formed as a by-product of smelting lead and other metals. [1235] Today, antimony is known to be responsible for estrogenic effects. "Leaching of antimony from PET containers may lead to endocrine-disrupting effects." [1236] Shotyk et al (2006) found antimony in up to 30 times higher concentrations in mineral water from PET compared to glass bottles and confirmed its leaching from PET. [1237]

"Endocrine disruptors, other than phthalates, specifically antimony, may also contribute to the endocrine-disrupting effect of water from PET containers." [1238]

"The trend of increasing antimony concentration leaching into water from PET bottles with temperature and time is a cause of concern because of its role as an endocrine disruptor." [1239]

Further, antimony is widely used in military technology and electronics, batteries and glass. [1240]

Lead in plumbing and fixtures is being replaced by less toxic, but still toxic metals (antimony, bismuth etc.). The WHO says that the most common way antimony enters drinking water is from metal plumbing and fittings dissolving.

Treatment

"For treatment of antimony poisoning, the agent of choice would be DMPS."[1241]

In rats, the most effective antidotes to acute antimony poisoning were the water-soluble vicinal dithiols: DMSA and sodium DMPS. Appreciably less effective, but still useful, was D-penicillamine. [1242]

Other studies corroborate DMSA has been shown to excrete antimony from children. [1243]

8.5 Aluminum (Al)

"For many years, aluminum was not considered harmful to human health because of its relatively low bioavailability. In 1965, however, animal experiments suggested a possible connection between aluminum and Alzheimer's disease." [1244]

And in the early 1970s, aluminum toxicity was first implicated in the pathogenesis of clinical disorders in patients with chronic renal failure involving bone (renal osteomalacia) or brain tissue (dialysis encephalopathy).

"Over-the-counter antacids (used to treat heartburn) are the most important source for human aluminum exposure from a quantitative point of view." Aluminum can act as a powerful neurological toxicant and provoke embryonic and fetal toxic effects in animals and humans after gestational exposure. [1245]

From 1999 onwards, Thimerosal, a mercury-based preservative of 90% mercury in vaccines was being replaced with aluminum-based adjuvants. [1246]

Aluminum is a pervasive heavy metal used as a food additive, in metal cookware, beverage cans, antacids and antiperspirants. "Aluminum has been associated with declining performance in attention, memory, and learning, as well as a number of other health concerns." [1247]

Aluminum in the human body has a half-life of 27 years, as it is deposited in the bones. After a large aluminum exposure, aluminum can be reliably detected in the blood for about 12 hours, after that it is either already deposited in the tissue or already excreted. [1248]

In the healthy body, "The kidney quickly eliminates aluminum from food and environmental sources in humans. However, aluminum salts in vaccine adjuvants are biologically active and accumulate in the nervous system. " [1249]

Aluminum reproductive toxicity:
Male Wistar rats exposed to aluminum trichloride had lower levels of testosterone and luteinizing hormone. [1250]
"Aluminum oxide nanoparticles-induce spermatotoxicity, oxidative stress and changes in reproductive hormones and testes histopathology in male rats." Glutathione has a possible protective effect. [1251]

Treatment aluminum
"The common chelator used therapeutically has been **desferrioxamine**. This chelator has proven effective in eliminating aluminum from the body; however, there are a number of toxic side effects associated with its use. [1252]
Calcium EDTA removed aluminum and improved brain damage symptoms in 2 trials on over 200 people with aluminum poisoning. [1253]

"Treatment of patients affected by Al burden with ten EDTA chelation therapies (EDTA intravenous administration once a week) was able to significantly reduce Al intoxication." [1254]
"Patients affected by neurodegenerative diseases (ND) - showing Al intoxication - benefit from short-term treatment with calcium disodium EDTA chelation therapy." [1255]
DMSA was useful as a clinical chelator for cases of chronic and remote aluminum toxicity. [1256]
Male symptomatic patients, employed in the aluminum industry, suffered from sinus infections, chronic fatigue, motor and sensory losses, ataxia (i.e., the loss of full control of bodily movements), vertigo, memory loss and chronic pain. All had a positive clinical response to treatment with DMSA in the usual treatment regimen of 900 mg bid for 19 days. [1257]
"Treatment with gallic acid was able to ameliorate myocardial injury of male SD rats induced by aluminum oxide (Al_2O_3) nanoparticles." [1258]

See also aluminum and breast cancer in 5.9.3

8.6 Arsenic (As)

More than 200 million individuals worldwide are exposed to arsenic-contaminated drinking water above the WHO's permissible limit of 10 µg/L. [1259]

"Arsenic is the only primary carcinogen in the skin following ingestion or topical exposure." [1260]

"Arsenic is a cytotoxic element, and exposure to this metal presents serious risks to human health. Contact with arsenic generally results from ingesting contaminated food and water, occupational exposure and environmental pollution." [1261]

Arsenic has been in use by man for thousands of years. It is infamous as a favored form of intentional poisoning and famous for being the first drug to cure syphilis. Today, arsenic is used in semiconductor manufacture and pesticides.

"It serves as a wood preservative in chromated copper arsenate (CCA). CCA-treated lumber products were banned as of 2004. CCA-treated lumber is a potential risk of exposure of children to arsenic in play-structures." [1262]

8.6.1 Arsenic in Groundwater

According to the WHO, "the greatest threat to public health from arsenic originates from contaminated groundwater. Inorganic arsenic is naturally present at high levels in the groundwater of a number of countries, including Argentina, Bangladesh, Cambodia, Chile, China, India, Mexico, Pakistan, the United States of America and Viet Nam." There is an increasing number of effective and low-cost options for removing arsenic from small or household supplies. [1263]

"Reverse osmosis systems are the only types of water filters certified to remove arsenic from water." [1264]

As mentioned above, in a Bangladesh study, 57.5% of the population had skin lesions caused by arsenic poisoning. [1265]

"Sporadic outbreaks of peripheral vascular gangrene known as blackfoot disease have occurred in Taiwan due to high levels of arsenic in the drinking water." [1266]

"Many adverse health effects of chronic arsenic exposure are evident in Bangladesh including arsenicosis, various types of cancers, neurological disorders, cardiovascular diseases, diabetes, respiratory diseases, renal and reproductive diseases as well as multi-organ pathologies. "

"In Bangladesh, the agricultural practices also largely depend on groundwater. Some natural and anthropogenic sources are considered as responsible for arsenic contamination in groundwater."

Groundwater wells have to be continuously drilled deeper due to overuse. [1267] The anthropogenic activities in Bangladesh, like the lowering of water table below the organic deposits, accelerate the oxidation process in the natural aquafers. It is hypothesized that in this way, "the origin of arsenic rich groundwater is man-made, which is a recent phenomenon." [1268]

In summary, even though the arsenic in the ground itself is present naturally, the mass poisoning is accelerated by land overexploitation, overpopulation and industrialization.

Rice and apple juice have been recognized as two common sources of arsenic exposure. [1269]

The major mechanism of As-related damage is oxidative stress. [1270]

Therapy/ chelation

"Dimercaprol (British anti Lewisite or BAL), was previously the most frequently recommended chelating agent for acute arsenic poisoning." [1271] "DMPS and DMSA, which have a higher therapeutic index than BAL and do not redistribute arsenic or mercury to the brain, offer advantages in clinical practice." [1272]

"In comparison to EDTA, DMSA chelation by equimolar concentration is better at extracting **lead** and **arsenic.**" [1273]

"Studies show that supplementation of antioxidants along with a chelating agent BAL, DMSA or DMPS prove to be a better treatment regime." [1274]

Gallic acid and MiADMSA reversed arsenic-induced oxidative/nitrosative damage in rat red blood cells. [1275]

8.7 Barium (Ba)

"Barium is a stable divalent earth metal and highly toxic upon acute and chronic exposure. Barium is present in many products and involved in a number of industrial processes."

"Orally administered **sulfate salts** to form insoluble barium sulfate in the intestinal tract and **potassium** supplementation have potential benefit." [1276]

Barium sulfate is widely used for gastroenterology [X-ray] imaging. Occasionally, retention of barium is observed in the appendix, causing barium-associated appendicitis. [1277]

"Barium is one of the most common metals implicated in kidney toxicity." [1278]
And it is associated with anxiety in pregnancy (see 4.7.1).

Treatment
EDTA attracts barium and beryllium. [1279]
The oral administration of ALA noticeably increased the urinary excretion of barium. [1280]
Potassium infusion is used clinically to reverse the toxic effects of barium. [1281] Calcium de-corporates barium.

8.8 Beryllium (Be)

Be is vital in the automotive, nuclear, space, medical, defense sectors and other consumer industries. "However, beryllium is considered the most toxic non-radioactive element on the planet. It is also a class one carcinogen and the cause of chronic beryllium disease (CBD)." [1282] CBC can also damage other organs, such as the heart. "In about 20% of all cases people die of this disease." [1283]

In susceptible individuals, a few particles of beryllium inhaled into the lungs can cause chronic, fatal CBD. In Lorain, Ohio, in the 1940s, workers and residents in the area of a beryllium plant were affected, even wives of workers came down with CBD from washing their husbands' work clothing. [1284]
"Chronic beryllium disease is typically considered only when there is known work exposure; however, CBD has also occurred in occupational and environmental settings where exposure was unexpected." [1285]
Occupational exposures to **silicon** or **beryllium** may also lead to lymphadenopathy. [1286]
"Beryllium exposure may produce acute pneumonitis or chronic interstitial pneumonia which can be histologically indistinguishable from sarcoidosis, an inflammatory disease." [1287]
"Beryllium induces some carcinogenic mechanism. The use of beryllium in the dental industry creates additional occupational risk for exposure." [1288]
Workplace beryllium exposure is linked to susceptibility to alcoholism and suicide risk. [1289] (see also 4.14).

Treatment

"Three experimentally known beryllium chelators are EDTA, NTP, and 10-HBQS, the complexes of EDTA were calculated to have the highest average binding energy." [1290]

In rats, tiron was found to be significantly more effective than CaNa(2)EDTA in reducing the beryllium concentration in the liver, kidney and lungs. [1291]

D-Penicillamine can chelate beryllium. [1292]

"Different rat biochemical and distribution studies reveal that DPA (D-penicillamine) + selenium was the most effective therapeutic agent to remove beryllium followed by DMPS + Se and GSH." [1293]

8.9 Bismuth (Bi)

"The Safe Drinking Water Act Amendment of 1996, which required that all new and repaired fixtures and pipes for potable water supply be lead free after August 1998, opened a wider market for bismuth as a metallurgical additive to lead-free pipe fittings, fixtures, and water meters." [1294]

Bismuth chelates (for example with DTPA as a chelating agent) are used as contrast agents for X-ray computed tomography. [1295]

Bismuth levels can be measured with a hair or urine elements analysis and can be used to corroborate Bi absorption for a period of days or a few weeks after the exposure. [1296]

Challenge urine tests with DMSA can reveal chronic bismuth toxicity.

Treatment
DMSA substantially increased excretion of **tin** and **bismuth**. [1297]

A study by Slikkerveer et al concluded: The dithiol compounds (DMPS, DMSA and BAL) were effective in most organs (especially in kidney and liver), resulting in a higher elimination of bismuth in urine by DMPS and BAL. BAL was the only chelator effective in lowering brain bismuth concentrations, whereas treatment with EDTA resulted in increased brain bismuth levels. [1298]

Ohio State University confirms "dimercaprol (BAL) is the only chelator that can lower the levels of bismuth in brain tissue." [1299]

DMPS and DMSA markedly reduced Bi levels in liver and kidneys, and increased Bi in urine in animal studies. [1300]

"Chelation therapy with d-penicillamine may also be indicated." [1301]

8.10 Bromine (Br; non-metal, toxic element)

Chronic oral exposure to liquid bromine results in dermal effects, changes in conditioned reflexes and blood indexes. [1302]
Survivors of serious poisoning caused by inhaling (breathing in) bromine may have long-term lung problems. People who survive serious bromine poisoning may also have long-term effects from damage done by what is called systemic poisoning, for example, kidney or brain damage from low blood pressure. [1303]
Treatment unknown

8.11 Cadmium (Cd)

According to the UNEP, "Cadmium is used in batteries, paints, plastics and electroplating, among other applications. It is released to the atmospheric environment from metals production and fossil fuel combustion. Phosphorous fertilizers and sewage sludges are also a major source of environmental releases of cadmium." [1304]
"Cadmium is a toxic metal characterized by extensive persistence in the environment. In addition, modern civilization processes contribute to an increase of Cd in environmental circulation, leading to its rising occurrence in the food chains." [1305]
Long-term exposure to cadmium is known to cause kidney disease and has been linked to lung cancer. Studies have shown an increase in all-cause mortality and cancer mortality in populations exposed to low levels of cadmium for long periods of time. [1306]

Cadmium kidney damage
"Several reports have shown that kidney damage and/or bone effects are likely to occur at lower kidney cadmium levels than the WHO limits. European studies have shown signs of cadmium induced kidney damage in the general population at urinary cadmium levels around 2–3 µg Cd/g creatinine." [1307]
CdMTs are released from the liver, enterocytes, and lungs into the systematic circulation. Thus, cadmium is transported primarily to the kidneys, where it accumulates. [1308] The half-life of renal Cd is 7–16 years or longer. [1309]
"Cd-induced nephrotoxicity is clearly the most important and the most frequently occurring ailment in humans as a result of chronic exposure to the metal." [1310]

"The various toxic effects induced by cadmium and other heavy metals in biological systems might be due to alterations in the antioxidant defense system." [1311]

The divalent Cd2+ is the main toxic form of cadmium that induces oxidative stress. "Other important targets for Cd2+ are the testes and cardiovascular system." [1312]

Cadmium impairs the blood-brain barrier and reduces levels of brain copper-zinc (Cu–Zn) superoxide dismutase (SOD). [1313]

"Tobacco smoke is one of the most common sources of Cd exposure." [1314]

Cadmium prenatal effects

Cadmium exerts a large number of adverse effects on ecosystems and human and animal health. "This metal is embryotoxic, causing different kinds of malformations and lethality in mammals as well as amphibians. It has an extremely long biological half-life (about 30 years) in both humans and experimental animals." [1315]

Subchronic exposure to cadmium causes persistent changes in the reproductive system in female Wistar rats. "The uterus is exceedingly sensitive to Cd toxicity." [1316]

As we saw above "Prenatal exposure within 281 women have revealed that Cd2+ at means of 0.22 µg/L in umbilical cord blood increase the risk of emotional problems to 1.53-fold greater within descending boys at the age of 7– 8 years for every doubling of cord blood Cd2+ concentration." [1317]

8.11.1 Treatment cadmium

"EDTA is the agent most widely accepted for clinical use." [1318]

"In acute cadmium poisoning, EDTA significantly increased urinary elimination of cadmium."

As a chelation protocol for acute cadmium poisoning: a normal dose of EDTA has been proposed to be 500 mg of Ca2+ EDTA in combination with 50 mg/kg of glutathione (GSH) via IV infusion over the next 24 hours and repeated over 12 consecutive days. [1319]

High concentrations of EDTA were effective in chelation of both **aluminum** and **cadmium**. [1320]

"DMSA mobilized Cd more efficiently than CaDTPA. The combined therapy with the two chelators gave generally better results." [1321]

It has been found that N-acetyl cysteine (NAC) and DMPS reduced **cadmium**- induced hepatic and renal metallothionein in rats. Cysteine or N-acetyl cysteine administration has a limited benefit on the efficacy of DMPS in the treatment of **cadmium** intoxication. [1322]

"In animal studies, the administration of cysteine alone to intoxicated animals reduces the amount of **cadmium** deposition in the kidney by 40%. " [1323]

N-acetylcysteine (NAC) administration improved oxidative stress markers with a concomitant chelator, monoisoamyl 2,3-dimercaptosuccinate (MiADMSA). [1324]

8.12 Cerium (Ce)

Cerium is a Rare Earth Metal contained, for instance, in electronic appliances or E-cigarettes.
Cerium levels in toenails have been associated with an increased risk of acute myocardial infarction (See 1.11).
In acute poisoning of rats with 141Ce (radioactive cerium), Ca-DTPA was effective in reducing retention. [1325]

8.13 Cesium (Cs)

Naturally occurring cesium is not radioactive and is referred to as stable cesium.
Prussian blue is the standard chelator for radioactive and non-radioactive cesium (see Prussian blue 8.41.4.).

8.14 Cobalt (Co) essential, but toxic in overload

"The use of cobalt in dental devices as crowns, bridges and removable partial prosthesis have now raised concern as cobalt is classified as a CMR (Carcinogenic, Mutagenic, toxic to Reproduction) substance."
The battery of an electric vehicle requires 10kg of cobalt,
75% of the global supply is mined by hand in the Kongo.
For a 100 kg person, the Median Lethal Dose LD50 would be about 20 grams. [1326]
Cobalt, used in making jet engines, may cause nausea, vomiting, lack of appetite (anorexia), ear ringing (tinnitus), nerve damage, respiratory diseases, an unusually large thyroid gland (goiter), and/or heart and/or kidney damage. [1327]

Exposure to **cobalt** metal dust is most common in the fabrication of **tungsten** carbide. Bone has the highest concentration of cobalt among the examined tissues, 0.036 µg per gram of fresh tissue on average. [1328]

Treatment

Chronic cobalt poisoning has occurred from ceramic-metal articular prosthesis and has led to almost complete loss of sight and hearing.

Treatment options in cases with chronic cobalt poisoning include chelation therapy with EDTA or BAL/DMPS. [1329]

Symptoms were gradually resolved with DMPS-enhanced decorporation of Co. "EDTA has been shown to be the most effective chelator for cobaltism." [1330]

N-Acetyl-cysteine reduces blood chromium and cobalt levels in metal-on-metal hip arthroplasty.

Prussian Blue binds Co2+ (see Prussian blue 8.41.4.).

8.15 Copper (Cu) essential but toxic in overload

"Over the past 30 years, excess copper or copper toxicity has become so common that it has affected the physical and psychological functioning of large numbers of people, especially teen-age girls and women." [1331]

"As girls reach puberty, the increase in estrogen levels tends to exacerbate the effects of copper excess because estrogen raises the level of copper in the body's cells and tissues. When this occurs, there is likely to be an increased risk for behavior and emotional disorders: mood swings, depression and suicidal tendencies, anxiety and panic disorder, irritability and aggression, running away, promiscuity, and eating disorders." [1332]

Sudden (acute) copper poisoning is rare. However, serious health problems from long-term exposure to copper can occur. [1333]

"Copper can leach into the water supply when copper pipes corrode. One of copper's roles in the body is to help produce dopamine, the neurotransmitter that provides alertness. However, too much copper creates an excess of dopamine leading to an excess of the neurotransmitter norepinephrine. High levels of these neurotransmitters lead to symptoms similar to ADHD symptoms: hyperactivity, impulsivity, agitation, irritability, and aggressiveness." [1334]

Treatment

"Wilson's disease can be treated with high doses of zinc." [1335]

Copper chelating agents available in the United States include penicillamine, trientine and dimercaprol. [1336]

D-Penicillamine has been widely used in copper overload, although DMSA or tetrathiomolybdate may be more suitable alternatives today.

Oral DMSA significantly increased the urinary copper excretion.

In copper-toxicity, a free radical scavenger might be recommended as adjuvant to the chelator therapy. [1337]

Trientine is given to treat Wilson disease. [1338]

8.16 Chromium (Cr) essential, but toxic in overload

Cr is abundant in the earth's crust, and its toxicity depends on its chemical state. It exists in divalent to hexavalent compounds, but only the trivalent and hexavalent compounds have significant biological toxicity. [1339]

Cr VI (hexavalent) compounds can cause mild to severe liver abnormalities. "Some Cr(VI) compounds, such as potassium dichromate and chromium trioxide, are caustic and irritating to gastrointestinal mucosal tissue. Ingestion of a lethal dose of chromate can result in cardiovascular collapse." [1340]

"There is limited published data on appropriate reference ranges for the metals released from prosthesis, which raises questions regarding the clinical utility of the data." It has been emphasized that elevated serum Co and Cr levels in the absence of corroborating symptoms do not independently predict prosthesis failure. [1341]

Cr compounds are usually found in industrial purposes such as chromite ore mining, pigment production, tanning of leather, formation of wood preservatives, and anticorrosive agents in cooking goods. Paint is a significant source of hexavalent Cr but is still used for industrial applications. [1342]

"High levels of hexavalent Cr in the bloodstream cause blood cell damage by oxidation and functional degradation of the liver and kidney." [1343]

Cr and Cr compounds mainly induce apoptosis, oxidative stress and DNA damage, diseases including lung cancer, skin allergy with dermatitis, and kidney diseases. [1344]

Treatment

In rat studies, combined chelation therapy results show that deferasirox and deferiprone are able to remove chromium (VI) ions from various tissues while iron concentration returned to normal levels and symptoms also decreased. [1345]

N-acetylcysteine proved to be an effective agent at increasing the excretion of chromium and boron and was also able to reverse the oliguria associated with these toxins in rats. [1346]

It has also been found that N- acetylcysteine (NAC) in combination with ascorbic acid show additive effects in reducing the chromium toxicity. [1347]

8.17 Gallium (Ga)

Breathing gallium can irritate the nose and throat causing coughing and wheezing. "Gallium and gallium compounds may damage the liver and kidneys, may cause metallic taste, dermatitis and depression of the bone marrow function." [1348]

Therapy

In rats, concentrations of gallium and arsenic in the brain tissue significantly decreased after chelating therapy with Desferrioxamine (DFO), Deferiprone (L1) and Deferasirox (Ex).
"The chelators are able to compensate learning and memory impairments. " [1349]

"After a single IP injection of gallium nitrate in mice the most effective chelating agents were: oxalic acid, malic acid, succinic acid and deferoxamine mesylate, in this order." [1350]

8.18 Gadolinium (Gd)

"Several MRI contrast agent clinical formulations are now known to leave deposits of the heavy metal gadolinium in the brain, bones, and other organs of patients." This persistent biological accumulation of gadolinium prompted the European Medicines Agency to recommend discontinuing the use of over half of the Gadolinium Based Contrast Agents (GBCAs) currently approved for clinical applications. [1351]

GBCAs have been widely used in diagnostic magnetic resonance imaging (MRI) for almost 3 decades and are pivotal for the diagnosis and monitoring of diseases. "In its injectable form the metal gets attached to chelating molecules to block its dangerous effects. In some cases, Ga in MRI is causing severe heavy metal poisoning." As a metal of the lanthanide series, Ga (a rare earth metal) is between Ba and Lu in the periodic table. [1352]

"The official recommendation is to use gadolinium-containing contrast media only in unavoidable examinations for now, also because acute to chronic kidney diseases have now been associated with gadolinium-containing contrast media. " [1353]

"In recent years, hyperintensity on unenhanced MRI scans and gadolinium (Gd) presence in some brain areas has been observed in patients with normal renal function after multiple contrast-enhanced MRI procedures." [1354]

"There is a high risk of nephrogenic systemic fibrosis in patients with chronic kidney disease at stage 5 due to exposure to gadodiamide during MRI." [1355]

"There is an increasing body of evidence from retrospective clinical and preclinical animal studies that MRI hyperintensity in the brain is primarily associated with repeated injections of linear GBCAs." [1356] Which means: some patients may not be so much hypersensitive to the magnetic fields of the machine, but rather to the accumulating toxic gadolinium. Some patients (even with normal renal function) have been severely injured by one single dose of GBCA. [1357]

"In 2010, the Food and Drug Administration issued a black box warning for all GBCM with the recommendation of kidney function screening before GBCM administration to identify patients with AKI or stage 4 or 5 CKD. [1358]

The Mayo Clinic says: "The type of gadolinium used in older contrast agents isn't safe for people with moderate or advanced chronic kidney disease. Older versions of contrast agents that contain gadolinium increase the risk of a rare but serious disease called nephrogenic systemic fibrosis."

"In patients with kidney impairment, conditions such as low clearance of the Gd-carrier complex, acid-base derangements, and high serum phosphorous can increase the presence of free Gd^{3+}, leading to a higher risk for toxicity." [1359]

Mechanism of action

Gadolinium has a high affinity for phosphate, citrate, and carbonate ions and will bind to proteins like serum albumin. [1360]

"Varying amounts [of GBCA] deposit in tissues of the brain, cardiac muscle, kidney, other organs and the skin, mainly depending on kidney function, structure of the chelates (linear or macrocyclic) and the dose administered." [1361]

"Gd3+, sitting exactly in the center of the lanthanide series, has an ionic radius of [0.094 nm]" [1362], very nearly equal to that of divalent Ca2+ [0.099 nm]. This is one of the reasons why Gd3+ is so toxic in biological systems - Gd3+ can compete with Ca2+ in all biological systems that require Ca2+ for proper function and, in doing so, the trivalent ion binds with much higher affinity. [1363]

"In the great majority of its compounds, like many rare-earth metals, gadolinium adopts the oxidation state +3. However, gadolinium can be found on rare occasions in the 0, +1 and +2 oxidation states." [1364]

Other rare earth metals are present in GBCAs. **Sc, Y, La, Ce, Pr, Nd, Eu, Tb, Tm, Dy, Ho,** and **Er** were present in all of 22 samples analyzed. "Terbium, Thulium, Europium, and Lanthanum were, on average, found in the highest amounts." [1365]

"Gadolinium-based contrast agents are not inherently radioactive" [1366]

Gadolinium has been deposited in the brain and bones and the diseases associated with gadolinium retention includes Nephrogenic Systemic Fibrosis (NSF). [1367]

Treatment gadolinium

DTPA is one of the chelators used in gadolinium-based contrast agents (GBCAs) for the initial use as a contrast agent. If the bond fails and Gd is retained in the patient, the same chelator is used in chelation therapy to attempt to remove the Gd from the body subsequently. (See DTPA, 11.10.). But that is only in the rare cases where gadolinium poisoning is recognized when MRI patients fall ill immediately after an MRI. In most cases where people become chronically ill gradually beginning weeks or months after the MRI, Gadolinium poisoning will not be suspected or tested for, and the affected persons, if they suffer from diverse degenerative illnesses, will never even hear the word Gadolinium.

"Patients with Gadolinium Deposition Disease following an MRI in which a gadolinium-containing contrast agent was utilized, were treated with DTPA. "They mostly experienced benefit after three paired Calcium-DTPA/Zinc-DTPA chelation treatments." [1368]

Routine practice involves an IV injection of 1g of DTPA for the first dose.

DTPA is approved as safe and effective by the federal Food and Drug Administration for the removal of certain radioactive heavy metals, has been in use for more than 60 years, is well tolerated, and has been safely used in three studies. [1369]

"Effects of DTPA are mediated exclusively by zinc deficiency; zinc supplementation negates developmental (and other) toxicity."

"DTPA does not possess intrinsic developmental toxic properties."

In regards to potential chelating agents, Rees et al 2018 found that the oral metal de-corporation agent 3,4,3-LI(1,2-HOPO) demonstrates superior efficacy at chelating and removing Gd from the body compared to DTPA. [1370] 1,2-HOPO is not yet available.

Subject for future studies: does Prussian blue assist the chelation of gadolinium?

There is some evidence suggesting that Prussian blue can chelate some of the GDd3+ ions.

The structure of gadolinium hexacyanoferrate Prussian blue analogue Gd[Fe(CN)6] · 4H2O was investigated.

The compound was prepared "by mixing the saturated aqueous solution of K3[Fe(CN)6] (soluble Prussian blue) with aqueous solution of Gd3+." The resulting precipitate was filtered, washed with water and ethanol and dried above KOH. [1371]

Now, as K3[Fe(CN)6] + Gd3+ (aqua) readily turns into Gd[Fe(CN)6] · 4H2O; or Prussian Blue releases K+ and exchanges it with Gd3+ in aqueous solution; can Prussian Blue also chelate Gd3+ from the body? Clinical studies are indicated.

8.19 Germanium

"Spirogermanium and propagermanium are examples of organic forms of germanium, that can build up in the body and cause serious side effects including kidney failure, multi-organ dysfunction, lung toxicity, and nerve damage." Inorganic (elemental) germanium is *Likely Unsafe*. [1372]

Seegarten Klinik, Switzerland uses EDTA for germanium chelation.

8.20 Gold (Au)

The signs and symptoms of gold toxicity may include: Inflammation of skin or dermatitis, kidney damage, damage to the platelet function causing thrombocytopenia purpura.

"Gold causes genetically determined autoimmune and immunostimulatory responses in mice." [1373]

Dental galvanism can be caused by "an amalgam restoration (mercury/silver) opposed or adjacent to a gold crown. These dissimilar metals, in conjunction with saliva, create an electric cell." This circuit can be shorted by contact or through the tissue, causing pain and accelerated erosion of the cathode (for instance mercury). "RCS (Ni–Cr) alloy was found to be highly susceptible to galvanic corrosion." [1374]

treatment

BAL is used principally to treat arsenic, **gold** and mercury poisoning. [1375]

"DMPS and bucillamine are very useful antidotes for gold toxicity." [1376] D-penicillamine and DMSA were used to chelate gold in rats. [1377]

8.21 Iron (Fe) essential, but toxic in overload

"A high content of tissue iron has been associated with several pathological conditions, including liver and heart diseases, cancer, neurodegenerative disorders, diabetes and immunological disorders." [1378]

"In rat studies, high iron-diet consumption caused brain iron accumulation, brain mitochondrial dysfunction, impaired brain synaptic plasticity and cognition, blood-brain-barrier breakdown, and brain apoptosis." Although both the iron chelator deferiprone (50 mg/kg) and n-acetyl cysteine (100 mg/kg) attenuated these deleterious effects, combined therapy provided more robust results.. [1379]

Hepatic fibrosis and cirrhosis are the major outcomes of chronic iron overload as well as to repeated blood transfusion. [1380]

Al increases expression of divalent metal transporter 1(DMT1), **causing Fe accumulation** and alteration of Fe homeostasis in the rat hippocampus. [1381]

As we have seen, "obsessive compulsive disorder patients have lower T2 values (suggesting higher iron content) in the globus pallidus (GP)." [1382]

Although extremely elevated ferritin levels may be associated with rheumatologic diseases, more often they are found in patients with other conditions such as malignancy or infection. In addition, extremely high ferritin levels can be found in patients with seemingly indolent disease or levels of chronic inflammation. [1383]

Treatment

"EDTA removes iron, but it is not specific to iron." [1384]

In the EDTA binding affinity table, it can be seen that EDTA binds Fe^{3+} more strongly than Pb^{2+}, Hg^{2+}, Co^{2+} or Cd^{2+}. [1385] see Fig. 6.)

It is this Fe^{3+} oxidation state that is mostly implicated in oxidative stress and chronic iron overload more so than Fe^{2+}.

For patients with different chronic illnesses, after 30 treatments with IV EDTA (3 gram per treatments) those with initial iron overload decreased their iron by 43%, while patients with initial low iron increased their iron content by 41%. [1386]

In this way, both patient groups improved in the direction of iron homeostasis.

"The important problems related to chronic Fe-overload observed in thalassemia (hemolytic diseases caused by faulty hemoglobin synthesis) patients can be overcome using chelating agents such as deferiprone, deferasirox, and deferoxamine." Deferiprone is used in oral treatment. [1387]

In 2005, deferasirox (DFX) became the first FDA-approved oral treatment for iron overload, and it was subsequently approved in the EU in 2006. [1388]

Deferasirox is also used in patients with non-transfusion-dependent thalassemia syndromes, and in patients with elevated liver iron concentration and serum ferritin. [1389]

Gallic acid has a chelating effect in cases of iron overload. [1390]

8.22 Lanthanum (La)

See Rare Earth Elements 1.11

8.23 Lead (Pb)

8.23.1 Epidemiological effects

A study by scientists of the University of Wales concluded in 2004: **"One out of a hundred** cases of disease worldwide, including AIDS, tuberculosis, cancer, allergies and all other diseases are **caused by environmental lead intoxication."**
"According to their assessments, the global environmental pollution with lead also has a significant responsibility in the defects in mental development and blood pressure related heart disease." [1391]
Recall a 2018 study published in The Lancet Public Health found that of the 2.3 million deaths every year in the US, about 412,000 **(or 18%)** are attributable to **lead** exposure, of which 250,000 are from cardiovascular disease. [1392]

According to the WHO, mild mental retardation and cardiovascular outcomes resulting from **exposure to lead amount to almost 1% of the global burden of disease**, with the highest burden in developing regions. [1393]
"There's no such thing as 'safe' or 'acceptable' lead levels," said Dr. Eswar Krishnan, of Stanford University School of Medicine in Palo Alto, California. [1394]
Recall that's also what the CDC says: "There is no safe amount of lead in the blood."
The CDC also defined a reference level of clinical concern at 3,5 mcg of lead per dL of blood. So, the CDC's or any other reference level is not safe by their own definition.
"To set a health goal value based on the loss of one IQ point, the EDA added a safety factor of three and assumed that water accounted for 20 percent of total lead exposures for a child." [1395]
Just before the release of the 2022 study, the CDC revised their level of concern (reference value) from >5.0 µg/dL to >3.5 µg/dL on May 14, 2021. Based on these values, 16% of US children, every third child globally, and every second adult in the USA are poisoned with Pb. [1396]

8.23.2 Leaded gasoline

From the 1930s to the 1990s (and still today in developing countries) the main exposure for the public to **lead** was from car exhausts, concentrating between the 1960s and the 1990s.

For most of the mid-twentieth century, lead gasoline was considered normal.

From 1923 onward, the lead additive solved a problem: it enabled engines to use higher compression ratios, which made cars more powerful and it decreased knocking of the engine. Engine knocking means combustion is triggered spontaneously by fuel compression, before the spark plug activation. This caused rotation irregularities as the pressure on the piston is at times applied in the reverse direction.

The first car that was non-hand-cranked (the Cadillac model 30 of 1911 with an electric starter) had higher compression ratios, prone to the said premature combustion and loud knocking.

Thomas Midgley, Jr. (1889 - 1944), an American chemist, developed the tetraethyl lead (TEL).

"On December 9, 1921, Midgley added the TEL to the fuel and started the one-cylinder test engine, the engine knock was gone. GM and Standard Oil of New Jersey (forerunner of Exxon) formed the Ethyl Corporation shortly thereafter in 1923 to produce TEL. The company's name was carefully chosen to avoid the use of the word "lead," but safeguards at the factory weren't as effective. Not long after it opened, workers at the Ethyl plant began suffering from lead poisoning. Two workers died from exposure to what the press called "loony gas." Midgley himself suffered from lead poisoning and took a vacation to "get a large supply of fresh air." "Ironically, Midgley would later develop freon, a refrigerant that cooled indoor air for nearly half a century." [1397]

This gas was later declared to have caused the ozone hole, which prompted journalists to call Midgley 'the men who killed more people than anyone else."

Researchers today are still puzzled why the petrol companies push tetraethyl lead instead of the much less toxic ethyl alcohol, which had much the same effect on the engines. I used to be puzzled myself until I came to realize the human inclination for stupidity and corruption. In a tragic irony, part of the stupidity that led to accepting this mass lead poisoning is due to the mass poisoning itself.

"Research has shown that lead exposure in children is linked to "a whole raft of complications later in life, among them lower IQ, hyperactivity, behavioral problems and learning disabilities." A significant body of research links lead exposure in children to violent crime. [1398]

The leaded gasoline catastrophe is even connected to prohibition in the US between 1920 and 1933. It turns out, the institutions who lobbied for the banning of alcohol were not really interested in reducing alcoholism.

"In 1906, the Free Alcohol bill was passed. The USA repeals the alcohol tax under Teddy Roosevelt. At 14 cents per US gallon, corn ethanol was cheaper than gasoline at 22 cents per US gallon. Bills pass that exempt farm stills from government control."

"In 1908, the Ford Model T is introduced. Early models had adjustable carburetors to run on ethanol with gasoline as an option."

"By the mid-1920s, ethyl alcohol would be blended with gasoline in every industrialized nation, and some blends are showing up as experiments in the United States, but the market was dominated by leaded gasoline." [1399]

In 1919, a few years before the launch of leaded gasoline, congress passed the 18th amendment for the prohibition of alcohol. At the time, most cars still ran on alcohol (ethanol from corn, potatoes, etc. and even seaweed).

Prohibition was initially used as one of the rationales to force tetra lead ethyl exposure and petrol gasoline onto everyone: The only alternative to prevent knocking of the emerging gasoline engines at the time was supposedly to add 20% ethanol, so alcohol, and due to prohibition, they couldn't use that, because some drunks would drink it before they could mix it into the gasoline. So, the entire industry was forced to change to mineral oil and toxic lead.

"Tetramethyl lead and tetraethyl lead as in leaded gasoline penetrate the skin easily."

These compounds may also cross the blood–brain barrier in adults, and thus adults may suffer from lead encephalopathy related to acute poisoning by organic lead compounds. [1400]

According to the EPA, the concentration was reduced to 1.7 gram of lead per gallon of gasoline in 1975. [1401]

In the US alone, vehicles using leaded gasoline deposited an estimated 4-5 million tons of lead in the environment across the country before the phase-out in the 1990s. [1402]

Total world lead production had been rising till the 1980s, when it reached over 3.8 million tons per year. [1403]

And thus, everyone (100%) of people in the US born between 1966 and 1975 had childhood levels of lead above the CDC safe levels.

From 1951- 1980, on average, 95,5% of all children had blood lead levels of clinical concern. This means, loosely speaking, most born

over these 3 decades are now less intelligent and physically and emotionally weaker than they should have been.
The estimated average reduction in intelligence was 6 IQ points. [1404]

While half of the US population living today was exposed to adverse lead levels in early childhood, last year the CDC level of concern was further lowered from 5 mcg/dL to 3,5 mcg /dL, which means things are even worse in this context, as more people alive today had childhood levels over the safe levels.

Table 2. US population estimates of BLLs above the current Centers for Disease Control and Prevention level of concern (>5 µg/dL) in early life by age in 2015

Birth cohort	Age in 2015	Population estimates > 5 µg/dL*	Percentage of population > 5 µg/dL*	Margin of error (80% confidence)	Total population
2011–2015	0–4	287,292	1.4	67,586	19,895,276
2006–2010	5–9	588,995	2.9	93,538	20,495,848
2001–2005	10–14	1,275,797	6.2	122,263	20,634,930
1996–2000	15–19	2,752,836	13.1	266,359	21,066,962
1991–1995	20–24	5,415,971	23.8	298,058	22,771,013
1986–1990	25–29	8,216,431	37.0	289,680	22,180,549
1981–1985	30–34	15,639,814	72.5	246,715	21,563,585
1976–1980	35–39	19,886,968	99.0	100,549	20,088,551
1971–1975	40–44	20,330,987	100.0	755,208	20,330,987
1966–1970	45–49	20,792,166	100.0	775,766	20,792,166
1961–1965	50–54	21,733,732	97.1	403,448	22,380,634
1956–1960	55–59	20,242,589	93.7	341,126	21,595,615
1951–1955	60–64	16,813,082	89.6	301,423	18,769,228
1946–1950	65–69	9,834,514	62.8	225,690	15,663,276
1940–1945	70–74	6,653,362	50.9	152,093	13,061,780

*The total population in 2015 was 318,479,402.
Estimates of early life BLLs by birth cohort. Exposure to elevated BLLs follows a "U"-shaped association with relatively low BLLs for cohorts born in the 1940s, increased dramatically for cohorts now middle aged, and decreased dramatically among younger cohorts.

Fig. 5 McFarland M. J. et al 2022: Half of US population exposed to adverse lead levels in early childhood; PROCEEDINGS OF THE NATIONAL ACADEMY OF SCIENCES; Vol. 119 | No. 11; March 15, 2022; PubMed: 35254913;; https://doi.org/10.1073/pnas.2118631119

Lead safety standards

In 2009, the California Office of Health Hazard Assessment set a public health goal for lead in drinking water to prevent IQ loss in children. The Environmental Working Group assumes that water accounted for 20 percent of total lead exposures for a child. [1405]
In 1976, Herbert Needleman, a psychiatrist at Harvard Medical School, suspected even trace amounts of lead ravaged children's brains. His study revealed that lead profoundly transformed children's brains, even at levels far below those considered dangerous. [1406]
A study in the coastal region of Semarang, Indonesia concluded that **"all school children** (8- 12 years old) had high blood lead levels (above the WHO cut off) and low zinc serum." Approximately 26.4% of children were anemic. [1407]

8.23.3 Mechanism of lead toxicity

"Blood lead is immediately available and relatively short-lived over a period of months. Once an individual is removed from current lead exposures, stored bone lead supplies lead into circulation, years for patella bone, and decades for tibia bone." [1408]

"Once absorbed, Pb is transported by the bloodstream mainly bound to erythrocytes and distributed to other tissues such as liver, kidneys, brain, lungs, spleen, teeth, and bones. More than 95% of Pb is deposited in skeletal bones, while in children, this percentage is lower, resulting in more Pb in soft tissues." [1409]

Unlike various other toxic metals, lead is able to substitute to calcium Ca2+ in many fundamental cellular signaling molecules. [1410]

Symptoms of elevated blood lead levels

"There are no pathognomonic signs of **lead** poisoning but the following may be seen:

A blue discoloration of gum margins - Mild anaemia. - Behavioral abnormalities (more marked in children) - irritability, restlessness, sleeplessness. Cognitive dysfunction. Impaired fine-motor coordination or subtle visual-spatial impairment. Chronic distal motor neuropathy with decreased reflexes and weakness of extensor muscles in adults." [1411]

In utero lead poisoning

"There is a strong correlation between maternal and umbilical cord blood lead levels, a fact which explains the transfer of **lead** from mother to fetus." [1412]

8.23.4 Lead and nutritional deficiencies

Already in 1979 it was established that **lead** toxicity was associated with nutritional deficiencies.

"Mineral deficiency has profound effects on lead toxicity, as the consequences of plumbism can be exaggerated by feeding diets low in calcium, phosphorus, iron, zinc, and, in some cases, copper." [1413]

Occupational lead exposure decreases selenium levels

In lead workers, blood levels of lead and zinc protoporphyrin (both are markers of lead exposure) were significantly elevated, while selenium levels were significantly decreased, compared to control groups. One of the major targets for lead toxicity is the thiol group of enzymes.

"The inhibition of ferrochelatase and ALAD by lead decreases heme synthesis which leads to anemia." [1414]

Children's underlying nutritional deficiencies, particularly iron deficiency, are associated with elevated BLLs. Lead **competes for absorption in the gut with several divalent metals**.

"These various divalent metal cations, such as magnesium ions ($Mg2+$), zinc ions ($Zn2+$), and copper ions ($Cu2+$), play vital roles in bone growth, modeling, and remodeling." [1415]

"Divalent metals play important roles in maintaining metabolism and cellular growth of both eukaryotic hosts and invading microbes. Both metal deficiency and overload can result in abnormal cellular function or damage." [1416]

In children, high blood lead levels are associated with low serum iron and ferritin. [1417]

"A longitudinal study of iron status at 2 clinic visits separated by approximately 1 **year suggests that iron deficiency increases lead absorption in children.**" Children without anemia who had depleted iron stores (low serum ferritin), experienced a decrease in BLLs following iron supplementation. [1418]

Further, animal studies documented increased gastrointestinal lead absorption in the presence of iron deficiency. [1419]

A 2005 study concludes Beethoven died from lead poisoning.

"The work, done at the Energy Department's Argonne National Laboratory outside of Chicago, confirms earlier hints that lead may have caused Beethoven's decades of poor health, which culminated in a long and painful death in 1827 at age 56." [1420]

Analyses of Beethoven's hair indicate an average lead exposure of 100 times the normal value. [1421]

It was suggested the lead came from wine sweetened with lead acetate. [1422]

"When Pope Clement II died in 1047, no one was exactly sure what killed him, but a 1959 examination of his remains clearly indicated lead poisoning." [1423]

8.23.5 Treatment for lead toxicity

The main treatment for chronic and acute **lead** toxicity is chelation therapy with DMSA, DMPS and EDTA.

"The accumulated data indicate that in **lead**-exposed workers, Fe, Zn, Se and Cu may reduce lead toxicity." [1424]

Gallic acid decreases oxidative stress in lead intoxicated rats.

8.24 Mercury (Hg)

"Tissue mercury levels in humans have increased during the past 50 years to an alarming concentration." [1425]

The EPA has determined the safe daily intake of mercury to be <0.1 µg/kg/d. [1426]

For a 60 kg person, that is 6 microgram (µg) per day.

However, it is estimated that one dental amalgam filling already releases about 3 µg to 17 µg of mercury vapor per day. The typical amalgam is composed of 50% **mercury**, 25% **silver**, and 25% **tin, copper,** and **nickel**. [1427]

So, one dental amalgam releases more than the EPA daily safe limit. Also, the EPA says dental amalgam are no health concern.

"Mercury accumulates during life so that the average 165-lb person has a total body burden of about 13 milligram (13,000 microgram) of mercury." [1428]

8.24.1 Sources of mercury pollution

The Environmental defense fund says "Mercury pollution from coal-fired power plants is extremely dangerous - it causes brain damage in babies and is associated with heart disease and many other serious health issues." [1429]

According to Harvard School of Public Health, coal-fired power plants continue to be the largest source of **mercury** pollution in the United States, accounting for approximately 8,800 pounds of mercury emissions in 2017 alone.

On the positive side, great progress has been made in recent years in reducing mercury emissions from power plants.

"There was a 90% reduction in mercury emissions from U.S. power plants between 2008 (26.8 Mg) and 2020 (2.8 Mg) totaling 24 Mg." [1430]

That's good news, but on the negative side, the mercury that has been dispersed in the soil, ground water and the food chain virtually lasts forever, and in the human body, mercury has a half-life of 30 years.

Other important sources of Hg exposure are the use of Hg in measuring instruments and as a disinfectant. Regulatory measures during the last decades have reduced the Hg emissions to the environment significantly. [1431]

Contact lens solutions often contain Thimerosal which is 90 % mercury by weight. Thimerosal used to be a main ingredient of vaccines. [1432]

227

in July 1999, the Public Health Service agencies, the American Academy of Pediatrics, and vaccine manufacturers agreed that thimerosal should be reduced or eliminated in vaccines as a precautionary measure. [1433]

Unfortunately, Thimerosal was replaced with aluminum compounds in most vaccines.

In Germany up to 0.007 % of thiomersal is allowed in cosmetic products (eye make-up and eye make-up remover [Directive 76/768/EE]). That's 0.07 grams per liter. [1434]

8.24.2 Minamata mass poisoning disaster

In Japan in Minamata Bay, in 1932, a chemical fertilizer factory, the Chisso factory, moved to Minamata, a quiet bay populated by a fishing community. The fishermen did not know anything about the plant's activities and did not know that its toxic poisons were going into their nets. Over the years, they witnessed a strange phenomenon. Cats that fed on the remains of human foods started displaying abnormal behaviors. Some even threw themselves into the sea. Then, in the 1950s, strange diseases also began to appear in the fishing families. Convulsions, tremors, involuntary movements, eye and hearing disorders, staggering gait, fatigue, etc. Mothers gave birth to children with severe disabilities. [1435] As of March 2001, 2,265 victims had been officially recognized as having Minamata disease and over 10,000 had received financial compensation from Chisso. More than 900 people died and 2 million suffered health problems from eating fish contaminated with mercury. [1436] Between 1932 and 1968, Chisso Corporation dumped an estimated 27 tons of mercury into Minamata bay.

8.24.3 Mercury health effects

"Mercury has a high affinity for sulfhydryl groups, inactivating numerous enzymatic reactions, amino acids, and sulfur-containing antioxidants (N-acetyl-L-cysteine, alpha-lipoic acid, L-glutathione), with subsequent decreased oxidant defense and increased oxidative stress. Mercury binds to metallothionein and substitute for zinc, copper, and other trace metals, reducing the effectiveness of metalloenzymes." [1437]

Adverse health effects from mercury exposure can be: tremors, impaired vision and hearing, paralysis, insomnia, emotional instability, developmental deficits during fetal development and attention deficit and developmental delays during childhood.

"Recent studies suggest that mercury may have **no threshold below which some adverse effects do not occur.**" [1438]
The overall vascular effects of mercury include increased oxidative stress and inflammation, reduced oxidative defense, thrombosis, vascular smooth muscle dysfunction, endothelial dysfunction, dyslipidemia, and immune and mitochondrial dysfunction. **Selenium and fish containing omega-3 fatty acids antagonize mercury.** [1439]
But inversely, mercury itself "diminishes the protective effect of fish and omega-3 fatty acids." [1440]
Geier et al (2013) found a statistically significant dose-dependent correlation between cumulative exposure to **dental amalgam** and urinary levels of an isozyme of glutathione-S-transferase (GST-α), which is considered a biomarker of **kidney damage.** [1441]

Antibiotics reduce excretion of mercury.
"High oral antibiotic usage is concerning because previous rat studies found that **oral antibiotics resulted in a near-total loss of the ability to excrete mercury.** " [1442]
In addition, there is a link between heavy metal contamination and increased **antibiotic resistance** (AR) in environmental bacteria.
The Almadén mining district (Ciudad Real, central Spain) is one of the environments with the highest **mercury** contamination worldwide. In this region, a total of 72% of soil Bacillus spp. showed resistance to two or more commonly used antibiotics. [1443]
Research has also shown that Hg vapor passes the placenta and is taken up by the fetus. The inorganic Hg concentrations in the placenta and umbilical cord have been found to correlate with the mother's number of amalgam fillings. [1444]
As we've already explored, dental personnel have a higher Hg body burden than unexposed individuals.

8.24.4 Neurological changes mercury

We have illustrated the negative psychological effects of chronic mercury poisoning which can manifest as erethism or "mad hatter syndrome" in 4.10.)
The brain and the kidneys are considered critical organs for Hg exposure. Other tissue targets include the retina, thyroid, heart, lungs, and liver. [1445]

Mercury as an endocrine disruptor
Mercury is well established as an endocrine disrupter (see 2.4.9).

229

As noted above, acute mercury exposure may give rise to lung damage. Chronic poisoning is characterized by neurological and psychological symptoms, such as tremor, changes in personality, restlessness, anxiety, sleep disturbance and depression. [1446]

Mercury, diverse cardiovascular diseases
"The clinical consequences of many pathophysiologic mechanisms explain the wide variety of cardiovascular diseases caused by mercury including CHD, MI, arrhythmias, abnormal heart rate variability, generalized atherosclerosis, sudden death, CVA, carotid artery stenosis, renal dysfunction, and hypertension." [1447]

8.24.5 Treatment mercury

Much like lead, "mercury does not last more than 48 hours in the blood and therefore in the urine." [1448]
"Clinical chelation therapy of mercury poisoning generally uses one or both of two drugs – DMSA and DMPS. " [1449]
In rats with acute mercury poisoning, treatment with DMPS significantly reduces kidney mercury and sharply increases urinary mercury excretion, at a higher capacity than BAL, APA, and CaEDTA. [1450]
"The methylmercury antidotes N-acetylcysteine and DMPS enhance urinary metal excretion and transport by the renal organic anion transporter." [1451]
796 patients suffering from a multitude of symptoms associated with metal exposure from dental amalgam and other metal alloys received a supportive antioxidant therapy plus removal of amalgam fillings. The researchers reported alleviation of symptoms and improvements in the quality of life in 70% of the patients. [1452]

8.25 Manganese (Mn) essential, but toxic in overload

Mn is necessary as a cofactor for many enzymes. "Humans obtain a sufficient amount of Mn through the diet and Mn deficiency is essentially unknown outside of the laboratory." [1453]
"Chronic manganism intoxication induces symptoms resembling Parkinson disease." [1454]
From the NIH we learn:
Some people have developed manganese toxicity by consuming water containing very high levels of manganese. Another cause of

manganese toxicity is inhaling large amounts of manganese dust from welding or mining work or battery manufacture. [1455]
The symptoms of manganese toxicity include tremors, muscle spasms, hearing problems, mania, insomnia, depression, loss of appetite, headaches, irritability, weakness, and mood changes, [1456] aggressiveness, and hallucinations. [1457] Manganism is further characterized by rigidity, a mask-like expression and gait disturbances. [1458]

Treatment
Current treatment of manganism is EDTA chelation; however, this treatment alone has shown limited efficacy. [1459]
Recent experiments have indicated that p-amino salicylate or para-Aminosalicylic Acid (PAS) plus CaEDTA may be a useful combination to remove Mn from binding sites in the CNS. [1460]
Additional data suggest that PAS likely acts as a chelating agent to mobilize and remove tissue Mn. [1461]

8.26 Molybdenum (Mo) essential, but toxic in overload

Molybdenum toxicity is very rare and is usually caused by occupational or environmental exposure.
"People exposed to high levels of molybdenum in the air and soil, such as miners and metalworkers, sometimes develop achy joints, gout-like symptoms, and high blood levels of uric acid. [1462]

Treatment
EDTA [in suppository form] has caused significant mobilization and secretion of cations (cadmium, copper, boron, lead, **molybdenum**, magnesium, and calcium). [1463]

8.27 Nickel (Ni) essential, but toxic in overload

"Ni has been added to the list of essential trace elements quite recently; however, by now, there exists a substantial list of Ni-required enzymes. It was considered as an essential element based on reports of Ni necessity for plants and deficiency in some animal species; however, the functional importance of Ni and its physiological relevance in humans yet remain unclear, and deficiency was never reported either." [1464]

The US Institute of Medicine has not confirmed that nickel is an essential nutrient for humans, so neither a Recommended Dietary Allowance (RDA) nor an Adequate Intake have been established. [1465]

In 1984, M. Anke found: nickel is necessary for the biosynthesis of the hydrogenase and carbon monoxide dehydrogenase. [1466]

"Nickel is used in most silver-colored cast metals for crowns, usually partially covered by porcelain. [1467]

In overload, dental nickel alloys can adversely affect the quantity of T-lymphocytes. [1468]

Skin contact with Ni compounds through contaminated water, air, and children's toys result in dermatitis and allergy. [1469]

Breathing in nickel-contaminated dust from nickel smelting, mining and tobacco smoking leads to significant damage to lungs and nasal cavities, resulting in occupational diseases such as lung cancer and nasal cancer in Ni refinery workers. [1470]

Kim et al 2015 discovered that various toxicity in lung, nose, skin, kidney and liver were induced by Ni. [1471]

Acute ingestion of nickel compounds may cause nausea, vomiting, diarrhea, headache, cough and shortness of breath. In severe cases, ingestion of large amounts of a nickel compound may cause death. [1472]

Treatment of nickel overload

"In animal models, zinc has shown some preemptive protective mechanisms against Ni toxicity." [1473]

The nickel -specific chelator dimethylglyoxime (DMG) has been used for many years to detect, quantitate or decrease Ni levels in various environments. "Nickel chelation therapy with DMG was applied as an approach to combat multi-drug resistant enteric pathogens."

In mice, oral delivery of nontoxic levels of DMG was effective in preventing fatal salmonellosis. [1474]

This chelator **DMG is dimethylglyoxime**, not the antioxidant dimethylglycine.

For the treatment of acute poisoning from the inhalation of nickel carbonyl, Dithiocarb has proved to be a specific antidote; Antabuse (see below) is effective to a lesser degree; BAL has a limited therapeutic value. [1475]

The oral administration of ALA noticeably increased the urinary excretion of nickel. [1476] DMSA also binds **nickel**. [1477]

232

A 2009 study showed in fish, CaNa2 EDTA is an effective chelating agent for the removal of nickel and it has proved efficient in restoring both the biochemical variables and pathological features immediately after a sub lethal exposure of nickel chloride. [1478]

After an i.p. dose of 62 mg/kg nickel acetate corresponding to LD90 or greater [acute nickel poisoning], Na2CaEDTA and DPA were the most effective antidotes. [1479]

Nickel chelators also include disulfiram and calcium carbonate. [1480] "Disulfiram (Antabuse, Wyeth-Ayerst, Philadelphia, PA) is a nonconventional pharmacologic agent used in therapy for nickel contact dermatitis. It is a chelating agent for metals such as nickel and cobalt, but its main use is as supportive therapy for alcohol addiction." [1481]

8.28 Osmium (Os)

"Chronic low-level inhalation exposures can lead to insomnia, digestive disturbance, and distress to the pharynx (back of the throat) and larynx (voice box). Prolonged contact with skin can lead to dermatitis (inflammation of the skin). Mild kidney damage has been observed in animals with long-term exposures." [1482]

Treatment unknown at time of publication.

8.29 Platinum (Pt)

Platinum compounds (e.g., halogenated salts) encountered in occupational settings can cause bronchitis and asthma after inhalational exposure and contact dermatitis after skin exposure. [1483]

Platinum-induced peripheral neurotoxicity (PIPN) is a common side effect of platinum-based chemotherapy. [1484]

Treatment

DMPS or DMSA caused a moderate reduction of platinum in kidney of rats. In comparison to controls, renal platinum concentration was significantly reduced in the DMSA and deferoxamine treated groups. However, significant deterioration occurred in the deferoxamine- treated group. [1485]

8.30 Palladium (Pd)

The German Health Ministry has been warning dentists since 1993 not to use palladium-copper alloys any longer. [1486]
Palladium can cause obstruction of important enzyme systems.

Treatment
Dimethylglyoxime (DMG) forms complexes with metals including nickel, **palladium, platinum** and cobalt. [1487]
"N-acetyl cystine and L-methionine are useful chelating agents for Pd. " [1488]

8.31 Polonium (Po)

All 25 isotopes of polonium are radioactive.
On 1 November 2006, Alexander Litvinenko was poisoned with radioactive polonium-210. He died on 23 November. Polonium-210 is found in tabaco smoke. [1489]

treatment
"DTPA (diethylenetriamine pentaacetate) is a potent chelator especially approved for radionuclide mobilization, including polonium and other actinides." [1490]
"Chelation therapy agents such as DMPS, DMSA and penicillamine have been used to bind polonium and eliminate it from the body." [1491]

8.32 Radium (Ra)

Radium is extremely toxic and radioactive; it is used in cancer treatment as targeted radionuclide therapy.
Glow in the dark watch dials used to be painted with radium till the 1970s.
Exposure to radium over a period of many years may result in an increased risk of some types of cancer, particularly lung and bone cancer. Higher doses of radium have been shown to cause effects on the blood (anemia), eyes (cataracts), teeth (broken teeth), and bones (reduced bone growth). [1492] Radium behaves similarly to calcium and displaces calcium in bones.
treatment

In acute poisoning, oral calcium reduces gastrointestinal absorption and increases urinary excretion. Alginates are also useful to reduce gastrointestinal absorption. [1493]

8.33 Radon

Radon is a decay product of radium which in turn is a decay product of uranium. Nearly one in 15 homes in the U.S. has a high level of indoor radon according to the EPA.

"Rainwater can be highly radioactive due to high levels of radon and its decay progenies 214Bi and 214Pb."

Radon is a major cause of cancer; it is estimated to contribute to ~2% of all cancer related deaths in Europe.

No treatment known at time of publication.

8.34 Rhodium (Rh)

"All rhodium compounds should be regarded as highly toxic and as carcinogenic. Compounds of rhodium stain the skin very strongly." [1494]

Rhodium represents an emerging cause of skin hypersensitivity.

Treatment

Chelation therapy trials show that: deferiprone(L1) and desferrioxamine (DFO) are able to remove rhodium ions from the body. [1495]

8.35 Ruthenium (Ru)

Here as well, "All ruthenium compounds should be regarded as highly toxic and as carcinogenic. Compounds of ruthenium stain the skin very strongly. It seems that ingested ruthenium is retained strongly in bones." [1496]

Treatment: DTPA and triethylenetetraaminehexaacetic acid, proved to be most effective for the removal of radioruthenium from the body. [1497]

8.36 Rubidium (Rb)

Rubidium has been used in alternative cancer treatments to raise pH. Toxicity studies in rats showed that rubidium chloride resulted in decreased growth, anaemia, and changes to liver cells, kidney cells, brain enzymes, and hepatic lipid composition. [1498]
Treatment: Prussian blue chelates rubidium. [1499]

8.37 Selenium (Se) essential, but toxic in overload

Selenium in the kidney can combine with mercury to form crystalloid inclusion bodies.
Overexposure to selenium can give the breath a characteristic garlic odor. [1500]
Currently, there is no known antidote or suitable chelator for Se toxicity.

8.38 Silver (Ag)

Dr. Klinghardt stated the silver content in amalgam fillings is more instrumental in causing autoimmune disease than the mercury content of said filling. [1501] Dental amalgam is roughly 50% mercury and 30% silver.
He further observes in clinical practice that in patients who had previously used colloidal silver as antibacterial agents, silver is excreted in challenge urine tests.
In mice, not only **mercury** but also **silver** accumulated in the spleen and kidneys after amalgam implantation. [1502]
Treatment with gold in the form of aurothiomaleate, silver or mercury in genetically susceptible mouse strains (H-2s) induces a systemic autoimmune condition. [1503]
Colloidal silver (silver nanoparticles) is also used as antiseptics in wound dressings.
"Colloidal solutions of SNPs directly bound to the solid surface of materials inhibiting the growth of highly multi-resistant bacteria." [1504]

"Silver nanoparticles (AgNP) are known to penetrate into the brain and cause neuronal death." AgNPs are able to induce cytotoxicity in human lung, skin and fibroblast cells. [1505]
In holistic medicine, colloidal silver (which are silver nanoparticles) in oral application is often used as a safer alternative to

pharmaceutical antibiotics, little consideration is given to the potential accumulation of silver in organs, particularly the brain.

"In vitro studies demonstrated that silver nanoparticles (SNPs) are toxic to brain cells. High levels of silver in plasma, erythrocytes and cerebro-spinal fluid along with epileptic seizures and coma after daily ingestion of colloidal silver have been reported." [1506]

Silver nanoparticles induced blood-brain barrier inflammation and increased permeability in primary rat brain microvessel endothelial cells. [1507]

Silver and gold (aurothiomaleate: Au) also induce anti-fibrillarin antibodies (AFA) in genetically susceptible strains. [1508]

Sub-chronic dermal exposure can cause considerable accumulation of silver nanoparticles in the liver and lungs: SNPs cause histopathologic abnormalities in spleen, liver and skin, and muscles also are target organs of SNP toxicity. [1509]

Besides argyria and argyrosis, exposure to soluble silver compounds may produce other toxic effects, including liver and kidney damage, irritation of the eyes, skin, respiratory, and intestinal tract, and changes in blood cells. [1510]

"Long-term human exposure to silver leads to argyria, a grey-blue pigmentation of the skin, particularly of regions exposed to light." Silver particles, diameter 30 - 100 nm, were found in the basement membrane of the glomerular capillary walls in kidneys from a patient with argyria. [1511]

Overexposure to silver may also cause a gray discoloration of hair and internal organs. Additional symptoms may include nausea, vomiting, and diarrhea. [1512]

Treatment

Silver has been excreted by DMSA and DMPS chelation. [1513]

"DMPS and ZnDTPA are used in clinical practice to chelate silver." [1514]

"Superoxide radical is the main product generated by nanosilver exposed mitochondria." Iron chelation has prevented the cell from nanosilver induced DNA damage and diminish nanosilver cytotoxicity. [1515]

8.39 Strontium (Sr)

The long-term, excess intake of strontium in aquatic products may cause adult rickets. [1516]

Treatment
CDTA, DTPA and ascorbic acid have been used for the chelation of strontium in mice. [1517]
The chelating agent calcium acetylamino propylidene diphosphonic acid (Ca-APDA), was shown to be effective in the removal of radioactive strontium (Sr-90) in rats (femur and whole body). [1518]
Further, "intravenous calcium gluconate may be indicated for inhaled radioactive strontium."
Oral Sodium Alginate and oral calcium de-corporates strontium. [1519]

8.40 Tellurium (Te)

Tellurium has been used in various industries including nanomaterial and solar panel manufacturing.
"Te is distributed to the kidneys, liver, bone, brain and testes. It has been reported that plants which accumulate selenium, can also accumulate Te." [1520]
Descriptions of human toxicity from tellurium ingestion are rare.
Clinical features included vomiting, black discoloration of the oral mucosa, and a garlic odor to the breath. [1521]
Even though it is rare, tellurium has the same toxicity level as cadmium (0.80 µg/g creatinine). [1522]
Famous chemist Linus Pauling said there were some chemists who managed to get "permanent" tellurium breath from being too careless when working with Te compounds and were then ostracized from society. Some apparently even committed suicide as a result. [1523]

Treatment
The successful use of BAL for chelation of 3 patients with inhalational tellurium toxicity has been reported. [1524] Ascorbic acid has been suggested to eliminate garlic odor.

8.41 Thallium (Tl)

This highly toxic element should be prioritized in metal toxicology for reasons explained below.
"Thallium is considered the most toxic non-radioactive element by weight." It is more toxic to humans than mercury, cadmium, lead, copper or zinc. [1525]

The LD50 of thallium sulfate is 16 mg/kg, (or 1.1 g for a 70 kg person). [1526]

Thallium has a crustal abundance of about 0.7 mg/ kg (ppm). Its toxicity is comparable to that of cyanide. Common sources of thallium are: Industrial sources, ceramic magnetic materials in microwave equipment, doping agents in lasers, diagnostic contrasting agents and (before 1984) pesticides. [1527]

"Because chronic thallium exposure mimics other diseases, cases of industrial thallium exposure may go unnoticed." [1528]

"Thallium has high bioaccumulation." [1529]

The CDC notes that "thallium disappears from the blood with a half-life of several days, representing distribution into other tissues. " [1530]

"Thallium may act as a cumulative poison with chronic intoxications and a sudden release from tissue stores may lead to acute toxic symptoms." [1531]

"A systematic risk characterization related to the long-term dietary exposure of the population to potentially toxic elements showed that the cumulative toxicity was mainly driven by **Tl and vanadium**." [1532]

A host of studies highlight that Tl exposure, **even at very low concentrations,** represents a threat to human health.

"Tl+ rapidly distributes in the various body compartments competing with K+, as confirmed by its diagnostic employment in imaging techniques. " [1533]

Mitochondria is a key intracellular target of thallium toxicity. [1534]

Thallium accumulates in tissues with high potassium concentrations such as muscle, heart, and central and peripheral nerve tissue. [1535]

"Delay in receiving treatment for thallium poisoning is associated with greater likelihood of lasting neurological problems." Reports of persistent peripheral neuropathy most commonly involve the feet and lower extremities. [1536]

"Thallium poisoning is easily misdiagnosed and is often accompanied by a series of serious sequelae." [1537]

"Thallium salts lack taste and odor, while also having the ability to completely dissolve in liquids, being absorbed at a fast speed and evade detection on routine toxicological reports. Such properties make it a perfect candidate for criminal poisonings." [1538]

239

"Because thallium is not a common environmental or workplace contaminant and is not readily available to the public, any thallium-poisoned patient should be **considered a victim of a criminal act** until proved otherwise." [1539]

Former KGB agent Alexander Litvinenko was initially believed to have been poisoned with thallium and was treated for it with Prussian blue in exile in London. It later turned out, Litvinenko had ingested polonium-210.

This illustrates how even in acute and fatal thallium poisoning, the element is difficult to diagnose, as it is quickly deposited in the nervous system.

In most Western countries, thallium has been removed from pesticides and rodenticides which, fortunately, has dramatically decreased the frequency of poisoning. "[Acute] thallium poisoning begins with a severe gastrointestinal illness." [1540]

The long-term intake of Tl in aquatic products may cause perifollicular (around hair follicles) atrophy. [1541]

8.41.1 Thallium (or cesium) as a "Trojan horse".

Thallium can interfere with a series of enzymes whose activation depend on **potassium** function.

"Thallium also appears to bind to sulfhydryl groups located on the mitochondrial membrane, hence interfering with its normal functions. This is illustrated by the acute hair loss, which could have been caused by thallium's ability to bind to cysteine sulfhydryl groups found in hair. "

"Moreover, thallium binds to **glutathione** which inhibits its activation and the inability to metabolize [other] heavy metals which causes their overaccumulation in the body." [1542]

Now, thallium is an element forming Tl3+ but also the more stable Tl+ ions (a rare property for an element of this group). So, although belonging to the boron group of earth metals, 'Tl exhibits alkali metal monocation properties.' The monovalent Tl+ form is more stable. It is a very dense heavy metal (between Pb and Hg) but it behaves more like the alkaline metals (monovalent) of the first group including the important essential Na and K. The most common toxic metals (including the Big Four) are most harmful in their 2+ oxidation state, thus the most common chelators primarily bind 2+ ions. In this way, as an example, someone may test positive for mercury and uses mercury chelators, but at the same time they were unaware that they also have elevated lead levels, the mercury chelation ideally also reduces the lead burden.

But differently, thallium, because of its rare 1+ oxidation property, can often go undetected and is not likely unintentionally chelated along with other metals.

In addition, due to this rare property, it can slip detection in common challenge urine tests, which are usually performed with EDTA and DMSA/ DMPS.

Element	Atomic Number	Symbol	Monovalent Ion	Ionic Radius of monovalent
Lithium	3	Li	Li^+	0.059- 0.092
Sodium	11	Na	Na^+	0.099- 0.139
Potassium	19	K	K^+	0.137-0.164
Copper	29	Cu	Cu^+	0.046- 0.077
Silver	47	Ag	Ag^+	0.067- 0.128
Caesium	55	Cs	Cs^+	0.167- 0.188
Gold	79	Au	Au^+	0.137
Rubidium	37	Rb	Rb+	0.152- 0.183
Thallium	81	Tl	Tl^+	0.15- 0.17
Frankium	87	Fr	Fr	0.18

Table 3: A list of some monovalent cations, the Ionic radius of the monovalent ion in nm depending on its coordination.

8.41.2 Mechanism of action

Thallium induces hydrogen peroxide generation by impairing mitochondrial function. [1543]

Further, thallium shows an affinity for melanin (in skin and eyes). [1544]

It has been taken up in the eye melanin of rabbits in vivo. [1545]

Thallium disrupts calcium homeostasis. [1546]

"Alopecia is a feature that should lead to suspicion of thallium toxicity." Chronic poisoning can lead to tiredness, headaches, depression, lack of appetite, leg pains, hair loss and disturbances of vision. [1547]

A Chinese study revealed that prenatal **thallium** exposure was related to shortened neonatal telomere length in the Chinese

population, pointing to the important role of thallium exposure in accelerating biological aging. [1548]
Thallium is also frequently found in firearm bullets (see also 14.3).

8.41.3 Treatment thallium

"Glutathione binds heavy metals, including **thallium**, through its SH group, inhibiting their toxicity. In addition, glutathione blocks the formation of ROS while maintaining the oxidant homeostasis of the plasma." [1549]
Under normal conditions, thallium in urine does not have to exceed 1 mg/g creatinine and can be detected after 1 h for up to 2 months after exposure. [1550] That is in an unprovoked urine test. With provocation, thallium toxicity from exposure years past can be detected. The biological half-life of thallium in the body has not been determined. One of the challenges is that the standard chelator, Prussian blue, eliminates thallium via feces, and Tl might avoid detection in a provoked urine test. Oral potassium chloride (salt substitute) can mobilize thallium prior to a test. The total amount of potassium in a 79 kg adult body is about 140g.
Deferasirox and **desferrioxamine** (DFO) were determined to be useful in chelation of thallium in rats. Both chelators were effective only at the higher dose level, while DFO was more effective than deferasirox in enhancing urinary thallium excretion.
"Not to be used, contraindicated in the treatment of thallium poisoning are BAL, EDTA, dithizone and diethyldithiocarbamate (dithiocarb)." [1551] The latter was contraindicated in patients with thallium poisoning due to redistribution to the brain. [1552]

8.41.4 Prussian blue for thallium chelation

"Prussian blue, also known as potassium ferric hexacyanoferrate, is used as a medication to treat poisoning with radioactive or non-radioactive thallium or radioactive cesium." [1553]
"Prussian blue is the treatment of choice for Tl exposure." [1554]
According to an EPA review "No data regarding the possible carcinogenicity of Prussian blue in humans were located."
Slightly different formulae are used for medical grade Prussian blue. "The common forms of Prussian Blue include:
- the insoluble ferric ferrocyanide $Fe4[Fe(CN)6]3$ used in the decorporation of internal radiocesium contamination,
- the soluble potassium ferric hexacyanoferrate(II) $KFe[Fe(CN)6]$ used as a therapeutic antidote to thallium poisoning,

- or the soluble ammonium ferric cyanoferrate NH4Fe[Fe(CN)6] used as a food additive in animal feed to prevent the transfer of dietary radiocesium to milk.[1555]

"Soluble" in the context of PB refers to colloidal PB.

Radiogardase® is the commercial drug made of insoluble PB (PB nanoparticles), used to treat patients after Tl intoxication or ^{137}Cs contamination. [1556]

This medical chelator Radiogardase is insoluble ferric hexacyanoferrate(II). Other formulae are: Fe4[Fe(CN)6]3. [1557]

"Prussian blue particles are very small and desirably are of a nanosize and can have the formula A4xFe4−x III[FeII(CN)6]3+x.nH2O wherein A comprises Li+, Na+, K+, Rb+, Cs+, NH4+ and Tl+, or any combination thereof, x is any number from 0 to about 1, and n is generally from about 1 to about 24." [1558]

The mechanism that causes thallium to be retained in the body even though it circulates in the intestines is this:

Thallium ions are excreted into the intestine and reabsorbed mainly in the colon into blood to be excreted again into the intestinal tract. "Prussian blue is administered orally; it exchanges potassium for cesium or thallium at the surface of the crystal in the intestinal lumen." [1559] This implies the potassium containing soluble form is meant here.

In acute poisoning, "rapidly administered PB reduces gastrointestinal Tl absorption, and later administration enhances fecal Tl elimination by blocking Tl reuptake during enteroherpatic Tl circulation." [1560]

"PB will bind preferentially to cesium, then thallium in respect to the essential metal ions potassium and sodium (it preferentially binds to ions with larger ionic radii). Therefore, a depletion of potassium and sodium is not likely [during chelation therapy]." Also rubidium (i.r. 0.148 nm) binds to Prussian blue (see table above). [1561]

In summary, Prussian blue preferentially binds to **Cs+, Tl+ or rubidium (Rb+) and more weekly to K+, Na+ and NH4+** (ammonium cation) and **NH3** (ammonia, which is toxic).

Although the size of divalent cations is quite different from that of Cs, in absence of Tl+ or Cs+, "PB can adsorb divalent cations, such as **Cu2+, Co2+, Ni2+, and Pb2+.**"

"By using magnetic PB, Uogintė et al showed the high capacity of sorption: **copper**, 138 mg/g, **cobalt**, 111 mg/g, **nickel**, 155 mg/g, and **Pb**, 778 mg/g. [1562]

Prussian Blue pigment has a higher adsorption capacity than common ammonia adsorbents. [1563] PB exhibits surprising adsorption properties of gaseous ammonia, up to double that of standard ammonia adsorbents.

Ammonium ion (NH4+) in itself is basically harmless, it is converted into poisonous ammonia (NH3) in alkaline solution (pH 8 or greater), not in gastric pH.

Therapeutic applications Prussian Blue

"Treatment with orally administered Prussian blue should begin as soon as the diagnosis [of acute thallium poisoning] is suspected."

In clinical use, "Prussian blue is administered orally in 2–4 divided doses and the normal, maximal dose is 150–250 mg/kg/day." This corresponds to the highest daily dose of 17.5 g of Prussian blue for a 70kg adult. [1564]

"In rats with acute thallium poisoning, Prussian blue-treated rats (50 mg/kg twice daily for 5 days) had 3.5 times higher survival rates and only half the whole-brain thallium concentrations compared to controls."

The researchers concluded " Prussian blue significantly reduces both **brain thallium concentrations** and mortality." [1565]

"The combined treatment of Prussian blue and metallothionein has proven to be a good antidotal option against thallotoxicosis." [1566]

In rats with thallium poisoning, treatment with a **combination** of D-penicillamine (DP) and Prussian blue (PB) decreased thallium content in all body organs, including kidney and brain regions. DP administration alone increased redistribution into the brain. [1567]

Thallium excretion via the kidney can also increase upon administration of diuretics. [1568]

Potassium chloride

In addition to Prussian blue, potassium chloride supplements are used to mobilize thallium from tissues and increase renal clearance. [1569]

"Treatment with orally administered potassium chloride effectively releases tissue thallium but aggravates symptoms by increasing plasma thallium content." [1570] Hence it should be used in combination with PB.

Independently from thallium toxicity, randomized trials have shown that increasing potassium intake lowers blood pressure. Both potassium chloride and potassium citrate lowered blood pressure from 151mm Hg to 140mm within one week. [1571]

Potassium chloride not only lowers blood pressure but also causes natriuresis [sodium excretion in the urine through the action of the kidneys] in older patients with hypertension. [1572]

In a Chinese study, among persons who had a history of stroke or were 60 years of age or older and had high blood pressure, the rates of stroke, major cardiovascular events and death from any cause were lower in people using salt substitute (potassium chloride) than in persons using regular salt (sodium chloride). [1573]

Cyanide release from Prussian Blue
Cyanide released from Prussian blue in gastric pH was formerly considered potentially problematic. However, it turned out to be negligible. At gastric pH of 1.0, the release is only (47.47 µg/g= 47.47 parts per million." The minimal adult lethal dose of cyanide is about 56 mg. 1g of PB releases no more than 47ug of cyanide (1/ 1100 of a lethal dose for a 70 kg person). In comparison, bitter almonds release 22 times more cyanide by weight than Prussian blue. The consumption of 50 bitter almonds (50 grams) is deadly for adults. [1574]

Prussian blue is thermodynamically stable but loses bound water following long- term storage. This loss of water does not affect the level of cyanide release. [1575]

Quality of Prussian blue products
Medical grade Prussian blue (such as RADIOGARDASE) is chemically the same as insoluble Prussian blue pigment as used in arts and industry, but the former is produced under strict control of quality and purity. Kremer Pigments claim their PB pigments are either potassium ferrocyanide (K4[Fe(CN)6]), [1576] which is the soluble form also used as a therapeutic antidote to thallium poisoning, or NH4Fe[Fe(CN)6] x 3H2O, which is a soluble form also used as animal feed additive to prevent cesium uptake. Even though Kremer Pigments produces highest quality PB pigments, theoretically the same as Radiogardase, the former is not medical grade PB.
Do not ingest factory grade Prussian blue pigments from unknown sources, they may contain undeclared chemicals and toxic metals.

8.42 Thorium (Th)

Thorium is a silvery, slightly radioactive metal. all forms are radioactive and are found at trace levels in soil, rocks, water, plants and animals.

Observed effects include liver disease, blood disorders, hematopoietic cancers, and bile duct and gall bladder cancers.
The NIH sites research evidence that inhaling thorium dust increases the risk of lung and pancreatic cancer. Individuals exposed to thorium also have an increased risk of bone cancer because thorium may be stored in bone. [1577]

In rat models, thorium decorporation was achieved with 3,4,3-LI(1,2-HOPO) and CaDTPA. [1578]

8.43 Tin (Sn)

"Overexposure to tin may damage the nervous system and cause psychomotor disturbances including tremor, convulsions, hallucinations, and psychotic behavior." [1579]
"Early signs of chronic organic tin excess can be: reduced sense of smell, headaches, fatigue and muscle aches, ataxia and vertigo. Hyperglycemia and glucosuria are reported." [1580]
The main results of toxicity are skin and eye irritation; cholangitis of the lower biliary tract, and later hepatotoxicity and neurotoxicity. [1581]

Recall tin is also associated with obesity.
"Single charged cations (of organotin compounds) are usually the most toxic." [1582]

Treatment
"A two- or three-fold increase in urine tin levels is not uncommon following administration of EDTA or with sulfhydryl agents (DMSA, D-penicillamine, DMPS) [in a provoked (challenge) urine test]."
Intravenous EDTA with a physiological saline solution (0.9% NaCL) at a very slow rate, has proven very effective for removing tin from the body. [1583]

8.44 Titanium (Ti)

Titanium particles concentrate in the spleen, lungs, heart, kidney and liver. [1584]
"Titanium toxicity can arise from arthroplasty joint replacement failure and from dental implants."
Corrosion and wear of implants can result in bone loss due to inflammatory reactions, which may lead to osseointegration failure

of the dental implant. These titanium ions and particles can also cause yellow nail syndrome. [1585]

Titanium toxicity can elicit a number of symptoms, including fatigue, headaches, blurring of vision, respiratory inflammation, lymphedema, and hyperpigmentation of the nails and skin. [1586]

Titanium in auto workers was associated with the buildup of plaque in the arteries of their necks, hearts and legs. [1587]

Treatment

EDTA has been shown to be the most effective chelator of Co, Cr, Ti and V. [1588]

8.45 Tungsten (W)

Tungsten has been declared an emerging toxicant, causing cardiovascular disease and cancer. [1589]

Symptoms of tungsten poisoning are lung diseases (pneumoconiosis, cancer), eczema, pruritus, folliculitis (infection and inflammation of hair follicles), and neurodermatitis. [1590]

As there remains a lack of toxicological data, tungsten was nominated as an emerging contaminant for further investigation by the US EPA and National Toxicity Program.

Cases of childhood leukemia were associated with industrial tungsten mining exposure in Fallon, NV, USA.

"Tungsten accumulates in bone but is neither labile nor inert once absorbed. Tungsten's relatively high cytosolic solubility and availability are problematic given its association with childhood lymphocytic leukemia. Persistence of tungsten in cortical bone tissue following removal of the source indicates that it is retained in an insoluble form." [1591] Tungsten can often augment the effects of other co-exposures or co-stressors, which could result in greater toxicity or more severe disease. [1592]

Tungsten has long been used to make medical implants. A 2008 review paper shows "that tungsten should not generally be used as a chronically implanted material." In the body, metallic tungsten will eventually dissolve into the soluble hexavalent form W^{6+}, typically represented by the orthotungstate WO_4^{2-}. [1593]

Treatment

Confirmatory tests for tungsten accumulation and exposure, respectively, are (DMPS/DMSA) urine provocation or Fecal Elements testing. [1594]

Tungsten has been associated with cardiovascular disease. EDTA chelates and allows excretion of this metal. [1595]
"EDTA chelation therapy is used in the treatment of tungsten toxicity." [1596]

8.46 Uranium (U)

"Uranium (U), like all elements with an atomic number greater than 82, has no stable isotopes", meaning all forms are radioactive.
Uranium is the heaviest naturally occurring element, certainly qualifying it as a heavy metal. "Depleted uranium (DU) is appreciably less radioactive – usually around 40 per cent less - than unprocessed uranium. "
Uranium acts as an environmental estrogen. [1597] C. A Dyer, 2007 proposes that uranium is a **potent estrogen mimic** at concentrations at or below the US EPA safe drinking water level. [1598]

In Iraq, smokers had 1.6 times the urinary uranium levels compared to non-smokers. In Switzerland, there was no difference between smokers and non-smokers as of 2017. [1599]
As mentioned in each corresponding paragraph above, uranium is associated with suicide, schizophrenia and insomnia.
"It is suggested that 5 g be provisionally considered the acute oral LD50 for uranium in humans."
After long-term, low-level uranium exposure to rats for up to 19 months, uranium accumulated in most organs, including teeth and brain that are not usually described as target organs. [1600]
Soluble uranium compounds (uranyl nitrate, uranyl fluoride, etc.) are more toxic than insoluble forms.

Treatment
Chelating agents that have been used for uranyl ion include citrate ion (citric acid and citrate salts, found in many fruits and vegetables,) and desferal (desferrioxamine B).
"Sodium citrate was as effective in uranium excretion when administered orally as when administered intravenously."
Uranium poisoned rats show increased excretion of citrate in urine without exogenous citrate administration. [1601]
EDTA was found to increase urinary excretion of uranyl ion, but was not effective at mobilizing uranium bound to bone. [1602]

I.V sodium bicarbonate (baking soda) de-corporates uranium, [1603] and is recommended by the National Council on Radiation Protection following uranium exposure.

In rats, intramuscular sodium bicarbonate protects against uranium-induced acute nephrotoxicity through uranium-decorporation by urinary alkalinization. [1604]

Oral sodium bicarbonate is disintegrated in stomach acid to salt, water and CO_2 and must therefore be administered IV, IM, or by rectal suppositories.

In animal trials, damage to target organs (short-term kidney and long-term bone damage) was avoided in a high percentage of animals treated with lethal doses of uranyl nitrate through the effective chelating action of a single dose of bisodic etidronate (EHBP). [1605] Animal study results found that this bisphosphonate ethane-1-hydroxy-1,1-bisphosphonate (EHBP) is a chelating agent capable of effectively neutralizing lethal uranium intoxication. [1606]

In uranium chelating trials, the main ligands forming complexes with uranium in the serum were estimated as follows: IP6 > EHBP > bioligands > DFO ≫ DTPA when the concentration ratio of the chelating agent to uranium was 10. [1607]

In a different study, sixteen chelating agents were tested for their efficacy as antidotes for acute uranium poisoning in mice, with eight producing significantly increased survival rates: Tiron, gallic acid, diethylenetriaminepentaacetic acid (DTPA), p-aminosalicylic acid, sodium citrate, EDTA, 5-aminosalicylic acid and ethylenebis (oxyethylenenitrilo) tetraacetic acid (EGTA). [1608]

Gallic acid can act as a protective agent against the adverse effects of uranyl acetate exposure on the liver (the latter is also used as a chemo-radiological agent). [1609]

Sodium citrate is freely available as a food additive (E331).

Gallic acid is prescription free, if taken orally, "GA is found to be non- toxic up to a dose of 5,000 mg/ kg b.w." [1610]

In mice with uranium poisoning, a significant decrease in the concentration of uranium in liver, spleen and bone was observed after administration of Tiron (sodium 4,5-dihydroxybenzene-1,3-disulfonate), whereas injection of gallic acid or DTPA resulted in a significant decrease in the concentration of the metal in the liver. The results show that Tiron was consistently the most effective chelator of those tested in the treatment of uranium poisoning after repeated daily administration of the metal. [1611]

8.47 Vanadium (Vi)

Vanadium is currently disputed as an essential element.
"Vanadium overload is damaging to the gastrointestinal, urinary and reproductive system and it affects fertility and causes fetuses malformations." [1612]
A synergistic effect with thallium has been established.
Vanadium is a trace mineral that can aggravate bipolar disorder and manic- depressive psychosis. [1613]
"An overload of **vanadium** is damaging to the reproductive system, affects fertility and it can cause fetuses malformations." [1614]

Treatment
In rat studies, vanadium overload has been effectively chelated with a combination of tiron + selenium and tiron + vitamin E + lipoic acid. [1615]
Other potential chelating antidotes for vanadium intoxication include desferrioxamine B, DMSA and DMPS. [1616]
"EDTA has been used to remove vanadium and lessen the symptoms of depression in bipolar patients." [1617]

8.48 Ytterbium (Yb)

See Rare Earth Elementes 1.11

8.49 Zinc (Zn) essential, but toxic in overload

Zinc deficiency is much more common than zinc overload.
Zinc is considered to be relatively nontoxic, particularly if taken orally. "However, manifestations of overt toxicity symptoms (nausea, vomiting, epigastric pain, lethargy, and fatigue) will occur with extremely high zinc intakes." [1618]
The long-term intake of Zn in aquatic products may reduce superoxide dismutase activity in red blood cells. [1619]

Treatment of overload
The most common extracellular zinc chelators in use today by the neuroscience community include EDTA; ethylene glycol-bis(2-aminoethylether)-N,N,N',N'-tetraacetic acid (EGTA); 1,2-bis(o-aminophenoxy)ethane-N,N,N',N'-tetraacetic acid (BAPTA); and ethylenediamine-N,N'-diacetic-N,N'-di-β-propionic (EDPA). [1620]

8.50 Elements of uncertain Human Requirement

"Little is known about the essentiality of some of the probably essential elements such as vanadium, boron and nickel in advanced organisms and humans' physiology and possibly treatment of diseases." [1621]

Here we look at evidence for benefits of adequate levels of the following 5 elements, and the symptoms of overload: **vanadium, boron, strontium, lithium** and **nickel**. No cases of deficiencies of these elements have been proven.

8.51 Boron (B)

Boron is officially considered non-essential. Evidence has been produced for boron having a positive effect in arthritis [1622] and to boost testosterone. [1623]

"Boron markedly reduces urinary calcium and magnesium loss, and increases calcium absorption. When compared with healthy bone, arthritic bone was associated with almost a 20-fold decrease in boron content."

Different boron compounds (BA, borax, colemanite and ulexite, 5-20 ppm) significantly reduced the genotoxic effects induced by low doses of heavy metals (**As, Bi, Cd, Pb** and **Hg**). [1624]

Boron overload

Boron has been known to be fatal when taking more than 20 grams in adults or 5 to 6 grams in children.

"No data are available on adverse effects of high boron intakes from food or water."

Boron toxicity can also cause "headache, hypothermia, restlessness, weariness, renal injury, dermatitis, alopecia, anorexia, and indigestion." [1625]

Treatment of overload

"NAC may be useful in intoxications with chromate and borate and is effective at reversing the oliguria associated with these intoxicants." [1626]

8.52 Lithium (Li)

There is currently no consensus on whether or to what extent lithium is an essential metal. It is used in high doses in acute psychosis and suicidal emergencies (see antidepressants 7.3.1). Further, "lithium protects brain cells against excess glutamate and calcium, and low levels cause abnormal brain cell balance and neurological disturbances. " [1627]

Dr. Timothy M. Marshall, PhD says:

"In high doses, lithium acts as a drug, accompanied by potentially serious and debilitating side effects. In low doses, lithium acts as a nutrient required for B12 and folate transport and uptake, neuromodulation, and the function of many biochemical processes in both humans and animals." Studies since the 1970s have shown the ability of lithium to stimulate the proliferation of stem cells. [1628]

"Lithium has been used as the gold standard in the treatment of major depressive and bipolar disorders for decades" (since 1949). [1629]

Studies have found low lithium levels common in learning disabled children, incarcerated violent criminals, and people with heart disease." [1630]

"Violent offenders and family abusers receiving lithium had significantly increased scores for mood, happiness, friendliness, and energy." [1631]

In a large Texas study, incidence of suicide, homicide, rape, robbery, burglary, theft, and drug use were significantly higher in counties with low lithium levels in drinking water. [1632]

Higher levels of natural lithium in drinking water in Japan was associated with lower suicide rates. [1633] Scientists say lithium should be added to drinking water to prevent suicides. [1634]

"It has been suggested that adding trace lithium to drinking water could be a safe and effective way to reduce suicide." [1635]

Toxicity

Chronic therapy with lithium can precipitate nephrogenic diabetes insipidus, which might elicit a cascade of symptoms and signs of lithium toxicity. This can be attributed to the diminished urinary concentrating capacity of the kidneys. [1636]

Further side effects include, renal tubular acidosis, chronic tubulointerstitial nephropathy, and minimal change disease. Although the former three adverse effects are well-known, minimal change disease is relatively rare. [1637]

Treatment of overload
Due to its narrow therapeutic index, lithium toxicity is a common clinical problem. [1638]
"As there is no specific antidote for lithium detoxification, the most effective treatment relies on minimizing exposure time to toxic lithium levels."
In cases of acute poisoning, hemodialysis is used. [1639]

8.53 Nickel (Ni)

See toxic metals of concern: nickel (8.27.)

8.54 Vanadium (V)

See toxic metals of concern: vanadium (8.54.)

8.55 Strontium (Sr)

See toxic metals of concern (8.39.)

Chapter 9
Nanoparticles (metals and non-metals)

Nanoparticles are a relatively new health hazard of hitherto undetermined severity having emerged in the past decade. In *Hormonageddon,* we explored how the biggest re-insurance company declared nanoparticles as one of the top three insurance topics for reliability claims of the next few years.

If we consider human gullibility and the example that we've known lead is toxic to all organs for 2,000 years, but then we try to use it anyways proficiently and carelessly again and again, this indicates that with nanoparticles, we opened yet another pandora's box.

Much like toxic metals, NP's are not biodegradable, and they keep being biochemically reactive without being consumed in a chemical reaction. Thus, they can stay in an organism and cause cell damage indefinitely.

"From current knowledge in the field of nanotoxicology, it has become evident that most, if not all NPs, are more toxic than bulk materials. " [1640]

"Similar to what occurs with NPs, heavy metal accumulation in the environment results from anthropogenic activities, in addition to some natural sources. These pollutants remain in the environment for long periods and have an impact on several organisms through different routes of exposure in soil, water and air. " [1641]

New research shows that nanoplastics - microscopic particles broken down from everyday plastic items such as polystyrene drinking cups - bind to proteins in the brain associated with Parkinson's disease and Lewy body dementia. "The most surprising finding was the tight bonds formed between the plastic and protein within neuron lysosomes." [1642]

EDX point spectrum (x-ray spectrographs) of particles found in Covid vaccines show a large peak in silver (Ag). [1643] Ag is not declared in the vaccine registration.

9.1.1 Graphene oxide (GO)

GO toxicity

"Several typical mechanisms underlying graphene-family nanomaterials (GFNs) toxicity have been revealed, for instance, physical destruction, oxidative stress, DNA damage, inflammatory response, apoptosis, autophagy, and necrosis." [1644]

"In animal studies, graphene oxide looked safe initially but eventually led to anti-body enhancement, which killed healthy cells and led to the death of every single tested animal." [1645]

Graphene nanoparticles have been shown to cross the blood-brain barrier, which has enormous implications for neurotoxicity. [1646]

"Reaction between graphene oxide and intracellular glutathione affects cell viability and proliferation." The reaction between GO and GSH provides a new perspective to explain the origin of GO cytotoxicity. [1647]

"Graphene oxide induces cell toxicity through plasma membrane damage, generation of reactive oxygen species (ROS), and DNA damage." Further, graphene oxide exposure elicits significant decreases in mitochondrial membrane potential and ATP synthesis. [1648]

Bacterial destruction

"Graphene has strong cytotoxicity toward bacteria." [1649]

While this could be applied in specific anti-bacterial treatment (of pathogenic bacteria infections), beneficial bacteria are eliminated as well. Further, graphene nanoparticles can penetrate cell walls and cannot be contained and securely excreted from the body after the desired reaction. "Most E. coli are harmless and actually are an important part of a healthy human intestinal tract."

"Incubation in graphene oxide medium significantly reduced the viability of 4 tested species of human bacteria (E. coli, S. aureus, E. faecalis and S. mutans)". The former three are endemic in the healthy body, only some strains of them are harmful, while S. mutans is associated with tooth decay. "It is widely accepted that GO damages the bacterial cell membrane." [1650]

"Both reduced GO (rGO) and GO show promising antibacterial properties with a broad antibacterial spectrum due to their special physicochemical properties and unique antibacterial mechanism." Metals such as silver and gold are often used as nanocomposites materials with GO and rGO to enhance the antibacterial activity of these structures. [1651]

9.1.2 Remedies for graphene oxide toxicity

Nanoparticles were declared an emerging health liability of vast proportions by the world's largest reinsurance company Swiss RE in 2013. Graphene oxide and other nano particles in the human body are a relatively new problem (of the last decade or so) and thus treatment experience is scarce. Hitherto recommended excretion agents are largely substances used in metal toxicity.

Graphene oxide provider shilpent.com proposes different substances to remove graphene oxide from the body: N-acetylcysteine, glutathione, zinc and high concentrations of vitamin D. [1652]

Other sources recommend intravenous vitamin C+ D, EDTA chelation, glutathione and NAC. [1653]

"N-acetyl cysteine (NAC) reduces graphene oxide (GO) at room temperature." NAC adheres to the reduced GO (rGO) surface and avoids GO-mediated oxidation of glutathione." [1654]

"Preclinical studies show that NAC reverses and prevents the oxidative damage caused by engineered nanoparticles." [1655] (see also Covid and NAC 12.6).

Can Prussian blue eliminate graphene oxide?

In aqueous medium at 60°C, iron(II) and glucose and graphene oxide were mixed with Prussian Blue $K_4Fe(CN)_6$, (without any toxic agents) to form PB modified rGO (G–rGO–PB). [1656] The resulting rGO- PB nanotubes could theoretically be excreted from the body. Further research is encouraged to see if the same reaction could be created in conditions conducive in the body (temperature and acidity outside the stomach) in order to safely eliminate GO.

In a similar process, a facile and green method for the synthesis of graphene oxide sheets (GOs)–Prussian blue nanocomposites has been presented via a spontaneous redox reaction in a aqueous solution containing $FeCl_3$, $K_3[Fe(CN)_6]$ and graphene oxide sheets. Electrochemical property investigation demonstrates PB nanocubes formed on the surface of GOs retain their excellent electrochemical activity. [1657]

Removal of GO from aqueous solutions by UV-light

"Direct UV-light irradiation without any catalysts or additional chemicals is a promising and green method to remove graphene oxide (GO) from aqueous solutions." UV-light induced a maximum removal rate of GO of 99.1% after 32 h irradiation without any additives.

"Under optimal conditions, GO was completely removed, with initial GO concentrations of 10 mg/L, while adjusting solution pH to 3 or adding Ca2+-containing salt." [1658]

GO was removed while it was transformed into photoreduced graphene oxide (prGO)

In comparison to GO, rGO shows high electrical conductivity. [1659]

In a different setting - namely wastewater treatment - GO was completely degraded to give CO2 within 28 days by Photo-Fenton (an advanced oxidation process that uses the hydroxyl radical to disinfect and decontaminate water). [1660]

Kaolin alleviates toxicity of graphene oxide

In a 2021 study, it was demonstrated that kaolin nanoclay significantly alleviates the toxicity of graphene oxide in aqueous environments. Importantly, the **toxicity** of graphene oxide coagulated with kaolin is **reduced** without the aggregated particles being removed from the environment. [1661]

The joint application of graphene oxide and planar kaolin nanoclay reduced the negative effects of graphene by almost 20%. [1662]

Chapter 10
Diagnosis

10.1 Testing limitations for Toxic Metals

"Checking blood for heavy metals is useful for current exposure but does not show past exposure or total body burden. Similarly, urine tests without provocation will show current toxic exposure, but provocation tests use a heavy metal mobilizing agent, such as oral DMSA or intravenous DMPS." [1663]

"Detoxifying heavy metals involves balancing mineral antagonists which dislodge the metals from the tissues into the blood with chelating agents that bind the metals in the blood and prevent them from being re-deposited somewhere else so the kidneys can excrete them; it is a specialist job. Regular detoxification techniques like fasting, the liver flush, kidney cleansers etc. do not work with heavy metals." [1664]

10.2 Challenge (provocation) urine test

The most common substances used by toxicologists and holistic practitioners as provocation agents are the same chelating agents most widely used for the subsequent actual chelation therapy (in case of a positive result), namely DMSA, DMPS or EDTA or a combination of several of the above. These three substances are available freely online in many countries. Make sure you comply with your country's laws before using these substances.

For examples of general applications of challenge (provoked) urine tests see Chapter 13.

Other more specific chelating agents are prescription drugs, administered only intravenously. In MRI examinations for instance, the chelator DTPA is used initially to bind the highly toxic gadolinium contrast agent so it will be excreted via the kidney. In cases where this bond fails and gadolinium is retained in the body, chelation with several doses of the same DTPA is used to remove the Gd subsequently.

10.2.1 Clinical (visual) Indicators

Cardiovascular disease and possible metal toxicity

There are several visually observable symptoms that are statistically associated with chronic cardiovascular disease. Some of these symptoms are independently associated with metal toxicity and overall, chronic cardiovascular disease is associated with metal toxicity.

These symptoms alone are not proof of heart disease or metal toxicity. It is important to not buy into premature conclusions of self-diagnoses. Only proper laboratory testing can confirm the types and quantity of certain metals in the body.

Such symptoms with associations to cardiovascular disease include:

- **Male pattern boldness**
- **Frank's sign**: a diagonal crease in the earlobe, it roughly runs from the upper front edge of the earlobe (face side) to the central bottom edge of the earlobe (in the general direction of the back of the neck). [1665] More than 50 studies confirm the relationship.
- **Loss of hair on the legs** - first the outer shins, then thighs - anterolateral leg alopecia; This may be a warning sign of peripheral artery disease in particular. (For the connection to metals see also alopecia 5.18.4).
- **Xanthelasma: yellow plaque** - fat deposits/ cholesterol on the eyelids.
- **Arcus senilis**, senile halo (corneal arcus) a bright ring seen around the iris. It develops around the edge of the cornea. It typically appears as an arc that affects the top and bottom of the cornea. (Cadmium exposure can cause conjunctivitis and damage the cornea).
- **Cyanosis**: Blueish or purple tone in skin.
Cyanosis is also listed as a symptom of **nickel** intoxication.
"Pseudo cyanosis is also caused by the ingestion of metals (such as **silver** or **lead**)," [1666] In the case of silver, the skin condition is called argyria.
- **Ulcers** – or sores that don't heal - on legs or feet.
"Exposure to chromium compounds can result in the formation of ulcers, which will persist for months and heal very slowly."
- **Swelling in the legs**, ancles and feet (oedema).
("toxic metals can target the vascular system, which contributes to edema"). [1667]

10.2.2 Fingernails

Fingernail samples are sometimes used for metal analysis with a similar efficacy as hair analysis, the process reveals acute, recent intoxication rather than chronic metal accumulation. Inhabitants of an Iranian region near a lead and zinc plant had 6 times more **lead** and 20 times more **arsenic** in their fingernails than controls in unpolluted regions. [1668]

Mees' lines (white spots or white lines in the fingernails) can appear after an episode of poisoning with **arsenic, thallium** or other heavy metals or **selenium**. [1669] They can also appear if the subject is suffering from kidney failure. [1670] Mees' lines may also be caused by heart failure or chemotherapy. [1671]

Further clinical signs in hands and fingernails in connection to different diseases (also non- metal related) are given by *Stanford Medicine in Examination of the Hand* (The Hand in Diagnosis). [1672]

Thought experiment: hands and personality

Do fortune tellers/ palm readers check for mees lines as an indicator for chronic arsenic poisoning to draw general conclusions on personality traits?

In Bangladesh, arsenic-affected people have "**poorer mental health**" (based on General Health Questionnaire). [1673] Plus **depression, weakness, restlessness, insufficient sleep, drowsiness and loss of appetite** among arsenicosis cases as compared to controls. [1674]

In *Hormonageddon*, a case was made that the finger length ratio of index and ring finger can be used to make statistically meaningful predictions about someone's personality. Men on average have a small, usually negative 2D:4D ratio, meaning the index finger is shorter than the ring finger. For the average woman the index is longer. Female athletes and self-described feminists are found to have more masculinized finger ratios. Homosexual men have a more feminized finger ratio. If fortune tellers or psychologists would be aware of this, they could use it to make general inferences of someone psychological profile by a look at someone's hand.

The same could be used for Mees' lines in the fingernails, they give a rough estimate of someone's arsenic, thallium or opioid intoxication levels and could be used to draw preliminary conclusions on mental states and personality.

Chapter 11
Treatment, Therapies

The American College for Advancement in Medicine says "all Americans should know about chelation therapy. In addition to helping rid the body of heavy metal pollution, which many experts believe is a cardiovascular risk, it also helps the body remove build-up in the cardiovascular (circulatory) system. Studies have shown EDTA has reduced atherosclerotic plaque and other mineral deposits throughout the cardiovascular system, especially the hardened arteries around the heart." [1675]

Again, prevention is the best cure for metal toxicity. As limited metal exposure is impossible to avoid in modern life, further, an overall healthy life style - including diet and exercise - can help to minimize metal accumulation and mitigate the negative effects of the poisoning, e.g., lower metal-induced oxidative stress. Highly trained long-distance runners have lower serum levels of As, Cd, and Pb and increased urine elimination of Cd and Pb compared to controls at equal dietary intake of these elements. [1676]

11.1 History of chelation agents

In 1920, Morgan and Drew suggested the term chelate, which originates from the Greek word *chele* (claw of a lobster). [1677]

"For more than a century, chelating agents were used by Ehrlich and Werner to decrease the toxicity of arsenic (As)-containing syphilis drugs." During 1920–1940, similar trials to reduce the toxicity of antimony drugs for schistosomiasis and trypanosomiasis were done by Voegtlin et al. [1678]

Chelation therapy in the modern sense can be traced back to 1935, when Ferdinand Munz, an Austrian chemist working for I.G. Farben in Germany, first synthesized ethylenediaminetetraacetic acid (EDTA).

[1679] Munz was looking for a replacement for citric acid as a water softener. The main purpose was to remove calcium ions from water in order to improve the dyeing process on fabrics.

The Germans used EDTA only for industrial applications, EDTA chelation therapy was introduced in the US in the days during and after WWII for lead poisoning (see history of EDTA,11.5.1).

BAL: The chemical war agent lewisite had already been used by the German military in WWI, but the remedy anti-lewisite (as BAL) was only available from WWII onward.
From what is officially known, in the first fortnight of the War (1939) fundamental research was initiated in the Oxford Department of Biochemistry by British scientist Rudolph Peters for the Chemical Defense Research Department. [1680]
BAL or dithiol 2,3 dimercaptopropanol combines with lewisite to form a stable ring, thus reducing the toxicity of the lewisite. The name became British Anti-Lewisite, BAL, although today it is also known as dimercaprol. [1681]
After World War II, BAL was found to offer therapeutic benefit for patients intoxicated by a variety of inorganic compounds containing metals such as **lead, arsenic, mercury, copper**, and **gold**, and possibly more uncommon acute poisonings involving others such as **bismuth** and **antimony**. [1682]
During the 1950s, DMSA (meso-dimercaptosuccinic acid) and DMPS (2,3-dimercapto-1-propanesulfonic acid) were used in China and the former Soviet Union. [1683]
In summary, the earliest useful chelating agents were invented in 1939 and onward. As far as conspiracies are concerned, there is no evidence that the people who forced the exhausts of leaded gasoline onto everyone, secretly had a remedy to protect themselves from chronic lead poisoning. Ethyl gasoline was launched in 1923.

11.2 Pharmaceutical chelating agents

Oral alpha-lipoic acid is a natural supplement - an essential omega-3 fatty acid - but it is listed in this section for it has shown effective chelating results similar to some of the pharmaceutical substances. Oral, over-the-counter EDTA is used therapeutically and has produced results comparable to intravenous (IV) EDTA, but on a slower time scale. IV EDTA must be administered by a health practitioner and is a prescription drug in most countries. EDTA is also contained in small quantities as a preservative in many processed foods.

Disclaimer:
No part of this book constitutes medical advice.
DMSA and DMPS are prescription medications in many countries, which may require the consultation of a medical doctor. Make sure you comply with your country's laws before you start using these substances.

Even though DMSA and DMPS can be purchased on the internet from outlets like living supplements in many countries, it is not recommended to undertake chelation without an authorized practitioner.
When you go to a general practitioner with a reasonable suspicion of chronic toxic metal overload, they will most likely take an unprovoked (non-challenge) blood, urine or hair test, and tell you that you have no heavy metal toxicity. They don't know that chronic, long-term heavy metal overload does usually not show up in the blood or urine without provocation agents.

11.3 DMSA (Meso-2,3-dimercaptosuccinic acid)

DMSA is a sulfhydryl-containing, water-soluble, **non-toxic**, orally administered metal chelator which has been in use as an antidote to heavy metal toxicity since the 1950s. [1684]
DMSA is used in the treatment of human inorganic poisoning with **Hg, Cd, Pb** and other metals.
It is considerably less toxic than the classical agent British anti-Lewisite (BAL, 2,3-dimercaptopropanol) and is the recommended agent in poisonings with **Pb** and organic **Hg**. Its toxicity is also lower than that of DMPS (dimercaptopropane sulfonate), although DMPS is the recommended agent in acute poisonings with Hg salts. [1685]
It has been shown that DMSA is not only effective to chelate **lead** and **mercury,** but also binds **aluminum, cadmium, arsenic, nickel** und other potentially toxic metals. [1686]
In comparison to EDTA, DMSA chelation by eqiumolar concentration is better at extracting **lead** and **arsenic**, comparable in extracting **aluminum**, and less efficient in extracting **cadmium**.
"Clearance of essential metals during chelation by 1g-3g of EDTA was increased over twenty-fold for **zinc** and **manganese**."
"Overall, these data suggest that the **agents EDTA and DMSA are essentially non- toxic.**" [1687]
"No significant loss of essential metals like zinc, iron, calcium and magnesium are observed." [1688]

The LD50 value of sodium salt of DMSA in mice is 2.4 gm/kg for the i.v., and 8.5 gm/kg for the oral route. [1689] For a 70 kg person, this would translate to an LD50 of oral 600g.

DMSA 30 mg/kg/day significantly increases urine **lead** elimination and significantly reduces blood lead concentrations in lead-poisoned patients.

Over a 5-day course, mean daily urine lead excretion exceeds baseline by between 5- and 20-fold and blood lead concentrations fall to 50% or less of the pretreatment concentration. Most symptomatic patients report improvement after 2 days of treatment. [1690]

Brain cells DMSA

The German Textbook of Clinical Metal toxicology states:
"DMSA is believed to pass the brain blood barrier and to detoxify brain centers." [1691]

"DMSA can remove **MeHg** and **Pb** from animal brains." [1692]

DMSA binds antimony

"DMSA greatly increased the excretion of **lead**, substantially increased excretion of **tin** and **bismuth**, and somewhat increased the excretion of **thallium, mercury, antimony,** and **tungsten**.

Only 1 round (9 doses: 10 mg/kg-dose, 3×/day, for 3 days. or 90mg/kg body weight) was sufficient to improve glutathione and platelets. "Overall, DMSA therapy seems to be reasonably safe, effective in removing several toxic metals (especially lead), **dramatically effective in normalizing RBC glutathione, and effective in normalizing platelet counts**. " [1693]

11.3.1 DMSA mechanism of action

Oral administration of DMSA may be limited by intestinal dysbiosis. Oral absorption is approximately 20%. [1694]

"About 95% of the absorbed drug bind to plasma proteins (albumin)." DMSA leaves its other SH group free to bind metals. Only 10%–25% of the oral application is excreted through urine. The other part is excreted via feces. [1695]

"DMSA has proven to be the least toxic but has a significant drawback in that it lacks the ability to cross cellular membranes and is distributed in the extracellular fluids only." [1696]

Administration

Between DMSA rounds of several days, on non-treatment days, a selenium supplement is recommended plus optionally chromium and zinc. [1697]

Blaurock-Busch recommends:

"In chronic toxicity, a maximum dose of 10- 30 mg/kg body weight [oral DMSA] is administered 1- 3 times per week. The dose depends on age, sensitive and weakened patients should begin with single doses of 100- 500 mg. " [translation mine]. [1698]

DMSA doses between 10 mg/kg body weight to 30mg/kg body weight have been administered without side effects or counterindications. [1699]

At a body weight of 70 kg, this would amount to:

10mg/kg = 700mg = 0.7 gram; 30mg/kg = 2100mg = 2.1 gram

"The US FDA approved a maximum DMSA label dose of 30mg/kg/day, that is typically used for less than a week at a time in children." [1700]

"Mild to moderate neutropenia is reported with DMSA." (neutropenia is a lack of neutrophils, a type of white blood cells). [1701]

In the Zamfara gold mining disaster 2008- 2010, where hundreds of children died from **lead** poisoning, treatment with oral DMSA (Succimer) reduced lead-related childhood mortality from 65% reported in the literature to 1.5%. [1702]

DMSA suppositories

Manufacturers claim "clinical experience has shown the rectal suppository absorption rate to be approximately 80-85%, " [1703] as opposed to 20% oral absorption rate.

11.4 DMPS (Dimercaptopropanesulfonate)

"DMPS is a powerful chelator especially beneficial during times of acute toxicity. It is a synthetic compound." Dr. Andy Cutler recommends oral DMSA for mercury chelation, especially for those that do not tolerate DMSA or ALA well.

"In different countries, DMPS can be prescribed as a drug in capsules for oral antidote treatment (one capsule Dimaval® contains 100 mg DMPS) or in ampoules for intravenous treatment (5 mL ampoule DMPS-Heyl® contains 250 mg DMPS)." In Germany, DMPS is a registered drug for treatments of Hg intoxication. [1704]

DMPS and its metabolites are rapidly eliminated from the body through the kidneys. "It is important to note that this drug does not redistribute **arsenic, lead,** or inorganic **mercury** to the brain. No major adverse effects following DMPS administration in humans or animals have been reported." [1705]

"DMPS oral absorption is approximately 39%, about double that of DMSA." [1706]

DMPS mercury

Approximately 50% of orally administered DMPS is detected in the urine. "Neither DMPS nor its metabolites are detected 12 hours after administration. In the brain, only very slight amounts are found." [1707]

One reviewed protocol involving the use of oral DMPS and oral DMSA in combination with intravenous glutathione and high-dose vitamin C for treatment of high-level mercury, yielded an average 69% reduction of urine **mercury** by provocation (challenge) analysis.

"Dr. P.J. Muran's protocol involves a 400mg oral dose of either DMPS or DMSA per day for 10 x 14 days, accompanied by sodium ascorbate, vitamins, minerals and intravenous glutathione. [1708]

11.5 EDTA (Ethylene-diaminetetraacetic acid)

11.5.1 History of EDTA

"EDTA is a hexadentate complexing agent. It forms particularly stable 1:1 chelate complexes with cations with a charge number of at least +2. Gerold Schwarzenbach performed pioneering work on EDTA in the 1940s at the Technical University ETH in Zurich." [Translation mine]. [1709]

"Researchers first started to notice EDTA in the days during and after World War II when men who worked in battery factories or painted ships with **lead**-based paint began coming down with lead poisoning from their high exposure in these jobs. EDTA was found to be extremely effective for removing the lead from the men's bodies, but what really made people sit up and take notice was an apparent reduction in symptoms of heart disease in many of these men." [1710]

Sodium calcium edetate (EDTA) came into medical use in the United States in 1953. [1711]

The first systematic study of EDTA in people with atherosclerosis was published in 1956. [1712]

When the researchers gave 20 patients with confirmed heart disease a series of 30 I.V. EDTA treatments, 19 of the patients experienced improvement, as measured by an increase in physical activity. [1713]

EDTA in clinical practice
In therapeutic use, EDTA is mostly administered intravenously, which is prescription based. When administered orally, only 2-18% of EDTA is absorbed (see below). However, effective chelation results have been achieved with oral EDTA, which is a freely available over-the-counter drug and food additive.

"The FDA has approved EDTA as a pharmaceutical agent for the treatment of **lead** and other heavy metal poisoning or exposure. In older literature, the FDA also approved EDTA as being "possibly effective in occlusive vascular disorders […] arrhythmias and atrioventricular induction defects […] and in the treatment of pathologic conditions to which calcium tissue deposits or hypercalcemia may contribute other than those listed above." [1714]
"These "possibly effective" indications were removed from FDA-approved literature in the late 1970s for unknown reasons." Today, the FDA has approved EDTA as a food additive that is generally recognized as safe. [1715]

11.5.2 EDTA cardiovascular disease (CVD)

"EDTA chelation therapy has recently been proposed for the treatment of patients affected by neurodegenerative (ND) or cardiovascular (CVD) diseases due to its efficacy in removing toxic metals that affect the functions of neurons and endothelial cells." [1716]

The efficacy of EDTA in neurodegenerative diseases (ND) may also depend on its ability to reach the central nervous system, which has been previously demonstrated by means of biodistribution of labeled EDTA." [1717]
Dr. Garry Gordon contends: "EDTA chelation may be one of the most effective, least expensive, and safest treatments for heart disease ever developed, yet it is practiced by perhaps only 2,000 physicians in the United States." [1718]

As we have seen in 5.10.4, the efficacy of EDTA in CVD is also supported by the protective effect against renal ischemia induced in rat models.

EDTA binding affinity
In the EDTA binding affinity table (Fig. 6), it can be seen that EDTA binds **FE3+** more strongly than **Pb2+, Hg2+, Co2+** or **Cd2+**. [1719]

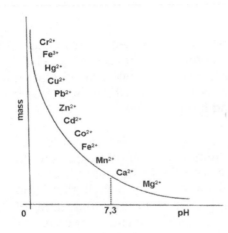

Fig. 6 In vitro affinity of EDTA for metal ions. The curve represents the affinity of EDTA for different metals, in relation with pH and mass; Image Corsello, Serafina et al. (2009). The usefulness of chelation therapy for the remission of symptoms caused by previous treatment with mercury-containing pharmaceuticals: A case report. Cases journal. 2. 199. http://doi.org/10.1186/1757-1626-2-199.

11.5.3 EDTA dosage and safety

"No noticeable toxicity of EDTA in very high doses has been shown in multiple safety testing in healthy animals, leading to the recommended safety doses for human use. In some animal studies, doses up to **2500 mg/kg** body weight have shown no toxicity." [1720]

The EU Risk assessment Report for EDETIC ACID (EDTA) 2004, concluded:

"No acute or chronic respiratory health effects have been observed in workers from exposure to EDTA. There is no valid indication for EDTA as a respiratory sensitizer."

"Thus, regarding repeated dose effects of the substance is **of no concern in relation to indirect exposure via the environment**." [1721]

In one safety assessment, "the lowest dose reported to cause a toxic effect in animals was 750 mg/kg/day." [1722]

For a 70 kg person, this would translate to 52.5 grams per day.

The acute oral Lethal Dose of Disodium EDTA was 3.7 g/kg for both male and female Wistar rats [1723] (or 260 grams for a 70 kg person). In comparison: The lethal dose of table salt is roughly 0.5-1g per kg of body weight. For a 70 kg person, that's 35- 70 grams. So theoretically, table salt is about 5 times more toxic (by lethal dose) than EDTA. [1724]

By the way, Americans eat on average about 3.4g of sodium per day.

Manufacturers of oral EDTA capsules (e.g. Arizona Natural) advice to take up to 1800 mg per day.

"Permissible levels of EDTA calcium disodium salt in food range from 25 to 800 ppm, and an acceptable daily intake of 2.5 mg/kg was established by the Joint FAO/WHO expert Committee on Food Additives (JECFA) in 1975." (For a 70 kg person, that's 175 mg per day only from food additives.) [1725]

The FDA states: EDTA (as Na2EDTA and CaNA2 EDTA) is widely used and FDA-approved as a direct food additive, as a preservative, processing aid, stabilizer and /or chelating agent (e.g. in canned soft drinks, canned vegetables, margarine, pickles) at 25-800ppm (CaNa2EDTA) or 36-500ppm (Na2EDTA). [1726]

The EU allows the same daily intake of 2.5 mg/kg. [1727]

So, for a 70 kg person, the acceptable daily intake from food is only 175mg/ per day, however, for oral EDTA supplements there are only recommendations, no regulations.

Carel Theo Jozef Wreesmann (2014) proposed that the maximum acceptable daily intake of EDTA can be raised to 4.4 or possibly up to 21.7 mg day−1 kgbw−1, which is 2.3–11.4 times higher than the current value.

"For a 5-kg infant, this regulatory change to a maximum ADI of EDTA of 14.9 µmol per day per kg body weight would allow a daily intake up to 5 mg Fe as iron EDTA rather than the currently permitted level of maximum 2.2 mg. With respect to the fortification of complementary foods for infants and young children aged 6–24 months, an addition level ensuring a daily intake of 5 mg Fe as iron EDTA is likely to be sufficient to allow adequate iron absorption and would be entirely safe." [1728]

For a 70 kg adult, the latter value would be 1500 mg per day.

11.5.4 Unintentional chelation therapy via processed foods?

So, the FDA allows 800 parts per million (0.08%) or 0.8 parts per 1000 permille of food can be EDTA.

In particular, the FDA allows 500 ppm (0.05%) in canned strawberry pie filling to "promote color retention", and 315 ppm (0.0315%) in ready-to-eat cereal products containing dried bananas. [1729]

Japan allows 0.25 grams/kg of CaNa2 EDTA in canned and bottled foods. At 2 kg of food consumption per day, that's 500 milligram per day alone from food. [1730]

"The average European consumes approximately 2.13 kg of food per day, or 777 kg /year" [1731]

So, let's put this together:

If you eat an average 2.1 kg of food per day and it's all processed and canned food, you might get up to 1,7 grams of EDTA already. For many with chronic metal toxicity (lead, mercury, cadmium and so on), this could theoretically be beneficial as an unwillingly performed daily "chelation therapy".

In this way, EDTA is one of the few artificial food additives, that can have potential inadvertent health benefits. But unfortunately, these overprocessed foods are rather laden with metals and other chemicals that are of no health benefits and potentially harmful. And ironically, EDTA, as the only synthetic food additive that is potentially beneficial to mitigate chronic diseases, is one of those that law makers and health experts are particularly warning against. EDTA is used as a common food preservative to prevent the oxidative degradation of bile salts into carcinogenic substances. [1732]

"Calcium disodium EDTA is also contained as a preservative in some brands of the following common foods:

Salad dressings, sauces and spreads, mayonnaise, pickled vegetables such as cabbage and cucumbers, canned beans and legumes, canned carbonated soft drinks, distilled alcoholic beverages, canned crab, clam and shrimp." [1733]

In Europe, calcium disodium EDTA may be declared on food labels as food additive E 385 (EU number).

11.5.5 Calcium depletion: Calcium disodium EDTA vs disodium EDTA

When administered intravenously in large doses, calcium disodium EDTA, Versinate, will not deplete calcium if given rapidly, while disodium EDTA will remove calcium through renal excretion in a life-threatening fashion if administered rapidly. [1734]

EDTA is acidic, CaNa2 EDTA is not, and is thus suitable for oral consumption.

"Calcium disodium EDTA (CaNa2 EDTA) is approved by the FDA for use in lead poisoning and has been the mainstay of treatment for childhood lead poisoning since the 1950s." The second drug, disodium EDTA (Na2 EDTA), is approved for use in patients with rhythm disorders from drug intoxication such as digitalis where there is hypercalcemia. [1735]

Chelation in cases of kidney insufficiency

Kidney insufficiency is generally considered a counterindication for chelation therapy. However, with appropriate monitoring, kidney health is often improved or restored by appropriate chelation (see 5.10.4).

In mice, EDTA administration improved renal function after a mechanical kidney injury, even when toxic metals were not evaluated (see 5.10.4).

11.5.6 EDTA administration

EDTA is usually administered intravenously or subcutaneously.
As already mentioned, "the bioavailability of [oral] CaNa2EDTA is low, about 5% of an oral dose is absorbed from the gastrointestinal tract. [1736] Some studies showed an oral absorption of only 2 to 5%,[1737] others of **5 to 18%**. [1738]

Because of the low absorption, oral administration of CaNa2EDTA was long believed to be not practical.

More recently, regiments for EDTA administrated via rectal suppository have been introduced (see below).

11.5.7 Oral EDTA trials

I.V. or oral EDTA?

"Most EDTA chelation therapy carried out today involves I.V. administration of EDTA, however, oral EDTA, which has a history at least as long as its I.V. cousin, is an option that is only now starting to be appreciated. Clinical experience suggests that oral chelation provides some, but not all, of the benefits of I.V. therapy. Overall, the difference in benefits is more one of degree and speed than of quality."

In 1955, a study on the effects of oral EDTA on patients with atherosclerosis and/ or hypertension was conducted on 10 patients. [1739]

"Some of these patients had hypertension, angina pectoris, peripheral vascular disease (intermittent claudication), and one was recovering from a heart attack. All were treated with one gram of **oral** EDTA daily for three months. "Seven of the ten patients experienced significant reductions in their cholesterol levels, and blood pressure was reduced in all ten. In the patient with intermittent claudication, cholesterol was halved." [1740]

And in 1956, in a series of 20 patients who suffered from hypercholesterolemia, hypertension, angina or peripheral vascular disease, one gram of EDTA was administered **orally** every day for 3 months. "During that short time, elevated cholesterol levels in nine of the patients dropped to within the normal range. No adverse results were experienced by any of the patients. Angina attacks were reduced in frequency and severity in five individuals." [1741]

11.5.8 Suppository EDTA

Two studies on magnesium Di-Potassium EDTA suppositories showed: "Liver enzymes remained unchanged (indicating no stress to the liver). BUN/creatinine ratios, bilirubin levels and prothrombin times all showed normalization towards optimal values whether initially high or low."

"92% of the subjects had an increase in blood CO_2 levels, indicating an increase of oxygenation and an increase in metabolic efficiency."

Dr. Bruce W. Halstead, M.D. estimated that approximately 90% or more of suppository EDTA is absorbed through the colon.

"Chelation with magnesium di-potassium EDTA in suppository form is both safe and effective and represents a valid alternative to intravenous chelation with Di-sodium EDTA." [1742]

In rat studies, the absolute bioavailability of CaNa2EDTA in blood following rectal dosing was 36.3% of the IV dose route (100%), "which confirmed that rectal dosing is an efficient method for delivering EDTA to tissues." Thus, theoretically, 3 rectal suppositories (even with regular oral CaNa2EDTA capsules) could replace 1 IV injection of the same dose. Both IV or rectal dosing showed negligible brain localization. "Moreover, the prostate showed greater absorption of suppositories than for IV administration (4x greater). The half-life of rectal administration was over 8 hours."

In human clinical practice "the use of rectal suppositories has proved to be an innovative, effective and simple approach, saving time and money for the patient, and its efficacy and safety have been validated in pre-clinical and clinical studies." [1743]

A patent has been filed for the use of potassium disodium EDTA suppositories. [1744] Absorption rates between 36 and 90 % were measured.

Challenge test dosing

A standard I.V. treatment for a challenge metal test is used regularly in the form of 1.5 grams CaNa2EDTA, (1.5 hours infusion time) plus oral 500 mg DMSA challenge, with a six-hour urine collection for heavy metal analysis. [1745]

11.5.9 Mechanism of action

"When EDTA is injected into the veins, it "grabs" heavy metals and minerals such as **lead, mercury, copper, iron, arsenic, aluminum** and **calcium** and removes them from the body." [1746]

Calcium is bound by EDTA, not by Ca2NaEDTA.

"Neuron protection provided by EDTA may explain the successful outcomes of toxic metal chelation therapy in neurodegenerative diseases." [1747]

"Studies have demonstrated the efficacy of CaNa(2)EDTA for reducing **lead** levels in blood and soft tissues, including brain."

EDTA forms especially strong complexes with **Mn(II), Cu(II), Fe(III) and Co(III)**. [1748]

EDTA: lead and liver

"Chronic exposure to **lead** causes lead to accumulate mainly in the liver." In one study, participants underwent chelation therapy with intravenous CaNa2EDTA for 2 days, followed by treatment with oral D-penicillamine for 90 days. "After chelation, the **mean Liver Stiffness significantly decreased**. Similarly, all of the inflammatory cytokines studied significantly decreased after chelation, and the mean glutathione (GSH) level increased significantly." [1749]

For **aluminum** removal, multiple low doses of Na-EDTA or Ca-EDTA were preferable to high doses, and Ca-EDTA was the better of the two antidotes. [1750]

11.6 Alpha-lipoic acid (ALA or AL)

ALA is an endogenous dithiol with antioxidant properties. [1751] As a supplement, it is prescription free, but it is included here because it has been proven to be effective in mobilizing and removing toxic metals and it is used in combination with DMSA or DMPS in different chelation regiments. ALA is lipophilic and can cross the blood brain barrier, it can remove lead and mercury from the brain. Alpha-lipoic acid is not alpha linolenic acid, sometimes the same abbreviation is used.

"Alpha-lipoic acid ((R)-5-(1,2-Dithiolan-3-yl) pentanoic acid, LA) is an organo-sulfur compound also known as thioctic acid. It is usually produced in the body, and it is essential for aerobic metabolism." It is a low molecular weight **dithiol** antioxidant and an important co-factor in several multienzyme complexes in the mitochondria. [1752]

The dithiol group makes it a "true" chelating agent according to the classification by Dr. Cutler"; (see below).

The reduced form of LA, called **dihydrolipoic acid (DHLA),** contains a pair of thiol groups. The R-enantiomer is the biologically and therapeutically active form. DHLA has high affinity to **Hg** and has been proposed as an effective Hg antidote. " [1753]

Under normal conditions in mammals, lipoic acid is converted rapidly by the cells to dihydrolipoic acid.

11.6.1 ALA chelation of lead

"Lipoic acid in combination with a chelator ameliorates **lead**-induced peroxidative damages in rat kidney." [1754]

In rodent studies, LA in combination with **thiol chelators** effectively chelated **lead** from the brain. "Alpha-lipoic acid has been reported to be highly effective in improving the thiol capacity of the cells and **in reducing lead induced oxidative stress."** [1755]

In a different study, treatment with alpha lipoic acid at three doses showed a significant decrease in blood **lead** levels. "These results confirm that LA is capable of removing lead from the bloodstream and target organs." [1756]

"LA seems to be a good candidate for therapeutic intervention of lead poisoning, in combination with a chelator, rather than as a sole agent." [1757]

Alpha-lipoic acid also has protective effects against **lead**-induced oxidative stress in erythrocytes of rats. [1758]

ALA mercury

"Clinical research confirmed ALAs extent of urinary excretion for the metals **arsenic, barium, manganese, mercury** and **nickel** following oral application." [1759]

"The α-LA compound is suggested for heavy metal detoxification, in particular for supporting the **mercury** detoxifying process." [1760]

Both ALA and DMSA show good bonding to **mercury**. While DMSA shows a stronger effect on **mercury** binding and urinary excretion, it is hydrophilic and therefore cannot pass the blood brain barrier (BBB). [1761]

"α-LA is readily absorbed from the diet and can easily cross the blood brain barrier." [1762]

Alpha-Lipoic Acid protects against neuro-, immuno- and male reproductive toxicity induced by co-exposure to **lead** and **zinc** oxide nanoparticles in rats. [1763]

"Since **oxidative stress is the source of almost all chronic disease and chronic pain,** ALA is an amazing adjunctive molecule to manage the symptoms of these problems." [1764]

"Germany allows ALA to be sold as a nutritional supplement, but also approved ALA as a drug for the treatment of diabetic neuropathy since 1966. "[1765]

11.7 BAL

BAL (British Anti-Lewisite) [2,3-dimercapto propanol] [Dimercaprol] is a dithiol- chelator, it was the predecessor to DMSA and DMPS. It is now used in rare cases due to its toxic side effects. BAL was the first true pharmaceutical chelator, it was developed in 1939 (see *history of chelation therapy*).

"Today BLA is given only in life-threatening cases (e.g., encephalopathy, coma, seizures or BLL >70 µg/dL) in intensive care settings, parenterally (deep intramuscular)."

Usually given only for initial 12–24 hours of therapy; - dissolved in peanut oil. [1766]

11.8 Desferrioxamine

It is also known as deferoxamine or desferal. Desferrioxamine has been the common chelator used therapeutically for **aluminum**. This chelator has proven effective in eliminating aluminum from the body; however, there are a number of toxic side effects associated with its use. [1767]

Deferasirox is also used to treat chronic **iron** overload caused by blood transfusions. It is further used in patients with non-transfusion-dependent thalassemia syndrome, and in patients with elevated liver iron concentration and serum ferritin. [1768] Desferrioxamine chelates **uranium.**

11.9 Disulfiram (Antabuse)

Diethyldithiocarbamate (DDTC) is the reduced form of disulfiram and a powerful chelator of transition divalent metal ions, including copper and zinc. [1769]

"Disulfiram (Antabuse) is a chelating agent used as a therapy for contact dermatitis for metals such as **nickel** and **cobalt**, but its main use is as supportive therapy for alcohol addiction." [1770]

11.10 DTPA (diethylenetriaminepentaacetic acid)

DTPA (diethylenetriaminepentaacetic acid or pentetic acid) is used to chelate, among other metals, gadolinium-based contrast agents (GBCAs) which are introduced to the body in MRI diagnostics. It is used mostly in the form of Zn- DTPA or Ca-DTPA.

According to the FDA, calcium-DTPA (Ca-DTPA) and zinc-DTPA (Zn-DTPA) are drug products that have been used for over 40 years to speed up excretion of the actinide elements plutonium, americium, and curium from the body. DTPA further increases the excretion of **Pb, Cd** and **Hg** but also of the essential metals Mn and Zn. [1771]

11.11 DMG (dimethylglyoxime, not dimethylglycine)

The **nickel** (Ni)-specific chelator dimethylglyoxime (DMG) has been used for many years to detect, quantitate or decrease Ni levels in various environments. [1772]

Dimethylglyoxime forms complexes with metals including **nickel, palladium, platinum** and **cobalt**. [1773]

"Accidental ingestion of the material may be harmful; animal experiments indicate that ingestion of less than 150 gram may be fatal or may produce serious damage to the health of the individual." [1774]

DMG is also known as 2,3-Butanedione dioxide and is also used as a reagent in analytical chemistry for the detection of nickel or palladium. "Further DMG inhibited activity of two Ni-containing enzymes, Salmonella hydrogenase and Klebsiella urease [1775] (see parasites).

11.12 DPA (D-penicillamine) (Cuprimine®)

"Chelating agents such as D-penicillamine and trientine are used as first-line therapies for symptomatic patients of Wilson disease." [1776]

"D-Penicillamine can chelate not only **copper**, but other divalent ions, such as **cadmium, lead, mercury, beryllium**, and **nickel**." [1777] This drug also chelates **iron, gold** [1778] and **zinc**. [1779]

11.13 Ethane-1-hydroxy-1,1-bisphosphonate (EHBP)

Used in uranium toxicity.

11.14 3,4,3-LI(1,2-HOPO)

Is used in uranium poisoning and experimentally in gadolinium poisoning.
"HOPO exhibits low acute toxicity in mice, is well-tolerated at high doses in rats, and shows good oral bioavailability. This is the most promising chelation against uranium toxicity and may be a candidate for clinical trials."

11.15 Prussian Blue (PB)

Prussian Blue is used to chelate non- radioactive and radioactive **thallium** as well as radioactive **cesium**, the latter is why it has been used on large scales after nuclear disasters (cesium 137). It also binds **Co** and **rubidium**.
See all the details on Prussian blue in the paragraph of thallium poisoning (8.41).

11.16 Trientine (copper chelation)

Trientine (triethylene tetramine dihydrochloride or trien) was introduced in 1969.

Copper chelators are a class of drugs used to treat an inherited disorder known as "Wilson's disease," a rare genetic metabolic disorder that causes an excess accumulation of copper in some parts of the body, particularly in the liver. These excess amounts of copper damage the organs which are affected. The only drug belonging to this class is **"trientine,"** a chelating agent used to remove toxic metals from the body (such as **lead, mercury**, or **copper**). [1780]

11.17 TPEN

TPEN, (N,N,N',N'-tetrakis(2-pyridinylmethyl) an uncharged polydentate ligand with nitrogens as donor atoms, 'has remarkably high affinity for a broad spectrum of metal ions, including **copper, iron** and **zinc**.' [1781]

11.18 Tiron, (4,5-dihydroxy-1,3-benzene disulfonic acid)

Tiron forms strong complexes with **titanium** and **iron**, it was use to successfully chelate **vanadium** and **beryllium** from rats. Further, it increases the excretion of **uranium**.

11.19 Citrate (trisodium Citrate or Sodium Citrate)

Citrate is a natural substance, freely available, for instance as sodium citrate (food additive E331) or potassium citrate. It is the dissociated anion of citric acid, a weak acid that is ingested in the diet and produced endogenously in the tricarboxylic acid cycle. [1782]

In mice with acute uranium poisoning, *sodium citrate* or gallic acid produced increased survival rates. [1783]

"Citrate is not only a powerful chelator of Al, but also powerful activator of reverse Na+/Ca2+ exchange in oubain-poisoning fibers." [1784]

In humans the normal plasma citrate concentration is within a range of ~100–150μM.

"The usual nutritional intake of citrate is approximately 4 grams per day and more than 95% of it is absorbed in the small intestine." [1785] Athletes performed better in fitness challenges when supplemented with sodium citrate 0.5 g/kg body mass 3 h prior the challenge. [1786]

11.20 Gallic Acid (3,4,5-trihydroxybenzoic acid)

Gallic acid is naturally found in a variety of plants.
Pharmaceutical grade gallic acid is prescription free, used to chelate **uranium**, it also binds **Al, U, As, Cd, Pb**, [1787] as well as **Hg**. [1788]

If taken orally, "GA is found to be non- toxic up to a dose of 5,000 mg/ kg b.w." [1789]
"Gallic acid can act as a protective agent against the adverse effects of uranyl acetate agent) exposure on the liver." [1790] Uranyl acetate is also used as a chemo-radiological agent.
Red wine contains gallic acid, up to 3,6 mg/100 ml, (comparable by weight with raw blackberries, 4.5mg/ 100 g). Raw chestnuts have 479 mg/100g, walnuts 15, rabbit eye blueberries 23 mg/100g. [1791]
"After oral administration, nearly 70% of GA is absorbed and then excreted via urine as 4-OMeGA."

Chemical name (Common names, abbreviations)	Elements chelated
DMSA 2,3-bis(sulfanyl)butanedioic acid (Dimercaptosuccinic acid; Succimer; Dimercaptosuccinic acid; **DMSA**; Suximer; Tin Salt; Succicaptal; Chemet)	Lead Arsenic Mercury Cadmium Silver Tin Copper Blaurock: Ni Mn Ba Cr Cs Sn Ti
DMPS Sodium 2,3-bis(sulfanyl)propane-1-sulfonate (Sodium Dimercaptopropanesulfonate; Unithiol; Dimaval; Unitiol; (+)-DMPS; (−)-DMPS)	Mercury Arsenic Lead Cadmium Tin Silver Copper Selenium, Zinc Magnesium

279

	Blaurock: Ni Cr Cs Sn Ti
EDTA 2-[2-[bis(carboxymethyl)amino]ethyl-(carboxymethyl)amino]acetic acid (Ethylenediaminetetraacetic acid; Edetic acid;; Edathamil; Endrate; Versene acid; Sequestrol; Titriplex; Havidote; Cheelox; Versene; Calcium Disodium Versenate (edetate calcium disodium injection, USP)	Lead Cadmium Zinc (Mercury)
(2S)-2-amino-3-methyl-3-sulfanylbutanoic acid (3-Sulfanyl-D-valine; **Penicillamine**; D-Penicillamine; Cuprimine; Depen; Penicillamine; Mercaptyl; Artamine; Cuprenil; Perdolat; Trolovol	Copper (Wilson's disease) Arsenic Zinc Mercury Lead
BAL Dimercaprol; British Anti-Lewisite; 2,3-bis(sulfanyl)propan-1-ol (;; 2,3-Dimercaptopropanol; Sulfactin; Dicaptol; Dimersol; Antoxol; Panobal; Dithioglycerine; Dithioglycerol)	Arsenic Gold Mercury Lead (BAL in combination with CaNa2EDTA)
Prussian Blue	Thallium, cesium,
DTPA Pentetic acid diethylenetriaminepentaacetic acid	Gadolinium, Lead, Gallium, Nickel, Silver, Bismuth, Tin

Table 4 Sears, M.E. et al 2013: Chelation: Harnessing and Enhancing Heavy Metal Detoxification—A Review; The Scientific World Journal; Hindawi.com https://www.hindawi.com/journals/tswj/2013/219840/tab1/

Chapter 12
Over-the-counter metal chelators

12.1 Natural metal binding agents

"True chelators are identified by the presence of two thiol groups."
Dr. Andy Cutler cautions "chlorella, cysteine, NAC and glutathione
are not true chelators in the chemical sense, as they do not contain
two or more binding groups (dithiol groups). Instead, they contain
only one thiol group making them ineffectual chelators. [1792]

DMSA, DMPS and EDTA are pharmaceutical chelation agents that
are freely available in many countries and sometimes advertised
as supplements (see each paragraph above).

In the following list, the substances are non- prescription, natural
agents that have the capacity to bind and excrete to a limited extent
heavy metals from the blood and tissue.
They primarily mobilize metals, but have a limited capacity to
excrete these metals. This can lead to unexpected problems of
metal redistribution from fat or bones into brain and other sensitive
organs.
Further, they can act against metal-induced oxidative stress.
These substances are most efficiently used as supplements to
chelation therapy with the above pharmaceutical chelating agents.

12.2 ALA (alpha lipoic acid)

See above (11.6.)

12.3 Citrates

See above 11.19.

12.4 Gallic acid

See above.

12.5 Glutathione

Glutathione is a tripeptide consisting of glutamate, cysteine, and glycine; the most abundant non-protein thiol that defends against oxidative stress. [1793] "In fact, it is a key player in metal-induced oxidative stress defenses." [1794]

"Glutathione is a potent chelator involved in cellular response, transport and excretion of metal cations and is a biomarker for toxic metal overload." [1795]

About 80% of the 8-10 grams glutathione produced daily is produced by the liver and distributed through the blood stream to the other tissues. [1796]

"Glutathione can function as a principal copper and zinc chelator in the cell because it can bind different transition metal ions with high affinity and is present in the cytosol at high concentrations." [1797]

Supplementation

Glutathione is produced by the healthy body in sufficient amounts to constantly detoxify and excrete the normal or natural toxic metal intake. In unnaturally high heavy metal toxicity, at levels that are the norm today, glutathione is sometimes administered therapeutically, in intravenous form.

Oral glutathione has a much lower bioavailability, for the three peptides are disintegrated in stomach acid. If intravenous administration is not an option, rectal suppository glutathione or orobuccal administration have a higher absorption rate.

"Compared to oral administration, whereby under 10% actually enters the blood stream, orobuccal administration (via buccal mucosa) leads to over 80% absorption directly into the systemic circulation." [1798]

"Glutathione need not be orally ingested in order to provide the beneficial effects noted. While the drug may be administered intravenously or parenterally, it may also be administered through mucous membranes, including sublingually, as a vaginal or rectal suppository, and by pulmonary inhaler, for topical applications to the alvcolar surface cells of the lungs to enhance pulmonary protection against unusual pneumonias. Systemic administration of glutathione may be used to concentrate glutathione in lymph nodes, and lymphoid tissues." [1799]

Glutathione levels can also be raised by oral supplementation of two of the 3 components, the peptides that make up glutathione. "Supplementing **glycine (as Dimethyl-glycine) and cysteine (as N-acetylcysteine)** (GlyNAC) in older adults improves glutathione deficiency, oxidative stress, mitochondrial dysfunction, inflammation, physical function, and aging hallmarks." [1800]

When healthy, non-smoking adults received oral reduced glutathione daily, glutathione levels increased significantly in whole blood and erythrocytes. "After 6 months, taking 1000mg glutathione per day increased glutathione levels by 31% in whole blood, by 35% in erythrocytes, and by 250% in buccal cells." [1801]

One recommendation involves a dose of 100 to 400 mg per day, in single or divided doses, for periods of between 10 and 12 weeks, administered by the orobuccal route, preferably using an oral dispersible film. [1802]

12.6 NAC (N-acetylcysteine)

NAC is a type of cysteine, one of the three peptides that constitute glutathione. "Cysteine is considered the rate-limiting factor in cellular glutathione biosynthesis due to its relatively little presence in foods." [1803]

"N-acetylcysteine proved to be an effective agent at increasing the excretion of **chromium** and **boron** and was also able to reverse the oliguria associated with these toxins in rats. " [1804]

A National Institute of Health article says:

"Some antioxidants, such as N-acetyl cysteine (NAC) chelate **lead** and remove it from the bloodstream, reducing blood lead levels in bipolar disorder and this may contribute to an improvement in symptoms." [1805]

"NAC may be useful as an adjuvant in treating various medical conditions, especially chronic diseases, including polycystic ovary disease, male infertility, sleep apnea, acquired immune deficiency syndrome, influenza, parkinsonism, multiple sclerosis, peripheral neuropathy, stroke outcomes, diabetic neuropathy, Crohn's disease, ulcerative colitis, schizophrenia, bipolar illness, and obsessive-compulsive disorder; it can also be useful as a chelator for **heavy metals and nanoparticles**." [1806]

Placebo-controlled trials conducted across a wide range of disease setting have further reported beneficial effects of oral NAC treatment, including in HIV, CF, colon cancer, protein energy malnutrition, Alzheimer disease and bronchitis. [1807]

As we have seen, most the above conditions can also be caused directly by heavy metal toxicity.

Nanoparticles may decrease DNA methylation. "Preclinical studies show that NAC reverses and prevents the oxidative damage caused by engineered nanoparticles." [1808] see also *Nanoparticles*, Chapter 9.).

Dr. Peter Smith says "NAC cysteine is reputedly effective at reducing mucus in the lungs and sinuses, this form of cysteine has been shown to have **antidepressant, antianxiety** and **anti-addiction affects.** " [1809]

NAC combination therapy with DMSA:

"NAC forms coordination bonds between metals and its thiol group. The thiol may also reduce free radicals." Combined administration of NAC and DMSA after **arsenic** exposure led to a significant reduction of oxidative stress biomarkers, as well as to removal of arsenic from organs. [1810]

Administration

In clinical trials, "Oral bioavailability of total NAC was 9.1%." [1811]

Manufacturers claim their NAC rectal suppositories provide 80-85% absorption. [1812]

"Eating high protein foods can provide your body with the amino acid cysteine, but you can also take NAC as a supplement to help treat certain conditions." The accepted daily [oral] supplement recommendation is 600–1,800 mg of NAC. [1813]

A clinical study on preterm infants with Meconium Ileus (small-bowel obstructions) concluded that orally administered n-acetyl cysteine is tolerable and as effective as rectal n-acetyl cysteine. [1814]

12.6.1 Covid and NAC:

"Despite greater baseline risk, use of NAC in COVID-19 patients was associated with significantly lower mortality." [1815"]

A 2021 Covid study published in *Infectious Diseases* looked at the effects of NAC supplementation. Researchers said "taking 600 mg NAC orally (by mouth) twice daily for 14 days led to: reduced disease progression, reduced need for intubation (breathing tube) and fewer deaths." [1816]

After decades of distribution as a supplement, the FDA declared in July 2020 that NAC was not a legal dietary ingredient because of its prior approval as a drug. [1817]

Which was a bit of an unfortunate timing considering the global vaccination efforts involving nanoparticles of a new generation.

NAC is available again for now.

12.7 DMG Dimethyl- glycine (not dimethylglyoxime)

DMG is not a chelator per se, but a methyl doner, glycine is a component of glutathione (see above). "When glycine availability is too low to sustain normal rates of glutathione synthesis, the consequent rise in tissue levels of gamma-glutamyl cysteine results in increased conversion of this compound to 5-L-oxoproline that is then excreted in the urine." [1818]

12.8 Chlorella

Do only take chlorella from strictly controlled production in fresh water tanks!
Chlorella vulgaris can cross the blood-brain barrier, but does not make a strong bond to metal ions due to having only one thiol group, and in this way, it may allow the re-distribution of toxic metals into the brain.
"Chlorella species are mainly freshwater algae and are particularly common in very nutrient-rich waters. They are also often found growing on soil." [1819]
The living chlorella algae absorbs toxic metals, and is used in this way to remediate soils. When used in this process, the plants must afterwards be disposed of, and must not be composted and reintroduced into agriculture. Chlorella is also used to remove toxic metals in water treatment. [1820]
Most studies on the efficacy of chlorella as a metal absorber are concerning removal of metals from soils and water, rather than from the human body. Most brands of dietary chlorella are produced in China in uncontrolled conditions, where they can absorb toxic metals from contaminated water as they grow, and can later inadvertently cause overall metal absorption into the body, rather than excretion.
"In rats previously fed **cadmium**, chlorella intake did not significantly facilitate renal and intestinal MT synthesis and urinary **Cd** excretion." [1821]
Seegarten Klinik, Switzerland warns of the unwarranted use of chlorella. In lab tests, 6 randomly selected brands of chlorella were all shown to contain **lead**, most contained various other toxic metals. [1822]

In acute poisoning, mice previously administered **thallium** and **strontium,** when subsequently treated with high doses of oral chlorella (1000 mg/70 kg), showed increased excretion of **strontium** (+46.40%) and **thallium** (+38.39%) through feces and urine. This does not allow conclusions about the excretion in cases of chronic, long-term metal poisoning. [1823]

The long-term algae extract (chlorella and fucus sp) and aminosulphurate supplementation modulate sod-1 activity and decrease heavy metals (**Hg++, Sn**) levels in patients with long-term dental **titanium** implants and **amalgam** fillings restorations. [1824]

Chlorella vulgaris extract (CVE, 1800 mg/day) over 6 weeks significantly improved physical and cognitive symptoms of depression as well as anxiety symptoms in patients who are receiving standard antidepressant therapy. [1825]

Supplementation with microalgae Chlorella vulgaris has beneficial effects in patients with non-alcoholic fatty liver disease (NAFLD): "Significant weight- reducing effects were measured after eight weeks. Moreover, C. vulgaris supplementation showed meaningful improvements in liver enzymes and reduction in C-reactive protein (CRP) values." [1826]

12.9 Coriander (Cilantro)

Coriander, like Chlorella, can cross the blood brain barrier, but does not make a strong bond to metal ions, and in this way, it may allow not only the removal from, but the redistribution of toxic metals into the brain.

Coriander is an annual herb in the family Apiaceae. It is also known as Chinese parsley, Vietnamese parsley, dhania, or cilantro. Coriandrum sativum is an herb belonging to Umbelliferae and is reported to have a protective effect against **lead** toxicity. [1827]

"Cilantro originated in the regions of Southern Europe, Northern Africa, and Southwest Asia. Cilantro has been cultivated and used by humans as medicine and in food for far longer than parsley, with descriptions of the herb found in texts as old as 1550 BC. The plant was even found preserved in Tutankhamen's tomb." [1828]

In rat studies, **lead** injection caused an increase in plasma lead levels while cilantro significantly reduced these levels. [1829]

Coriander (corindrum sativum) was also shown to have a protective effect against **lead** toxicity in rabbits. [1830]

12.9.1 Wild Bear's Garlic (Allium ursinum)

Wild Bear's Garlic extracts are used in holistic medicine to mobilize mercury and to ideally facilitate their excretion (Dr. Klinghardt). Here as well, due to weak bonds, metals can in some cases be redistributed instead of excreted.

Like chlorella, wild Bear's Garlic can absorb toxic metals not only in the body, but also from the soil and water during growth. Its bioaccumulation factor (BAF) is high for K, Ca, Zn, **As**, and medium for Mg, **Cu, B, Ni**, Na, **Pb**. [1831] When plants are gathered from contaminated locations (near cities, near former industrial zones), more metals may be introduced into the body than are excreted from it.

12.10 Zeolite

Zeolite is a volcanic mineral that has some ability to absorb metals. In ideal circumstances, oral medical grade zeolite can absorb some toxic metals from the body, but primarily from the digestive tract.

A more effective use of zeolite is in remediation of agricultural soil. Natural zeolite has been used for heavy-metal remediation as a single additional phase to polluted soil or combined with other minerals.It can restrain **lead** uptake by plants in lead contaminated soils. The appropriate zeolite dose to significantly reduce soluble lead is ≥10 g/kg. [1832] Zeolite can absorb lead in the soil, even when the zeolite is taken up by the plant and the plant is consumed by humans, **lead** absorption can be limited; some of the lead is excreted with the zeolite.

"Such remediation technologies are based on heavy metal immobilization through processes of stabilization/solidification (S/S)." [1833]

"A reason for concern in human supplementation is the leakage of **lead** from clinoptilolite, which the mineral can previously absorb from the ground." At pH 3 and higher, the Pb leakage was less than 1%, while at pH 1, the leakage was observed up to 20% of the initial lead content. [1834]

In unfavorable conditions, this could introduce mor lead into the body than is extracted from it.

One study on healthy men aged 36 to 70 years, did show that the use of the above mentioned naturally occurring zeolite, clinoptilolite, significantly increased the urinary excretion **of**

aluminum, antimony, arsenic, bismuth, cadmium, lead, mercury, nickel and **tin** as compared to placebo controls. [1835]

In the human body, "data from longer-term studies suggest that zeolite supports the mobilization of some heavy metals (e.g., **lead**) from storage pools including bone tissue." However, mobilization is not equal to excretion.

"In long-term supplementation trials, zeolite diminished essential **Na** and **Ca** in osteoporosis patients. In the short- and long-term supplementation trials, increased levels of **lead** were observed in zeolite-supplemented subjects." [1836]

12.11 Modified Citrus Pectin (MCP)

Published clinical studies demonstrate that the supplement Modified Citrus Pectin (MCP), a highly bio-available form of pectin, safely removes toxic metals such as **lead, mercury**, and **arsenic** from the body without disrupting essential minerals.

"In addition to its cancer-inhibiting effects, modified citrus pectin shows promise in chelating toxic heavy metals that can be damaging to overall health." [1837] In one study, there was a 150% increase in the excretion of **cadmium** and a 560% increase in **lead** excretion on day six.

"In a case study report, five patients with different illnesses were given MCP or an MCP/alginate complex for up to seven months. patients had a 74% average decrease in toxic heavy metals and positive clinical outcomes after treatment. [1838]

In a 2008 pilot study at the Children's Hospital of Zhejiang University, Hangzhou, China, seven children hospitalized with toxic **lead** levels, aged five to 12, were given 15 grams of MCP (PectaSol®) per day in three divided dosages. All of the children had a significant increase in urinary excretion of lead. [1839]

Magnesium - Lead treatment experimental
Rats that were fed high amounts of **lead** compounds in the diet, when also given magnesium, had significantly lower lead levels of bones than those given lead alone. With magnesium, also enzyme levels approached normal values at 106 days. [1840]

12.12 Zinc

Zinc supplementation has beneficial effects during chelation treatment of **lead** intoxication in rats. [1841]

"When Zn2+ is administered with **Cd2+** during chronic Cd2+ exposure, it prevents the development of renal dysfunction and Fanconi syndrome." [1842]

Zinc supplementation protects against **cadmium** accumulation and cytotoxicity in madin-darby bovine kidney cells. [1843]

"Zinc is one of the most well studied essential metals for the alleviation of heavy metal toxicity." [1844]

"Zinc in zinc supplements can be in the form of zinc sulfate, zinc gluconate, zinc acetate, or zinc citrate, all water-soluble zinc salts." (For more on the interaction of essential minerals and toxic metals see also 1.9.)

12.12.1 Antioxidant nutrients and lead toxicity

Antioxidant nutrients, including **vitamin E, vitamin C, vitamin B6, β-carotene, zinc,** and **selenium** are proposed to have a beneficial role in **lead**-induced oxidative stress. [1845]

Different studies corroborate N-acetylcysteine (NAC), zinc, vitamins B6, C and E, selenium, taurine, and alpha-lipoic acid have been shown to interrupt or minimize the damaging effects of **lead** and improve the effects of pharmaceutical chelating agents. [1846]

"Vitamin E and melatonin can prevent the majority of metal-mediated (**iron, copper, cadmium**) damage both in vitro systems and in metal-loaded animals." [1847]

"Administration of natural and synthetic antioxidants like quercetin, catechin, taurine, captopril, gallic acid, melatonin, N-acetyl cysteine, α- lipoic acid and others have been recognized in the disease prevention and clinical recovery against heavy metal intoxication." [1848]

For all the above-mentioned substances, check the daily allowable value.

Chapter 13
Common protocols of diagnosis and chelation therapies

The first action to be taken against metal toxicity should always be avoidance. Some unusual and preventable sources can often be identified and eliminated, such as old lead paint in a house, using metal cookware, smoking, workplace toxins etc.

But in the modern world, a limited exposure and life- long accumulation is unavoidable. Once the source is removed, the chronic body burden may persist for years, often decades without proper chelation treatment.

Mercury in air, soil and food, thallium and arsenic in vegetables, aluminum in skincare products, lead in drinking water and so on.

So there is little benefit in contemplating whether or not you have been exposed to some levels of toxic metals. Most people (especially adults) have some toxic metal burden, with a solid potential to affect their health.

The only way of knowing your baseline toxicity is adequate laboratory testing (For preliminary clinical, visual indicators - which can easily be checked - see 10.2.1).

One simple and cheap measure for improving overall health, with and without metal toxicity, is adequate mineral and vitamin supplementation (see below).

The following does not constitute medical advice!

In cases of suspected metal toxicity, here are two possible procedures for laboratory metal diagnosis:

Option 1: Find a certified metal toxicologist (medical doctor) or holistic therapist who performs a challenge (provoked) urine test for the most relevant metals (15 – 40 elements or preferably more) and if indicated, chelation with the appropriate pharmaceutical chelating agents (EDTA, DMSA etc.) They will probably also suggest a complete blood count. They may recommend a normal (unprovoked) blood metal test as well to get a better picture of the difference between acute metal accumulation and long-term metal storage.

In cases of chronic metal poisoning, unprovoked tests alone are not conclusive and can only give general indications for some metals to be interpreted by an experienced practitioner. If a holistic practitioner only offers an unprovoked urine-, blood- or hair test or no laboratory test at all and claims to detox heavy metals with natural agents, then these claims are unsubstantiated and the treatment is likely ineffective or even dangerous.

Professional help is advised in cases where chelation is applied for metals which are still present in the body as solid foreign objects. For instance, if amalgam fillings are not removed, mercury chelation must not be performed. Cobalt chelation is sometimes performed with cobalt prostheses in the body, lead chelation is sometimes performed with lead bullet fragments still in the body, and so on.

Option 2: not recommended by general practitioners:
Some people with suspected metal toxicity have performed their own protocol of a challenge test at home using a certified heavy metal urine test available online, which is sent into the lab for diagnostic processing (challenge urine tests are generally not for children). Small doses of oral EDTA (1800mg) and oral DMSA (150-300 mg) have been safely administered, and the urine was subsequently collected for 4- 24 hours (see 13.1.4.).

Mail-in urine tests with a home-collection kit are available for around 100 USD, they ideally cover a broad range of toxic metals. In central Europe for instance, the German lab Medivere [1849] covers 17 of the most relevant metals (essential and non- essential). In the US, Doctor's Data is the standard test lab for home collection urine metal tests (they test for 38 non-essential and essential elements, ca. 200 USD). [1850] In Germany, practitioners have access to a Biovis Diagnostik heavy metal urine test for 38 metals, test results are calibrated to the prior administration of a chelating agent (provoked urine test).

Most tests and the interpretation of the results provided by the test labs are not intended by the manufacturers for challenge tests, but are frequently and effectively used as such by practitioners and metal toxicologists. Your health practitioner outside the US might offer a lab test covering more than 38 metals (the more the better) as long as it is a provoked (challenge) urine test.

13.1 Treatment/ chelation therapy

Some metals are chelated by toxicologists and holistic practitioners with chelating agents that are freely available in many countries.
In most cases, IV administration is more effective, but sometimes practitioners preferer non-IV administration in the form of oral capsules (often used with DMSA and DMPS, sometimes with EDTA), rectal suppositories (EDTA), or buccal mucosa administration (EDTA).
Some patients with a thorough understanding of their medical situation and their challenge test results have successfully chelated their toxic metals with specific chelating agents, which are available prescription-free online.
The choice of the prescription-free chelating agents or combinations thereof could be evaluated according to the test results using a list such as the one provided above of the *Toxic Metals of Concern* and their appropriate chelating agents (Chapter 8). In this list, each element has a treatment paragraph at the end.

In the case of EDTA chelation, if intravenous (IV) EDTA is not an option, it can be substituted with rectal suppositories or oral mucosal administration of regular NaCa2 EDTA vegan capsules for better absorption than swallowed oral NaCa2EDTA. Oral mucosal administration means letting capsules dissolve slowly between the gums and the buccal mucosa.
IV EDTA is supposed to have up to 100% bioavailability. For rectal suppositories, it is up to 36%. An established protocol for rectal EDTA has been used with 750 mg, 3 times per week for 6 months. [1851]

Orally swallowed EDTA is absorbed only 5- 18 % and doses of more than 1800 mg per day over longer times can be harmful to the stomach or kidney (see EDTA dosage and safety).
Manufacturers of oral EDTA capsules (e.g. Arizona Natural) advice to take 1800 mg per day.

Oral DMSA in capsules of up to 100 mg or DMPS 5 mg have been purchased online, they are available in many countries, for instance at mandimart dot eu, and maybe consumed according to the labels. **Buyers must make sure to comply with their countries' laws and regulations!**
CaNa2 EDTA by brands like Arizona Natural have been purchased for instance from iherb dot com in 600 mg capsules.

When toxic metals are diagnosed which are not effectively chelated with freely available chelators such as EDTA or DMSA, then a health practitioner with access to the appropriate chelators may be the only option. Examples are DTPA for gadolinium, DMG (DMGlyoxime) for nickel, medical grade Prussian blue for thallium and cesium, cobalt etc. Most of these chelating agents must also be administered IV or subcutaneously.

Medical grade Prussian blue is prescription based.
Companies like Kremer Pigments produce high-quality industrial grade Prussian blue pigments, which are technically the same as medical grade Radiogardase. But Prussian blue pigments from unknown sources should not be used for chelation therapy, as the manufacturing process is not monitored.
Do not ingest factory grade Prussian blue pigments from unknown sources, they may contain undeclared chemicals and toxic metals.

Mucosal or rectal suppositories (for better bioavailability than oral administration) are therapeutically used not only for EDTA, but also for DMSA, glutathione and NAC (see oral bioavailability of each substance in 12.1.)
Sodium citrate and **gallic acid** are natural compounds used against uranium poisoning. Both are prescription free. Gallic acid chelates **Al, Cd, Pb** and **U**. Gallic acid has a chelating effect in cases of **iron** overload and is effective against **arsenic** induced oxidative stress.

13.1.1 Essential metals/ mineral supplementation

DMSA causes not only excretion of toxic metals, but also of essential minerals, chromium and potassium, which must be supplemented subsequently within the daily upper limit of each mineral. [1852] "EDTA chelation therapy may decrease levels of certain vitamins and minerals in the body, including vitamin C, magnesium, iron, and calcium." [1853] Here, Ca is not excreted with CaNa2 EDTA. "If [DMPS] 100 mg is applied for a longer period, it may affect the mineral balance, primarily of the elements zinc and copper." [1854]
Monitoring of the urinary excretion of the toxic metals and of essential trace elements should be carried out regularly during long-term therapy.

293

All essential metals (at least the primary 11 minerals) should be orally supplemented in sufficient amounts with at least the recommended daily value (even without chelation therapy). In fact, two different mechanisms make almost all people mineral deficient in one way or another, independently from metal toxicity: 1.) As our food and drinking water contains only half of the minerals it did in the 1940s, it is very likely that even healthy people who eat a natural diet are mineral deficient nowadays. 2. Toxic metals and other toxins prevent proper uptake of present minerals. (See also *Lack of essential Minerals*, 1.9.)

Supplementing the daily value of all essential minerals independently of any symptoms is an easy, safe precaution to improve or maintain overall health.
This can be done with, for instance, an all-in-one mineral and vitamin supplement mixture: 13 vitamins, 11 minerals, most products contain only 13 vitamins and 10 minerals (potassium not included). The primary 10 comprise:
Magnesium, calcium, iron, copper, zinc, manganese, molybdenum, iodine, selenium and **cobalt.**
Potassium, (if not contained in an all-in-one supplement) can be added in the form of potassium chloride (as salt substitute, not more than 1/8 of a teaspoon per day).
Sodium **(Na)** and phosphate **(P)** are essential elements, but deficiency is extremely rare; due to table salt intake, overload of Na is more common.
Disputed essential elements are **V, Li, B, Ni** and **Sr**. They were demonstrated to have biological roles, but no cases of deficiency of these elements were proven, so supplementation is generally not recommended.

Essential metals that did not show the required body store (deficiency) according to the challenge urine test, have been supplemented with higher doses than the recommended daily value (but within the upper limit for daily intake).
Various essential metals can have different upper limits of daily intake. For instance, for zinc, up to 2.6 times the recommended daily value (minimum amount) can be consumed per day. For magnesium it is 1x, meaning the recommended daily value is the same as the upper limit. One should get it just right.
Values for all essential elements (minerals) are shown in Table 5.

Nutrient (mineral/ Vitamin)	The Daily Value, as in food labels; it is mostly the same as the Recommended Dietary Allowance (RDA)	UL (Tolerable Upper Intake Levels, USA) for food and suppl. combined. Or SUL*	Ratio Safe UL/ Daily Value
The essential 11 Minerals			
Calcium	1000 mg	2500 mg	2.5x
Magnesium	400 mg	400 mg*	**1x**
Selenium	70 mcg	400 mcg	5.7x
Zinc	15 mg	40 mg	2.6x
Copper	2 mg	10 mg	5x
Chromium	120 mcg	10,000 mcg*	83x
Iodine	150 mg	1100mg	7.3x
Iron	18 mg	45 mg	2.5x
Manganese	2 mg	11 mg	5.5
Molybdenum	75 mcg	200mcg	2.6x
Potassium	3500 mg	3700 mg*	1.2x
Disputed Essential Min.			
Vanadium	-	1.8mg	-
Nickel	-	1000 mcg	-
Boron	-	20 mg	-
Vitamin C	60 mg	2000 mg	33x
Vitamin D	10 mcg (400 IU)	100 mcg	10x
Vitamin E (alpha-tocopherol)	20 (30 IU) mg	1000 mg	50x

Table 5 The Daily Value is what is on food labels; it is mostly the same as the Recommended Dietary Allowance (RDA) USA. - UL = Tolerable Upper Intake Level (UUSA); Ratio Save UL/Daily Value = (an adult can take this many times the Daily Value without exceeding the UL; for instance: an adult should not take more than 5.7 times the recommended daily amount of selenium; Data by C. Alan Titchenal, PhD, CNS. Originally published in: NASM Certified Personal Trainer Course Manual, 2004, pp. 632-633; Copyright ©: National Academy of Sports Medicine - www.nasm.org http://www.nutritionatc.hawaii.edu/UL.htm

Apart from vitamins and minerals, a common deficiency that can often be corrected with supplements is omega-3 fatty acids.

13.1.2 Combination chelation therapy

In mice with acute **lead** poisoning, when undergoing EDTA monotherapy, lead was reduced in kidneys. Combined treatment with EDTA plus DMSA reduced lead in kidneys, brain and femur. Urine lead elimination was increased by EDTA monotherapy 10 times, and by combined treatments 14–15 times. [1855]

"In lead-treated rats, a DMSA and CaNa2EDTA combination was superior to either drug on its own, in depleting organ and bone **lead**, normalizing lead-sensitive biochemical measures with no redistribution of lead to any other organ. DMSA was the only drug that resulted in decreased brain lead levels." [1856]

"EDTA- DMSA compared to EDTA results in a greater reduction in blood **Pb** during chelation therapy." [1857]

13.1.3 Additional supplements

As mentioned above, sodium citrate and gallic acid are over the counter natural compounds effectively used to chelate uranium. Gallic acid also chelates Al, Cd, Pb, As and Fe.

For the support of pharmaceutical chelation agents such as DMPS, DMSA, EDTA or medical grade Prussian blue, over-the-counter supplements and antioxidants have been used by patients according to their labels. When any of them turned out to be symptomatically beneficial, they have been continued. The following over- the-counter substances can reduce oxidative stress caused by toxic metals or have metal- chelating abilities themselves:

Alpha Lipoic Acid (ALA), N-Acetyl-Cysteine (NAC), Dimethyl-Glycine (DMG), sodium citrate, sodium bicarbonate, gallic acid, glutathione and modified citrus pectin.

(Oral glutathione bioavailability is low, orobuccal or rectal suppositories have a higher efficacy): As we saw above, "Compared to oral administration, whereby under 10% actually enters the blood stream, orobuccal administration leads to over 80% absorption directly into the systemic circulation."

Non pharmaceutical, natural chelation agents such as **chlorella, cilantro (coriander) or zeolite** have been recommended by leading metal toxicologists for limited absorption of metals (mostly gastrointestinal).

Take chlorella only from controlled quality production in water tanks! As chlorella can absorb limited amounts of metals from the body, it readily absorbs toxic metals from water and soil during production, before it is used.

Potassium chloride is used as table salt substitute to lower blood pressure in general and also as a metal mobilizer (mostly in assistance for thallium and cesium chelation with Prussian blue).

13.1.4 Examples of typical provocation test protocols:

"There is no standard, validated challenge [urine] test." Government agencies often site this as evidence that challenged urine tests are not valid. state and medical industry argue: 'We have regulated safe limits of (unprovoked) urine metal concentrations and blood metal concentrations. So, what are the recommended safe limits for challenged urine metal concentrations?'

Well, the CDC declared there is no safe level of **lead** in the body, therefore the safe limits for urine lead concentration is ZERO. So also challenged urine lead should be zero.

DMSA

A typical provocation test protocol is being used by Autism Research Institute to test children with autism for **mercury, lead** and **cadmium** toxicity: 9-doses of DMSA are given over the course of 3 days; 1 dose =10 mg/kg. Just before administering the last dose, void the bladder, and then collect all urine for the next 8- 10 hours. "Bradstreet et al have established a reference range for typical children, based on a study of 18 typical children vs. 221 children with autism. Using Doctor's Data Laboratory, they reported levels of 1.29 mcg **Hg**/g-creatinine, 15.0 mcg **Pb**/g-creatinine, and 0.46 mcg **Cd**/g-creatinine in typical children given DMSA. Children with autism had, on average, 3x higher levels of **Hg** excretion." [1858] **In general, 3 days before test sample collection:** "Stop supplements with creatinine, vitamin C, any minerals that are on the list being tested and seafood."

"Other advocates prefer to simplify dosing recommendations. They suggest a dosage for toxic metal detection in adults to be 2x 500 mg of DMSA, as a challenge substance, taken 4 hours apart. The 2x 500 mg is considered a conservative, but effective dose for adults weighing between 40 and 80 kg. This protocol may be done following 1-2 days of DMSA at similar doses to allow greater time for re-equilibration of body pools." [1859]

"Take 2 tabs of 250 mg DMSA (500 mg total) and then collect your urine in the provided container for the next 6 hours. This must be kept in the refrigerator during the entire 6 hour period." [1860]

EDTA+ DMSA challenge test protocol

These are the recommendations by the commercial test provider Zetpil test kit. When these products are taken as a suppository, DMSA (260 mg) are inserted first, followed by two suppositories of CaNa(2)EDTA (2x 850 mg). [1861]

DMPS
P.J. Muran M.D. reported DMPS provocation using oral DMPS 10 mg/kg body weight up to a maximum of 500 mg as a one-time dose. The next 6-hour cumulative urine was collected, mixed well, and sent to Doctors Data, Inc, for analysis. [1862]

Chapter 14
Less prevalent Sources of toxic Metals

14.1.1 Naturopathic medicine/ Medicinal herbs

In holistic medicine, various herbal remedies are sometimes marketed as heavy metal detox methods. Unfortunately, some (not all) of these preparations contain more toxic metals than they can extract from the body. A wide range of "alternative" medicines contain dangerous loads of toxic metals. Just as arsenic used to be prescribed for syphilis, because it can briefly mitigate symptoms, as long as the devastating long-term effects of chronic arsenic poisoning are ignored. In this way, ayurvedic and other medicine are proclaimed by many as a safe alternative to pharmaceutics without any awareness of the accompanying long-term metal toxicity.

"It is estimated that about 70–80% of the world's population relies on non-conventional medicine, mainly of herbal origin. However, owing to the nature and sources of herbal medicines, they are sometimes contaminated with toxic heavy metals such as **lead, arsenic, mercury** and **cadmium.**" [1863]

In medicinal plants which are widely consumed in Brazil, 16 different non-essential, toxic metals were found. [1864]

"**Cadmium, lead** and other toxic metals are commonly found in high doses in medicinal herbs in India." [1865]

"Some Ayurvedic medicines and other traditional medicines may contain harmful heavy metals including **mercury** and **arsenic**." [1866]

"A recent study found that one out of every five Ayurvedic medications purchased online contained **lead, mercury**, or **arsenic**." [1867]

"One study showed that 64% of samples of traditional Indian remedies collected in India contained significant amounts of **lead.** (64% contained **mercury,** 41% **arsenic** and 9% **cadmium).**" [1868]

In a Boston study, 20% of locally available traditional Indian herbal medicine products contained harmful levels of **lead, mercury** and/or **arsenic**. [1869]

In Germany, ayurvedic medicine products from India, sold on the internet globally were found to contain 95,000 times the amount of

mercury allowed in Germany. 6 different products contain concentrations of **lead** 70 times and **cadmium** 111 times over the legal limit. [1870]

Some Chinese therapeutic foods and herbs frequently consumed by people in both the East and West were found to contain heavy metals above the FDA safe limits. [1871]

"The FDA also warns of disturbingly high levels of heavy metals found in kratom products," said FDA Commissioner Scott Gottlieb, M.D. [1872] Kratom is an herbal extract supplement that is sold as an energy booster, mood enhancer, pain reliever and antidote for opioid withdrawal.

Albert M. Li proposed: "Even though still relatively rare, heavy metal poisoning with Chinese medicinal herbs (CMH) should always be suspected if a previously healthy child develops unusual symptoms, especially those involving the central nervous system." [1873]

Cd, Ni, and **Pb** were accumulated in different parts of the medicinal plant Mentha piperita (the most common medicinal plant in Romania). [1874]

14.1.2 Ritual use of toxic metals

"Ritual use of **mercury** is common in much of the United States." [1875]

"In some cultures, occult rituals represent an important source for exposure and poisoning with elemental **mercury**. " [1876]

In 1997, the New York Times reported hundreds of children in the South Bronx had to be tested for poisoning by **mercury**, a toxic substance that researchers say is used in some homes in religious and mystic rituals by immigrants from the West Indies and Latin America. "Studies in Chicago and New York found that believers in the magic powers of **mercury** use a few drops to clean their floors or mix it in their bath water or in their perfume. Some swallow it, put it under the bed in a cup of water, pour it in a candle and then burn it." [1877]

The US task force on ritualistic uses of **mercury** reports:

"In many urban areas in the United States, religious supply stores known as botanicas sell a variety of herbal remedies and religious items used in certain Latino and Afro-Caribbean traditions, including Santería, Palo, Voodoo, and Espiritismo. The involved religions evolved from native faiths brought to the New World by African slaves." [1878]

In Romania, occult practices involving elemental **mercury** imply mostly drinking liquids with mercury in order to protect marriage or to have good luck and money. "Traditional Romanian witchcraft which implies putting **mercury** in hidden places of the house is used to curse one's enemies." [1879]

At the National Poisoning Centre in Romania alone, about 200 cases of related acute **mercury** poisoning are admitted to ERs. [1880] Subsequent disease and deaths due to chronic poisoning (the majority of cases) go unreported.

Some Romani claim "Gypsies could create spells ordering **mercury** to kill a target." [1881]

If someone places mercury in the enemy's house (where it will evaporate to be inhaled by the occupants), that's attempted murder or manslaughter, if they place it in their own house, that's self-deletion.

CaEDTA was used to avoid damage from acute **Pb** poisoning in an infant who received traditional Omani medicine (which was found to contain high **Pb**) for constipation. [1882]

A 15- year- old American boy injected mercury into his forearms because he wanted to "become a Marvel superhero." The resulting ulcers and infections could be treated; the liquid mercury was removed - at least the visible droplets - and skin grafts were placed. The surgeons say there was no systemic mercury poisoning and the incident was brushed off as a lucky recovery. The media treated it as a joke. However, the long-term consequences could turn out to be devastating, since provoked testing and chelation therapy was not initiated. In this case, only serum- and unprovoked urine tests were performed. [1883]

14.2 Vegan diet and heavy metals

"People on primarily plant-based diets (including vegans, vegetarians and even flexitarians) are likely to consume more heavy metals than people consuming primarily animal-based food products." A published study from Slovak Medical University in the Czech Republic (2006), found in healthy adults that the vegetarian group had significantly higher blood **cadmium** levels than those who were non-vegetarian. [1884]

Other studies corroborate that a vegetarian diet possesses higher levels of **cadmium** compared to a nonvegetarian diet. [1885] "The levels were high enough in some vegans to raise the concern of the researchers." [1886]

Protein powders

The *vegan review* warns: "The biggest concern of all protein powders, whether they are whey or plant-based, are heavy metals." [1887]

The most concerning four metals are again the "Big Four".

Studies from the Clean Label Project 2018 tested 134 top-selling protein powders. More than 75% of plant-based protein powders had measurable levels of **lead**. [1888]

Here are some results from this study: Organic protein powders had on average 2x the heavy metals of conventional ones.

Egg protein was the cleanest with the least heavy metals/toxins.

Plant-based powders were, on average, the most toxic. [1889]

Vegetarians and vegans are more likely to be depressed than meat eaters. A collation of 18 studies involving 160,257 people, concluded that people who did not eat meat had significantly higher rates of depression, anxiety and self-harm.

"In fact, it was suggested that turning to vegetarianism or veganism could itself be a 'behavioral marker', meaning that these individuals were already experiencing poor mental health." [1890]

"Men who go vegetarian are more likely to have serious depression. Vegetarian men have more depressive symptoms after adjustment for socio-demographic factors." [1891]

Further, toxic metals and other endocrine disrupting chemicals can cause suppression of sex-hormone regulation and depression. Depression, anxiety and oversensitivity may cause some people to become vegetarians in the first place. And then everybody is angry at each other: depression, anxiety and anorexia may cause some people to go vegan, the metals are not excreted despite all the "detoxing", they keep losing weight. And then obese people (who might have thyroid under function from chronic arsenic toxicity) tell vegans to get some meet on their bones, and then they accuse people of average weight of "fat shaming". And some average weight people are indeed mean to either obese or anorexic people and accuse them of having low self-control. Some people go vegan and gain weight and so on.

And so everybody is screaming at each other while suffering from hormonal imbalance, dismissing the probable contributors to body dysmorphia and abnormal BMI: metal toxicity and other toxins that cause chronic oxidative stress and hormonal damage.

Even people on gluten-free diets have higher heavy metal toxicity.

In an analysis of data collected from NHANES, persons on a GFD had significantly higher urine levels of total **arsenic** and blood levels of **mercury, lead** and **cadmium** than persons not avoiding gluten. [1892] Here again, we combine this with the fact that chronic heavy metal toxicity is associated with allergies. Cause and effect may not be clearly distinguished here either.

14.2.1 The "Soy Boys" insult

Some natural foods, such as soy, have endocrine disrupting properties, they are endocrine disrupting substances, but are technically not counted as EDCs.

Many young men are becoming vegetarian or vegan these days - as is promoted heavily by politicians, the media and the technocrat establishment – and they then resort to soy as protein substitution. This led to the derogative term of the "Soy Boy".

And it doesn't help that virtually all the soy is of heavy pesticide GMO production and extensively processed.

In Japan, many young men (purportedly 50%) are vegans and also uninterested in sex or marriage, they are referred to as "*grass eaters* (soshokukei danshi) in the wake of the continuing 20-year-long Japanese economic impotency." They supposedly lack adequate testosterone." [1893]

As soy and testosterone are concerned, cause and effect may be partly mix up here as well. The rapid increase in veganism and soy consumption might be partly caused by testosterone disruption in males, rather than vice versa. Hypogonadism, whether caused by toxic metals or other chemicals - and subsequently low testosterone - can lead to depression, oversensitivity and irritability which may have contributed to the exorbitant increase in veganism in recent years.

When I turned vegetarian 30 years ago, most people, and especially other young men, were laughing at the idea. The past couple years that I've been eating meat again and coincidently restored my health, the same people are suddenly lecturing me on the evils of meat eating, as they see it in every TV show, political movement and youth culture pushed by celebrities. What's more, even people who eat meat themselves demand more government control to reduce meat consumption (for the climate, for justice).

Well-meaning people become vegans or vegetarians for ideological reasons, but it is usually overlooked that evolution is a slow process, even though in modern humans, major genetic changes take place every 400 years, compared to every 10,000

Chapter 14

years in non-human animals. Whether we like it or not, hunter-gatherer tribes are observed to generally eat a lot of meat (see below). Meat consumption is an important part of every culture and ethnicity globally and is regarded as a crucial prerequisite in the evolution of hominin and human brains. Which means to change humanity to a fully vegan lifestyle would be an unprecedented artificial selection process, with those who have a possible genetic anomaly to be able to perform and work over a life-time on a vegan diet will survive and procreate and everybody else would die out. At this stage of the process, the opposite trend is observed: vegans have lower fertility and fewer children.

As seen above, analysis by Loren Cordain et al showed that "whenever and wherever it was ecologically possible, hunter-gatherers consumed high amounts (45– 65% of energy) of animal food. Most (73%) of the worldwide hunter-gatherer societies derived >50% (≥56–65% of energy) of their subsistence from animal foods, whereas only 14% of these societies derived >50% (≥56–65% of energy) of their subsistence from gathered plant foods."

"No hunter-gatherer population is entirely or largely dependent (86–100% subsistence) on gathered plant foods, whereas 20% (n = 46) are highly or solely dependent (86–100%) on fished and hunted animal foods." [1894]

As for modern men and soy, more decisive for the testosterone levels of a young man than his own current soy consumption is his soy intake in childhood (which is determined by the parents) on the one hand, and the soy intake of the mother during pregnancy, on the other. I'm opposed to derogative and insulting terms for well-meaning, empathetic people, especially if these terms are not leading to problem solutions, but since the term 'Soy Boys' is being used, technically, the phenomenon may be more accurately called "sons-of-soy-mothers".

"Endocrine disruption by dietary phyto-oestrogens has an impact on dimorphic sexual systems and behaviours. Because soya is a hormonally active diet, soya can be endocrine disrupting, particularly when exposure occurs during development."

"Consumption by infants and small children is of particular concern. Their susceptibility to the endocrine-disrupting activities of soya phyto-oestrogens may be especially high. " [1895]

Girls are affected as well. "Early-life soy exposure was associated with less female-typical play behavior in girls at 42 months of age.

304

Soy exposure was not significantly associated with play behavior in boys at the same age. " [1896]

A video series has cherry picked promoters of vegan lifestyle from the internet to put vegans in a bad light, the portrayed vegans having indeed suffered from extreme weight loss and degenerative health conditions during the years of their vegan journey, from anorexia to mental illness and tooth decay. [1897]
Most of the apparent symptoms are consistent with oxidative stress and possible chronic metal toxicity. Some of the portrayed influencers are severely anorexic and still believe they have to "detox" more from all the meat they used to eat. In reality, some might simply need to properly chelate toxic metals in order to improve mental and physical health and then they can eat more of what they want. Similar thought patterns are observable in promoters of meat- centered diets. For instance, if someone has iron deficiency from chronic lead toxicity, they may believe they need even more meat to "replenish iron" and "to not turn into a soy boy".

14.3 Metal Poisoning from Retained Bullet Fragments

"Lead poisoning from intraarticular bullets has been recognized since 1867." [1898]
The CDC came a bit late to recognize lead toxicity from bullet fragments, about 150 years. "In 2017, the CDC released its first report linking lead toxicity to bullet fragments." [1899]
"Overall, only 0.3% of cases of adults with elevated blood **lead** levels were caused by retained bullet fragments. However, for those with the highest blood lead levels, nearly 5% of cases could be linked to bullets. [1900]
Recall that according to the CDC "There are no safe levels of lead in the human body." [1901]
"Spectrographic analysis of **lead** bullets shows the presence of other elements in traces: **copper, bismuth, silver** and **thallium**." [1902] In a forensic study, out of 26 compositional groups of bullets and shotgun **lead** samples, **copper, arsenic, silver, antimony, thallium** and **bismuth** were found in all compositional groups. [1903]
In Botswana shooting ranges, **Cd** accumulation from ammunition posed the highest pollution risk to the biota. [1904]

In standard ammunition of the Canadian forces, **lead, antimony** and **arsenic** are found. [1905]

"Many studies have demonstrated the toxic effects of metal fragments on brain tissue." [1906]

When a **lead** ball is implanted in the brains of rats, 28 days after surgery, the concentration of lead in the brain increased with time after implantation of the lead ball.

"Expression of metallothionein protein increased significantly with time. Metallothionein detoxifies lead and its overexpression is a known method of protection against lead neurotoxicity." [1907]

"Lead intoxication (plumbism) from retained bullets may be fatal if unrecognized."

"It is important to employ chelation therapy prior to any operative intervention. This will reduce the mobilization of **lead** from bone during or following the surgical procedure." [1908]

"It was also reported that increased **Pb** concentration provoked a reduction in **iron** and **calcium** concentrations altering the ratios of Fe/copper, Fe/zinc, and Ca/Zn not only in blood, but also in hair."

"In patients with retained bullet fragments in proximity to bones and joints, element levels within blood and serum can be within acceptable ranges; while element levels within the tissues show pronounced **lead** intoxication in the proximity of the metallic body, inducing significant damage to nearby neural elements. [1909]

A study on gunshot victims presenting for care at the King/Drew Medical Center in Los Angeles, California, demonstrated that blood **lead** tends to increase with time after injury in patients with projectile retention, and that the increase in significant part depended on the presence of a bone fracture caused by the gunshot. [1910] In Rio de Janeiro/ Brazil, victims of gunshot lesions with metallic fragments retained for more than 6 months had on average 4.5 times higher blood lead levels than the control group.

"In patients with retained **lead** fragments in the body, although the mean lead levels found were lower than the current laboratory references, even low levels have been associated with both rising morbidity and mortality." [1911]

"Surveillance of blood **lead** levels in all cases of extra-articular retained missiles (EARMs) is warranted." [1912]

"Retained intra-articular (outside of or other than a joint) bullets frequently cause arthritis." Twelve out of 14 patients had radiographic findings characteristic of lead synovitis. The lead was deposited extracellularly in the subsynovial layer and within the marrow spaces of subarticular and periarticular bone. [1913]

"The degree of the arthropathy is directly related to the amount of time the bullet has been retained in the tissue." [1914]

A systematic review and meta-analysis of studies published between1988 and 2018 recommended that patients with bony fractures or multiple retained bullet fragments, who are at higher risk of elevated BLL, should be monitored for BLL in intervals of 3 months within the first year of injury. [1915] Which is only a temporary solution, for after 3 months, the lead is dispersed into bone and other tissue, rather than being excreted. Therefore, regular challenge urine tests are required.

As we've seen, police officers and fire arm instructors have higher **lead** and **antimony** levels. [1916] Metal dust is abrased from the exiting bullet and inhaled in a shooting range. Lead is being replaced by less toxic, but still toxic metals (**antimony, bismuth** etc.).

14.4 Even expensive wines contain toxic metals

Only a few exclusive wines are produced organically, but most (even expensive) wines contain not only excess levels of **Cu, Fe, chromium, manganese** and **zinc** but also non-essential toxic metals such as **aluminum, arsenic, cadmium, nickel** and **lead.**

"Wine quality depends greatly on its metal composition. Moreover, metals in wine may affect human health." Consumption of wine can also have potentially toxic effects if metal concentrations are not kept under allowable limits. "The main focus is set on **aluminum, arsenic, cadmium, chromium, copper, iron, manganese, nickel, lead** and **zinc**, as these elements most often affect wine quality and human health." [1917]

Analyses during winemaking in Romania showed **Ni, Fe** (white wine) and **Cr, Ni, Fe** (red wine) concentrations increased during winemaking. [1918]

French wine grown near an industrial region in Bordeaux, exceeded maximum admissible levels of **lead** about two times. [1919]

In 2008, U.K. researchers found: Red and white wines from most European nations carry potentially dangerous doses of at least seven heavy metals. [1920]

Wealthy people seem not to be concerned too much about heavy metal intake, including from wine. You can test this for yourself. You can go to the most expensive wine dealer in your region and ask for certified organic wines in the 200+ USD prize range and you will find there aren't more than in the median segment. The most expensive wines are non- organic.

The same is true for expensive foods: in European food stores, organic foods are marketed to an urban middleclass customer base, while in very exclusive food stores and the most expensive restaurants, organic is not much of an issue.

This is in line with the presumption that very wealthy and well-informed people don't have the health issues related to chronic heavy metal overload and don't need to care much about what they eat. If 'good' doctors and health retreats regularly cleanse the toxic metals with low dose chelation treatment before they become a burden. If a person starts from a theoretical clean slate from conception and birth onward, and is not exposed to excess workplace or environmental heavy metal loads, a regular light and harmless chelation regiment can continuously extract most metals from the bloodstream, before they are deposited in the tissue.

14.4.1 Moonshine, arsenic and lead in illicit alcohol.

Drinkers of illicitly distilled alcohol are at risk for exposure to a variety of toxic substances, including **lead, copper, arsenic,** and **methanol**. A high percentage of ER patients who reported moonshine consumption had elevated blood **lead** levels. [1921]

In one study of cases of **arsenic** poisoning, contaminated illicit whiskey (moonshine) appeared to be the source in approximately 50% of the patients. [1922]

14.4.2 Illicit drugs

The level of **lead** in pregnant women taking illegal drugs is higher than that of the control group who do not have a history of illegal drug abuse. [1923]

Aghababae et al suggest "The toxic metals and/or bacterial contaminants in illicit drugs are the main health problems in drug users worldwide." **Lead, cadmium** and **chromium** exposure as well as bacterial contamination could be the major threats for drug users. [1924]

In 26 female injection heroin users, mean (standard deviation (SD)) tibial **lead** concentration was 1.8 times higher than in other women. Interaction effects of tibial lead concentration and selected cognitive functions on frequency with which heroin was used were significant. [1925]

Very high blood **lead** levels were also found in marijuana users in Leipzig, Germany. "Of five hundred ninety-seven marijuana consumers, 27.3% had lead levels above the HBM-II threshold, 12.2% had concentrations that required monitoring." [1926]
New research confirms that adults who consumed marijuana had significantly higher levels of **lead** and **cadmium** in blood and urine. [1927]

"Thallium (Tl) intoxication has been identified in drug abuse and cigarette smoking, leading to various signs and symptoms." [1928]
Lead was found in opium, burned opium, cracker Afghani and heroin as opium products in Iran. [1929] "In Iran, adulterated opium is one of the new sources of exposure to **lead** and has precipitated an increase in lead-poisoned cases owing to the widespread use of opium." [1930]
Although the presence of **lead** in street-level heroin, marijuana, and amphetamines has been reported from some countries previously, recently, several reports suggested lead poisoning in Iranian opium addicts. [1931] The **lead** poisoning among opium users was declared an emerging health hazard. [1932]

14.4.3 Smoking

Toxic metals such as **aluminum, cadmium, chromium, copper, lead, mercury, nickel** and **zinc** are not only found in tobacco, but in cigarette papers, filters, and cigarette smoke. [1933]
Among Chinese smokers it was found: Cigarette smoking is associated with depression and insomnia. Active smokers have significantly higher cerebrospinal fluid levels of **magnesium, zinc, iron, lead, lithium** and **aluminum** than controls. Scores for Depression (BDI) are associated with **zinc, iron, lead** and **aluminum** and are also significantly higher in active smokers than nonsmokers. [1934]
Tobacco contains minute quantities of radioactive isotopes of **uranium, lead** and **thorium** series (^{210}Pb, ^{210}Po and ^{226}Ra), which are radioactive carcinogenics. "In a number of studies, inhalation of some naturally occurring radionuclides via smoking has been considered to be one of the most significant causes of lung cancer." [1935]

"Drago et al found that smoking in enclosed spaces was associated with elevated levels of suspended particles measuring less than 2.5 µm (PM 2.5) of **cerium, lanthanum, cadmium**, and **thallium** which were associated with a higher probability of respiratory symptoms among adolescents and children. [1936]

In autopsy studies, renal **cadmium** levels were higher in cigarette smokers and increased to middle age. [1937]
The average cigarette (weighs 1 g) in 2009 contained the following amounts of metals: **arsenic** = 0.17, **cadmium** = 0.86, **chromium** = 2.35, **nickel** = 2.21, and **lead** 0.44 µg/g (microgram per gram). [1938] At a rate of one pack a day, that's 6,200 micrograms or 6 milligrams of **cadmium** in one year. In 30 years of smoking, that's 188 milligrams or 0.188 grams. The half-life of cadmium in the body is 20-40 years. [1939]

Vaping/ E-cigarettes
Things are apparently even worse for vaping: E-cigarettes are a source of toxic and potentially carcinogenic metals.
In a study by the American Chemical Society, with the exception of **cadmium**, e-cigarette users had more of all metals studied in their bodily fluids than smokers did. [1940]
"In recent research, CDPH found that vape aerosol and e-liquids can contain a greater concentration of certain toxic heavy metals compared to cigarettes, **including chromium, nickel, manganese** and **lead.**" [1941] Other studies also found **cadmium**. [1942]

A systematic review including 24 studies on metals/metalloids in e-liquid and e-cigarettes identified metals/metalloids in all products. 4 studies reported metal/metalloid levels in human biosamples (urine, saliva, serum, and blood) of e-cigarette users. [1943]
Ana María Rule, Ph.D. from Johns Hopkins University confirms E-cigarette devices can expose users to toxic metals such as **arsenic, chromium, nickel** and **lead**. [1944]

Puffing rare earth elements
When comparing non-smokers, cigarette smokers and electronic cigarettes smokers, it was shown that: Cigarette smokers had the highest levels of **copper, molybdenum, zinc, antimony** and **strontium**. E-cigarette users had 25 times higher **beryllium** rates than cigarette smokers. E-cigarette users also had increased **europium** and **lanthanides** and the highest concentrations of **selenium, silver** and **vanadium**.
The number of detected other rare earth elements was also higher among e-cigarette users (11.8% of them showed more than 10 different elements). Serum levels of **cerium** and **erbium** increased as the duration of the use of e-cigarettes was longer. The study concluded that smoking is mainly a source of [common] heavy

metals while the use of e-cigarettes is a potential source of rare earth elements (REE). [1945]
Recall **beryllium** is associated with alcohol addiction and suicide. At this point, it can be assumed that the toxic metals in tobacco and similar products are more addictive than the nicotine itself.

The loss of life years due to smoking tobacco is sometimes sited to be only 7 years. However, that doesn't take into consideration that most smokers quit before the age of 30. For long-term smokers, the loss is closer to 18 years, not including the years of terminal illness prior to death. Researchers at 'Action on Smoking and Health' have reported that a 30-year-old smoker can expect to live about 35 more years, whereas a 30-year-old non-smoker can expect to live 53 more years. [1946]

Smokeless tobacco (snuff or chewing) also contains heavy metals such as **lead, chromium, cobalt, nickel** and **mercury,** of course. [1947]

14.4.4 Tattoos

According to the Washington Post, a survey of tattooed people in New York concluded that more than ten percent of those questioned reported skin conditions stemming from their injections. [1948]

"There are more than 200 colorants and additives used to produce tattoo inks. Most standard tattoo ink colors are derived from heavy metals, including **antimony, beryllium, lead, cobalt-nickel, chromium** and **arsenic.**" [1949]
Tattoo ink particles can spread into lymph nodes.
"Studies demonstrated simultaneous transport of organic pigments, heavy metals and **titanium** dioxide from skin to regional lymph nodes." [1950]
Additional research has revealed that tattoo ink particles (including **aluminum, chromium, iron, nickel** and **copper**) can be responsible for a chronic enlargement of the lymph nodes and a breakdown in the immune system. [1951]

Even if the heavy metal-based pigments remain stable without dispersing into tissue, during the tattooing process, **mercury** containing antiseptics are introduced as part of the solvent of the ink.

Importantly, after laser removal of a tattoo, the pigments are broken up and dispersed throughout the body. "A 2019 study in Lasers in Surgery and Medicine found that laser irradiation of tattoo pigments released heavy metals, including **nickel** and **chromium**, into the surrounding tissue. Post-mortem analyses of people with tattoos have revealed heavy metal deposits in various organs and tissues, suggesting systemic absorption." [1952]

Chelation therapy is the only known mechanism to effectively remove these heavy metals after laser treatment. So chelation must be started before laser removal. Also without laser removal, it is wise for anyone with a lot of tattoos to get a challenge heavy metal test.

"People with tattoos are more likely to also have mental health issues." [1953] It has only been 30 years since the medical consensus suggested 'Finding a tattoo on physical examination should alert the physician to the possibility of an underlying psychiatric condition.' [1954]

14.4.5 Criminal poisoning with toxic metals

Acts of criminal poisoning with toxic metals are occasionally identified and investigated, only 500 cases of homicidal poisoning are reported annually in the US. [1955] In cases where intentional metal poisoning led to gradual health decline, chronic disease and early death (years or decades after the event), poisoning is rarely suspected, just as in unintentional metal toxicity. [1956] From the nature of the few cases that are brought to trial, it can be concluded that the dark number could be 10, possibly 100 times that of the reported number.

Among the historically 10 or so most used poisons are the elements **mercury, arsenic** and **thallium**.

It is extremely problematic that many of the most toxic elements can be obtained legally and illegally.

Occasionally, criminal cases of attempted murder with mercury are prosecuted. [1957]

See also: thallium poisoning (8.41.)

Ground Zero

Uniformed service personnel and residents of lower Manhattan who were exposed to the air at Ground Zero following September 11, 2001, had at least eight health complaints.

The authors reported that of those tested for heavy metal toxicity using a challenge urine test, **85% had excessively high levels of**

lead and mercury. Chelation for heavy metals using DMSA was the primary treatment prescribed. After three to four months of treatment, the first cohort of 100 individuals reported significant (greater than 60%) improvement in all symptoms. [1958]

14.4.6 Nauru, the most obese Nation on Earth

Nauru, a 10 km small Pacific Island state has the highest BMI in the world. [1959] The following reasons have been proposed: general wealth from former phosphate mining, and therefore lack of exercise or "laziness", - fatty junk food, - pacific islander genetics. While many other pacific islands share all the above problems, including some of the highest national BMIs worldwide, one probable contributor has not been considered for Nauru:

Not the wealth, but rather the pollution from **phosphate** mining which is a prominent source of **arsenic** and **cadmium** pollution. [1960] Arsenic and cadmium are both known contributors to obesity (see obesity 5.15.3).

This **phosphate** mining is what once made the Island rich and prosperous, which led to the perception that the islanders must be lacy and sedentary. The wealth is long gone, but the environmental pollution remains.

"The Nauru rock phosphate is produced by strip mining since 1907, it has considerable value as an agricultural nutrient," most of the island surface was turned into a desert, only the outer coastline retains the natural vegetation and is inhabited. "The mining surface contains high concentrations of the toxic metal **cadmium**. Nauru phosphate deposits have a **cadmium** content between 100 and 1,000 times the average lithosphere concentration." [1961]

"Phosphogypsum (PG) produced during phosphoric acid production contains significant amounts of **arsenic** and can potentially cause adverse environmental and health effects." [1962]

For comparison, in the Gafsa-Metlaoui phosphate mining area, Tunisia, both sediments and tailings showed higher-than-background concentrations of potentially toxic metals (mainly of **Cd, Zn** and **Cr**). [1963] "Phosphate rock (from international samples) is a source of heavy metal pollution [**Cd, Cu, Cr, Ni, Pb, Zn**] of air, soil, water, the food chain etc. " [1964]

14.4.7 Animal fertility studies and heavy metals

Panda extinction

The fertility of the endangered Panda is of great concern to China and the people of the West, our own human infertility and approaching extinction is not.

It has been a longstanding mystery why pandas refuse to breed, they even refuse trying, which is puzzling from an evolutionary view. For humans in complex societies, it is possible to change sexual behavior within centuries via cultural development and a process of 'self-domestication', which gradually changes the gene pool. But there is no explanation why other mammals should just stop copulating, if this behavior is not chemically induced.

It now appears the pandas might suffer a similar fate as humans, environmental pollution of hydrocarbon chemicals and heavy metals are causing them to suffer from their own version of "*Hormonageddon*", including infertility as well as sexual inactivity, on a path to extinction, much like us.

Four heavy metals (**As, Cd, Cr** and **Pb**), PCDD/Fs and polychlorinated biphenyls (PCBs) were detected in blood drawn from captive Qinling pandas. Time spent in captivity was a better predictor of toxicant concentration accumulation than was panda age. "The proportion of live sperm was significantly lower and the aberrance ratio of sperm was significantly greater for captive pandas than for wild ones." [1965]

Studies showed that not only captive but also wild pandas were exposed to toxins in their diet of bamboo, but the ultimate origin of these toxins had long been unknown. "Chen et al, 2018 showed that atmospheric deposition is the origin of **heavy metals** and persistent organic pollutants (POPs) in the diets of captive and wild Qinling giant pandas." [1966]

One year later it was found that the concentrations of **Cu, Zn, Mn, Pb, Cr, Ni, Cd, Hg** and **As** in soil samples collected from sites along a major highway bisecting the panda's habitat in the Qinling Mountains were elevated. "The study has confirmed that traffic does contaminate roadside soils and poses a potential threat to the health of pandas."

Concentrations of all metals except arsenic exceeded background levels. Topsoil up to 300 m away from the highway was extremely contaminated with **Cd**. [1967]

A health risk assessment by the hazard index (HI) showed a potential to strong risk for giant pandas exposed to **Pb, As** and **Hg**. In addition, the concentrations of heavy metals in feces showed a higher exposure risk for captive giant pandas than wild giant pandas. [1968]

What the above studies hadn't considered, is "some bamboo species have a high ability to adapt to metalliferous environments and a high capacity to **absorb heavy metals**." [1969]

Now we compare the toxic elements in pandas and in their food with the associations of these metals to infertility in humans and other mammals as listed in 2.4. And we might get some idea of what could be happening here.

Could this (partly) solve the mystery of the panda reproduction hiatus? If so, you're welcome.

14.5 Historic and prehistoric metal toxicity

14.5.1 Lead poisoning and the end of the Roman Empire

Both the ancient Greek and then especially Roman elites were suffering from lead and other heavy metal toxicity and in the context of societal developments, they underwent a process of "*Hormonageddon*" to the point of self-extinction: low birth rates, infertility, psychoses, nihilism, sexual obsession, abortion, low ethnocentrism.

Already the Greek elites exposed themselves to high levels of **lead**. Even the Egyptian used it in small quantities: "Galena (argentiferous lead ore, PbS), was used as eye-paint in Egypt during the prehistoric Baderian period, about 5,000 years B.C. The practice of using galena for eye-paint survives to the present day, particularly in India, where it is known as surma." [1970]

The Greek philosopher Nikander of Colophon in 250 BC already reported on the colic and anemia resulting from **lead** poisoning.

Hippocrates related gout to the food and wine, the association between gout and lead poisoning was not recognized during this period (450-380 BC), although he did described colic, or upset stomach, in metal workers. [1971]

"The role of manufacturing sugar lead goes all the way back to the Greeks, but the Romans popularized it". [1972]

In the first century A.D., Dioscorides, another Greek physician, noticed that exposure to lead could cause paralysis and delirium in addition to intestinal problems and swelling. [1973]

"During the Roman period, gout was prevalent among the upper classes of Roman society and is believed to be a result of the enormous lead intake." [1974] According to Encyclopedia Romana,

"Nriagu estimates the aristocracy of Rome to have consumed two liters of wine a day or almost three bottles (which would seem to make alcoholism more suspect than lead poisoning [for the decline of the Roman elite]) and the resulting lead intake to have averaged 180 µg daily. He further estimates the total amount of lead absorbed from all sources to be 250 µg per day and lead concentration in the blood to be 50 µg/dL, at least for the gluttonous and bibulous (as he phrases it) and those with an appetite for adulterated wines and sweetened dainties—who he presumes most Roman emperors to have been." [1975]

"Pliny, in his Natural Histories, wrote about the noxious fumes that emanated from lead furnaces, he also wrote that sapa and onion are effective elements towards inducing abortions." [1976] (The sweetener *sapa* was a sirup prepared from boiling grapes in lead pots). Vitruvius and Celsus were aware of the toxicity of lead and advised against its usage. [1977]

Joanna Moore et al argued that lead also contributed to the high infant mortality rates within Roman populations. [1978]

Lead enhanced one-fifth of the 450 recipes in the Roman *Apician Cookbook*, a collection of first through fifth century recipes attributed to gastrophiles associated with Apicius, the famous Roman gourmet. [1979]

Other than cognitive decline, fatigue and sterility, the main deteriorating effect of the aristocrats' lead poisoning seems to have been lack of resolve and hormonal confusion, enhancing oikophobia and anti- ethnocentrism.

As we see, according to their lifestyle, the Roman aristocracy would have received a much higher steady dose than the lower classes, which could have contributed to the circumstance that these upper classes were more affected by the reluctance to have children, by low fertility, by low ethnocentrism and high levels of oikophobia. Meanwhile, the general public had a hard time understanding what was wrong with their rulers.

"Ancient Rome featured a myriad of, what could be understood, both then and now, as experiences that transcended sex and gender norms." [1980] Most famously, Elagabalus was a controversial teenage emperor who shook Roman society to its core with radical sexual promiscuity transforming from a boy to a woman, marrying once a sacred female priestess, then a young man. He was married 5 times in his short life of 18 years (He reigned from 218 - 222 AD). "According to Dio Cassius, castration was one of Elagabalus' fondest desires, not out of religion but out of "effeminacy". [1981]

"Dio says that Elagabalus prostituted himself in taverns and brothels. Some writers suggest that Elagabalus may have identified as female or been transgender, and may have sought sex reassignment surgery. Dio says Elagabalus delighted in being called Hierocles's mistress, wife, and queen." [1982]

He was killed by the Pretorian Guard and thrown into the Tiber. [1983]

"Roman men [citizens] were free to enjoy sex with other males without a perceived loss of masculinity or social status as long as they took the dominant or penetrative role." [1984]

Roman writers did note that "*Indeed, those who eat the least expensive foods are the strongest. Thus, slaves are generally stronger than their masters, country folk are stronger than city folk, and the poor are stronger than the rich. Furthermore, those who eat inexpensive food can work harder, are less fatigued by working, and are sick less often than those who eat expensive food. Also, they are better able to tolerate cold, heat, lack of sleep, and so forth.*" (trans. King, 2010) [1985]

Apart from the lead poisoning via wine cauldrons, alcohol itself disrupts testosterone. [1986]

14.6 Global lead pollution from the Greco-Roman era to today.

F.P. Retief calculated that lead production in the Graeco-Roman era in Europe and the Mediterranean area during the 2nd millennium BC increased tenfold, reaching a peak in the 1st millennium BC and the period up to AD 500, after which it dropped dramatically until AD 1000 to levels comparable with those of the 3rd millennium BC.

"**Lead** contamination in the ice layers of Greenland dating from the period 500 BC to AD 300 must have been caused by atmospheric pollution from the ore furnaces of ancient Rome (and Greece). "

"The burden of lead in the ice is equivalent to 15% of the 20th century's ice pollution due to leaded petrol." [1987]

Lead bone records also mirror atmospheric **Pb** pollution recorded in a local peat archive at the edge of the Roman Empire in NW Iberia. Over a 700-year period, rural Romans incorporated two times more **mercury** and **lead** into their bones than post-Romans inhabiting the same site, independent of sex or age. [1988]

As we've seen above, children in ancient Rome often suffered from rickets, a common symptom of chronic lead poisoning (see 5.13.4).

Mercury

Beyond the well documented lead poisoning of the Roman elite, "mercury concentration was on average 3.5-fold greater in ancient Roman compared to post-Roman inhabitants, even on the edge of the Roman Empire." [1989] As we know, **mercury** poisoning can cause anxiety, depression, insomnia and other symptoms. [1990] And mercury is also a strong endocrine disruptor, of course. [1991] Cinnabar and vermilion (mercury sulfide pigments) were used in objects collected at The New York Met by almost two dozen cultures, on many continents, dating from at least the third millennium B.C. to the mid-19th century A.D. [1992]

Antimony

More recently, it has been suggested that another heavy metal, **antimony**, may have done the main job of dissolving the Roman empire. [1993]

If true, it is noteworthy that antimony from drinking water is a neurotoxin more effective than lead, and it also acts as an endocrine disruptor. As we saw, today, **antimony** is known to be responsible for estrogenic effects." [1994]

Thought Experiment: Were the Venetian nobility lead poisoned? The Doce Palace (Palazzo Ducale), the adjacent basilica San Marco and the administration buildings across the street are all covered with **lead** roofing, much like the Notre Dame in Paris.

The Venice drinking water was provided from rainwater run-off from roofs running onto the squares and courtyards where it was filtered through a sand bed underground. The water ran into special gutters on the squares, and was collected and harvested in the center well or 'pozzo'.

Two large wells or 'pozzi' are in the courtyard of the Doce Palace, surrounded by the lead roofs of the palazzo and basilica, so most of the water harvested there had run off from lead roofs. It is not clear how many of the Venetian nobility drank of the water from the wells or whether they brought their own from their own palazzi's courtyard's, their palazzi had tiled roofs. However, all of the 1,000 noblemen (patricians) of Venice were regularly gathered for days at the Palazzo Ducale for sessions and the Doce himself and most higher officials worked there fulltime. If a large number of the Venetian elite drank enough leaded rainwater, it could have driven the government into stupidity and mental illness, together with lead sweetened whine - just as the ancient Romans - both would have indeed contributed to the decline and fall of the Venetian Empire.

Meanwhile the noblewomen used copious amounts of Venetian *ceruse* as skin whiteners - a white lead carbonate - sourced from Venice.

14.6.1 Further historic toxic metal pollution

14.6.2 Mercury in the Americas

Datasets of mercury contents of soils and sediments contemporaneous with the Classic Maya Period at ten sites confirm that at (or near) ancient Maya settlements, elevated **mercury** (often many times greater than the toxic effect threshold, TET) has been preserved in environmental materials.

In one of the dominant Mayan centers of the Late Classic period, the city of Tikal, located in present day northern Guatemala, most samples taken today contain mercury above the TET, many over 20-fold. Cinnabar (a red mercury sulfide mineral) was found in multiple architectural contexts. [1995]

Large quantities of **mercury** were found under the ruins of a Mexican pyramid in Teotihuacan in a discovery that could shed light on the city's mysterious leader. "An archaeologist has discovered liquid mercury at the end of a tunnel beneath a Mexican pyramid, a finding that could suggest the existence of a king's tomb or a ritual chamber far below one of the most ancient cities of the Americas." [1996]

14.6.3 Prehistoric metal pollution

14.6.4 Prehistoric lead

In some estimates, in the 20th century, most humans carried concentrations of **lead** 100 times higher than their prehistoric ancestors, based on analyses of ancient skeletons." [1997]

Researchers at the California Institute of Technology published a study assessing that average bone **lead** levels today are even **1,000 times** higher than a few hundred years ago. [1998]

Comparison of prehistoric animal bones from 20- 50,000 years old to contemporary bones, showed a drastic increase in toxic metals. "In Europe and Peru in the late Middle Ages, the concentration of **lead** in human bones increased by one order of magnitude (10-fold)." [1999]

Cadmium in prehistoric bones

"The concentration of **Cd** has increased in human bones in the 20th century, to about ten times above the pre-industrial level." [2000]

As we have seen, both **lead** and **cadmium** exposures derive not only from industrialization and certain habits - such as cigarette smoking in the case of cadmium – but also from natural sources.

Bones of prehispanic inhabitants of Gran Canaria, prehispanic domestic animals (sheep, goat and pigs) from island, modern individuals and modern domestic animals were analyzed for **lead** and **cadmium** content.

Modern individuals showed 6-fold higher bone **cadmium** values than prehistoric ones (values of prehistoric individuals did not differ from those of the prehistoric animals but were higher than those of the modern animals).

In the same way, modern individuals and modern animals showed approximately 7-fold higher bone **lead** than ancient individuals and ancient animals. [2001]

Here it must be pointed out that the Canary Islands in the Atlantic never had any heavy industry to speak of, low population density, prevailing sea winds and thus relatively low heavy metal toxicity from air pollution. The increased **cadmium** load as compared to prehistoric people must be expected to be even higher in continental industrial regions.

Despite these favorable conditions, contemporary inhabitants of the Canary Islands also have 4 to 5 times higher bone **lead** contents than did their predecessors of the 18th century living in the same locations. [2002]

Analysis of caves in the Iberian Peninsula indicate a long-term exposure of Homo to heavy metals like **copper** and **zinc**, via fires, fumes and their ashes, which could have played certain roles in environmental-pollution tolerance, a hitherto neglected influence. [2003]

The End

Notes

[1] Harvard Social Impact Review: Stem the Tsunami of Suffering From Metabolic Disease – Limit Ultra-Processed Foods in Our Food Supply; Virginia Gleason; https://www.sir.advancedleadership.harvard.edu/articles/stem-tsunami-suffering-metabolic-disease-limit-ultra-processed-foods#:~:text=A%202019%20study%20revealed%20that,the%20quality%20of%20their%20lives.

[2] Araujo, J. et al 2019: Revalence of Optimal Metabolic Health in American Adults: National Health and Nutrition Examination Survey 2009-2016 https://doi.org/10.1089/met.2018.0105

[3] Prescription Drugs; Health Policy Institute; https://hpi.georgetown.edu/rxdrugs/#:~:text=Three%2Dquarters%20of%20those%20age,older%20(see%20Figure%201).

[4] Ho, Jessica Y. 2023: Life Course Patterns of Prescription Drug Use in the United States Demography (2023) 60 (5): 1549–1579. https://doi.org/10.1215/00703370-10965990

[5] CDC: Managing Chronic Health Conditions; Page last reviewed: October 20, 2021. https://www.cdc.gov/healthyschools/chronicconditions.htm#:~:text=In%20the%20United%20States%2C%20more,%2C%20and%20behavior%2Flearning%20problems.

[6] CDC: Physical Activity Helps Prevent Chronic Diseases; Last Reviewed: May 8, 2023 Source: (NCCDPHP) https://www.cdc.gov/chronicdisease/resources/infographic/physical-activity.htm#:~:text=Regular%20physical%20activity%20helps%20improve,depression%20and%20anxiety%2C%20and%20dementia.

[7] Lanphear BP, Rauch S, Auinger P, Allen RW, Hornung RW. Low-level lead exposure and mortality in US adults: a population-baseno a cohort study. Lancet Public Health.; 2018;3(4):E177-E184 https://www.researchgate.net/publication/323742199_Low-level_lead_exposure_and_mortality_in_US_adults_A_population-based_cohort_study

[8] Buchholz, Ernst W. (editer), 1955: Bevoelkerungs-Ploetz; Raum und Bevoelkerung in der Weltgeschichte, Ploetz, Wuerzburg, 23

[9] Mehrheit der Jugend braucht finanzielle Hilfe. Zdf heute. 10.08.2023; https://www.zdf.de/nachrichten/wirtschaft/erwerbslosigkeit-jugend-finanzen-abhaengigkeit-deutschland-100.html

[10] Alvaro, P. K., Roberts, R. M., & Harris, J. K. (2014). The independent relationships between insomnia, depression, subtypes of anxiety, and chronotype during adolescence. Sleep Medicine, 15(8), 934–941. https://pubmed.ncbi.nlm.nih.gov/24958244/

[11] Grandjean, Philippe et al. 2014: Neurobehavioural effects of developmental toxicity The Lancet Neurology, Volume 13, Issue 3, 330 – 338; 2014 https://www.thelancet.com/journals/laneur/article/PIIS1474-4422(13)70278-3/fulltext

[12] Soisungwan Satarug editor, 2022: Toxic Metals, Chronic Diseases and Related Cancers; Journal Toxins; https://mdpi-res.com/bookfiles/book/5706/Toxic_Metals_Chronic_Diseases_and_Related_Cancers.pdf?v=1707161676

[13] Lanphear BP, Rauch S, et al: 2018. Low-level lead exposure and mortality in US adults: a population-based cohort study. Lancet Public Health.; 2018;3. https://www.thelancet.com/journals/lanpub/article/PIIS2468-2667(18)30025-2/fulltext

[14] https://embodywellness.com/services/chelation-therapy/

[15] McFarland M. J. et al 2022: Half of US population exposed to adverse lead levels in early childhood; PROCEEDINGS OF THE NATIONAL ACADEMY OF SCIENCES; Vol. 119 | No. 11; March 15, 2022; https://www.pnas.org/doi/10.1073/pnas.2118631119

[16] Bouchard MF, Bellinger DC,et al 2009: Blood lead levels and major depressive disorder, panic disorder, and generalized anxiety disorder in US young adults. Arch Gen; Psychiatry. 2009 Dec;66 https://www.ncbi.nlm.nih.gov/pmc/articles/PMC2917196/

[17] Gollenberg AL, et al: 2010: Association between lead and cadmium and reproductive hormones in peripubertal U.S. girls. Environ Health Perspect. 2010 Dec;118(12) https://www.ncbi.nlm.nih.gov/pmc/articles/PMC3002200/

[18] Warniment C, Tsang K, Galazka SS. Lead poisoning in children. Am Fam Physician. 2010 Mar 15;81(6):751-7. https://www.azdhs.gov/documents/preparedness/epidemiology-disease-control/lead-poisoning/lead-poisoning-in-children.pdf

Notes

[19] Canfield RL, Henderson CR Jr, Cory-Slechta DA, Cox C, Jusko TA, Lanphear BP. Intellectual impairment in children with blood lead concentrations below 10 microg per deciliter. N Engl J Med. 2003 Apr https://pubmed.ncbi.nlm.nih.gov/12700371/

[20] Dyer,C. A.2007; Heavy Metals as Endocrine-Disrupting Chemicals; 2007/01/01; 111; 133; 978-1-58829-830-0;; 10.1007/1-59745-107-X_5; Endocrine-Disrupting Chemicals: From Basic Science to Clin. Practice http://eknygos.lsmuni.lt/springer/631/111-133.pdf

[21] Tabb MM, Blumberg B. New modes of action for endocrine-disrupting chemicals. Mol Endocrinol 2006; 20:475–82. https://academic.oup.com/mend/article/20/3/475/2738085

[22] Medici N, Minucci S, Nigro V, Abbondanza C, Armetta I, Molinari AM, Puca GA. 1989: Metal binding sites of the estradiol receptor from calf uterus and their possible role in the regulation of receptor function. Biochemistry 1989; 28:212–19.

[23] Gay, Flaminia; Laforgia, Vincenza; et al Chronic Exposure to Cadmium Disrupts the Adrenal Gland Activity of the Newt Triturus carnifex (Amphibia, Urodela) https://www.hindawi.com/journals/bmri/2013/424358/

[24] Philippe Grandjean & Clair C. Patterson (1988) Ancient Skeletons as Silent Witnesses of Lead Exposures in the Past, CRC Critical Reviews in Toxicology, 19:1, 11-21, http://doi.org/10.3109/10408448809040815

[25] Jennrich, Peter, 2007: Schwermetalle - Ursache für Zivilisationskrankheiten; Company'MED-Verlag-Ges., 2007 SBN; 3934672264, 9783934672260

[26] Jaishankar M, et al 2014:Toxicity, mechanism and health effects of some heavy metals. Interdiscip Toxicol. 2014 Jun;7(2):60-72. http://doi.org10.2478/intox-2014-0009.

[27] James, John T. PhD. A New, Evidence-based Estimate of Patient Harms Associated with Hospital Care. Journal of Patient Safety 9(3):p 122-128, September 2013. | https://journals.lww.com/journalpatientsafety/Fulltext/2013/09000/A_New,_Evidence_based_Estimate_of_Patient_Harms.2.aspx

[28] CDC: Childhood Lead Poisoning Prevention; Page last reviewed: September 2, 2022; https://www.cdc.gov/nceh/lead/prevention/default.htm

[29] Gorini, F., Muratori, F. & Morales, M.A. The Role of Heavy Metal Pollution in Neurobehavioral Disorders: a Focus on Autism. Rev J Autism Dev Disord 1, 354–372 (2014). https://doi.org/10.1007/s40489-014-0028-3

[30] Smith, AH; Arroyo, AP; Mazumdar, DN. Arsenic-induced skin lesions among Atacameno people in northern Chile despite good nutrition and centuries of exposure. Environ. Hea. Perspect 2000, 108, 617–620. https://europepmc.org/article/med/10903614

[31] Ilieva, I. .et al 2020: Toxic Effects of Heavy Metals (Lead and Cadmium) on Sperm Quality and Male Fertility; Acta morphologica et anthropologica, 27 (3-4) Sofia, 2020; http://www.iempam.bas.bg/journals/acta/acta27b/61-73.pdf

[32] Jain M, Kalsi AK, et al 2016: High Serum Estradiol and Heavy Metals Responsible for ffggdHuman Spermiation Defect-A Pilot Study. J Clin Diagn Res. 2016 Dec;10(12):. https://www.ncbi.nlm.nih.gov/pmc/articles/PMC5296528/

[33] Our World in data: Around one-in-three children globally suffer from lead poisoning. What can we do to reduce this?; Hannah Ritchie; January 25, 2022; https://ourworldindata.org/reducing-lead-poisoning

[34] Dyer, C.A. 2007: Heavy Metals as Endocrine-Disrupting Chemicals; 2007/01/01; 111; 133; 978-1-58829-830-0;; 10.1007/1-59745-107-X_5; Endocrine-Disrupting Chemicals: From Basic Science to Clinical Practice http://eknygos.lsmuni.lt/springer/631/111-133.pdf

[35] Hsueh, YM., Lee, CY., et al. Association of blood heavy metals with developmental delays and health status in children. Sci Rep https://doi.org/10.1038/srep43608

[36] Pan S, Lin L, Zeng F, et al 2017: Effects of lead, cadmium, arsenic, and mercury co-exposure on children's intelligence quotient in an industrialized area of southern China. Environ Pollut. 2018 Apr. https://pubmed.ncbi.nlm.nih.gov/29274537/

[37] McFarland M. J. et al 2022: Half of US population exposed to adverse lead levels in early childhood; PROCEEDINGS OF THE NATIONAL ACADEMY OF SCIENCES; Vol. 119 | No. 11; March 15, 2022; https://doi.org/10.1073/pnas.2118631119

[38] Shoshan, Michal S 2022:; Will Short Peptides Revolutionize Chelation Therapy? Zurich Open Repository and Archive; Univ. of Zurich; https://www.zora.uzh.ch/id/eprint/230581/1/ZORA_5418.pdf

[39] UNICEF; The toxic truth; Children's exposure to lead pollution undermines a generation of future potential; Publication date July 2020; https://www.unicef.org/reports/toxic-truth-childrens-exposure-to-lead-pollution-2020

[40] Pan S, Lin L, et 2018: Effects of lead, cadmium, arsenic, and mercury co-exposure on children's intelligence quotient in an industrialized area of southern China. Environ Pollut. 2018 Apr; 235:47-54. https://pubmed.ncbi.nlm.nih.gov/29274537/

[41] Clarkson TW, Magos L (2006). The toxicology of mercury and its chemical compounds. Critical Reviews in Toxicology 36: 609–662. https://pubmed.ncbi.nlm.nih.gov/16973445/

[42] Arinola G, Idonije B, Akinlade K, Ihenyen O. 2010: Essential trace metals and heavy metals in newly diagnosed schizophrenic patients and those on anti-psychotic medication. J Res Med Sci. 2010 Sep;15(5):245-9.
https://www.researchgate.net/publication/51082705_Essential_trace_metals_and_heavy_metals_in_newly_diagnosed_schizophrenic_patients_and_those_on_anti-psychotic_medication

[43] Navas-Acien A, Guallar E, Silbergeld EK, Rothenberg SJ. Lead exposure and cardiovascular disease--a systematic review. Environ Health Perspect. 2007 Mar;115(3):472-82. http://doi.org/10.1289/ehp.9785.

[44] Jennrich; Peter; 05/08: Quecksilber und Blei machen es ihrem Herz schwer; Well-Aging http://tierversuchsfreie-medizin.de/download/Quecksilber-und-Blei_Herz.pdf

[45] Ansarihadipour H, Bayatiani M. Influence of Electromagnetic Fields on Lead Toxicity: A Study of Conformational Changes in Human Blood Proteins. Iran Red Crescent Med J. 2016 May 31;18(7):e28050.
https://www.researchgate.net/publication/303710327_Influence_of_Electromagnetic_Fields_on_Lead_Toxicity_A_Study_of_Conformational_Changes_in_Human_Blood_Proteins

[46] Amara S, Douki T, et al 2011: Effects of static magnetic field and cadmium on oxidative stress and DNA damage in rat cortex brain and hippocampus. Toxicol Ind Health. 2011 Mar;27(2):99-106. https://pubmed.ncbi.nlm.nih.gov/20837562/

[47] Sanders AP, et al: Perinatal and Childhood Exposure to Cadmium, Manganese, and Metal Mixtures and Effects on Cognition and Behavior: A Review of Recent Literature. Curr Envir. Health Rep. 2015 Sep;2(3) https://www.ncbi.nlm.nih.gov/pmc/articles/PMC4531257/

[48] Govarts, Eva, Sylvie Remy et al. 2016. "Combined Effects of Prenatal Exposures to Environmental Chemicals on Birth Weight" International Journal of Environmental Research and Public Health 13, no. 5: 495. https://doi.org/10.3390/ijerph13050495

[49] Singh, Nitika et al 2017: Synergistic Effects of Heavy Metals and Pesticides in Living Systems; Front. Chem., 11 October 2017; Sec. Cellular Biochemistry ; Volume 5 - 2017 | https://doi.org/10.3389/fchem.2017.00070

[50] Minxue Shen, Chengcheng Zhang, 2001: Association of multi-metals exposure with intelligence quotient score of children: A prospective cohort study, Environment Internat., V.155, 2021 (https://www.sciencedirect.com/science/article/pii/S0160412021003172)

[51] Craftsmanship; Issue: Spring 2022: The Vegetable Detective; by TODD OPPENHEIMER https://craftsmanship.net/the-vegetable-detective/

[52] Faith Ngwewa et al 2022: Effects of Heavy Metals on Bacterial Growth, Biochemical Properties and Antimicrobial Susceptibility; Journal of Applied & Environmental Microbiology, 2022, Vol. 10, No. 1, 9-16 http://doi.org/10.12691/jaem-10-1-2

[53] Rowland IR, Robinson RD, Doherty RA. Effect of diet on mercury metabolism and excretion in mice given methylmercury: role of gut flora. Arch Env Health. 1984;39:401–408. https://europepmc.org/article/med/6524959

[54] Seko Y, Miura T, Takahashi M, Koyama T. Methyl mercury decomposition in mice treated with antibiotics. Acta Pharmacol Toxicol (Copenh). 1981 Oct;49(4):259-65. http://doi.org/10.1111/j.1600-0773.1981.tb00903.x.

[55] Pamphlett, Roger et al 2023: The toxic metal hypothesis for neurological disorders; ; Front. Neurol., 23 June 2023; V. 14 – 2023; https://doi.org/10.3389/fneur.2023.1173779

[56] Blumer, W., and Cranton, E. 1989, "Ninety Percent Reduction in Cancer Mortality after Chelation Therapy With EDTA", J. of Advancement in Medicine, Vol 2, No, 1/2, Spring/Summer 1989. https://oradix.com/ninety-percent-reduction-in-cancer-mortality-after-chelation-therapy-with-edta-the-famous-swiss-study/

[57] Hancke C and Flytlie K 1993: Benefits of EDTA chelation therapy in arteriosclerosis: a retrospective study of 470 patients. J Adv Med 6(3):161,1993.
https://www.researchgate.net/publication/265322766_Benefits_of_EDTA_Chelation_Therapy_in_Arteriosclerosis_A_Retrospective_Study_of_470_Patients

[58] Hancke C and Flytlie K 1993: Benefits of EDTA chelation therapy in arteriosclerosis: a retrospective study of 470 patients. J Adv Med 6(3):161,1993.
https://www.researchgate.net/publication/265322766_Benefits_of_EDTA_Chelation_Therapy_in_Arteriosclerosis_A_Retrospective_Study_of_470_Patients

[59] American College for Advancement in Medicine: Why All Americans Should Know About Chelation Therapy; Posted By Guest Post by Malissa Stawicki of Natural Medicine & Detox, Friday, September 13, 2019; https://www.acam.org/blogpost/1092863/331320/Why-All-Americans-Should-Know-About-Chelation-Therapy

Notes

[60] CDC; Case Studies in Environmental Medicine: Lead Toxicity; U.S. Department of Human Services, Public Health Service, Agency for Toxic Substance and Disease Registry; Publication date: 09/01/1992
https://wonder.cdc.gov/wonder/prevguid/p0000017/p0000017.asp
image: CDC guidelines for management in children:
Madhusudhanan, M., & Lall, S.B. (2007). Acute lead poisoning in an infant. Oman medical journal, 22 3, 57-9 .

[61] Hopf G. M 2016: Those Who Remain: A Postapocalyptic Novel (The New World Series Book 7) Kindle Edition;

[62] Swiss Medical detox: PUBLICATIONS; 18 January 2019; Environmental diseases The chelation, an indispensable therapy with a future;
http://www.swissmedicaldetox.ch/en/publications-2/

[63] Healing partnership: Dr.Bryan Stern Heavy Metals and Chronic Disease;
https://www.healingpartnership.com/articles/heavy-metals-and-chronic-disease/

[64] Sanders AP, Claus Henn B, Wright RO. Perinatal and Childhood Exposure to Cadmium, Manganese, and Metal Mixtures and Effects on Cognition and Behavior: A Review of Recent Literature. Curr Environ Health Rep. 2015 Sep;2(3)
https://www.ncbi.nlm.nih.gov/pmc/articles/PMC4531257/

[65] Sears CG, Zierold KM. Health of Children Living Near Coal Ash. Glob Pediatr Health. 2017
https://www.ncbi.nlm.nih.gov/pmc/articles/PMC5533260/

[66] Li, H., Li, H., Li, Y. et al. Blood Mercury, Arsenic, Cadmium, and Lead in Children with Autism Spectrum Disorder. Biol Trace Elem Res 181, 31–37 (2018).
https://doi.org/10.1007/s12011-017-1002-6

[67] Mohamed Fel B, Zaky EA, El-Sayed AB, et al 2015: Assessment of Hair Aluminum, Lead, and Mercury in a Sample of Autistic Egyptian Children: Environmental Risk Factors of Heavy Metals in Autism. Behav Neurol. https://www.ncbi.nlm.nih.gov/pmc/articles/PMC4609793/

[68] Children's Health Defense: Robert F. Kennedy, Jr;; Studies Link Heavy Metals to the Explosion of Neurodevelopmental Disorders and Declining IQ in American Children; By. SEPTEMBER 13, 2017; https://childrenshealthdefense.org/news/studies-link-heavy-metals-to-the-explosion-of-neurodevelopmental-disorders-and-declining-iq-in-american-children/

[69] Larsson SC, Wolk A. Urinary cadmium and mortality from all causes, cancer and cardiovascular disease in the general population: systematic review and meta-analysis of cohort studies. Int J Epidemiol. 2016 Jun; https://pubmed.ncbi.nlm.nih.gov/25997435/

[70] Grandjean, Philippe et al. 2014: Neurobehavioural effects of developmental toxicity The Lancet Neurology, Volume 13, Issue 3, 330 – 338; 2014
https://www.thelancet.com/journals/laneur/article/PIIS1474-4422(13)70278-3/fulltext

[71] Soisungwan Satarug editor, 2022: Toxic Metals, Chronic Diseases and Related Cancers; Journal Toxins; https://mdpi-res.com/bookfiles/book/5706/Toxic_Metals_Chronic_Diseases_and_Related_Cancers.pdf?v=1707161676

[72] CDC: Childhood Lead Poisoning Prevention; Page last reviewed: September 2, 2022;
https://www.cdc.gov/nceh/lead/prevention/default.htm

[73] Gorini, F., Muratori, F. & Morales, M.A. The Role of Heavy Metal Pollution in Neurobehavioral Disorders: a Focus on Autism. Rev J Autism Dev Disord 1, 354–372 (2014).
https://doi.org/10.1007/s40489-014-0028-3

[74] CDC; Case Studies in Environmental Medicine: Lead Toxicity; U.S. Department of Human Services, Public Health Service, Agency for Toxic Substance and Disease Registry; Publication date: 09/01/1992
https://wonder.cdc.gov/wonder/prevguid/p0000017/p0000017.asp
image: CDC guidelines for management in children:
Madhusudhanan, M., & Lall, S.B. (2007). Acute lead poisoning in an infant. Oman medical journal, 22 3, 57-9 .

[75] Soisungwan Satarug editor, 2022: Toxic Metals, Chronic Diseases and Related Cancers; Journal Toxins; https://mdpi-res.com/bookfiles/book/5706/Toxic_Metals_Chronic_Diseases_and_Related_Cancers.pdf?v=1707161676

[76] Khan, Naser et al,. 2023. "Synergistic Effect of Multiple Metals Present at Slightly Lower Concentration than the Australian Investigation Level Can Induce Phytotoxicity" Land 12, no. 3: 698. https://doi.org/10.3390/land12030698

[77] Govarts, Eva, Sylvie Remy et al. 2016. "Combined Effects of Prenatal Exposures to Environmental Chemicals on Birth Weight" International Journal of Environmental Research and Public Health 13, no. 5: 495. https://doi.org/10.3390/ijerph13050495

[78] Nitika Singh et al 2017: Synergistic Effects of Heavy Metals and Pesticides in Living Systems; Front. Chem., 11 October 2017; Sec. Cellular Biochemistry ; Volume 5 - 2017 | https://doi.org/10.3389/fchem.2017.00070

[79] Jayasumana, C., Gunatilake, S. & Siribaddana, S. Simultaneous exposure to multiple heavy metals and glyphosate may contribute to Sri Lankan agricultural nephropathy. BMC Nephrol 16, 103 (2015). https://doi.org/10.1186/s12882-015-0109-2

[80] Minxue Shen, Chengcheng Zhang, 2001: Association of multi-metals exposure with intelligence quotient score of children: A prospective cohort study, Environment Internat., V.155, 2021 (https://www.sciencedirect.com/science/article/pii/S0160412021003172)

[81] Francesco Esposito, Antonio Nardone, et al 2018: A systematic risk characterization related to the dietary exposure of the population to potentially toxic elements through the ingestion of fruit and vegetables from a potentially contaminated area. A case study: The issue of the "Land of Fires" area in Campania region, Italy, Environmental Pollution, Volume 243, Part B, 2018, https://doi.org/10.1016/j.envpol.2018.09.058.
(https://www.sciencedirect.com/science/article/pii/S0269749118322668)

[82] Craftsmanship; Issue: Spring 2022: The Vegetable Detective; by TODD OPPENHEIMER https://craftsmanship.net/the-vegetable-detective/

[83] Jain, R.B. 2019: Synergistic impact of co-exposures to toxic metals cadmium, lead, and mercury along with perfluoroalkyl substances on the healthy kidney function, Environmental Research, Volume 169, 2019, https://doi.org/10.1016/j.envres.2018.11.037.

[84] Adeleye, A.T., et al. The Unseen Threat of the Synergistic Effects of Microplastics and Heavy Metals in Aquatic Environments: A Critical Review. Curr Pollution Rep (2024). https://doi.org/10.1007/s40726-024-00298-7

[85] Flora, Swaran J.S., and Vidhu Pachauri. 2010. "Chelation in Metal Intoxication" International Journal of Environmental Research and Public Health 7, no. 7: 2745-2788. https://doi.org/10.3390/ijerph7072745;

[86] https://embodywellness.com/services/chelation-therapy/

[87] Wax PM. Current use of chelation in American health care. J Med Toxicol. 2013 Dec;9(4):303-7. https://pubmed.ncbi.nlm.nih.gov/24113860/

[88] Ferrero, Maria Elena 2016: Rationale for the Successful Management of EDTA Chelation Therapy in Human Burden by Toxic Metals; Hindawi; Volume 2016 | https://pubmed.ncbi.nlm.nih.gov/27896275/

[89] AETNA Chelation Therapy; Number: 0234 ; Last Reviewopens in a new browser pop-up window 01/19/2023 https://www.aetna.com/cpb/medical/data/200_299/0234.html

[90] The History of the Thalidomide Tragedy https://www.thalidomide-tragedy.com/the-history-of-the-thalidomide-tragedy

[91] Fort Wayne; IV Chelation Lounge; https://www.fwivlounge.com/blog/chelation

[92] Jaishankar M, Tseten T, Anbalagan N, Mathew BB, Beeregowda KN. Toxicity, mechanism and health effects of some heavy metals. Interdiscip Toxicol. 2014 Jun;7(2):60-72. https://pubmed.ncbi.nlm.nih.gov/26109881/

[93] Abernethy, D.R., DeStefano, A.J., Cecil, T.L. et al. Metal Impurities in Food and Drugs. Pharm Res 27, 750–755 (2010). https://doi.org/10.1007/s11095-010-0080-3

[94] Dyer, C.A.2007; Heavy Metals as Endocrine-Disrupting Chemicals; 2007/01/01; 111; 133; 978-1-58829-830-0; Endocrine-Disrupting Chemicals: From Basic Science to Clinical Practice; http://eknygos.lsmuni.lt/springer/631/111-133.pdf

[95] Pourret, O. & Hursthouse, A. It's Time to Replace the Term "Heavy Metals" with "Potentially Toxic Elements" When Reporting Environmental Research. Int. J. Environ. Res. Public Health 16. https://www.ncbi.nlm.nih.gov/pmc/articles/PMC6887782/

[96] Water for Health: Do you need to detoxify heavy metals to reduce the impact of EMFs?; Written on August, 13 2021; https://www.water-for-health.co.uk/our-blog/2021/08/do-you-need-to-detoxify-heavy-metals-to-reduce-emf-impact/

[97] Theresa Dale, PhD, CCN, NP Heavy Metal Toxicity Increases Your Risk of Electromagnetic Sensitivity; https://www.wellnesscenter.net/resources/Heavy_Metal_Toxicity.htm

[98] Ansarihadipour H, et al Influence of Electromagnetic Fields on Lead Toxicity: A Study of Conformational Changes in Human Blood Proteins. Iran Red Crescent Med J. 2016 https://www.researchgate.net/publication/303710327_Influence_of_Electromagnetic_Fields_on_Lead_Toxicity_A_Study_of_Conformational_Changes_in_Human_Blood_Proteins

[99] Amara S, Douki T, et al 2011: Effects of static magnetic field and cadmium on oxidative stress and DNA damage in rat cortex brain and hippocampus. Toxicol Ind Health. 2011 Mar;27(2):99-106. https://pubmed.ncbi.nlm.nih.gov/20837562/

[100] Mortazavi, S. M. J., Paknahad, M., Khaleghi, I., & Eghlidospour, M. (2018). Effect of radiofrequency electromagnetic fields (RF-EMFS) from mobile phones on nickel release from

Notes

---

orthodontic brackets: An in vitro study. International Orthodontics. https://www.cochranelibrary.com/central/doi/10.1002/central/CN-01915145/full

[101] Mortazavi SM, Daiee E, et al 2008: Mercury release from dental amalgam restorations after magnetic resonance imaging and following mobile phone use. Pak J Biol Sci. 2008 Apr 15;11(8):1142-6. https://pubmed.ncbi.nlm.nih.gov/18819554/

[102] Shahidi SH, et al 2009. Effect of magnetic resonance imaging on microleakage of amalgam restorations: an in vitro study. Dentomaxillofac Radiol 2009;. https://pubmed.ncbi.nlm.nih.gov/19767518/

[103] Mortazavi SM, et al 2014: High-field MRI and mercury release from dental amalgam fillings. Int J Occup Environ Med. 2014 Apr;5(2):101-5. https://www.researchgate.net/publication/261613339_High-Field_MRI_and_Mercury_Release_from_Dental_Amalgam_Fillings

[104] Dr. Lam coaching: Heavy Metal Poisoning, Copper Overload, and Adrenal Fatigue By: Michael Lam, https://www.drlamcoaching.com/adrenal-fatigue/complications/heavy-metal-poisoning-copper-overload/

[105] Water for Health: Do you need to detoxify heavy metals to reduce the impact of EMFs?; Written on August, 13 2021; https://www.water-for-health.co.uk/our-blog/2021/08/do-you-need-to-detoxify-heavy-metals-to-reduce-emf-impact/

[106] Mariea T, Carlo G. Wireless radiation in the etiology and treatment of autism: Clinical observations and mechanisms. I Aust Coll Nutr & Env Med. 2007; 28(2): 3-7. https://studylib.net/doc/14162533/wireless-radiation-in-the-etiology-and-treatment-of-autis

[107] TAMARA MARIEA AND GEORGE CARLO (2007) "Wireless Radiation in the Etiology and Treatment of Autism: Clinical Observations and Mechanisms." https://static1.squarespace.com/static/58aca709cd0f6853031b4d1b/t/61197f33a80a3404d7c1539e/1629060915367/Excerpt+-+EMF+-+heavy+metals+and+other+synergistic+effects.pdf

[108] Juutilanen J, Kumlin T, Naarala J. Do extremely low frequency magnetic fields enhance the effects of environmental carcinogens? A meta-analysis of experimental studies. Ing J Radiat Biol. 2006; 82: 1-12. https://pubmed.ncbi.nlm.nih.gov/16546898/

[109] Amara S, Abdelmelek H, Carrel C, et al. Zinc supplementation ameliorates static magnetic field-induced oxidative stress in rat tissues. Environ Toxic& Pharmacol. 2007; 23(2): 193-197. https://pubmed.ncbi.nlm.nih.gov/21783757/

[110] Yurekli A, Ozkan M, Kalkan T, et al. GSM base station electromagnetic radiation and oxidative stress in rats. Elearomagn Biol Med. 2006; 25(3): 177-188.

[111] The Free Library. S.v. Interaction between electromagnetic radiation and toxic metals.." Retrieved May 21 2023 https://www.thefreelibrary.com/Interaction+between+electromagnetic+radiation+and+toxic+metals.-a0276901131

[112] Vecchia, Paolo; et al 2009: Exposure to high frequency electromagnetic fields, biological effects and health consequences (100 kHz-300 GHz) ETH Zürich; International Commission on Non-Ionizing Radiation Protection 2009 https://www.emf.ethz.ch/fileadmin/redaktion/public/downloads/4_wissen/externes_material/ICNIRP_effekte_RFReview.pdf

[113] Swiss Medical detox: Publications; 18 January 2019; Environmental diseases The chelation, an indispensable therapy with a future; http://www.swissmedicaldetox.ch/en/publications-2/

[114] Robyn Correll, MPH How Lead Poisoning Is Diagnosed; on July 07, 2021; Medically reviewed by Michael Menna, DO; verywellhealth.com https://www.verywellhealth.com/how-lead-poisoning-is-diagnosed-4160774

[115] Markowitz ME, Bijur PE, Ruff H, Rosen JF. Effects of calcium disodium versenate (CaNa2EDTA) chelation in moderate childhood lead poisoning. Pediatrics. 1993 Aug;92(2):265-71. https://pubmed.ncbi.nlm.nih.gov/8337028/

[116] Centers for Medicare & Medicaid Services: Heavy Metal Testing; A58628 https://www.cms.gov/medicare-coverage-database/view/article.aspx?articleId=58628&ver=5

[117] Wikipedia: Poisoning of Alexander Litvinenko; 14. 03. 2023 https://en.wikipedia.org/wiki/Poisoning_of_Alexander_Litvinenko

[118] Jennrich, Peter, 2007: Schwermetalle - Ursache für Zivilisationskrankheiten; 9783934672260 Company'MED-Verlag-Ges., 2007 https://www.zvab.com/products/isbn/9783934672260/30353487175

[119] Kern, Janet & Geier, David & Bjorklund, et al (2014). Evidence supporting a link between dental amalgams and chronic illness, fatigue, depression, anxiety, and suicide. Neuro endoc letters. 35. https://www.researchgate.net/publication/271536688_Evidence_supporting_a_link_between_dental_amalgams_and_chronic_illness_fatigue_depression_anxiety_and_suicide

[120] Koizumi N, Hatayama F, Sumino K. Problems in the analysis of cadmium in autopsied tissues. Environ Res. 1994 Feb;64(2):192-8. http://doi.org/10.1006/enrs.1994.1015.

[121] N. Zoeger,et al 2006: Lead accumulation in tidemark of articular cartilage; Generative AI: New policies, opportunities, and risks; VOLUME 14, ISSUE 9, P906-913, SEPT, 2006 https://doi.org/10.1016/j.joca.2006.03.001

[122] Smith, AH; Arroyo, AP; Mazumdar, DN. Arsenic-induced skin lesions among Atacameno people in northern Chile despite good nutrition and centuries of exposure. Environ. Hea. Perspect 2000, 108, 617–620. https://europepmc.org/article/med/10903614

[123] M S Islam, EuroAquae (2005-2007), Arsenic Contamination In Groundwater In Bangladesh: An Environmental And Social Disaster; Hydro Informatics and Water Management Program, University of Newcastle upon Tyne, Department Of Civil Engineering and Geosciences; https://www.iwapublishing.com/news/arsenic-contamination-groundwater-bangladesh-environmental-and-social-disaster

[124] Gabrielli, Paolo et al 2020: Early atmospheric contamination on the top of the Himalayas since the onset of the European Industrial Revolution; PNAS; February 10, 2020; 117 (8) 3967-3973; https://doi.org/10.1073/pnas.1910485117

[125] Houde M, Krümmel EM, et al 2022: Contributions and perspectives of Indigenous Peoples to the study of mercury in the Arctic. Sci Total Environ. 2022 Oct 1;841: https://pubmed.ncbi.nlm.nih.gov/35697218/

[126] Ebinghaus, R, Tripathi, R M, et al 1998: Natural and anthropogenic mercury sources and their impact on the air-surface exchange of mercury on regional and global scales. Germany: N. p., 1998. https://www.osti.gov/etdeweb/servlets/purl/351472

[127] Valera B, Dewailly E, Poirier P. Environmental mercury exposure and blood pressure among Nunavik Inuit adults. Hypert. 2009 Nov; https://pubmed.ncbi.nlm.nih.gov/19805642/

[128] Anjali Gopakumar, Julia Giebichenstein, Evgeniia Raskhozheva, Katrine Borgå, Mercury in Barents Sea fish in the Arctic polar night: Species and spatial comparison, Marine Pollution Bulletin, V. 169, 2021, (https://www.sciencedirect.com/science/article/pii/S0025326X2100535X)

[129] Muir DC, Wagemann R, Hargrave BT, Thomas DJ, Peakall DB, Norstrom RJ. Arctic marine ecosystem contamination. Sci Total Environ. 1992 Jul 15;122(1-2):75-134. https://pubmed.ncbi.nlm.nih.gov/1514106/

[130] Dastoor, Ashu; Wilson, S.J., et al 2022: Arctic atmospheric mercury: Sources and changes, Science of The Total Environment, Volume 839, 2022, 156213, (https://www.sciencedirect.com/science/article/pii/S0048969722033101)

[131] Lead pollution beat Amundsen and Scott to the South Pole by 20 years; July 28, 2014: https://theconversation.com/lead-pollution-beat-amundsen-and-scott-to-the-south-pole-by-20-years-29800

[132] Gworek, B., Dmuchowski, W. & Baczewska-Dąbrowska, A.H. Mercury in the terrestrial environment: a review. Environ Sci Eur 32, 128 (2020). https://doi.org/10.1186/s12302-020-00401-x

[133] Gabrielli, Paolo et al 2020: Early atmospheric contamination on the top of the Himalayas since the onset of the European Industrial Revolution; PNAS; February 10, 2020; 117 (8); https://doi.org/10.1073/pnas.1910485117

[134] Sundseth K, Pacyna JM, et al 2017: Global Sources and Pathways of Mercury in the Context of Human Health. Int J Environ Res Public Health. 2017 . https://www.ncbi.nlm.nih.gov/pmc/articles/PMC5295355/

[135] Heng YY, Asad I, Coleman B, et al 2022: Heavy metals and neurodevelopment of children in low and middle-income countries: A systematic review. PLoS One. 2022 Mar 31;17(3). https://www.ncbi.nlm.nih.gov/pmc/articles/PMC8970501/

[136] A Tribute to Karen Wetterhahn; Dartmouth Toxic Metals Superfund Research Program https://sites.dartmouth.edu/toxmetal/about-us/a-tribute-to-karen-wetterhahn/

[137] Gosselin RE, Smith RP, Hodge HC, eds. Clinical toxicology of commercial products. 5th ed. Baltimore: Williams & Wilkins, 1984. https://hero.epa.gov/hero/index.cfm/reference/details/reference_id/594545

[138] Los Angeles Times: Scientist's Death Helped Increase Knowledge of Mercury Poisoning; BY HELEN O'NEILL; SEPT. 14, 1997 ; https://www.latimes.com/archives/la-xpm-1997-sep-14-mn-32049-story.html

[139] Medpagetoday: Tiny Organic Mercury Spill Did This to Scientist's Brain A big lesson in lab safety and protocol; by Chubbyemu July 11, 2019; https://www.medpagetoday.com/publichealthpolicy/generalprofessionalissues/80958

[140] David W. Nierenberg, M.D.,1998: Delayed Cerebellar Disease and Death after Accidental Exposure to Dimethylmercury; une 4, 1998; N Engl J Med 1998; 338:1672-1676; https://www.nejm.org/doi/full/10.1056/nejm199806043382305

[141] Los Angeles Times: Scientist's Death Helped Increase Knowledge of Mercury Poisoning; BY HELEN O'NEILL; SEPT. 14, 1997 ; https://www.latimes.com/archives/la-xpm-1997-sep-14-mn-32049-story.html

[142] David W. Nierenberg, M.D.,1998: Delayed Cerebellar Disease and Death after Accidental Exposure to Dimethylmercury; une 4, 1998; N Engl J Med 1998; 338:1672-1676; https://www.nejm.org/doi/full/10.1056/nejm199806043382305

[143] Barnes: The cities most sought after by the wealthy: Miami 1st, Paris rises to 5th place; MARCH 17, 2022 https://www.barnes-miami.com/en/global-property-handbook-2022-miami-the-1st-city-sought-after-by-the-wealthy/

[144] Barnes international New 2023 edition of the GLOBAL PROPERTY HANDBOOK; Perspective; 06/03/2023; https://www.barnes-international.com/en/2023/new-2023-edition-of-the-global-property-handbook-1577-643-0-0

[145] Lead contamination lessons from the Notre Dame fire; By Sean M. Scott and Briana C. Scott | October 15, 2021; https://www.propertycasualty360.com/2021/10/15/lead-contamination-lessons-from-the-notre-dame-fire/?slreturn=20230208123143

[146] CBC news: Notre Dame fire spewed lead dust over Paris, with no rules for safe levels; The Associated Press · Posted: Dec 22, 2019 11:04 AM EST | Last Updated: December 8, 2022; https://www.cbc.ca/news/world/lead-dust-notre-dame-paris-1.5406214

[147] Gollenberg AL, Hediger ML, Lee PA, Himes JH, Louis GM. Association between lead and cadmium and reproductive hormones in peripubertal U.S. girls. Environ Health Perspect. 2010 Dec;118(12):1782-7. https://pubmed.ncbi.nlm.nih.gov/20675266/

[148] CDC: Childhood Lead Poisoning Prevention; Page last reviewed: September 2, 2022; https://www.cdc.gov/nceh/lead/prevention/default.htm

[149] Lanphear BP, Rauch S, Auinger P, Allen RW, Hornung RW. Low-level lead exposure and mortality in US adults: a population-baseno d cohort study. Lancet Public Health.; 2018;3(4):E177-E184. https://www.researchgate.net/publication/323742199_Low-level_lead_exposure_and_mortality_in_US_adults_A_population-based_cohort_study

[150] Choi HS, Suh MJ, Hong SC, Kang JW. The Association between the Concentration of Heavy Metals in the Indoor Atmosphere and Atopic Dermatitis Symptoms in Children Aged between 4 and 13 Years: A Pilot Study. Children (Basel). 2021 Nov 3;8(11):1004. https://www.ncbi.nlm.nih.gov/pmc/articles/PMC8625560/

[151] Blumer, W., and Cranton, E. 1989, "Ninety Percent Reduction in Cancer Mortality after Chelation Therapy With EDTA", J. of Advancement in Medicine, Vol 2, No, 1/2, Spring/ Summer 1989. https://oradix.com/ninety-percent-reduction-in-cancer-mortality-after-chelation-therapy-with-edta-the-famous-swiss-study/

[152] BBC: Notre-Dame fire lead pollution endangered life, lawsuit claims; Published; 6 July 2021; https://www.bbc.com/news/world-europe-57733690

[153] France 24 English: Concern over lead poisoning after Notre-Dame Cathedral fire; https://www.youtube.com/watch?v=UMm1WKKA0y0

[154] NYT: Notre-Dame's Toxic Fallout; By Elian Peltier, James Glanz, Weiyi Cai and Jeremy White; Sept. 16, 2019; https://www.nytimes.com/interactive/2019/09/14/world/europe/notre-dame-fire-lead.html

[155] Where does Paris water come from?; https://www.eaudeparis.fr/en/where-does-the-water-come-from-paris

[156] France 24 English: Concern over lead poisoning after Notre-Dame Cathedral fire; https://www.youtube.com/watch?v=UMm1WKKA0y0

[157] Daily Mail: PICTURED: Moment Michelle Obama's idyllic Parisian river cruise turns sour as the former First Lady and other revelers realize Notre Dame is on fire; EMILY CRANE FOR DAILYMAIL.COM PUBLISHED: 19:18 GMT, 16 April 2019; https://www.dailymail.co.uk/news/article-6928937/Michelle-Obama-Paris-cruise-Notre-Dame-caught-fire.html

[158] The Worst NASCAR Driver ; https://www.youtube.com/watch?v=i537kMchN44&t=50s

[159] Danica Patrick on detoxing from heavy metals https://www.youtube.com/watch?v=jPfgQ0le1u0&t=7s

[160] MERCURY EMISSIONS FROM MOTOR; 2004 International Emissions Inventory Conference 1 VEHICLES Clearwater, Florida Air Toxics Session June 7-10; https://www3.epa.gov/ttn/chief/conference/ei13/toxics/baldauf_pres.pdf

[161] Race Fuel 101: Lead and Leaded Racing Fuels https://www.sunocoracefuels.com/tech-corner/article/race-fuel-101-lead-leaded-racing-

fuels#:~:text=Lead%20is%20used%20in%20racing,P%2D51%20Mustang%20legendary%20perf
ormers!

[162] Mercury Toxicity & How Dr. Vane Treats Her Own Autoimmune Symptoms
https://www.youtube.com/watch?v=CsF8hwbdkNk

[163] Zhai Q, Narbad A, Chen W. Dietary strategies for the treatment of cadmium and lead toxicity.
Nutrients. 2015 Jan 14;7(1):552-71. http://doi.org/10.3390/nu7010552.

[164] Oregon State University: 2018; Micronutrient Inadequacies in the US Population: an
Overview; https://lpi.oregonstate.edu/mic/micronutrient-inadequacies/overview

[165] science.drinklmnt POTASSIUM DEFICIENCY (AND HOW TO GET ENOUGH POTASSIUM);
Robb Wolf; https://science.drinklmnt.com/electrolytes/potassium-
deficiency/#:~:text=Over%2097%25%20of%20Americans%20are,daily%20target%20of%204.7%
20grams.

[166] Anne-Marie Berenice Mayer, Liz Trenchard & Francis Rayns (2022) Historical changes in the
mineral content of fruit and vegetables in the UK from 1940 to 2019: a concern for human
nutrition and agriculture, International Journal of Food Sciences and Nutrition, 73:3,
https://www.tandfonline.com/doi/full/10.1080/09637486.2021.1981831#:~:text=The%20overall%2
0longer%2Dterm%20comparison,%25)%20and%20Mg%20(10%25).

[167] The Guardian: Mineral levels in meat and milk plummet over 60 years; Felicity Lawrence Thu
2 Feb 2006 https://www.theguardian.com/uk/2006/feb/02/foodanddrink

[168] Rangan, A., Jenkins, A., Murthy, D., & Cunningham, J. (2023). Temporal changes in mineral
content of fruit, vegetables and grains in Australian food composition databases. Proceedings of
the Nutrition Society, 82(OCE2), E91. https://www.cambridge.org/core/journals/proceedings-of-
the-nutrition-society/article/temporal-changes-in-mineral-content-of-fruit-vegetables-and-grains-
in-australian-food-composition-databases/0C23BA5457DFEDEA9753261900963E6E

[169] deannaminich.com: How Essential Minerals Protect Against Heavy Metals by dminich | Sep
15, 2021; https://deannaminich.com/metals-and-minerals/

[170] Schwalfenberg, Gerry, 2015: Vitamin D, essential Minerals, and Toxic Elements: Exploring
Interactions between Nutrients and Toxicants in Clinical Medicine; The Scientific World Journal;
http://doi.org/10.1155/2015/318595

[171] Moon J. The role of vitamin D in toxic metal absorption: a review. J Am Coll Nutr. 1994
Dec;13(6):559-64. http://doi/org/10.1080/07315724.1994.10718447.

[172] Better Health Channel https://www.betterhealth.vic.gov.au/health/healthyliving/Vitamins-and-
minerals

[173] chemistryworld.com ; Glyphosate persistence raises questions, BY REBECCA TRAGER25
FEBRUARY 2016; https://www.chemistryworld.com/news/glyphosate-persistence-raises-
questions/9510.article

[174] Demirci et al. (2020) Toxic Effects of Glyphosate-Based Herbicide on Melanopsis praemorsa,
ADYU J SCI, 10(1), 10- 21 https://dergipark.org.tr/en/download/article-file/1167268

[175] Piera M. Cirillo, et al 2021: Grandmaternal Perinatal Serum DDT in Relation to
Granddaughter Early Menarche and Adult Obesity: Three Generations in the Child Health
and Development Studies Cohort. Cancer Epidemiol Biomarkers Prev 1 August 2021; 30
(8): 1480–1488. https://doi.org/10.1158/1055-9965.EPI-20-1456

[176] USA Today: EPA finds no safe level for two toxic 'forever chemicals,' found in many U.S. water
systems; KYLE BAGENSTOSE; https://eu.usatoday.com/story/news/2022/06/15/epa-no-safe-
level-toxic-pfas-thousands-water-systems/7632524001/

[177] Cousins, Ian T. et al 2022: Outside the Safe Operating Space of a New Planetary Boundary
for Per- and Polyfluoroalkyl Substances (PFAS) Environ. Sci. Technol. 2022,
https://doi.org/10.1021/acs.est.2c02765

[178] wbur.org: Tracing the path of toxic 'forever chemicals' inside the body; February 16, 2023;
Gabrielle Emanuel; https://www.wbur.org/news/2023/02/16/pfas-biology-blood-new-hampshire

[179] Pennsylvania Departement of Health Revised January 30, 2023; Per- and polyfluoroalkyl
substances (PFAS) (also known as perflurochemicals, PFCs)
https://www.health.pa.gov/topics/Documents/Environmental%20Health/PFAS%20Fact%20Sheet.
pdf

[180] Emily Beglarian et al 2023: Exposure to perfluoroalkyl substances and longitudinal changes
in bone mineral density in adolescents and young adults: A multi-cohort study
https://doi.org/10.1016/j.envres.2023.117611

[181] Emily Beglarian, et al 2023: Exposure to perfluoroalkyl substances and longitudinal changes
in bone mineral density in adolescents and young adults: A multi-cohort study, Environmental
Research, Volume 244, 2024, https://doi.org/10.1016/j.envres.2023.117611.

[182] 'NBC Forever chemicals' stay in the air and water permanently. But scientists have found a
new way to destroy them. Aug. 18, 2022, By Aria Bendix

Notes

https://www.nbcnews.com/health/health-news/new-way-destroy-pfas-forever-chemicals-rcna43528

[183] Li, Jianqiu et al 2020: Coherent toxicity prediction framework for deciphering the joint effects of rare earth metals (La and Ce) under varied levels of calcium and NTA, Chemosphere, Volume 254, 2020, https://doi.org/10.1016/j.chemosphere.2020.126905.

[184] University of Strathclyde; ELECTRIC VEHICLE PARADIGM SHIFT; Rare Earth Elements: https://www.esru.strath.ac.uk/EandE/Web_sites/17-18/paradigmev/

[185] Electric vehicles: motors and magnets?; https://thundersaidenergy.com/downloads/electric-vehicles-motors-and-magnets/#:~:text=The%20average%20EV%20in%20our,much%20as%2015%20g%2FkW.

[186] Ramos-Ruiz A, et al 2017: Leaching of cadmium and tellurium from cadmium telluride (CdTe) thin-film solar panels under simulated landfill conditions. J Hazard Mater. 2017 http://doi.org/10.1016/j.jhazmat.2017.04.052.

[187] DHEC; scdhec.gov ; Whining some light on solar panels; https://scdhec.gov/sites/default/files/Library/OR-1695.pdf

[188] L.C. Su, H.D. Ruan, et al Release of metal pollutants from corroded and degraded thin-film solar panels extracted by acids and buried in soils, Applied Geochemistry, Volume 108, 2019, https://doi.org/10.1016/j.apgeochem.2019.104381.

[189] Aik Doulgeridou et al 2020: Review of Potentially Toxic Rare Earth Elements, Thallium and Tellurium in Plant-based Foods; efsa Journal; 26 November 2020; Volume 18, Issue S1; https://doi.org/10.2903/j.efsa.2020.e181101

[190] Antonios Apostolos Brouziotis 2022: Toxicity of rare earth elements: An overview on human health impact; Front. Environ. Sci., 07 September 2022; Sec. Toxicology, Pollution and the Environment ; Volume 10 - 2022 | https://doi.org/10.3389/fenvs.2022.948041

[191] Liu, Y., Wu, M., et al. (2019). Prenatal exposure of rare Earth elements cerium and ytterbium and neonatal thyroid stimulating hormone levels: Findings from a birth cohort study. Environ. Int. 133, https://www.sciencedirect.com/science/article/pii/S0160412019320720?via%3Dihub

[192] Antonios Apostolos Brouziotis 2022: Toxicity of rare earth elements: An overview on human health impact; Front. Environ. Sci., 07 September 2022; Sec. Toxicology, Pollution and the Environment; Volume 10 - 2022 | https://doi.org/10.3389/fenvs.2022.948041

[193] Li, Mengshi;, 2021: Association between exposure of light rare earth elements and outcomes of in vitro fertilization-embryo transfer in North China, Science of The Total Environment, Volume 762, 2021, 143106, https://doi.org/10.1016/j.scitotenv.2020.143106.

[194] Hu, Xin & Ding,et al (2002). Bioaccumulation of lanthanum and cerium and their effects on the growth of wheat (Triticum aestivum L.) seedlings. Chemosphere. 48. https://doi.org/10.1016/S0045-6535(02)00109-1.

[195] Aik Doulgeridou et al 2020: Review of Potentially Toxic Rare Earth Elements, Thallium and Tellurium in Plant-based Foods; efsa Journal; 26 November 2020; Volume 18, Issue S1; https://doi.org/10.2903/j.efsa.2020.e181101

[196] Brouziotis. AA et al 2022: Toxicity of rare earth elements: An overview on human health impact https://www.frontiersin.org/articles/10.3389/fenvs.2022.948041/full

[197] Flegal A. R. Smith D. R. 1992 Current needs for increased accuracy and precision in measurements of low levels of lead in blood. Environ Res. Aug; 58 2 125 33 .

[198] Dyer,C.A.2007; Heavy Metals as Endocrine-Disrupting Chemicals; 2007/01/01; 111; 133; 978-1-58829-830-0;; Endocrine-Disrupting Chemicals: From Basic Science to Clinical Practice; http://eknygos.lsmuni.lt/springer/631/111-133.pdf

[199] Grison, H., Petrovsky, E., Stejskalova, S., and Kapicka, A. (2015), Magnetic and geochemical characterization of Andosols developed on basalts in the Massif Central, France, Geochem. Geophys. Geosyst., 16, 1348– 1363, https://agupubs.onlinelibrary.wiley.com/doi/full/10.1002/2015GC005716

[200] British Geological Survey; Living with volcanoes; Discovering Geology — Volcanoes; https://www.bgs.ac.uk/discovering-geology/earth-hazards/volcanoes/living-with-volcanoes/

[201] Freire, Sergio, Aneta J. Florczyk, Martino Pesaresi, and Richard Sliuzas. 2019. "An Improved Global Analysis of Population Distribution in Proximity to Active Volcanoes, 1975–2015" ISPRS International Journal of Geo-Information 8, no. 8: 341. https://doi.org/10.3390/ijgi8080341

[202] Ermolin MS, Fedotov PS, Malik NA, Karandashev VK. Nanoparticles of volcanic ash as a carrier for toxic elements on the global scale. Chemosphere. 2018 Jun;200:16-22. https://pubmed.ncbi.nlm.nih.gov/29471164/

[203] Peña-Ocaña, Betsy-Anaid & Velázquez-Ríos,et al (2020). Changes in the Concentration of Trace Elements and Heavy Metals in El Chichón Crater Lake Active Volcano. Polish Journal of Environmental Studies. 30. http://www.pjoes.com/Changes-in-the-Concentration-of-Trace-Elements-nand-Heavy-Metals-in-El-Chichon-Crater,121045,0,2.html

[204] Ilyinskaya, E., Mason, E., Wieser, P.E. et al. Rapid metal pollutant deposition from the volcanic plume of Kīlauea, Hawai'i. Commun Earth Environ 2, 78 (2021). https://doi.org/10.1038/s43247-021-00146-2

[205] Ma Q, Han L, Zhang J, Zhang Y, Lang Q, Li F, Han A, Bao Y, Li K, Alu S. Environmental Risk Assessment of Metals in the Volcanic Soil of Changbai Mountain. Int J Environ Res Public Health. 2019 https://www.ncbi.nlm.nih.gov/pmc/articles/PMC6604000/

[206] Jianzhou Yang, Yanling Sun, et al 2022: Heavy metal pollution in agricultural soils of a typical volcanic area: Risk assessment and source appointment, Chemosphere, Volume 304, 2022, (https://www.sciencedirect.com/science/article/pii/S0045653522018331)

[207] Paula Silva Linhares, D., Ventura Garcia, P., & dos Santos Rodrigues, A. (2021). Trace Elements in Volcanic Environments and Human Health Effects. Trace Metals in the Environment - New Appr and Recent Adv. https://www.intechopen.com/chapters/70730

[208] Malandrino, Pasqualino,et al. 2020. "Increased Thyroid Cancer Incidence in Volcanic Areas: A Role of Increased Heavy Metals in the Environment?" International Journal of Molecular Sciences 21, no. 10: 3425. https://doi.org/10.3390/ijms21103425

[209] Several Site-specific Cancers are Increased in the Volcanic Area in Sicily MARCO RUSSO, PASQUALINO MALANDRINO, et al 2015: Anticancer Research, Jul 2015, 35 (7) 3995-4001; https://ar.iiarjournals.org/content/35/7/3995

[210] Malandrino, Pasqualino,et al. 2020. "Increased Thyroid Cancer Incidence in Volcanic Areas: A Role of Increased Heavy Metals in the Environment?" International Journal of Molecular Sciences 21, no. 10: 3425. https://doi.org/10.3390/ijms21103425

[211] Vigneri R, Malandrino P, Giani F, Russo M, Vigneri P. Heavy metals in the volcanic environment and thyroid cancer. Mol Cell Endocrinol. 2017 Dec 5;457:73-80. https://pubmed.ncbi.nlm.nih.gov/27794445/

[212] Ramos A, Quintana PJ, Ji M. Hair mercury and fish consumption in residents of O'ahu, Hawai'i. Hawaii J Med Public Health. 2014 Jan;73(1):19-25.: 24470983; https://www.ncbi.nlm.nih.gov/pmc/articles/PMC3901168/

[213] Brook RD, Brook JR, Tam EK. Volcanic smog and cardiometabolic health: Hawaiian hypertension? J Clin Hypertens (Greenwich). 2019 Apr;21(4):533-535. https://www.ncbi.nlm.nih.gov/pmc/articles/PMC8030391/

[214] Hlodversdottir H, Petursdottir G, Carlsen HK, et al Long-term health effects of the Eyjafjallajökull volcanic eruption: a prospective cohort study in 2010 and 2013 BMJ Open 2016;6:e011444. https://bmjopen.bmj.com/content/6/9/e011444.citation-tools

[215] Blumer, W., and Cranton, E. 1989, "Ninety Percent Reduction in Cancer Mortality after Chelation Therapy With EDTA", J. of Advancement in Medicine, Vol 2, No, 1/2, Spring/ Summer 1989. https://oradix.com/ninety-percent-reduction-in-cancer-mortality-after-chelation-therapy-with-edta-the-famous-swiss-study/

[216] EDTA Chelation Therapy UK & Europe; EDTA Chelation Studies Chelation Therapy Trials & Studies; https://cardiorenew-europe.com/studies/

[217] Die Deutsche Apotheker Zeitung (DAZ) Wie beeinflusst Übergewicht das Krebsrisiko? STUTTGART - 10.03.2021; https://www.deutsche-apotheker-zeitung.de/news/artikel/2021/03/10/wie-beeinflusst-uebergewicht-das-krebsrisiko

[218] Kontoghiorghes GJ, Efstathiou A, et al: Chelators controlling metal metabolism and toxicity pathways: applications in cancer prevention, diagnosis and treatment. Hemoglobin. 2008; https://pubmed.ncbi.nlm.nih.gov/18274999/

[219] Hancke C and Flytlie K 1993: Benefits of EDTA chelation therapy in arteriosclerosis: a retrospective study of 470 patients. J Adv Med 6(3):161,1993. https://www.researchgate.net/profile/Claus-Hancke/publication/265322766_Benefits_of_EDTA_Chelation_Therapy_in_Arteriosclerosis_A_Retrospective_Study_of_470_Patients/links/551fa6110cf2a2d9e1407b4a/Benefits-of-EDTA-Chelation-Therapy-in-Arteriosclerosis-A-Retrospective-Study-of-470-Patients.pdf

[220] Lamas GA, Goertz C, Boineau R, et al. Effect of Disodium EDTA Chelation Regimen on Cardiovascular Events in Patients With Previous Myocardial Infarction: The TACT Randomized Trial. JAMA. 2013 https://jamanetwork.com/journals/jama/fullarticle/1672238

[221] Enbody Wwellness: Chelation Therapy; What is Chelation Therapy? https://embodywellness.com/services/chelation-therapy/

[222] S. J. Cobbina, et al 2015: Low concentration toxic metal mixture interactions: Effects on essential and non-essential metals in brain, liver, and kidneys of mice on sub-chronic exposure, Chemosphere, 2015, https://doi.org/10.1016/j.chemosphere.2015.03.013.

[223] Gilani SR, Zaidi SR, et al. 2015: Report: Central nervous system (CNS) toxicity caused by metal poisoning: Brain as a target organ. Pak J Pharm Sci. 2015 Jul;28(4):1417-23. https://pubmed.ncbi.nlm.nih.gov/26142507/

Notes

[224] Morris LS, McCall JG, Charney DS, Murrough JW (21 July 2020). "The role of the locus coeruleus in the generation of pathological anxiety". Brain Neurosci. Adv. (4:2398212820930321). https://pubmed.ncbi.nlm.nih.gov/32954002/

[225] mhanational.org; What is Noradrenaline? https://mhanational.org/what-noradrenaline#:~:text=Noradrenaline%20(also%20called%20%22norepinephrine%22,brings%20on%20symptoms%20of%20depression.

[226] Pamphlett, R., Kum Jew, S. 2013: Heavy metals in locus ceruleus and motor neurons in motor neuron disease. acta neuropathol comm. https://doi.org/10.1186/2051-5960-1-81

[227] Pamphlett R, et al (2018): Age-related accumulation of toxic metals in the human locus ceruleus. PLoS ONE 13(9): e0203627. https://doi.org/10.1371/journal.pone.0203627

[228] Pamphlett, Roger et al 2023: The toxic metal hypothesis for neurological disorders; Front. Neurol., 23 June 2023; Vol. 14 – 2023; https://doi.org/10.3389/fneur.2023.1173779

[229] Pamphlett R, Mak R, Lee J, et al. (2020) Concentrations of toxic metals and essential trace elements vary among individual neurons in the human locus ceruleus. PLoS ONE 15(5): e0233300. https://doi.org/10.1371/journal.pone.0233300

[230] Pamphlett R, Mak R, Lee J, et al. (2020) Concentrations of toxic metals and essential trace elements vary among individual neurons in the human locus ceruleus. PLoS ONE 15(5): e0233300. https://doi.org/10.1371/journal.pone.0233300

[231] https://pubmed.ncbi.nlm.nih.gov/20329590/

[232] Shaw, William, 2010: The Unique Vulnerability of the Human Brain to Toxic Chemical Exposure and the Importance of Toxic Chemical Evaluation and Treatment in Orthomolecutar Psychiatry. Journal of Orthomolecular Medicine . 2010, Vol. 25 Issue 3, p125-134. 10p. https://isom.ca/wp-content/uploads/2013/01/The-Unique-Vulnerability-of-the-Human-Brain-to-Toxic-Chemical-Exposure-and-the-Importance-of-Toxic-Chemical-Evaluation-and-Treatment-in-Orthomolecular-Psychiatry-25.3.pdf

[233] López-Berenguer,G.; Peñalver,J.; E. Martínez-López, A critical review about neurotoxic effects in marine mammals of mercury and other trace elements, Chemosphere, Volume 246, 2020, (https://www.sciencedirect.com/science/article/pii/S0045653519329285)

[234] "Lead Linked to Premature Deaths in Adults: Early Exposure = 46% Higher Mortality." Source: TheBaltimore Sun. Quoted from the CDC.

[235] HAO, Z. et al 2015: association between longevity and element levels in food and drinking water of typical chinese longevity area; J Nutr Health Aging; September 30, 2015; http://www.igsnrr.cas.cn/news/kyjz/202011/P020201102589581781988.pdf

[236] Deng Q, Chen L, Wei Y, Li Y, Han X, Liang W, Zhao Y, Wang X, Yin J. Understanding the Association between Environmental Factors and Longevity in Hechi, China: A Drinking Water and Soil Quality Perspective. Int J Environ Res Public Health. 2018 Oct 16;15(10):2272. https://www.ncbi.nlm.nih.gov/pmc/articles/PMC6210010/

[237] R Lacatusu Radu,1996: Soil-plant-man relationships in heavy metal polluted areas in Romania,; Ap. Geochem., V. 11 1–2, 1996, https://doi.org/10.1016/0883-2927(95)00101-8.)

[238] Hormonesbalance.com: Top 4 Heavy Metals that Cause Hormone Imbalance, Fatigue, and Weight Gain; October 11th, 2019; Posted In Articles, Thyroid https://hormonesbalance.com/articles/heavy-metals-that-cause-hormone-imbalance-fatigue-weight-gain/--

[239] Iavicoli I, Fontana L, Bergamaschi A. The effects of metals as endocrine disruptors. J Toxicol Environ Health B Crit Rev. 2009 Mar; https://pubmed.ncbi.nlm.nih.gov/19466673/

[240] Sengupta, P. et al 2014: Metals and female reproductive toxicity; Human and Exp. Tox. 2015, V. 34 https://journals.sagepub.com/doi/pdf/10.1177/0960327114559611

[241] Vaiserman, Alexander, 2014: Early-life Exposure to Endocrine Disrupting Chemicals and Later-life Health Outcomes: An Epigenetic Bridge? Aging Dis. 2014 Dec; 5(6): https://www.ncbi.nlm.nih.gov/pmc/articles/PMC4249811/

[242] Fleisch AF, Wright RO, Baccarelli AA. 2012 : Environmental epigenetics: a role in endocrine disease? J Mol Endocrinol. 2012 Aug 30;49(2):R61-7. https://europepmc.org/article/med/22798698

[243] Genet, H. M. 2015: Geome-wide association study of toxic metals and trace elements reveals novel associations

[244] Gencer, B., Bonomi, M., Adorni, M.P. et al. Cardiovascular risk and testosterone – from subclinical atherosclerosis to lipoprotein function to heart failure. Rev Endocr Metab Disord 22, (2021). https://doi.org/10.1007/s11154-021-09628-2

[245] Dyer, C.A.2007; Heavy Metals as Endocrine-Disrupting Chemicals; 2007/01/01; 111; 133; 978-1-58829-830-0;; 10.1007/1-59745-107-X_5; Endocrine-Disrupting Chemicals: From Bas. Science to Clin Prac http://eknygos.lsmuni.lt/springer/631/111-133.pdf

[246] McGregor AJ, Mason HJ. Occupational mercury vapour exposure and testicular, pituitary and thyroid endocrine function. Hum Exp Toxicol. 1991;10(3): https://pubmed.ncbi.nlm.nih.gov/1678950/

[247] Doumouchtsis KK, Doumouchtsis SK, Doumouchtsis EK, Perrea DN. 2009: The effect of lead intoxication on endocrine functions. J Endocrinol Invest. 2009 Feb;32(2): https://pubmed.ncbi.nlm.nih.gov/19411819/

[248] Gerhard I, Waibel S, Daniel V, Runnebaum B. Impact of heavy metals on hormonal and immunological factors in women with repeated miscarriages. Hum Reprod Update. 1998 May-Jun;4(3): https://pubmed.ncbi.nlm.nih.gov/9741713/

[249] Camoratto, AM; White, LM; Berry, W; Moriarty, CM 1992: Effect of Heavy Divalent Metals on Anterior Pituitary Growth Hormone and Prolactin Release In Vitro Journal In Vitro Toxicology; Journal of Molecular and Cellular Toxicology; Issue 1 https://hero.epa.gov/hero/index.cfm/reference/details/reference_id/4971414

[250] Lafuente A; Esquifino, Ana I 1999: Cadmium effects on hypothalamic activity and pituitary hormone secretion in the male, Toxicology Letters, Volume 110, Issue 3, 1999, (https://www.sciencedirect.com/science/article/pii/S0378427499001599)

[251] Kalsi, A.K.,Halder,A.Jain,M.Srivastava,A.(2020).Association of Cadmium, Chromium, Manganese and Lead with Hyperprolactinemia: A Pilot Study,J Clin of Diagn Res. 14(1), QC04-QC07. https://www.doi.org/10.7860/JCDR/2020/42690/13439.

[252] hellomotherhood.com 4 Parts of the Brain Not Protected by the Blood Brain Barrier; By: Michele Noonal; 05 December, 2018; https://www.hellomotherhood.com/4-parts-of-the-brain-not-protected-by-the-blood-brain-barrier-4113369.html

[253] Kosta L, Byrne AR, Zelenko V. Correlation between selenium and mercury in man following exposure to inorganic mercury. Nature. 1975 Mar 20;254(5497):238-9.. https://pubmed.ncbi.nlm.nih.gov/1113885/

[254] Rana, S.V.S. 2014: Perspectives in Endocrine Toxicity of Heavy Metals—A Review. Biol Trace Elem Res 160, 1–14 (2014). https://doi.org/10.1007/s12011-014-0023-7

[255] Berger M, Gray JA, Roth BL. 2009 The expanded biology of serotonin. Annu Rev Med. 2009;60:355-66. https://www.ncbi.nlm.nih.gov/pmc/articles/PMC5864293/

[256] Carlsen E, Giwercman A, Keiding N, Skakkebaek NE. Evidence for decreasing quality of semen during past 50 years. BMJ. 1992 Sep 12;305(6854): https://pubmed.ncbi.nlm.nih.gov/1393072/

[257] Zeng L, Zhou J, Wang X, Zhang Y, Wang M, Su P. Cadmium attenuates testosterone synthesis by promoting ferroptosis and blocking autophagosome-lysosome fusion. Free Radic Biol Med. 2021 Nov 20;176:176-188. https://pubmed.ncbi.nlm.nih.gov/34610361/

[258] Yao Q, Zhou G, Xu M, Dai J, Qian Z, Cai Z, Zhang L, Tan Y, Hu R. 2019: Blood metal levels and serum testosterone concentrations in male and female children and adolescents: NHANES 2011-2012. PLoS One. 2019 Nov 7;14(11):e0224892. https://www.ncbi.nlm.nih.gov/pmc/articles/PMC6837506/

[259] Surampudi PN, Wang C, Swerdloff R. Hypogonadism in the aging male diagnosis, potential benefits, and risks of testosterone replacement therapy. Int J Endocrinol. 2012;2012:625434. https://pubmed.ncbi.nlm.nih.gov/22505891/

[260] Psychologytoday; Charles Harper Webb; TESTOSTERONE; How Testosterone Is the Jekyll and Hyde of Hormones; December 20, 2022; https://www.psychologytoday.com/us/blog/drawing-the-curtains-back/202211/how-testosterone-is-the-jekyll-and-hyde-of-hormones#:~:text=Testosterone%20increases%20muscle%20mass%20and,i.e.%2C%20adventurousness)%20and%20competition.

[261] Pluchino, Nicola & Carmignani, Arianna & Cubeddu, Alessandra & Santoro, Anna & Cela, Vito & Errasti, Tania. (2013). Androgen therapy in women: For whom and when. Archives of gynecology and obstetrics. 288. https://www.researchgate.net/publication/255177615_Androgen_therapy_in_women_For_whom_and_when

[262] Lucchini R, Albini E, 2000: Assessment of neurobehavioral performance as a function of current and cumulative occupational lead exposure Neurotoxicology 2000 21(5):805-11. https://pubmed.ncbi.nlm.nih.gov/11130286/

[263] Ronchetti SA, Miler EA, Duvilanski BH, Cabilla JP, Cadmium mimics estrogen-driven cell proliferation and prolactin secretion from anterior pituitary cells PloS One 2013 8(11):e8110 1https://doi.org/10.1371/journal.pone.0081101

[264] Luo, Qiong; Zhao, Hao; et al 2020: Association of blood metal exposure with testosterone and hemoglobin: A cross-sectional study in Hangzhou Birth Cohort Study,: Env. Int., Vol 136 (https://www.sciencedirect.com/science/article/pii/S0160412019331332)

Notes

[265] Đurđica Marić, et al (2022) Puzzling relationship between levels of toxic metals in blood and serum levels of reproductive hormones: Benchmark dose approach in cross-sectional study, All Life, 15:1, https://doi.org/10.1080/26895293.2022.2128439

[266] Dyer, C. A., 2007; Heavy Metals as Endocrine-Disrupting Chemicals; 2007/01/01; 111; 133; 978-1-58829-830-0;; 10.1007/1-59745-107-X_5; Endocrine-Disrupting Chemicals: From Basic Science to Clinical Practice http://eknygos.lsmuni.lt/springer/631/111-133.pdf

[267] Waalkes MP, Liu J, Chen H, Xie Y, Achanzar WE, Zhou YS, Cheng ML, Diwan BA. 2004: Estrogen signaling in livers of male mice with hepatocellular carcinoma induced by exposure to arsenic in utero. J Natl Cancer Inst 2004; https://academic.oup.com/jnci/article/96/6/466/2606744

[268] Jana K, Jana S, Samanta PK. Effects of chronic exposure to sodium arsenite on hypothalamo- pituitary-testicular activities in adult rats: possible an estrogenic mode of action. Reprod Biol Endocrinol 2006; 4:9. https://pubmed.ncbi.nlm.nih.gov/16483355/

[269] Meeker JD, Rossano MG, Protas B, et al 2008: Environmental exposure to metals and male reproductive hormones: circulating testosterone is inversely associated with blood molybdenum. Fertil Steril. 2010 https://www.ncbi.nlm.nih.gov/pmc/articles/PMC2823119/

[270]

[271] Hagai Levine, Niels Jørgensen, et al 2022: Temporal trends in sperm count: a systematic review and meta-regression analysis of samples collected globally in the 20th and 21st centuries, Human Reproduction, https://doi.org/10.1093/humupd/dmac035

[272] Karina M. Shreffler et al 2016: Infertility and fertility intentions, desires, and outcomes among US women: ; DEMOGRAPHIC RESEARCH; VOLUME 35, ARTICLE 39, PAGES 1149–1168 PUBLISHED 20 OCTOBER 2016 https://www.demographic-research.org/volumes/vol35/39/35-39.pdf

[273] Jennifer J. Yland, Michael L. Eisenberg, Elizabeth E. Hatch, Kenneth J. Rothman, Craig J. McKinnon, et al 2021: A North American prospective study of depression, psychotropic medication use, and semen quality, Fertility and Sterility, Volume 116, Issue 3, 2021, Pages 833-842, , https://doi.org/10.1016/j.fertnstert.2021.03.052.

[274] Jamalan M, Ghaffari MA, Hoseinzadeh P, Hashemitabar M, Zeinali M. Human Sperm Quality and Metal Toxicants: Protective Effects of some Flavonoids on Male Reproductive Function. Int J Fertil Steril. 2016 https://www.ncbi.nlm.nih.gov/pmc/articles/PMC4948074/

[275] Magda Carvalho Henriques, et al 2019: Exposure to mercury and human reproductive health: A systematic review, Reproductive Toxicology, Volume 85, 2019, https://doi.org/10.1016/j.reprotox.2019.02.012.

[276] López-Botella A et al 2021: Impact of Heavy Metals on Human Male Fertility-An Overview. Antioxidants (Basel). 2021 Sep 15; https://www.researchgate.net/publication/354621612_Impact_of_Heavy_Metals_on_Human_Male_Fertility-An_Overview

[277] Ilieva, I. .et al 2020: Toxic Effects of Heavy Metals (Lead and Cadmium) on Sperm Quality and Male Fertility; Acta morphologica et anthropologica, 27 (3-4) Sofia • 2020; http://www.iempam.bas.bg/journals/acta/acta27b/61-73.pdf

[278] Wilk A, Szypulska-Koziarska et al 2017: The toxicity of vanadium on gastrointestinal, urinary and reproductive system, and its influence on fertility and fetuses malformations. Postepy Hig Med Dosw (Online). 2017 Sep 25 https://pubmed.ncbi.nlm.nih.gov/29039350/

[279] Dekker Marcel, 1978: Hypogonadism in Chronically Lead -Poisoned Men; UCLA School of Medicine, Los Angeles, California 90048 and Reproductive Research Branch National Institute of Child Health; Infertility, 1(1), 33-51 (1978)

[280] Ilieva, I. .et al 2020: Toxic Effects of Heavy Metals (Lead and Cadmium) on Sperm Quality and Male Fertility; Acta morphologica et anthropologica, 27 (3-4) Sofia • 2020; http://www.iempam.bas.bg/journals/acta/acta27b/61-73.pdf

[281] Lin S, Hwang SA, Marshall EG, Stone R, Chen J. Fertility rates among lead workers and professional bus drivers: a comparative study. Ann Epidemiol. 1996 May;6(3):201-8. http://doi.org/10.1016/1047-2797(96)00010-5.

[282] Wani AL, Ara A, Usmani JA. Lead toxicity: a review. Interdiscip Toxicol. 2015 Jun;8(2):55-64. http://doi.org/10.1515/intox-2015-0009.

[283] Hertz-Picciotto, I. (2000), The evidence that lead increases the risk for spontaneous abortion. Am. J. Ind. Med.. https://doi.org/10.1002/1097-0274(200009)38:3<300::AID-AJIM9>3.0.CO;2-C

[284] Osmel La Llave León and José M. Salas Pacheco, 2020: Effects of Lead on Reproductive Health; Published: April 15th 2020; http://doi.org/10.5772/intechopen.91992

[285] Braunstein GD, Dahlgren J, Loriaux DL. Hypogonadism in chronically lead-poisoned men. Infertility. 1978;1(1):33-51..

[286] Doumouchtsis KK, Doumouchtsis SK, Doumouchtsis EK, Perrea DN. The effect of lead intoxication on endocrine functions. J Endocrinol Invest. 2009 Feb;32(2):175-83. http://doi.org/10.1007/BF03345710.

[287] Gollenberg AL, Hediger ML, Lee PA, Himes JH, Louis GM. Association between lead and cadmium and reproductive hormones in peripubertal U.S. girls. Environ Health Perspect. 2010 Dec;118(12):1782-7. http://doi.org/10.1289/ehp.1001943.

[288] Dickinson H, Parker L. Do alcohol and lead change the sex ratio. J Theor Biol 1994; 169:313–15 https://pubmed.ncbi.nlm.nih.gov/7967623/

[289] Dyer, C. A., 2007; Heavy Metals as Endocrine-Disrupting Chemicals; 2007/01/01; 111; 133; 978-1-58829-830-0;; 10.1007/1-59745-107-X_5; Endocrine-Disrupting Chemicals: From Basic Science to Clinical Practice http://eknygos.lsmuni.lt/springer/631/111-133.pdf

[290] Doumouchtsis KK, Doumouchtsis SK, Doumouchtsis EK, Perrea DN. 2009: The effect of lead intoxication on endocrine functions. J Endocrinol Invest. 2009 Feb;32(2). https://pubmed.ncbi.nlm.nih.gov/19411819/

[291] Pollack AZ, Schisterman EF,et al 2011: Cadmium, lead, and mercury in relation to reproductive hormones and anovulation in premenopausal women. Environ Health Perspect. 2011 Aug;119(8); https://www.ncbi.nlm.nih.gov/pmc/articles/PMC3237358/

[292] Jain M, Kalsi AK, et al 2016: High Serum Estradiol and Heavy Metals Responsible for Human Spermiation Defect-A Pilot Study. J Clin Diagn Res. 2016 Dec;10(12):. https://www.ncbi.nlm.nih.gov/pmc/articles/PMC5296528/

[293] Ali, H. M. et al 2019: "Effect of Some Heavy Metals on Testosterone Hormone in Infertile Men", JUBPAS, vol. 27, no. 6, pp. 368–377, Dec. 2019. https://www.journalofbabylon.com/index.php/JUBPAS/article/view/3169

[294] Enehizena, O.O.; Emokpae, M.A. 2022: Toxic Metal Concentrations in Drinking Water and Possible Effect on Sex Hormones among Men in Sabongida-Ora, Edo State, Nigeria. Medicines 2022,9,4. https://doi.org/10.3390/medicines9010004

[295] Igharo, O. G., Anetor, J. I.,et al . (2018). Endocrine disrupting metals lead to alteration in the gonadal hormone levels in; Nigerian e-waste workers. Universa Medicina, 37(1 https://doi.org/10.18051/UnivMed.2018.v37.65-74

[296] Wirth, Julia J &. Mijal, Renée S (2010) Adverse Effects of Low Level Heavy Metal Exposure on Male Reproductive Function, Systems Biology in Reproductive Medicine, https://web.archive.org/web/20190226110907id_/http://pdfs.semanticscholar.org/6c65/7853005e4c14fc1f0dd987fca769e213d1cf.pdf

[297] David, M., Jahan, S., Hussain, J. et al. Biochemical and reproductive biomarker analysis to study the consequences of heavy metal burden on health profile of male brick kiln workers. Sci Rep 12, 7172 (2022). https://doi.org/10.1038/s41598-022-11304-7

[298] Togawa, Kayo et al (2016). Parental Occupational Exposure to Heavy Metals and Welding Fumes and Risk of Testicular Germ Cell Tumors in Offspring: A Registry-Based Case-Control Study. Cancer Epidemiology Biomarkers & Prevention. 25. Http://doi.org/10.1158/1055-9965.EPI-16-0328.

[299] Sharma, T., B. D. Banerjee, et al. Heavy metal levels in adolescent and maternal blood: association with risk of hypospadias. – ISRN Pediatr., 2014, 714234. https://pubmed.ncbi.nlm.nih.gov/24729887/

[300] Ilieva, I. .et al 2020: Toxic Effects of Heavy Metals (Lead and Cadmium) on Sperm Quality and Male Fertility; Acta morphologica et anthropologica, 27 (3-4) Sofia, 2020; http://www.iempam.bas.bg/journals/acta/acta27b/61-73.pdf

[301] Ashrap P, Sánchez BN, et al 2019: In utero and peripubertal metals exposure in relation to reproductive hormones and sexual maturation and progression among girls in Mexico City. Environ Res. 2019 Oct https://pubmed.ncbi.nlm.nih.gov/31421446/

[302] Heidari, Amir Hassan, et al 2021: Detrimental effects of long-term exposure to heavy metals on histology, size and trace elements of testes and sperm parameters in Kermani Sheep, Ecotoxicology and Environmental Safety, Volume 207, 2021, 111563, (https://www.sciencedirect.com/science/article/pii/S0147651320314007)

[303] Al-Hasawi, Z.M. Adverse Impacts of Toxic Metal Pollutants on Sex Steroid Hormones of Siganus rivulatus (Teleostei: Siganid ae) from the Red Sea. Fishes 2022, 7, 367. https://doi.org/10.3390/fishes7060367

[304] Anyanwu, BO,et al 2020: Low-dose heavy metal mixture (lead, cadmium and mercury)-induced testicular injury and protective effect of zinc and Costus afer in wistar albino rats. Andrologia. 2020; 52:e13697. https://doi.org/10.1111/and.13697

[305] Nasiadek, M., Danilewicz, M., Sitarek, K. et al. The effect of repeated cadmium oral exposure on the level of sex hormones, estrous cyclicity, and endometrium morphometry in female rats. Environ Sci Pollut Res 25, 2018 https://doi.org/10.1007/s11356-018-2821-5

[306] Lafuente A; Esquifino, Ana I 1999: Cadmium effects on hypothalamic activity and pituitary hormone secretion in the male, Toxicology Letters, Volume 110, Issue 3, 1999, (https://www.sciencedirect.com/science/article/pii/S0378427499001599)

Notes

[307] Dyer, C. A., 2007; Heavy Metals as Endocrine-Disrupting Chemicals; 2007/01/01; 111; 133; 978-1-58829-830-0;; 10.1007/1-59745-107-X_5; Endocrine-Disrupting Chemicals: From Basic Science to Clin. Pract. http://eknygos.lsmuni.lt/springer/631/111-133.pdf

[308] Alsberg, C. L., & Schwartze, E. W. (1919). Pharmacological action of cadmium. J Pharmacol Exp Ther, 13, 504-505 .

[309] Chiquoine Ad. Observations On The Early Events Of Cadmium Necrosis Of The Testis. Anat Rec. 1964. https://www.ncbi.nlm.nih.gov/pmc/articles/PMC2752624/#R2

[310] Pant N, Upadhyay G, Pandey S, Mathur N, Saxena DK, Srivastava SP: Lead and cadmium concentration in the seminal plasma of men in the general population: correlation with sperm quality. Reprod Toxicol. 2003, 17: 447-450. http://doi.org/10.1016/S0890-6238(03)00036-4.

[311] Henson MC, Chedrese PJ: 2004: Endocrine disruption by cadmium, a common environmental toxicant with paradoxical effects on reproduction. Exp Biol Med. 2004, 229: 383-392. https://doi.org/10.1177/1535370204229005

[312] Ilieva, I. .et al 2020: Toxic Effects of Heavy Metals (Lead and Cadmium) on Sperm Quality and Male Fertility; Acta morphologica et anthropologica, 27 (3-4) Sofia, 2020; http://www.iempam.bas.bg/journals/acta/acta27b/61-73.pdf

[313] Dyer, C. A., 2007; Heavy Metals as Endocrine-Disrupting Chemicals; 2007/01/01; 111; 133; 978-1-58829-830-0;; 10.1007/1-59745-107-X_5; Endocrine-Disrupting Chemicals: From Basic Science to Clinical Practice http://eknygos.lsmuni.lt/springer/631/111-133.pdf

[314] Ilieva, I. .et al 2020:Toxic Effects of Heavy Metals (Lead and Cadmium) on Sperm Quality and Male Fertility; Acta morphologica et anthropologica, 27 (3-4) Sofia • 2020; http://www.iempam.bas.bg/journals/acta/acta27b/61-73.pdf

[315] NIH: ClinicalTrials.gov Role of the Toxic Metal Cadmium in the Mechanism Producing Infertility With a Varicocele; Identifier: NCT00044369; Information provided by National Institute of Environmental Health Sciences (NIEHS) Last Update Posted: 2006-09-04 ; https://beta.clinicaltrials.gov/study/NCT00044369

[316] Georgescu B. et. al. 2011: Heavy Metals Acting as Endocrine Disrupters/Scientific Papers: Animal Science and Biotechnologies, 2011, 44 (2); https://www.researchgate.net/publication/267725054_Heavy_Metals_Acting_as_Endocrine_Disrupters

[317] Castellini, Cesareet al. (2009). In vitro toxic effects of metal compounds on kinetic traits and ultrastructure of rabbit spermatozoa. Reproductive Toxicology. 27. https://pubmed.ncbi.nlm.nih.gov/19126427/

[318] Georgescu B. et. al. 2011: Heavy Metals Acting as Endocrine Disrupters/Scientific Papers: Animal Science and Biotechnologies, 2011, 44 (2); https://www.researchgate.net/publication/267725054_Heavy_Metals_Acting_as_Endocrine_Disrupters

[319] Mohamed MK, Burbacher TM, Mottet NK: Effects of methylmercury on testicular functions in Macaca fasicularis monkeys. Pharmacol Toxicol. 1987, 60:. https://pubmed.ncbi.nlm.nih.gov/3562387/

[320] Choy CM, Yeung QS, et al 2002: Relationship between semen parameters and mercury concentrations in blood and in seminal fluid from subfertile males in Hong Kong. Fertil Steril. 2002, 78: https://pubmed.ncbi.nlm.nih.gov/3562387/

[321] Dickerson EH, Sathyapalan T, Knight R, Maguiness SM, Killick SR, Robinson J, Atkin SL. 2011: Endocrine disruptor & nutritional effects of heavy metals in ovarian hyperstimulation. J Assist Reprod Genet. 2011 Dec;28(12):1223-8. https://www.researchgate.net/publication/51788741_Endocrine_disruptor_nutritional_effects_of_heavy_metals_in_ovarian_hyperstimulation

[322] Söderström-Anttila V, et al Surrogacy: outcomes for surrogate mothers, children and the resulting families-a systematic review. Hum Reprod Update. 2016 Mar-Apr;22(2):260-76. doi: http://10.1093/humupd/dmv046.

[323] Mills KC. Serotonin syndrome – a Clinical update. Med Toxicol. 1997;13:763-783. https://pubmed.ncbi.nlm.nih.gov/9330840/

[324] Phys.org; Study results suggest wild birds suffer personality disorders due to ingestion of heavy metals; by Bob Yirka , MARCH 26, 2018; https://phys.org/news/2018-03-results-wild-birds-personality-disorders.html

[325] NATIONAL GEOGRAPHIC NEWS: Mercury Poisoning Makes Birds Act Homosexual BY CHRISTINE DELL'AMORE ; PUBLISHED DECEMBER 5, 2010; https://www.nationalgeographic.com/science/article/101203-homosexual-birds-mercury-science

[326] Jabi Zabala, Joel C. Trexler,et al 2020: Early Breeding Failure in Birds Due to Environmental Toxins: A Potentially Powerful but Hidden Effect of Contamination Environm. Science & Technology 2020 https://pubs.acs.org/doi/10.1021/acs.est.0c04098

[327] Grunst AS, Grunst ML, Thys B, Raap T, Daem N, Pinxten R, Eens M. Variation in personality traits across a metal pollution gradient in a free-living songbird. Sci Total Environ. 2018 July https://www.researchgate.net/publication/323523365_Variation_in_personality_traits_across_a_metal_pollution_gradient_in_a_free-living_songbird

[328] Grunst, AS. et al 2019: An Important Personality Trait Varies with Blood and Plumage Metal Concentrations in a Free-Living Songbird; Environ. Sci. Technol. 2019, 53, 17, 10487–10496; August 2, 2019 https://pubs.acs.org/doi/abs/10.1021/acs.est.9b03548

[329] Chauhan V, Srikumar S, et al 2017: Methylmercury Exposure Induces Sexual Dysfunction in Male and Female Drosophila Melanogaster. Int J Environ Res Public Health. 2017 https://www.ncbi.nlm.nih.gov/pmc/articles/PMC5664609/

[330] Tan SW, Meiller JC, Mahaffey KR. The endocrine effects of mercury in humans and wildlife. Crit Rev Toxicol. 2009;39(3):228–269. https://pubmed.ncbi.nlm.nih.gov/19280433/

[331] Rice KM, Walker EM Jr, Wu M, Gillette C, Blough ER. Environmental mercury and its toxic effects. J Prev Med Public Health. 2014 Mar;47(2):74-83. https://www.ncbi.nlm.nih.gov/pmc/articles/PMC3988285/

[332] Rana, S.V.S. 2014: Perspectives in Endocrine Toxicity of Heavy Metals—A Review. Biol Trace Elem Res 160, 1–14 (2014). https://doi.org/10.1007/s12011-014-0023-7

[333] Smith SW 2013: The role of chelation in the treatment of other metal poisonings. Journal of Medical Toxicology: 2013, https://doi.org/10.1007/s13181-013-0343-6

[334] Rezaei M, et al 2019: Thyroid dysfunction: how concentration of toxic and essential elements contribute to risk of hypothyroidism, hyperthyroidism, and thyroid cancer. Environ Sci Pollut Res Int. 2019 Dec;26(35):35787-35796.. https://pubmed.ncbi.nlm.nih.gov/31701424/

[335] osewellness ; 6 Toxins That Threaten Thyroid Health March 12, 2021 ; https://rosewellness.com/toxins-threaten-thyroid-health/#:~:text=Heavy%20Metals%20–%20Most%20people%20have,children%27s%20toys%20can%20contain%20lead.

[336] Stojsavljević, A., Rovčanin, B., Krstić, Đ. et al. Risk Assessment of Toxic and Essential Trace Metals on the Thyroid Health at the Tissue Level: The Significance of Lead and Selenium for Colloid Goiter Disease. Expo Health 12, 255–264 (2020). https://doi.org/10.1007/s12403-019-00309-9

[337] Malandrino, Pasqualino,et al. 2020. "Increased Thyroid Cancer Incidence in Volcanic Areas: A Role of Increased Heavy Metals in the Environment?" International Journal of Molecular Sciences 21, no. 10: 3425. https://doi.org/10.3390/ijms21103425

[338] Livestrong.com What Happens When Your Body Uses Protein Instead of Fat? Angela Brady; https://www.livestrong.com/article/526008-what-happens-when-your-body-uses-protein-instead-of-fat/

[339] Libretexts medicine: 6.4: Protein Digestion and Absorption, https://med.libretexts.org/Bookshelves/Nutrition/An_Introduction_to_Nutrition_(Zimmerman)/06%3A_Proteins/6.04%3A_Protein_Digestion_and_Absorption

[340] Libretexts medicine: Protein Digestion and Absorption; https://med.libretexts.org/Bookshelves/Nutrition/An_Introduction_to_Nutrition_(Zimmerman)/06%3A_Proteins/6.04%3A_Protein_Digestion_and_Absorption#:~:text=Just%20as%20some%20plastics%20can,referred%20to%20as%20protein%20turnover.

[341] Markus J. Tamás, et al 2014: Heavy Metals and Metalloids As a Cause for Protein Misfolding and Aggregation; Biomolecules. 2014 Mar; 4(1): 252–267. ; Published online 2014 Feb 25. https://www.ncbi.nlm.nih.gov/pmc/articles/PMC4030994/

[342] Jessica Briffa, Emmanuel Sinagra, Renald Blundell, 2021: Heavy metal pollution in the environment and their toxicological effects on humans, Heliyon, Volume 6, Issue 9, 2020, (https://www.sciencedirect.com/science/article/pii/S2405844020315346)

[343] Olivier Barbier, Grégory Jacquillet, Michel Tauc, Marc Cougnon, Philippe Poujeol; Effect of Heavy Metals on, and Handling by, the Kidney. Nephron Physiology 1 April 2005; 99 (4): p105–p110. https://doi.org/10.1159/000083981

[344] Witkowska, Danuta & Słowik, Joanna & Chilicka-Hebel, Karolina. (2021). Heavy Metals and Human Health: Possible Exposure Pathways and the Competition for Protein Binding Sites. Molecules (Basel, Switzerland). 26. http://doi.org/10.3390/molecules26196060.

[345] Markus J. Tamás, et al 2014: Heavy Metals and Metalloids As a Cause for Protein Misfolding and Aggregation; Biomolecules. 2014 Mar; 4(1): 252–267. ; Published online 2014 Feb 25. https://www.ncbi.nlm.nih.gov/pmc/articles/PMC4030994/

[346] Markus J. Tamás, et al 2014: Heavy Metals and Metalloids As a Cause for Protein Misfolding and Aggregation; Biomolecules. 2014 Mar; 4(1): 252–267. ; Published online 2014 Feb 25. https://www.ncbi.nlm.nih.gov/pmc/articles/PMC4030994/

Notes

347 Sandeep K. Sharma, et al 2008: , Heavy metal ions are potent inhibitors of protein folding, Biochemical and Biophysical Research Communications, Volume 372, Issue 2, 2008, (https://www.sciencedirect.com/science/article/pii/S0006291X08009522)

348 Tewari, P.C., Jain, V.K., et al. (1986). Influence of protein deficiency on cadmium toxicity in rats. Arch. Environ. Contam. Toxicol. 15, https://doi.org/10.1007/BF01066408

349 D.J. Millward, Protein: Requirements, Editor(s): Benjamin Caballero, Paul M. Finglas, Fidel Toldrá, Encyclopedia of Food and Health, Academic Press, 2016, https://doi.org/10.1016/B978-0-12-384947-2.00573-0.

350 How much protein do you need every day? Harvard Health Publications; https://www.health.harvard.edu/blog/how-much-protein-do-you-need-every-day-201506188096

351 CDC news: What you need to know about protein supplements, and if you need them; Stephanie Dubois, CBC News, Feb 25, 2023 https://www.cbc.ca/radio/whitecoat/what-you-need-to-know-about-protein-supplements-and-if-you-need-them-1.6756834

352 Mayo Clinic, Heath services; SPEAKING OF HEALTH FRIDAY, APRIL 29, 2022; Are you getting too much protein? https://www.mayoclinichealthsystem.org/hometown-health/speaking-of-health/are-you-getting-too-much-protein

353 Deer RR, Volpi E. Protein Requirements in Critically Ill Older Adults. Nutrients. 2018 Mar 20;10(3):378. http://doi.org/10.3390/nu10030378.

354 HEALTHLINE.com Protein Intake — How Much Protein Should You Eat per Day? https://www.healthline.com/nutrition/how-much-protein-per-day#muscles-strength

355 EU; EFSA sets population reference intakes for protein; 9 February 2012; https://www.efsa.europa.eu/en/press/news/120209#:~:text=According%20to%20collated%20national%20food,g%20per%20day%20for%20women).

356 Loren Cordain, et al 2000: Plant-animal subsistence ratios and macronutrient energy estimations in worldwide hunter-gatherer diets12, The American Journal of Clinical Nutrition, Volume 71, Issue 3, 2000, (https://www.sciencedirect.com/science/article/pii/S0002916523070582)

357 Kious, Brent M. 2002: Hunter-gatherer Nutrition and Its Implications for Modern Societies; Nutrition Noteworthy, 5(1); https://escholarship.org/content/qt4wc9g8g4/qt4wc9g8g4.pdf

358 Scientificamerican; The Exercise Paradox; BY HERMAN PONTZER; FEBRUARY 1, 2017; https://www.scientificamerican.com/article/the-exercise-paradox/#:~:text=Hadza%20men%20ate%20and%20burned,fat%20percentage%2C%20age%20and%20sex.

359 Harman D. Free radical theory of aging: history. EXS. 1992;62:1-10. http://doi.org/10.1007/978-3-0348-7460-1_1.

360 Pham-Huy LA, He H, Pham-Huy C. Free radicals, antioxidants in disease and health. Int J Biomed Sci. 2008 Jun;4(2): https://www.ncbi.nlm.nih.gov/pmc/articles/PMC3614697/

361 Orisakwe OE. 2014. The role of lead and cadmium in psychiatry. N Am J Med Sci. 2014 Aug;6(8):370-6. https://www.ncbi.nlm.nih.gov/pmc/articles/PMC4158644/

362 Dumont, M.P. 1989; Psychotoxicology: The return of the mad hatter; Social Science & Medicine, Volume 29, Issue 9, 1989, Pages 1077-1082,; https://doi.org/10.1016/0277-9536(89)90019-1 .

363 What is mad hatter's disease? Medically reviewed by Heidi Moawad, M.D. — By Veronica Zambon on June 8, 2020; https://www.medicalnewstoday.com/articles/mad-hatters-disease

364 Ayuso-Álvarez, A.; Simón, L. et al 2019: Association between heavy metals and metalloids in topsoil and mental health in the adult population of Spain, Environ. Research, Volume 179, (https://www.sciencedirect.com/science/article/pii/S001393511930581X)

365 Bouchard, M. F., Bellinger, D. C., Weuve, J., Matthews-Bellinger, J., Gilman, S. E., Wright, R. O., Schwartz, J., & Weisskopf, M. G. (2009). Blood lead levels and major depressive disorder, panic disorder, and generalized anxiety disorder in US young adults. Archives of general psychiatry, 66(12), https://doi.org/10.1001/archgenpsychiatry.2009.164

366 Bouchard MF, Bellinger DC, 2009 Blood lead levels and major depressive disorder, panic disorder, and generalized anxiety disorder in US young adults. Arch Gen Psychiatry. 2009 Dec;66(12):1313-9.. https://www.ncbi.nlm.nih.gov/pmc/articles/PMC2917196/

367 Rhodes, Daniel MD, MPH; Spiro,2003: Relationship of Bone and Blood Lead Levels to Psychiatric Symptoms: The Normative Aging Study. Journal of Occupational and Envir. Medicine: November 2003 – V. 45 – Is.11 https://www.jstor.org/stable/44996906

368 Bouchard MF, Bellinger DC, 2009 Blood lead levels and major depressive disorder, panic disorder, and generalized anxiety disorder in US young adults. Arch Gen Psychiatry. 2009 Dec;66(12):1313-9. https://www.ncbi.nlm.nih.gov/pmc/articles/PMC2917196/

[369] Nord rarediseases.org: Heavy Metal Poisoning;: March 28, 2008; https://rarediseases.org/rare-diseases/heavy-metal-poisoning/

[370] Renzetti, S., Cagna, G., Calza, S. et al. 2021: The effects of the exposure to neurotoxic elements on Italian schoolchildren behavior. Sci Rep 11, 9898 (2021). https://doi.org/10.1038/s41598-021-88969-z

[371] Greenblatt, James M., M.D. The Role Of Heavy Metals In Psychiatric Disorder; Wednesday, June 28, 2017; The Great Plains Laboratory

[372] Mfem CC, Seriki SA, Oyama SE. 2021: Effects of Heavy Metal Toxicity on Anxiety Disorder. J Biomed Res Environ Sci. https://www.jelsciences.com/articles/jbres1294.php

[373] Marlowe M, Errera J, Jacobs J. 1983: Increased lead and mercury levels in emotionally disturbed children. Journal of Orthomolecular Psychiatry 1983; 12: 260-267; & Journal of Abnormal Psychology 1983; 93:386-9. https://psycnet.apa.org/record/1983-21305-001

[374] Akert RM, Aronson E, Wilson TD: Social Psychology, 7th Edition. Upper Saddle River, NJ, Prentice Hall, 2010

[375] Yıldız S, Gözü Pirinççioğlu A, Arıca E (January 17, 2023) Evaluation of Heavy Metal (Lead, Mercury, Cadmium, and Manganese) Levels in Blood, Plasma, and Urine of Adolescents With Aggressive Behavior. Cureus 15(1): https://www.cureus.com/articles/130878-evaluation-of-heavy-metal-lead-mercury-cadmium-and-manganese-levels-in-blood-plasma-and-urine-of-adolescents-with-aggressive-behavior#!/

[376] Cory-Slechta, D. Relationships between lead-induced learning impairments and changes in dopaminergic, cholinergic, and glutamatergic neurotransmitter system functions. Annu. Rev. Pharm. Toxicol. 35, 391–415 (1995). https://www.annualreviews.org/doi/10.1146/annurev.pa.35.040195.002135

[377] Needleman, H. Lead poisoning. Annu. Rev. Med. 55, 209–222 (2004). https://www.annualreviews.org/doi/10.1146/annurev.med.55.091902.103653

[378] Takeuchi, H., Taki, Y., Nouchi, R. et al. Lead exposure is associated with functional and microstructural changes in the healthy human brain. Commun Biol 4, 912 (2021). https://doi.org/10.1038/s42003-021-02435-0

[379] Smithsonian: Leaded Gas Was a Known Poison the Day It Was Invented; Kat Eschner; December 9, 2016; https://www.smithsonianmag.com/smart-news/leaded-gas-poison-invented-180961368 /

[380] Barrett, Kimberly L.; January 2013; Assessing the Relationship Between Hotspots of Lead and Hotspots of Crime; University of South Florida, Criminology and Criminal Justice Commons.

[381] Wani AL, Ara A, Usmani JA. Lead toxicity: a review. Interdiscip Toxicol. 2015 Jun;8(2):55-64. http://doi.org/10.1515/intox-2015-0009.

[382] Araújo GCSd, Mourão NT, Pinheiro IN, Xavier AR, Gameiro VS (2015): Lead Toxicity Risks in Gunshot Victims. PLoS ONE 10(10): https://doi.org/10.1371/journal.pone.0140220

[383] Bouchard, M. F., Bellinger, D. C., Weuve, J., Matthews-Bellinger, J., Gilman, S. E., Wright, R. O., Schwartz, J., & Weisskopf, M. G. (2009). Blood lead levels and major depressive disorder, panic disorder, and generalized anxiety disorder in US young adults. Archives of general psychiatry, 66(12), https://doi.org/10.1001/archgenpsychiatry.2009.164

[384] Edetanlen B, Saheeb B. Effect of bone fracture(s) on blood lead levels from retained lead pellets in craniomaxillofacial region. Human & Experimental Toxicology. 2019;38(12):1378-1383. https://journals.sagepub.com/doi/10.1177/0960327119862019

[385] Miao D, Young SL, Golden CD. A meta-analysis of pica and micronutrient status. Am J Hum Biol. 2015 Jan-Feb;27(1) https://www.ncbi.nlm.nih.gov/pmc/articles/PMC4270917/

[386] Eppright TD,et al 1996. ADHD, infantile autism, and elevated blood level: a possible relationship. Mo Med 1996; https://pubmed.ncbi.nlm.nih.gov/8867271/

[387] McFarland M. J. et al 2022: Half of US population exposed to adverse lead levels in early childhood; PROCEEDINGS OF THE NATIONAL ACADEMY OF SCIENCES; Vol. 119 | No. 11; March 15, 2022; https://doi.org/10.1073/pnas.2118631119

[388] Crime and Heavy Metal; Air Date: Week of June 6, 1997; https://www.loe.org/shows/segments.html?programID=97-P13-00023&segmentID=1

[389] H.R. Casdorph, Toxic Metal Syndrome, Avery Publishing Group, 1995 & S.E. Levick, Yale Univ. School of Medicine, New England Journal of Med; July 17, 1980.

[390] Worldwide Health Center; Effects of Toxic Metals on Learning and Behaviour George Georgiou 10/04/2017; https://www.worldwidehealthcenter.net/effects-toxic-metals-learning-behaviour/

[391] Gottschalk LA, et al, Abnormalities in hair trace elements as indicatores of aberrant behavior. Compr Psychiatry 1991; 32(3): 229-37.

[392] Menon AV, Chang J, Kim J. 2016: Mechanisms of divalent metal toxicity in affective disorders. Toxicology. 2016 Jan https://www.ncbi.nlm.nih.gov/pmc/articles/PMC4724313/

Notes

393 https://www.youtube.com/watch?v=ra4-gmQT_50

394 CDC: Understanding the Pandemic's Impact on Children and Teens; March 22, 2022 https://www.cdc.gov/nssp/partners/Understanding-the-impact.html

395 Addiitutemag: TikTok Tics: What's Causing a Surge in Tic Disorders Among Teens?; By Carole Fleck; February 6, 2023 https://www.additudemag.com/tiktok-tics-adhd-teens-tic-disorders/

396 Schneider SA, Hennig A, Martino D. 2021: Relationship between COVID-19 and movement disorders: A narrative review. Eur J Neurol. 2022 Apr;29(4):1243-1253. https://pubmed.ncbi.nlm.nih.gov/34918437/

397 Pringsheim, T., Ganos, C., McGuire, J.F., Hedderly, T., Woods, D., Gilbert, D.L., Piacentini, J., Dale, R.C. and Martino, D. (2021), Rapid Onset Functional Tic-Like Behaviors in Young Females During the COVID-19 Pandemic. Mov Disord, 36: 2707-2713. https://doi.org/10.1002/mds.28778

398 Geier DA, Kern JK, Hooker BS, King PG, Sykes LK, Homme KG, Geier MR. Thimerosal exposure and increased risk for diagnosed tic disorder in the United States: a case-control study. Interdiscip Toxicol. 2015 Jun;8 http://doi.org/10.1515/intox-2015-0011.

399 Polanczyk G., de Lima M.S., Horta B.L., Biederman J., Rohde L.A. The worldwide prevalence of ADHD: A systematic review and metaregression analysis. Am. J. Psychiatry. 2007;164:942–948. https://ajp.psychiatryonline.org/doi/full/10.1176/ajp.2007.164.6.942

400 Christensen, D. L. et al. (2016). Prevalence and characteristics of autism spectrum disorder among children aged 8 years—Autism and developmental disabilities monitoring network, 11 sites, United States, 2012. MMWR Surveill. Summ. 65, 1–23. https://doi.org/10.15585/mmwr.ss6503a1

401 Polanczyk GV, Willcutt EG, Salum GA, Kieling C, Rohde LA: ADHD prevalence estimates across three decades: an updated systematic review and meta-regression analysis. Int J Epidemiol. 2014, https://www.ncbi.nlm.nih.gov/pmc/articles/PMC4817588/

402 Norwegian Institute of Public Health : Heavy metals and essential minerals during pregnancy and associations with ADHD and autism in children; Research findings Published 08.04.2021; https://www.fhi.no/en/news/2021/heavy-metals-pregnancy-adhd/

403 Cho, Sung-Yun et al 2012: Analysis of Heavy Metals in the Hair of Children with Attention-Deficit Hyperactivity Disorder and Tourette's Syndrome; Journal of the Korean Academy of Child and Adolescent Psychiatry; Volume 23 Issue 2 / http://www.koreascience.or.kr/article/JAKO201222350106484.page

404 Baum Hedlund Aristei & Goldman; Heavy Metals in Baby Food and ADHD; https://www.baumhedlundlaw.com/toxic-baby-food-lawsuit-autism-adhd/heavy-metals-and-adhd/

405 Sudha R Raman et al 2018:,Trends in attention-deficit hyperactivity disorder medication use: a retrospective observational study using population-based databases; Lancet psychiatry; articles| volume 5, issue 10, p824-835, October 01, 2018; https://www.thelancet.com/journals/lanpsy/article/PIIS2215-0366%2818%2930293-1/fulltext#articleInformation

406 Cheuk, D & Wong, Virginia. (2006). Attention-Deficit Hyperactivity Disorder and Blood Mercury Level: a Case-Control Study in Chinese Children. Neuropediatrics. 37. 234-40. http://doi.org/10.1055/s-2006-924577.

407 Li, Y., Cha, C., Lv, X. et al. Association between 10 urinary heavy metal exposure and attention deficit hyperactivity disorder for children. Environ Sci Pollut Res 27, 31233–31242 (2020). https://doi.org/10.1007/s11356-020-09421-9

408 Boucher O, Jacobson SW, et al 2012: Prenatal methylmercury, postnatal lead exposure, and evidence of attention deficit/hyperactivity disorder among Inuit children in Arctic Québec. Environ Health Perspect. 2012 Oct;120(10):1456-61. https://www.ncbi.nlm.nih.gov/pmc/articles/PMC3491943/

409 WHO 2007: Health risks of heavy metals from long-range trasboundery air pollution. ; https://www.euro.who.int/__data/assets/pdf_file/0007/78649/E91044.pdf

410 Richard Malter : Copper Excess (Toxicity): Psychological Implications for Children, Adolescents, and Adults; April, 1984 June, 2001 https://nutritionalbalancing.org/center/htma/science/articles/copper-excess

411 Russo AJ. Decreased Serum Cu/Zn SOD Associated with High Copper in Children with Attention Deficit Hyperactivity Disorder (ADHD). J Cent Nerv Syst Dis. 2010 May http://doi.0rg/10.4137/jcnsd.s4553. .

412 GREENBLATT, JAMES, MD; The Role Of Heavy Metals And Environmental Toxins In Psychiatric Disorders; July 10, 2017: file:///Users/sachadobler/Desktop/The%20Role%20of%20Heavy%20Metals%20and%20Environmental%20Toxins%20in%20Psychiatric%20Disorders%20—%20%20Great%20Plains%20Laboratory.html

413 Nayak S, Sahu S, Patra S, et al. (December 25, 2021) Assessment of Copper and Zinc Levels in Hair and Urine of Children With Attention Deficit Hyperactivity Disorder: A Case-Control

Study in Eastern India. Cureus 13(12): https://www.cureus.com/articles/79204-assessment-of-copper-and-zinc-levels-in-hair-and-urine-of-children-with-attention-deficit-hyperactivity-disorder-a-case-control-study-in-eastern-india#!/

[414] Ciesielski T, Bellinger DC, Schwartz J, Hauser R, Wright RO. 2013: Associations between cadmium exposure and neurocognitive test scores in a cross-sectional study of US adults. Env. Health. 2013 https://ehjournal.biomedcentral.com/articles/10.1186/1476-069X-12-13

[415] Lee MJ, Chou MC, Chou WJ, Huang CW, Kuo HC, Lee SY, Wang LJ. Heavy Metals' Effect on Susceptibility to Attention-Deficit/Hyperactivity Disorder: Implication of Lead, Cadmium, and Antimony. Int J Environ Res Public Health. 2018 Jun 10;15(6):1221. https://www.ncbi.nlm.nih.gov/pmc/articles/PMC6025252/

[416] Tuthill RW. 1996: Hair lead levels related to children's classroom attention- deficit behavior. Arch Environ Health 1996; https://doi.org/10.1080/00039896.1996.9936018

[417] Choi WJ, Kwon HJ, Lim MH, Lim JA, Ha M. 2016: Blood lead, parental marital status and the risk of attention-deficit/hyperactivity disorder in elementary school children: A longitudinal study. Psychiatry Res. 2016 Feb 28; https://www.sciencedirect.com/science/article/abs/pii/S0165178115300810

[418] Said Yousef, Abdu Adem, Taoufik Zoubeidi, Melita Kosanovic, Abdel Azim Mabrouk, Valsamma Eapen, Attention Deficit Hyperactivity Disorder and Environmental Toxic Metal Exposure in the United Arab Emirates, Journal of Tropical Pediatrics, Volume 57, Issue 6, December 2011, https://doi.org/10.1093/tropej/fmq121

[419] Sioen et al. (2013). Prenatal exposure to environmental contaminants and behavioural problems at age 7–8years. Envir. Internat, 59, https://pubmed.ncbi.nlm.nih.gov/23845936/

[420] Braun et al (2006). Exposures to environmental toxicants and attention deficit hyperactivity disorder in U.S. children. Environmental Health Perspectives, 114(12),. https://www.ncbi.nlm.nih.gov/pmc/articles/PMC1764142/

[421] Kim et al. (2010). Association between blood lead levels (< 5 µg/dL) and inattention-hyperactivity and neurocognitive profiles in school-aged Korean children. Science of the Total Environment, 408(23), https://www.sciencedirect.com/science/article/abs/pii/S0048969710008119?via%3Dihub

[422] Fredrick, Randi, Ph.D; Chelation Therapy and Mental HealthMentalhelp.net; https://www.mentalhelp.net/blogs/chelation-therapy-and-mental-health/

[423] Medicalmedium; Obsessive Compulsive Disorder (OCD); 30-May-2017 https://www.medicalmedium.com/blog/obsessive-compulsive-disorder

[424] HTMA testing,; Copper Toxicity and Obsessive Compulsive Disorder ; © Alternative Health Experts LLC 2009-2023.https://www.htmaexperts.com/copper-toxicity-and-obsessive-compulsive-disorder/

[425] metabolichealing.com; Michael McEvoy; THE COPPER TOXICITY EPIDEMIC: TOP 10 HEALTH CONDITIONS, STRATEGIES & SOLUTIONS; https://metabolichealing.com/copper-toxicity-major-epidemic/#:~:text=Copper%20toxicity%20and%20deranged%20ceruloplasmin,compulsive%20disorder)%20(6).

[426] Osman Virit et al 2006: High ceruloplasmin levels are associated with obsessive compulsive disorder: a case control study: Behavioral and Brain Functions 2008, https://behavioralandbrainfunctions.biomedcentral.com/counter/pdf/10.1186/1744-9081-4-52.pdf

[427] Correia S, Hubbard E, Hassenstab J, Yip A, Vymazal J, Herynek V, Giedd J, Murphy DL, Greenberg BD. Basal ganglia MR relaxometry in obsessive-compulsive disorder: T2 depends upon age of symptom onset. Brain Imaging Behav. 2010 Mar;4(1):35-45. https://www.ncbi.nlm.nih.gov/pmc/articles/PMC3018344/

[428] Vanderbilt University Medical Center. (2009, January 29). New Role For Serotonin 'Ironed Out'. ScienceDaily. Retrieved April 29, 2023 from www.sciencedaily.com/releases/2009/01/090127123009.htm

[429] Serotonin Levels Linked to Iron Buildup in Dopamine Brain Region Steve Bryson, PhD avatar; by Steve Bryson, PhD | December 29, 2021; https://parkinsonsnewstoday.com/news/serotonin-levels-linked-iron-buildup-substantia-nigra-study-finds/

[430] True Cause of OCD - Obsessive Compulsive Disorder; https://www.medicalmedium.com/blog/true-cause-of-ocd-obsessive-compulsive-disorder

[431] Melendez, Luana et al.,2013: Aluminium and Other Metals May Pose a Risk to Children with Autism: Spectrum Disorder: Biochemical and Behavioural Impairments: Clin Exp Pharmacol 2013, 3:1; http://doi.org/10.4172/2161-1459.1000120

[432] Canadian Lyme disease foundation; AUTISM-A TYPE OF LYME DISEASE Medical Hypothosis Kathy Blanco December 15, 2004 Copywrite 2004; http://wellnesspharmacy.com/wp-content/uploads/2015/01/autism-lyme-disease.pdf

Notes

[433] Jafari T, Rostampour N, Fallah AA, Hesami A. The association between mercury levels and autism spectrum disorders: A systematic review and meta-analysis. J Trace Elem Med Biol. 2017 Dec;44:289-297. http://doi.org/10.1016/j.jtemb.2017.09.002.

[434] Treatment Options for Mercury/Metal Toxicity in Autism and Related Developmental Disabilities: Consensus Position Paper; February 2005; AUTISM RESEARCH INSTITUTE; p. 6 https://vce.org/mercury/merctreat.pdf

[435] Li, H., Li, H., Li, Y. et al. Blood Mercury, Arsenic, Cadmium, and Lead in Children with Autism Spectrum Disorder. Biol Trace Elem Res 181, 31–37 (2018). https://doi.org/10.1007/s12011-017-1002-6

[436] Mohamed Fel B, et al 2015: Assessment of Hair Aluminum, Lead, and Mercury in a Sample of Autistic Egyptian Children: Environmental Risk Factors of Heavy Metals in Autism. Behav Neurol. https://www.hindawi.com/journals/bn/2015/545674/

[437] Kern, Janet & Geier, David & Bjorklund, et al (2014). Evidence supporting a link between dental amalgams and chronic illness, fatigue, depression, anxiety, and suicide. Neuro endocrinology letters. 35. https://www.researchgate.net/publication/271536688_Evidence_supporting_a_link_between_dental_amalgams_and_chronic_illness_fatigue_depression_anxiety_and_suicide

[438] Canadian Lyme disease foundation; AUTISM-A TYPE OF LYME DISEASE Medical Hypothosis Kathy Blanco December 15, 2004 Copywrite 2004; http://wellnesspharmacy.com/wp-content/uploads/2015/01/autism-lyme-disease.pdf

[439] Homme, K., Kern, J. K., Geier, D. A., Bjørklund, G., King, P. G., Homme, K. G., ... Geier, M. R. (2014). Amalgams and Chronic Illness, Fatigue, Depression, Anxiety, and Suicide. Academic Press.

[440] Lahouaoui, H.; et al 2019: Depression and Anxiety Emerging From Heavy Metals: What Relationship? Source Title: Handbook of Research on Global; Environmental Changes and Human Health; Pages: 17 https://www.researchgate.net/publication/330635466_Depression_and_Anxiety_Emerging_From_Heavy_Metals_What_Relationship

[441] Theorell, T., Hammarström, A., Aronsson, G. et al. A systematic review including meta-analysis of work environment and depressive symptoms. BMC Public Health 15, 738 (2015). https://doi.org/10.1186/s12889-015-1954-4

[442] Shih RA, Glass TA, Bandeen-Roche K, et al. 2006: Environmental lead exposure and cognitive function in community-dwelling older adults. Neurology. 2006;67:1556-1562. https://www.researchgate.net/publication/6818756_Environmental_lead_exposure_and_cognitive_function_in_community-dwelling_older_adults

[443] Siblerud RI. 1989: The relationship between mercury from dental amalgam and mental health. Am J Psychother. 1989;43:575-587. https://pubmed.ncbi.nlm.nih.gov/2132561/

[444] Xia F, Li Q, Luo X, Wu J. Machine learning model for depression based on heavy metals among aging people: A study with National Health and Nutrition Examination Surv. 2017-2018. Fr. Pub. H. 2022 https://www.frontiersin.org/articles/10.3389/fpubh.2022.939758/full

[445] Brunswick Health Clinic: Essential Minerals and Mood Disorders;; HAIR TESTING ANALYSIS; 2020; https://hairtestinganalysis.com.au/essential-minerals-and-mood-disorders.html

[446] Shiue, I. (2015). Urinary heavy metals, phthalates and polyaromatic hydrocarbons independent of health events are associated with adult depression: USA NHANES, 2011–2012. Environmental Science and Pollution Research International, 22(21), 17095–17103. https://core.ac.uk/download/pdf/74228649.pdf

[447] Fu, Xihang; Li, Huiru; et al 2023: Association of urinary heavy metals co-exposure and adult depression: Modification of physical activity, NeuroToxicology, Volume 95, 2023, (https://www.sciencedirect.com/science/article/pii/S0161813X23000165)

[448] World Health Organization. Mental Health: New Understanding, New Hope. Geneva, Switzerland: World Health Organization; 2001. World health report. https://apps.who.int/iris/handle/10665/42390

[449] Lamtai, M. , et al (2018) Effect of Chronic Administration of Cadmium on Anxiety-Like, Depression-Like and Memory Deficits in Male and Female Rats: Possible Involvement of Oxidative Stress Mechanism. Journal of Behavioral and Brain Science, 8, 240-268. https://www.scirp.org/journal/paperinformation.aspx?paperid=84469

[450] Scinicariello F, Buser MC. Blood cadmium and depressive symptoms in young adults (aged 20-39 years). Psychol Med. 2015 https://www.ncbi.nlm.nih.gov/pmc/articles/PMC4571450/

[451] Nguyen, D., Oh, H., Hoang, N.H.M. et al. 2022: Environmental science and pollution research role of heavy metal concentrations and vitamin intake from food in depression: a national cross-sectional study (2009–2017). Environ Sci Pollut Res 29, (2022). https://doi.org/10.1007/s11356-021-15986-w

[452] Sciarillo, W. G., Alexander, G., & Farrell, K. P. (1992). Lead exposure and child behavior. American Journal of Public Health, 82 https://pubmed.ncbi.nlm.nih.gov/1415859/

[453] Sioen, I., Den Hond, E., Nelen, V., Van de Mieroop, E., Croes, K., Van Larebeke, N., ... Schoeters, G. (2013). Prenatal exposure to environmental contaminants and behavioural problems at age 7-8years. Environment International, 59, 225–231. https://www.sciencedirect.com/science/article/pii/S0160412013001323?via%3Dihub 6

[454] Siblerud, R. L., Motl, J., & Kienholz, E. (1994). Psychometric evidence that mercury from silver dental fillings may be an etiological factor in depression, excessive anger, and anxiety. Psychological Reports, 74(36), http://orthomolecular.org/library/jom/1998/articles/1998-v13n01-p031.shtml

[455] Kern, Janet & Geier, David & Bjorklund, et al (2014). Evidence supporting a link between dental amalgams and chronic illness, fatigue, depression, anxiety, and suicide. Neuro endocrinology letters. 35. 537-552. https://www.researchgate.net/publication/271536688_Evidence_supporting_a_link_between_dental_amalgams_and_chronic_illness_fatigue_depression_anxiety_and_suicide

[456] Siblerud, R. L., Motl, J., & Kienholz, E. (1994). Psychometric evidence that mercury from silver dental fillings may be an etiological factor in depression, excessive anger, and anxiety. Psychological Reports, 74(1), 67–80. https://doi.org/10.2466/pr0.1994.74.1.67

[457] Jarup, Lars 2013: Hazards of heavy metal contamination; British Medical Bulletin, Volume 68, Issue 1, December 2003, https://doi.org/10.1093/bmb/ldg032

[458] Mercury Fillings: Dental Amalgam Side Effects and Reactions; The International Academy of Oral Medicine and Toxicology; https://iaomt.org/resources/dental-mercury-facts/dental-mercury-amalgam-side-effects/#_edn1

[459] Bernhoft, R. A. (2012). Mercury toxicity and treatment: A review of the literature. Journal of Environ- mental and Public Health, 2012, 1–10. https://downloads.hindawi.com/journals/jeph/2012/460508.pdf

[460] Lahouaoui, H.; et al 2019: Depression and Anxiety Emerging From Heavy Metals: What Relationship? Source Title: Handbook of Research on Global; Environmental Changes and Human Health; Pages: 17 https://www.researchgate.net/publication/330635466_Depression_and_Anxiety_Emerging_From_Heavy_Metals_What_Relationship

[461] Mills KC. Serotonin syndrome. Med Toxicol. 1997;13:763-783. https://pubmed.ncbi.nlm.nih.gov/9330840/

[462] Bouchard MF, Bellinger DC,et al 2009: Blood lead levels and major depressive disorder, panic disorder, and generalized anxiety disorder in US young adults. Arch Gen; Psychiatry. 2009 Dec;66 https://www.ncbi.nlm.nih.gov/pmc/articles/PMC2917196/

[463] Rhodes, Daniel MD, MPH; Spiro, Avron III PhD; Aro, Antonio PhD; Hu, Howard MD, MPH, ScD. Relationship of Bone and Blood Lead Levels to Psychiatric Symptoms: The Normative Aging Study. Journal of Occupational and Environmental Medicine: November 2003 - Volume 45 - Issue 11 - http://doi.org/10.1097/01.jom.0000094995.23808.7b

[464] Rhodes, Daniel MD, MPH; Spiro, et al 2003: Relationship of Bone and Blood Lead Levels to Psychiatric Symptoms: The Normative Aging Study. Journal of Occupational and Environmental Medicine: November 2003 - Volume 45 - Issue 11 - p 1144-1151 https://www.jstor.org/stable/44996906

[465] Päivi Leino, Guido Magni, 1993: Depressive and distress symptoms as predictors of low back pain, neck-shoulder pain, and other musculoskeletal morbidity: a 10-year follow-up of metal industry employees, Pain, Volume 53, Issue 1, 1993, Pages 89-94, (https://www.sciencedirect.com/science/article/pii/0304395993900603)

[466] Mfem CC, Seriki SA, Oyama SE. 2021: Effects of Heavy Metal Toxicity on Anxiety Disorder. J Biomed Res Environ Sci. 2021 Aug 13; 2(8): 660-668. https://www.jelsciences.com/articles/jbres1294.php

[467] Bridges of Recovery. Beverly hills: 5 Ways to Tell the Difference Between Stress and Anxiety: When to Get Help March 18, 2020, Mary Ellen EllisBridges to RecoveryLOGO; https://www.bridgestorecovery.com/blog/5-ways-to-tell-the-difference-between-stress-and-anxiety-when-to-get-help/

[468] Bouchard MF, Bellinger DC,et al 2009: Blood lead levels and major depressive disorder, panic disorder, and generalized anxiety disorder in US young adults. Arch Gen; Psychiatry. 2009 Dec;66 https://www.ncbi.nlm.nih.gov/pmc/articles/PMC2917196/

[469] Alvaro, P. K., Roberts, R. M., & Harris, J. K. (2014). The independent relationships between insomnia, depression, subtypes of anxiety, and chronotype during adolescence. Sleep Medicine, 15(8), 934–941. https://pubmed.ncbi.nlm.nih.gov/24958244/

Notes

[470] Mfem CC, Seriki SA, Oyama SE. 2021: Effects of Heavy Metal Toxicity on Anxiety Disorder. J Biomed Res Environ Sci. 2021 Aug 13; 2(8): 660-668. https://www.jelsciences.com/articles/jbres1294.php

[471] Levin-Schwartz, Yuri; Whitney Cowell et al, 2022: Metal mixtures are associated with increased anxiety during pregnancy, Environmental Research, Volume 204, Part C, 2022, (https://www.sciencedirect.com/science/article/pii/S0013935121015772)

[472] rezilirhealth.com: Heavy Metal Toxic Exposure Can Severely Affect Brain Health By Susan Luck, RN, BS, MA, HN-BC, CCN, HWNC-BC; https://rezilirhealth.com/brain-health-heavy-metal-toxic-exposure/

[473] Guo G, Ma H, Wang X. [Psychological and neurobehavioral effects of aluminum on exposed workers]. Zhonghua Yu Fang Yi Xue Za Zhi. 1998 Sep;32(5):292-4. Chinese. https://pubmed.ncbi.nlm.nih.gov/10322775/

[474] Lahouaoui, H.; et al 2019: Depression and Anxiety Emerging From Heavy Metals: What Relationship? Source Title: Handbook of Research on Global; Environmental Changes and Human Health; |Pages: 17; https://www.researchgate.net/publication/330635466_Depression_and_Anxiety_Emerging_From_Heavy_Metals_What_Relationship

[475] Jurczak A; Brodowska, A,et al. 2018: Influence of Pb and Cd levels in whole blood of postmenopausal women on the incidence of anxiety and depressive symptoms. Ann Agric Environ Med. 2018; 25(2): 219–223. https://pubmed.ncbi.nlm.nih.gov/29936823/

[476] Shvachiy, Liana, Ângela Amaro-Leal,et al 2022. "From Molecular to Functional Effects of Different Environmental Lead Exposure Paradigms" Biology 11, no. 8: 1164. https://doi.org/10.3390/biology11081164

[477] Flora SJ, Mittal M, Mehta A. 2008: Heavy metal induced oxidative stress & its possible reversal by chelation therapy. Indian J Med Res. 2008 Oct;128(4):501-23. https://www.researchgate.net/publication/23688119_Flora_SJS_Mittal_M_Mehta_A_Heavy_metal_induced_oxidative_stress_its_possible_reversal_by_chelation_therapy_Indian_J_Med_Res_128_501-523

[478] Steenkamp, Lisa R. et al 2017: Severity of Anxiety– but not Depression– is Associated with Oxidative Stress in Major Depressive Disorder; J Affect Disord. 2017 Sep; 219: 193–200. NIHMSID: NIHMS880258 https://www.ncbi.nlm.nih.gov/pmc/articles/PMC5550320/

[479] Bouayed J, Rammal H, Soulimani R. Oxidative stress and anxiety: relationship and cellular pathways. Oxid Med Cell Longev. 2009 Apr-Jun;2(2):63-7. https://downloads.hindawi.com/journals/omcl/2009/623654.pdf

[480] Anbrin Masood, Ahmed Nadeem, S. Jamal Mustafa and James M. O'Donnell 2008: Reversal of Oxidative Stress-Induced Anxiety by Inhibition of Phosphodiesterase-2 in Mice Journal of Pharmacology and Experimental Therapeutics August 2008, 326 (2) https://doi.org/10.1124/jpet.108.137208

[481] Player, M. S., & Peterson, L. E. (2011). Anxiety Disorders, Hypertension, and Cardiovascular Risk: A Review. The International Journal of Psychiatry in Medicine, 41(4), 365–377. https://doi.org/10.2190/PM.41.4.f;

[482] Yu Pan, et al 2015: Association between anxiety and hypertension: a systematic review and meta-analysis of epidemiological studies; Neuropsychiatr Dis Treat. 2015; 11: 1121–1130. Published online 2015 Apr 22. https://www.researchgate.net/publication/275720146_Association_between_anxiety_and_hypertension_A_systematic_review_and_meta-analysis_of_epidemiological_studies

[483] Ekerdt DJ, Sparrow D, Glynn RJ, Bossé R. Change in blood pressure and total cholesterol with retirement. Am J Epidemiol. 1984 Jul;120(1):64-71. https://pubmed.ncbi.nlm.nih.gov/6741924/

[484] Juraschek SP, Woodward M, Sacks FM, Carey VJ, Miller ER 3rd, Appel LJ. Time Course of Change in Blood Pressure From Sodium Reduction and the DASH Diet. Hypertension. 2017 Nov;70(5):923-929. https://pubmed.ncbi.nlm.nih.gov/28993451/

[485] Cheung BM, Au T, Chan S, Lam C, Lau Sh, Lee R, Lee S, Lo W, Sin E, Tang M, Tsang H. The relationship between hypertension and anxiety or depression in Hong Kong Chinese. Exp Clin Cardiol. 2005 Spring;10(1):21-4. https://www.ncbi.nlm.nih.gov/pmc/articles/PMC2716224/

[486] Gerstner HB, Huff JE (1977). Clinical toxicology of mercury. Journal of Toxicology and Environmental Health 2: 491–526 https://pubmed.ncbi.nlm.nih.gov/321797/

[487] Darja Kobal Grum, et al 2006: Personality Traits in Miners with Past Occupational Elemental Mercury Exposure; Environmental Health Perspectives 114:2 CID: https://doi.org/10.1289/ehp.7863

[488] Kern, Janet & Geier, David & Bjorklund, et al (2014). Evidence supporting a link between dental amalgams and chronic illness, fatigue, depression, anxiety, and suicide. Neuro endocrinology letters. 35. 537-552.

https://www.researchgate.net/publication/271536688_Evidence_supporting_a_link_between_den
tal_amalgams_and_chronic_illness_fatigue_depression_anxiety_and_suicide
[489] Figgs LW, Holsinger H, et al 2011: Increased suicide risk among workers following toxic metal
exposure at the Paducah gaseous diffusion plant from 1952 to 2003: a cohort study. Int J Occup
Environ Med. 2011 Oct;2(4) https://pubmed.ncbi.nlm.nih.gov/23022839/.
[490] The Guardian: Leyland Cecco in Victoria
Thu 20 Jul 2023; https://www.theguardian.com/world/2023/jul/20/canada-mercury-poisoning-first-
nations-indigenous-youth-suicides
[491] Gronek I, Kolomaznik M. Urove'n tsinka v syvorotke krovi pri nekotorykh psikhicheskikh
rasstroĭstvakh [Serum zinc levels in various mental disorders]. Zh Nevropatol Psikhiatr Im S S
Korsakova. 1989;89(10):126-7. Russian. https://pubmed.ncbi.nlm.nih.gov/2618218/
[492] Seattle Times; Rising number of suicide attempts among young children worries NW
physicians, poison centers ; May 31, 2022 By Hannah Furfaro;
https://www.seattletimes.com/seattle-news/mental-health/rising-number-of-suicide-attempts-
among-young-children-worries-physicians-poison-centers/
[493] CDC; NIOSH Backgrounder: Alice's Mad Hatter & Work-Related Illness; March 4, 2010;
https://www.cdc.gov/niosh/updates/upd-03-04-10.html
[494] Clarkson TW, Magos L (2006). The toxicology of mercury and its chemical compounds.
Critical Reviews in Toxicology 36: 609–662. https://pubmed.ncbi.nlm.nih.gov/16973445/
[495] Wikipedia Erethism: 12.24.2022: https://en.wikipedia.org/wiki/Erethism
[496] https://www.oldsaltblog.com/2014/03/terrible-tilly-and-other-killer-lighthouses/
[497] The Old Salt Blog: Mad as a Lighthouse Keeper — Not the Solitude, but the Mercury
Posted on March 20, 2014 by Rick Spilman; https://www.oldsaltblog.com/2014/03/mad-as-a-
lighthouse-keeper-not-the-solitude-but-the-mercury/
[498] Split Rock Lighthouse; Lighthouse Technology;
https://www.mnhs.org/splitrock/learn/technology
[499] The Dark Side of Lighthouses Mouthfuls of molten lead, wild weather, and insanity: the
occupational hazards of an early lighthouse keeper. by Amorina Kingdon; November 18, 2016;
https://hakaimagazine.com/article-short/dark-side-lighthouses/
[500] History of Medicine Days; Lighthouse Keeper's Madness: Folk Legend Or Something More
Toxic? By Michaela Walter; Paskowitz M D, Richard A. Paskowitz
Soldier Joker the Legacy; Lulu.com, 23 Jul 2008,
[501] Twin Light lighthouse: Lighthouse Keepers In The Early 1900s: A Difficult Job; November 4,
2022 by Scott; https://www.twinlightslighthouse.com/lighthouse-keepers-in-the-early-1900s-a-
difficult-job/
[502] The Mirror: Inside island where lighthouse keeper driven mad and then raped and executed
neighbours; 15 Jul 2022 https://www.mirror.co.uk/news/weird-news/inside-island-lighthouse-
keeper-driven-27430237
[503] Duplinsky TG, Cicchetti DV (2012). The health status of dentists exposed to mercury from
silver amalgam tooth restorations. International Journal of Statistics in Medical Research 1:
https://www.lifescienceglobal.com/pms/index.php/ijsmr/article/view/433/pdf
[504] Dr. Matthew Carpenter; 2018, Austin All Natural; TO CHELATE, OR NOT TO CHELATE;
https://www.tdhtx.com/articles/to-chelate-or-not-to-chelate
[505] Hollins DM, McKinley MA, et al 2009: Beryllium and lung cancer: A weight of evidence
evaluation of the toxicological and epidemiological literature. Critical Reviews in Toxicology.
https://pubmed.ncbi.nlm.nih.gov/19384680/
[506] Fireman E, Kramer MR, Priel I, Lerman Y. Chronic beryllium disease among dental
technicians in Israel. Sarcoidosis Vasc Diffuse Lung Dis. 2006.
https://pubmed.ncbi.nlm.nih.gov/18038921/
[507] Hilt B, Svendsen K, et al. 87 (2009). Occurrence of cognitive symptoms in dental assistants
with previous occupational exposure to metallic mercury. Neurotox. 30:
https://pubmed.ncbi.nlm.nih.gov/19427330/
[508] Duplinsky TG, Cicchetti DV (2012). The health status of dentists exposed to mercury from
silver amalgam tooth restorations. International Journal of Statistics in Medical Research 1: 1–
15. https://www.lifescienceglobal.com/pms/index.php/ijsmr/article/view/433/pdf
[509] Goodrich JM, Wang Y, Gillespie B, Werner R, Franzblau A, Basu N. Methylmercury and
elemental mercury differentially associate with blood pressure among dental professionals. Int J
Hyg Environ Health. 2013 Mar;216(2):195-201.
https://www.ncbi.nlm.nih.gov/pmc/articles/PMC3727420/ .
[510] Bjørklund, G, Hilt, B, Dadar, M, Lindh, U, Aaseth, J. 2019: Neurotoxic effects of mercury
exposure in dental personnel. Basic Clin Pharmacol Toxicol. 2019; 124:.
https://onlinelibrary.wiley.com/doi/full/10.1111/bcpt.13199

[511] Waalkes MP, Liu J, Chen H, Xie Y, Achanzar WE, Zhou YS, Cheng ML, Diwan BA. Estrogen signaling in livers of male mice with hepatocellular carcinoma induced by exposure to arsenic in utero. J Natl Cancer Inst 2004; 96:466–74.

[512] Chattopadhyay S, Ghosh S, Chaki S, Debnath J, Ghosh D. Effect of sodium arsenite on plasma levels of gonadotrophins and ovarian steroidogenesis in mature albino rats: duration-dependent response. J Toxicol Sci 1999; 24:425–31.

[513] Kern, Janet & Geier, David & Bjorklund, et al (2014). Evidence supporting a link between dental amalgams and chronic illness, fatigue, depression, anxiety, and suicide. Neuro endocrinology letters. 35. 537-552.
https://www.researchgate.net/publication/271536688_Evidence_supporting_a_link_between_den tal_amalgams_and_chronic_illness_fatigue_depression_anxiety_and_suicide

[514] Knobeloch L, Steenport D, Schrank C, Anderson H. Methylmercury exposure in Wisconsin: A case study series. Environ Res. 2006 May;101(1):113-22.
https://www.researchgate.net/publication/7567458_Methylmercury_exposure_in_Wisconsin_A_c ase_study_series

[515] Substance Use Disorders Among Dentists; J. William Claytor Jr., DDS, MAGD On Oct 11, 2021 https://decisionsindentistry.com/article/substance-use-disorder-among-dentists/

[516] Curtis EK. (2011) "When dentists do drugs: A prescription for prevention." Today's FDA. 23: 28. http://www.dentistwellbeing.com/pdf/DentistsDoDrugs.pdf.

[517] Robb ND. Alcoholism and the dentist. Br J Addict. 1990 Apr;85(4):437-9.
https://pubmed.ncbi.nlm.nih.gov/2189510/

[518] Arnetz BB, Hörte LG, Hedberg A, Malker H (1987). Suicide among Swedish dentists. A ten-year follow-up study. Scandinavian Journal of Social Medicine 15: 243–246
https://pubmed.ncbi.nlm.nih.gov/3500511/

[519] Elizabeth Meyer: Stress, burnout, substance abuse and impairment amongst members of the dental profession; INTERNATIONAL DENTISTRY – AFRICAN EDITION VOL.11, NO. 1
https://www.moderndentistrymedia.com/moderndentistrymedia/wp-content/uploads/2021/02/meyer.pdf

[520] Cooper C, Watts J and Kelly M. Job satisfaction, mental health, and job stressors among general dental practitioners in the UK. Br Dent J 1987; 162: 77-81.
https://scirp.org/reference/referencespapers.aspx?referenceid=3054984

[521] Westgarth D. Mental health in dentistry: Has the profession opened up through the years? BDJ In Pract. 2022;35(6) https://www.ncbi.nlm.nih.gov/pmc/articles/PMC9168629/ .

[522] Robb ND. Alcoholism and the dentist. Br J Addict. 1990 Apr;85(4):437-9.
https://pubmed.ncbi.nlm.nih.gov/2189510/

[523] investopedia 2022: 25 Highest Paid Occupations in the US;
https://www.investopedia.com/personal-finance/top-highest-paying-jobs/

[524] Lohnanalyse, Zahnarzt/Zahnärztin in der Schweiz;
https://www.lohnanalyse.ch/ch/loehne/details/zahnarztzahnaerztin.html

[525] Bush DM, Lipari RN. Substance use and substance use disorder by industry. Substance Abuse and Mental Health Services Administration. Center for Behavioral Health Statistics and Quality. 2015.

[526] Chris Carberg; Last updated: June 14, 2023
https://www.addictionhelp.com/addiction/statistics/#:~:text=Percent%20of%20People%20with%2 0a,of%20people%2026%20and%20older

[527] WebMD: Doctors' Suicide Rate Highest of Any Profession; May 8, 2018; Written by Pauline Anderson; https://www.webmd.com/mental-health/news/20180508/doctors-suicide-rate-highest-of-any-profession

[528] punemirror.com ; Doctor dies earlier than a normal citizen: IMA study; By PuneMirror Bureau Vicky PathareWed, 11 Jul 2018; https://punemirror.com/pune/civic/doctor-dies-earlier-than-a-normal-citizen-ima-study/cid5133648.htm

[529] Gul N, Khan S, Khan A, Ahmad SS. Mercury health effects among the workers extracting gold from carpets and dusted clays through amalgamation and roasting processes. Environ Sci Pollut Res Int. 2015 Nov;22(22) https://pubmed.ncbi.nlm.nih.gov/26169819/

[530]Forum; Schmutziger Goldrausch; So finden Sie faires Gold; https://www.forum-csr.net/News/10279/Schmutziger-Goldrausch.html

[531] tamararubin.com: Gold wedding set (c. 2016): 5,527 ppm Mercury, 1,214 ppm Arsenic (+ Gold, Silver, Titanium & Copper). https://tamararubin.com/2017/01/gold-wedding-set-c-2016-5527-ppm-mercury-1214-ppm-arsenic-gold-silver-titanium-copper/

[532] Monger, A. et al 2020 : Lead and Mercury Exposure and Related Health Problems in Metal Artisan Workplaces and High-Risk Household Contacts in Thimphu, Bhutan; Hindawi the Scientific World Journal; Volume 2020, Article ID 9267181,
https://downloads.hindawi.com/journals/tswj/2020/9267181.pdf

[533] Mercury in Our Waters: The 10,000-Year Legacy of California's Gold Rush; By Alexandria Herr; September 30, 2020 https://www.kcet.org/shows/earth-focus/mercury-in-our-waters-the-10-000-year-legacy-of-californias-gold-rush

[534] Mercury Contamination: Toxic Legacy of the Gold Rush; Assembly Natural Resources Committee March 24, 2014 Hearing Background Paper; https://antr.assembly.ca.gov/sites/antr.assembly.ca.gov/files/hearings/Background%20paper0324 14.pdf

[535] Mercury in Our Waters: The 10,000-Year Legacy of California's Gold Rush; By Alexandria Herr; September 30, 2020 https://www.kcet.org/shows/earth-focus/mercury-in-our-waters-the-10-000-year-legacy-of-californias-gold-rush

[536] Malm O. Gold mining as a source of mercury exposure in the Brazilian Amazon. Environ Res. 1998 May;77(2):73-8. https://pubmed.ncbi.nlm.nih.gov/9600798/

[537] Gworek, B., Dmuchowski, W. et al Mercury in the terrestrial environment: a review. Environ Sci Eur 32, 128 (2020). https://doi.org/10.1186/s12302-020-00401-x

[538] Drasch G, Böse-O'Reilly S, Beinhoff C, Roider G, Maydl S. The Mt. Diwata study on the Philippines 1999--assessing mercury intoxication of the population by small scale gold mining. Sci Total Environ. 2001 Feb 21;267 https://pubmed.ncbi.nlm.nih.gov/11286210/

[539] Böse-O'Reilly S, Drasch G, et al 2003: The Mt. Diwata study on the Philippines 2000-treatment of mercury intoxicated inhabitants of a gold mining area with DMPS (2,3-dimercapto-1-propane-sulfonic acid, Dimaval). Sci Total Environ. 2003 May 20;307(1-3):71-82. https://pubmed.ncbi.nlm.nih.gov/12711426/

[540] Mary Jean Brown, Alan D. Woolf, Chapter 1.8 - Zamfara gold mining lead poisoning disaster—Nigeria, Africa, 2010, Editor(s): Alan D. Woolf, In History of Toxicology and Environmental Health, History of Modern Clinical Toxicology, Academic Press, 2022, https://doi.org/10.1016/B978-0-12-822218-8.00012-0.

[541] Theresa Dale, PhD, CCN, NP Heavy Metal Toxicity Increases Your Risk of Electromag Sensitivity; https://www.wellnesscenter.net/resources/Heavy_Metal_Toxicity.htm

[542] University of Alaska, Fairbanks: Powerful Radio Signals add Free Soundtrack February 09, 1995 / Ned Rozell https://www.gi.alaska.edu/alaska-science-forum/powerful-radio-signals-add-free-soundtrack

[543] Snopes: Did Lucille Ball's Fillings Help Capture Japanese Spies? Was a memorable episode of 'Gilligan's Island' an inadvertent re-creation of what Lucille Ball experienced in real life?; David Mikkelson; Published Jul 24, 1999; https://www.snopes.com/fact-check/lucille-ball-fillings-spies/

[544] bradfordfamilydentist; How Lucille Ball Heard Spies Through Her Dental Fillings; Jesse Chai Dentistry; https://www.bradfordfamilydentist.ca/lucille-ball-heard-spies-dental-fillings/

[545] American radio Archives: Can You Hear Radio Through Fillings? NOVEMBER 10, 2022; https://www.americanradioarchives.com/can-you-hear-radio-through-fillings/

[546] Boza RA, Liggett SB. Pseudohallucinations: radio reception through shrapnel fragments. Am J Psychiatry. 1981 Sep;138(9). https://pubmed.ncbi.nlm.nih.gov/7270748/

[547] Kelly R Smith, Jack R Nation, Developmental exposure to cadmium alters responsiveness to cocaine in the rat, Drug and Alcohol Dependence, Volume 72, Issue 1, 2003, https://doi.org/10.1016/S0376-8716(03)00170-4.

[548] Nation JR, Smith KR, Bratton GR. Early developmental lead exposure increases sensitivity to cocaine in a self-administration paradigm. Pharmacol Biochem Behav. 2004 Jan;77(1):127-35. http://doi.org/10.1016/j.pbb.2003.10.009.

[549] Douglas C. Jones, Gary W. Miller: 2008: The effects of environmental neurotoxicants on the dopaminergic system: A possible role in drug addiction, Biochemical Pharmacology, Volume 76, Issue 5, 2008, https://doi.org/10.1016/j.bcp.2008.05.010.

[550] Robert L. Siblerud, Eldon Kienholz, John Motl, 1999: Evidence that mercury from silver dental fillings may be an etiological factor in smoking, Toxicology Letters, Volume 68, Issue 3, 1993, Pages 307-310, , https://doi.org/10.1016/0378-4274(93)90022-P. (https://www.sciencedirect.com/science/article/pii/037842749390022P)

[551] Li, Y, Wu, F, Mu, Q, et al. 2022: Metal ions in cerebrospinal fluid: Associations with anxiety, depression, and insomnia among cigarette smokers. CNS Neurosci Ther. 2022; 28: 2141- 2147. https://onlinelibrary.wiley.com/doi/full/10.1111/cns.13955

[552] Figgs LW, Holsinger H, et al 2011: Increased suicide risk among workers following toxic metal exposure at the Paducah gaseous diffusion plant from 1952 to 2003: a cohort study. Int J Occup Environ Med. 2011 Oct;2(4):199-214. https://www.researchgate.net/publication/231612549_Increased_Suicide_Risk_among_Workers

following Toxic Metal Exposure at the Paducah Gaseous Diffusion Plant From 1952 to 2
003 A Cohort Study
[553] Are you toxic from beryllium? Natural health Group,
https://www.naturalhealthgroup.com.au/heavy-metal-toxicity/are-you-toxic-from-beryllium/
[554] Antonella Tammaro; et al; Topical and Systemic Therapies for Nickel Allergy DISCLOSURES
Dermatitis. 2011;22(05) https://www.medscape.com/viewarticle/753985_7
[555] M. M. Brzóska, J. Moniuszko-Jakoniuk, M. Jurczuk, M. Gałażyn-Sidorczuk, J. Rogalska,
EFFECT OF SHORT-TERM ETHANOL ADMINISTRATION ON CADMIUM RETENTION AND
BIOELEMENT METABOLISM IN RATS CONTINUOUSLY EXPOSED TO CADMIUM, Alcohol
and Alcoholism, Volume 35, Issue 5, September 2000, https://doi.org/10.1093/alcalc/35.5.439
[556] Prystupa A, Błażewicz A, Kiciński P, Sak JJ, Niedziałek J, Załuska W. Serum Concentrations
of Selected Heavy Metals in Patients with Alcoholic Liver Cirrhosis from the Lublin Region in
Eastern Poland. Int J Environ Res Public Health. 2016 Jun 13;13(6):582..
https://www.ncbi.nlm.nih.gov/pmc/articles/PMC4924039/
[557] EPA: Health & Environmental Research Online (HERO); Flora, SJS; Dube, SN; 1994;
Modulatory effects of alcohol ingestion on the toxicology of heavy metals; Indian Journal of
Pharmacology https://hero.epa.gov/hero/index.cfm/reference/details/reference_id/8381010
[558] Wallace DR, Hood AN. Human dopamine transporter function following exposure to heavy
metals and psychostimulants. Toxicol Forensic Med Open J. 2018; 3(1): 1-13.
https://openventio.org/wp-content/uploads/Human-Dopamine-Transporter-Function-Following-
Exposure-to-Heavy-Metals-and-Psychostimulants-TFMOJ-3-124.pdf
[559] Nechifor M. Magnesium in drug abuse and addiction. In: Vink R, Nechifor M, editors.
Magnesium in the Central Nervous System [Internet]. Adelaide (AU): University of Adelaide
Press; 2011. Available from: https://www.ncbi.nlm.nih.gov/books/NBK507260/
[560] Ciubotariu, D., et al 2015: Zinc involvement in opioid addiction and analgesia – should zinc
supplementation be recommended for opioid-treated persons?. Subst Abuse Treat Prev Policy
10, 29 (2015). https://doi.org/10.1186/s13011-015-0025-2
[561] Stanley PC, Wakwe VC. Toxic trace metals in the mentally ill patients. Niger Postgrad Med J.
2002 Dec;9(4):199-204. https://pubmed.ncbi.nlm.nih.gov/12690679/
[562] Naylor GJ. Vanadium and Manic Depressive Psychosis. Nutrition and Health. 1984;3(1-2):79-
85. https://www.ncbi.nlm.nih.gov/pmc/articles/PMC9697979/
[563] Ma J, Yan L, Guo T, et al 2019: Association of Typical Toxic Heavy Metals with Schizophrenia.
Int J Environ Res Public Health. 2019 Oct 30;16(21):4200.. https://www.mdpi.com/1660-
4601/16/21/4200
[564] Modabbernia, A., Velthorst,et al. (2016). Early-life metal exposure and schizophrenia: A proof-
of-concept study using novel tooth-matrix biomarkers. European Psychiatry, 36, 1-6.
https://www.cambridge.org/core/journals/european-psychiatry/article/earlylife-metal-exposure-
and-schizophrenia-a-proofofconcept-study-using-novel-toothmatrix-
biomarkers/658656D61088118338D6A40FCAA8811C/share/a6738bc8c59c9f99dfd1d007bb5f76
56a8b5dbeb
[565] Arinola G, Idonije B, Akinlade K, Ihenyen O. 2010: Essential trace metals and heavy metals in
newly diagnosed schizophrenic patients and those on anti-psychotic medication. J Res Med Sci.
2010 Sep;15(5):245-9.
https://www.researchgate.net/publication/51082705_Essential_trace_metals_and_heavy_metals
_in_newly_diagnosed_schizophrenic_patients_and_those_on_anti-psychotic_medication
[566] Jiahui Ma, Bin Wang, Xi Gao, Hao Wu, Dongfang Wang, Nan Li, Jiping Tan, Jingyu Wang,
Lailai Yan, 2018: A comparative study of the typical toxic metals in serum by patients of
schizophrenia and healthy controls in China, Psychiatry Research, Volume 269, 2018,
(https://www.sciencedirect.com/science/article/pii/S0165178118306188)
[567] Worldwide Health Center; Effects of Toxic Metals on Learning and Behaviour; Bernard
Windham; 10/04/2017; https://www.worldwidehealthcenter.net/effects-toxic-metals-learning-
behaviour/
[568] Annau Z, Cuomo V. et al 1988: Mechanisms of neurotoxicity and their relationship to
behavioral changes. Toxicology 1988; 49(2-3): 219-25.
[569] Lee MJ, Chou MC, Chou WJ, Huang CW, Kuo HC, Lee SY, Wang LJ. Heavy Metals' Effect on
Susceptibility to Attention-Deficit/Hyperactivity Disorder: Implication of Lead, Cadmium, and
Antimony. Int J Environ Res Public Health. 2018 Jun 10;15(6):1221..
https://www.mdpi.com/1660-4601/15/6/1221
[570] Yue Sun, Yanwen Wang, et al 2023: Exposure to metal mixtures may decrease children's
cognitive flexibility via gut microbiota, Environmental Technology & Innovation, Volume 29, 2023,
https://doi.org/10.1016/j.eti.2023.103012.

[571] Worldwide Health Center; Effects of Toxic Metals on Learning and Behaviour; Bernard Windham; 10/04/2017; https://www.worldwidehealthcenter.net/effects-toxic-metals-learning-behaviour/

[572] Payton M, Riggs KM, Spiro A, et al. 1998: Relations of bone and blood lead to cognitive function: the VA Normative Aging Study. Neurotoxicol Teratol. 1998; 201: 19–27. https://pubmed.ncbi.nlm.nih.gov/9511166/

[573] EPA; Learn About Lead Designations; LAST UPDATED ON JUNE 30, 2022; https://www.epa.gov/lead-designations/learn-about-lead-designations

[574] Canfield, R. L. ed al,2003: Intellectual impairment in children with blood lead concentrations below 10 microg per deciliter. N Engl J Med. 2003;348(16):1517-1526. https://www.nejm.org/doi/full/10.1056/NEJMoa022848

[575] Pan S, Lin L, Zeng F, et al 2017: Effects of lead, cadmium, arsenic, and mercury co-exposure on children's intelligence quotient in an industrialized area of southern China. Environ Pollut. 2018 Apr;235:47-54. https://pubmed.ncbi.nlm.nih.gov/29274537/

[576] Heidari S, et al 2022: The effect of lead exposure on IQ test scores in children under 12 years: a systematic review and meta-analysis of case-control studies. Syst Rev. 2022 https://www.ncbi.nlm.nih.gov/pmc/articles/PMC9150353/

[577] Minxue Shen, Chengcheng Zhang, 2001: Association of multi-metals exposure with intelligence quotient score of children: A prospective cohort study, Environment Internat, V. 155, 2021, (https://www.sciencedirect.com/science/article/pii/S0160412021003172)

[578] Jedrychowski WA, et al: Depressed height gain of children associated with intrauterine exposure to polycyclic aromatic hydrocarbons (PAH) and heavy metals: the cohort prospective study. Environ Res. 2015 Jan; http://doi.org/10.1016/j.envres.2014.08.047.

[579] Bair, Emily 2022: A narrative Review of Toxic Heavy Metal content of Infant and Toddler Foods and Evaluation of United States Policy. Front. Nutr., 27 June 2022; Sec. Clinical Nutrition; Volume 9 - 2022 | https://doi.org/10.3389/fnut.2022.919913

[580] Jiehua Ma, Shijie Geng, 2023: Exposure to metal mixtures and young children's growth and development: A biomonitoring-based study in Eastern China, Ecotox. a. Environ. Safety, V 268, 2023 https://www.sciencedirect.com/science/article/pii/S0147651323012307

[581] Renee M. Gardner, et al 2011: Environmental Exposure to Metals and Children's Growth to Age 5 Years: A Prospective Cohort Study, American Journal of Epidemiology, Volume 177, Issue 12, 15 June 2013, , https://doi.org/10.1093/aje/kws437

[582] Jiaolong Ma, Hongling Zhang, et al 2022: Exposure to metal mixtures and hypertensive disorders of pregnancy: A nested case-control study in China, Environmental Pollution, Volume 306, 2022, 119439, https://doi.org/10.1016/j.envpol.2022.119439. (https://www.sciencedirect.com/science/article/pii/S0269749122006534)

[583] Oritsemuelebi B, Frazzoli C, Eze EC, Ilo CE, Nwaogazie IL, Orisakwe OE. Levels of toxic and essential metals in maternal cord blood and anthropometry at birth: a pilot study. Journal of Global Health Reports. 2021;. http://doi.org//10.29392/001c.29888

[584] Björkman L, Lygre GB, Haug K, Skjærven R. Perinatal death and exposure to dental amalgam fillings during pregnancy in the population-based MoBa cohort. PLoS One. 2018 Dec 7;13(12):e0208803. https://pubmed.ncbi.nlm.nih.gov/30532171/

[585] Mayumi Tsuji, Eiji Shibata, et al 2018: The association between whole blood concentrations of heavy metals in pregnant women and premature births: The Japan Environment and Children's Study (JECS), Environmental Research, Volume 166, 2018, https://doi.org/10.1016/j.envres.2018.06.025.

[586] Gustin K, Vahter M, Barman M, Jacobsson B, Skröder H, Filipsson Nyström H, Sandin A, Sandberg AS, Wold AE, Kippler M. Assessment of Joint Impact of Iodine, Selenium, and Zinc Status on Women's Third-Trimester Plasma Thyroid Hormone Concentrations. J Nutr. 2022 Jul 6;152(7):1737-1746. https://openarchive.ki.se/xmlui/handle/10616/47973

[587] Yu XD, Yan CH,et al 2011: Prenatal exposure to multiple toxic heavy metals and neonatal neurobehavioral development in Shanghai, China. Neurotoxicol Teratol. 2011 Jul-Aug;33(4):437-43. https://pubmed.ncbi.nlm.nih.gov/21664460/

[588] Van Brusselen D, Kayembe-Kitenge T, et al 2020: Metal mining and birth defects: a case-control study in Lubumbashi, Democratic Republic of the Congo. Lancet Planet Health. 2020 https://www.thelancet.com/journals/lanplh/article/PIIS2542-5196(20)30059-0/fulltext

[589] Worldwide Health Center; Effects of Toxic Metals on Learning and Behaviour; Bernard Windham; 10/04/2017; https://www.worldwidehealthcenter.net/effects-toxic-metals-learning-behaviour/

[590] Heng YY, Asad I, Coleman B, Menard L, Benki-Nugent S, Hussein Were F, Karr CJ, McHenry MS. 2022: Heavy metals and neurodevelopment of children in low and middle-income countries: A systematic review. PLoS One. 2022 Mar 31;17(3):e0265536. https://www.ncbi.nlm.nih.gov/pmc/articles/PMC8970501/

Notes

[591] Worldwide Health Center; Effects of Toxic Metals on Learning and Behaviour
George Georgiou 10/04/2017; https://www.worldwidehealthcenter.net/effects-toxic-metals-learning-behaviour/
[592] Choi J, Chang JY, Hong J, Shin S, Park JS, Oh S. 2018: Low-Level Toxic Metal Exposure in Healthy Weaning-Age Infants: Association with Growth, Dietary Intake, and Iron Deficiency. Int J Environ Res Public Health. 2017 Apr 6;14(4):388.
https://www.ncbi.nlm.nih.gov/pmc/articles/PMC5409589/
[593] Greatplainslaboratory; JAMES GREENBLATT 2017: The Role Of Heavy Metals And Environmental Toxins In Psychiatric Disorders; July 10, 2017 Toxic Chemicals, Metals Resources, GPL-TOX Resources, Hormones, Copper + Zinc Resources;;
https://www.greatplainslaboratory.com/articles-1/2017/7/10/the-role-of-heavy-metals-and-environmental-toxins-in-psychiatric-disorders
[594] Sciarillo, W. G., Alexander, G., & Farrell, K. P. (1992). Lead exposure and child behavior. American Journal of Public Health, 82(10), 1356–1360.
[595] Gonzalez-Cossio T, Peterson KE, Sanin LH et al: Decrease in birth weight in relation to maternal bone-lead burden. Pediatrics, 1997; https://pubmed.ncbi.nlm.nih.gov/9346987/
[596] Gomaa A, Hu H, Bellinger D, Schwartz J, Tsaih SW, Gonzalez-Cossio T, Schnaas L, Peterson K, Aro A, Hernandez-Avila M. Maternal bone lead as an independent risk factor for fetal neurotoxicity: a prospective study. Pediatrics. 2002 Jul;110(1 Pt 1):110-8..
https://pubmed.ncbi.nlm.nih.gov/12093955/
[597] Braun JM, Wright RJ,et al. 2014: Relationships between lead biomarkers and diurnal salivary cortisol indices in pregnant women from Mexico City: a cross-sectional study. Environ Health. 2014 Jun 10;13(1):50.
https://www.researchgate.net/publication/263014956_Relationships_between_lead_biomarkers_and_diurnal_salivary_cortisol_indices_in_pregnant_women_from_Mexico_City_a_cross-sectional_study
[598] Marlowe, Mike et al 1993: Hair Element Concentrations and Young Children's Classroom and Home Behavior Journal of Orthomolecular Medicine Vol. 8, No. 2, 1993 https://isom.ca/wp-content/uploads/2020/01/JOM_1993_08_2_05_Hair_Element_Concentrations_and_Young_Childrens-.pdf
[599] Nigg, J. T. et al. Low blood lead levels associated with clinically diagnosed attention-deficit/hyperactivity disorder and mediated by weak cognitive control. Biol Psychiatry. 63, 325–331 (2008). https://www.ncbi.nlm.nih.gov/pmc/articles/PMC2818788/
[600] Department of Statistics, Ministry of the Interior (Taiwan, ROC); 2011–2013.
[601] Mikirova, Nina et al 2011: Efficacy of oral DMSA and intravenous EDTA in chelation of toxic metals and improvement of the number of stem/ progenitor cells in circulation; TRANSLATIONAL BIOMEDICINE; 2011 Vol. 2 No. 2:2 https://www.transbiomedicine.com/translational-biomedicine/efficacy-of-oral-dmsa-and-intravenous-edta-in-chelation-of-toxic-metals-and-improvement-of-the-number-of-stem-progenitor-cells-in-circulation.pdf
[602] Andersen, H. R., Nielsen, J. B., & Grandjean, P. (2000). Toxicologic evidence of developmental neurotoxicity of environmental chemicals. Toxicology, 144(1–3), 121–127.
https://pubmed.ncbi.nlm.nih.gov/10781879/
[603] Adinolfi, M. (1985). The development of the human blood-CSF-brain barrier. Developmental Medicine and Child Neurology, 27(4), 532–537. https://pubmed.ncbi.nlm.nih.gov/4029526/
[604] Bellinger, D. C. Very low lead exposures and children's neurodevelopment. Curr Opin Pediatr. 20, 172–177 (2008). https://pubmed.ncbi.nlm.nih.gov/18332714/
[605] Geoffrey T. Wodtke, et al 2022; Toxic Neighborhoods: The Effects of Concentrated Poverty and Environmental Lead Contamination on Early Childhood Development. Demography 1 August 2022; 59 (4) https://doi.org/10.1215/00703370-10047481
[606] DeSoto, M. C., & Hitlan, R. T. (2010). Sorting out the spinning of autism: heavy metals and the question of incidence. Acta Neurobiologiae Experimentalis (Warsaw), 70(2), 165–176.
https://pubmed.ncbi.nlm.nih.gov/20628440/
[607] Gorini, F., Muratori, F. & Morales, M.A. The Role of Heavy Metal Pollution in Neurobehavioral Disorders: a Focus on Autism. Rev J Autism Dev Disord 1, 354–372 (2014).
https://doi.org/10.1007/s40489-014-0028-3
[608] Kjell Vegard F. Weyde et al 2023: Association between gestational levels of toxic metals and essential elements and cerebral palsy in children; Front. Neurol., 17 August 2023; Sec. Pediatric Neurology ; Vol. 14,2023 https://doi.org/10.3389/fneur.2023.1124943
[609] Hsueh, YM., Lee, CY., Chien, SN. et al. Association of blood heavy metals with developmental delays and health status in children. Sci Rep 7, 43608 (2017). https://doi.org/10.1038/srep43608
[610] Hsueh, YM., Lee, CY., Chien, SN. et al. Association of blood heavy metals with developmental delays and health status in children. Sci Rep 7, 43608 (2017). https://doi.org/10.1038/srep43608

[611] Rodríguez-Barranco, M. et al. Cadmium exposure and neuropsychological development in school children in southwestern Spain. Environ Res. 134, 66–73 (2014). https://www.sciencedirect.com/science/article/abs/pii/S0013935114002229

[612] Capel ID, Pinnock MH, Dorrell HM, Williams DC, Grant EC. Comparison of concentrations of some trace, bulk, and toxic metals in the hair of normal and dyslexic children. Clin Chem 1981 Jun;27(6):879-81. https://www.researchgate.net/publication/15960867_Comparison_of_concentrations_of_some_trace_bulk_and_toxic_metals_in_the_hair_of_normal_and_dyslexic_children

[613] Qi Xue, Yu Zhou, et al, 2020: Urine metals concentrations and dyslexia among children in China, Environment International, Volume 139, 2020, (https://www.sciencedirect.com/science/article/pii/S016041201934810X)

[614] Capel ID, Pinnock MH, Dorrell HM, Williams DC, Grant EC. Comparison of concentrations of some trace, bulk, and toxic metals in the hair of normal and dyslexic children. Clin Chem. 1981 Jun;27(6):879-81. https://pubmed.ncbi.nlm.nih.gov/7237768/

[615] Huang A, Zhang J, Wu K, Liu C, Huang Q, Zhang X, Lin X, Huang Y. 2022: Exposure to multiple metals and the risk of dyslexia - A case control study in Shantou, China. Environ Pollut. 2022 Aug 15;307:119518. . https://pubmed.ncbi.nlm.nih.gov/35618141/

[616] Hye Seon Choi: Relationships of Lead, Mercury and Cadmium Levels with the Timing of Menarche among Korean Girls; Child Health Nurs Res. 2020 Jan; 26(1): 98–106. Published online 2020 Jan 31. http://doi.org/10.4094/chnr.2020.26.1.98

[617] Surabhi Shah-Kulkarni, Seulbi Lee, et al, 2020: Prenatal exposure to mixtures of heavy metals and neurodevelopment in infants at 6 months, Environmental Research, Volume 182, 2020, https://doi.org/10.1016/j.envres.2020.109122.

[618] Fløtre CH, Varsi K, Helm T, Bolann B, Bjørke-Monsen AL. Predictors of mercury, lead, cadmium and antimony status in Norwegian never-pregnant women of fertile age. PLoS One. 2017 Dec 5;12(12): https://www.ncbi.nlm.nih.gov/pmc/articles/PMC5716542/

[619] Gamila S. M. El-saeed and Soheir A Abdel et al; 2016: Mercury toxicity and DNA damage in patients with Down syndrome, Medical Research Journal; 2016; volume15; pp. 22–26; https://content.iospress.com/articles/journal-of-alzheimers-disease-reports/adr170010

[620] Timesofindia: Arsenic-Down syndrome link found By – TNN Jayanta Gupta: Jul 9, 2016, https://timesofindia.indiatimes.com/life-style/health-fitness/health-news/Arsenic-Down-syndrome-link-found/articleshow/53126940.cms

[621] Malakooti N, Pritchard MA, Adlard PA, Finkelstein DI. Role of metal ions in the cognitive decline of Down syndrome. Front Aging Neurosci. 2014 Jun 23;6:136. doi: 10.3389/fnagi.2014.00136. https://www.ncbi.nlm.nih.gov/pmc/articles/PMC4066992/

[622] Grabeklis AR, Skalny AV, Skalnaya AA, Zhegalova IV, Notova SV, Mazaletskaya AL, Skalnaya MG, Tinkov AA. Hair Mineral and Trace Element Content in Children with Down's Syndrome. Biol Trace Elem Res. 2019 Mar;188(1):230-238. https://www.researchgate.net/publication/327617621_Hair_Mineral_and_Trace_Element_Content_in_Children_with_Down%27s_Syndrome

[623] El-saeed, G.S., Abdel Maksoud, S.A., et al (2016). Mercury toxicity and DNA damage in patients with Down syndrome. Medical Research Journal, 15, 22–26. https://www.researchgate.net/publication/305954666_Mercury_toxicity_and_DNA_damage_in_patients_with_Down_syndrome

[624] Moore PB, Edwardson JA , Ferrier IN , Taylor GA , Tyrer SP , Day JP , King SJ , Lilley JS ((1997)) Gastrointestinal absorption of aluminum is increased in Down's syndrome. Biol Psychiatry 41:, 488–492. https://pubmed.ncbi.nlm.nih.gov/9034543/

[625] The conscious pod: METALS AND MINERALS IN DOWN SYNDROME; http://www.theconsciouspod.com/metals-and-minerals-in-down-syndrome/

[626] TOP 10; MEDICAL ERRORS THAT LEAD TO DEATH; Law Offices of Dr. Michael M. Wilson, M.D., J.D; https://www.wilsonlaw.com/fatal-medical-errors/

[627] James, John T. PhD. A New, Evidence-based Estimate of Patient Harms Associated with Hospital Care. Journal of Patient Safety 9(3):p 122-128, September 2013. https://journals.lww.com/journalpatientsafety/Fulltext/2013/09000/A_New,_Evidence_based_Estimate_of_Patient_Harms.2.aspx

[628] Welt online: Der Tod kommt immer öfter auf Rezept; 24.10.2007 | Lesedauer: 3 Minuten; Elke Bodderas; https://www.welt.de/wissenschaft/article1293472/Der-Tod-kommt-immer-oefter-auf-Rezept.html

[629] Welt online: Der Tod kommt immer öfter auf Rezept; 24.10.2007 | Lesedauer: 3 Minuten; Elke Bodderas; https://www.welt.de/wissenschaft/article1293472/Der-Tod-kommt-immer-oefter-auf-Rezept.html

Notes

[630] Li, X., Zhang, D., Zhao, Y. et al. 2023: Correlation of heavy metals' exposure with the prevalence of coronary heart disease among US adults: findings of the US NHANES from 2003 to 2018. Environ Geochem Health 45, https://doi.org/10.1007/s10653-023-01670-0

[631] Avila, Maria D.; Escolar, Esteban; Lamas, Gervasio A.. Chelation therapy after the Trial to Assess Chelation Therapy: results of a unique trial. Current Opinion in Cardiology 29(5):p 481-488, September 2014. | http://doi.org/10.1097/HCO.0000000000000096

[632] Rajiv Chowdhury et al 2018: Environmental toxic metal contaminants and risk of cardiovascular disease: systematic review and meta-analysis; BMJ 2018;362:k3310; https://doi.org/10.1136/bmj.k3310 (Published 29 August 2018)

[633] Navas-Acien A, Guallar E, Silbergeld EK, Rothenberg SJ. Lead exposure and cardiovascular disease--a systematic review. Environ Health Perspect. 2007 Mar;115(3):472-82. http://doi.org/10.1289/ehp.9785.

[634] Jennrich; Peter; 05/08: Quecksilber und Blei machen es ihrem Herz schwer; Well-Aging http://tierversuchsfreie-medizin.de/download/Quecksilber-und-Blei_Herz.pdf

[635] Jennrich, Peter, 2009: die medizinische bedeutung chronischer metallbelastungen – ein Überblick umwelt·medizin·gesellschaft | 22 | 3/2009; http://tierversuchsfreie-medizin.de/download/chronische_Metallbelastungen_Ueberblick.pdf

[636] Johns Hopkins Bloomberg School of Public Health ; Mercury Associated With Risk of Heart Attack; November 27, 2002; https://publichealth.jhu.edu/2002/fish-mercury

[637] Barregard L, et al 2021: Cadmium Exposure and Coronary Artery Atherosclerosis: A Cross-Sectional Population-Based Study of Swedish Middle-Aged Adults. Environ Health Perspect. 2021 Jun; https://www.ncbi.nlm.nih.gov/pmc/articles/PMC8221368/

[638] Borné Y, Barregard L, Persson M, et al 2015: Cadmium exposure and incidence of heart failure and atrial fibrillation: a population-based prospective cohort study BMJ Open 2015;5:e007366. https://bmjopen.bmj.com/content/5/6/e007366

[639] Dugi, Daniel; Takemoto, Arnold 2002: The Role of Heavy Metal Detoxification in Heart Disease and Cancers : A Pilot Study in Detoxification of Heavy Metals; Presented at the WESCON Biomedicine and Bioengineering Conference Anaheim Convention Center The Future of Medicine Afternoon Session; September 24, 2002 Anaheim, California USA

[640] Lanphear BP, Rauch S, Auinger P, Allen RW, Hornung RW. Low-level lead exposure and mortality in US adults: a population-baseno d cohort study. Lancet Public Health.; 2018;3(4):E177-E184. https://www.researchgate.net/publication/323742199_Low-level_lead_exposure_and_mortality_in_US_adults_A_population-based_cohort_study

[641] Ai-Min Yang, Kenneth Lo, et al 2020: Environmental heavy metals and cardiovascular diseases: Status and future direction, Chronic Diseases and Translational Medicine, Volume 6, Issue 4, 2020, https://doi.org/10.1016/j.cdtm.2020.02.005.

[642] Tomášek A, et al 2023: Metals and Trace Elements in Calcified Valves in Patients with Acquired Severe Aortic Valve Stenosis: Is There a Connection with the Degeneration Process? J Pers Med. 2023 Feb 13;13(2):320. https://www.mdpi.com/2075-4426/13/2/320

[643] Frustaci, Andrea et al 1999: Marked elevation of myocardial trace elements in idiopathic dilated cardiomyopathy compared with secondary cardiac dysfunction; Journal of the America College of Cardiology; Volume 33, Issue 6, Pages 1578-1583 https://www.sciencedirect.com/science/article/pii/S0735109799000625

[644] Skalny,A.V.; Kopylov, P.Y: et al 2021: Hair Lead, Aluminum and Other Toxic Metals in Normal-Weight and Obese Patients with Coronary Heart Disease. Int. J. Environ. Res. https://www.ncbi.nlm.nih.gov/pmc/articles/PMC8345938/

[645] BMJ. (2018, December 11). Workplace exposure to pesticides and metals linked to heightened heart disease risk. ScienceDaily. Retrieved April 17, 2023 from www.sciencedaily.com/releases/2018/12/181211190008.htm

[646] Bulka CM, Daviglus ML, Persky VW, et al Association of occupational exposures with cardiovascular disease among US Hispanics/Latinos Heart 2019; https://heart.bmj.com/content/105/6/439

[647] Al-Mubarak, A.A., Grote Beverborg, N., Zwartkruis, V. et al. Micronutrient deficiencies and new-onset atrial fibrillation in a community-based cohort: data from PREVEND. Clin Res Cardiol (2023). https://doi.org/10.1007/s00392-023-02276-3

[648] Gianpaolo Guzzi, Anna Ronchi, Paolo D. Pigatto. Mercury overexposure and atrial fibrillation. Anatol J Cardiol. 2016; 16(1): 68-68; Anatol J Cardiol. 2016; 16 https://jag.journalagent.com/anatoljcardiol/pdfs/AJC_16_1_68.pdf

[649] WebMD: AFib: Prognosis and Life Expectancy; Written by Stephanie Watson Medically Reviewed by James Beckerman, MD, FACC on November 05, 2022 https://www.webmd.com/heart-disease/atrial-fibrillation/atrial-fibrillation-prognosis-life-expectancy

[650] bu.edu : Framingham Heart Study Will Examine Aging with New $38 Million Funding.

April 19, 2019; https://www.bu.edu/sph/news/articles/2019/framingham-heart-study-will-examine-aging-with-new-38-million-funding/

[651] Buhari O, Dayyab FM, Igbinoba O, Atanda A, Medhane F, Faillace RT. The association between heavy metal and serum cholesterol levels in the US population: National Health and Nutrition Examination Survey 2009-2012. Hum Exp Toxicol. 2020 Mar;39(3):355-364. http://doi.org/10.1177/0960327119889654.

[652] M. Ghayour-Mobarhan, A.et al 2009: The relationship between established coronary risk factors and serum copper and zinc concentrations in a large Persian Cohort, J. of Trace Elements in Medicine and Biology, Volume 23, Issue 3, 2009, (https://www.sciencedirect.com/science/article/pii/S0946672X09000340)

[653] Malamba-Lez, Didier, et al 2021: "Concurrent Heavy Metal Exposures and Idiopathic Dilated Cardiomyopathy: A Case-Control Study from the Katanga Mining Area of the Democratic Republic of Congo" International Journal of Environmental Research and Public Health 18, https://doi.org/10.3390/ijerph18094956

[654] Li Q, Yang Y, Reis C, et al. Cerebral Small Vessel Disease. Cell Transplantation. 2018;27(12):1711-1722. https://journals.sagepub.com/doi/10.1177/0963689718795148

[655] Patwa, Jayant, and Swaran Jeet Singh Flora. 2020. "Heavy Metal-Induced Cerebral Small Vessel Disease: Insights into Molecular Mechanisms and Possible Reversal Strategies" International Journal of Molecular Sciences 21, no. 11: 3862. https://doi.org/10.3390/ijms21113862;

[656] Dev P et al 2022: A. Systematic Review and Meta-analysis of Environmental Toxic Metal Contaminants and the Risk of Ischemic Stroke. Ann Indian Acad Neurol. 2022 Nov-Dec;25(6):1159-1166. https://doi.org/10.21203/rs.3.rs-1540330/v1

[657] Edmunds LH, Stephenson LW, Edie RN, Ratcliffe MB. Open-heart surgery in octogenarians. N Engl J Med. 1988; https://pubmed.ncbi.nlm.nih.gov/3386692/

[658] CASS Principal Investigators and the Associates. Myocardial infarction and mortality in the Coronary Artery Surgery Study randomized trial. N Engl J Med. 1984; https://pubmed.ncbi.nlm.nih.gov/6608052/

[659] Ravalli, Filippo; Parada, Xavier Vela; et al 2022: Chelation Therapy in Patients With Cardiovascular Disease: A Systematic Review Originally published Mar 2022 J. of the American Heart Association. https://doi.org/10.1161/JAHA.121.024648

[660] Houston, M.C. (2011), Role of Mercury Toxicity in Hypertension, Cardiovascular Disease, and Stroke. J.of Clin H.., 13: https://doi.org/10.1111/j.1751-7176.2011.00489.x

[661] Jennrich, Peter, 2009: die medizinische bedeutung chronischer metallbelastungen – ein Überblick umwelt·medizin·gesellschaft | 22 | 3/2009; http://tierversuchsfreie-medizin.de/download/chronische_Metallbelastungen_Ueberblick.pdf

[662] Houston MC. 2007: The role of mercury and cadmium heavy metals in vascular disease, hypertension, coronary heart disease, and myocardial infarction. Altern Ther Health Med. 2007 Mar-Apr;13(2) https://pubmed.ncbi.nlm.nih.gov/17405690/

[663] whoop: Everything You Need to Know About Heart Rate Variability (HRV) AUGUST 11, 2021; https://www.whoop.com/thelocker/heart-rate-variability-hrv/#:~:text=Is%20it%20better%20to%20have,respond%20effectively%20to%20different%20stressors.

[664] Salonen JT, et al 2000: Mercury accumulation and accelerated progression of carotid atherosclerosis: a population-based prospective 4-year follow-up study in men in eastern Finland. Atherosclerosis. 2000 Feb;148(2) https://pubmed.ncbi.nlm.nih.gov/10657561/

[665] Maria Grau-Perez, Maria J. Caballero-Mateos et al 2021: Toxic Metals and Subclinical Atherosclerosis in Carotid, Femoral, and Coronary Vascular Territories: The Aragon Workers Health Study; 9 Dec 2021 Arteriosclerosis, Thrombosis, and Vascular Biology. 2022;42:87–99 https://doi.org/10.1161/ATVBAHA.121.316358

[666] American Heart Association News: Low-level toxic metal exposure may raise the risk for clogged arteries;: December 9, 2021; https://www.heart.org/en/news/2021/12/09/low-level-toxic-metal-exposure-may-raise-the-risk-for-clogged-arteries

[667] World Health Organization Global health risks: mortality and burden of disease attributable to selected major risks. [Accessed January, 19 2015]. Available from: http://www.who.int/healthinfo/global_burden_disease/GlobalHealthRisks_report_full.pdf.

[668] WHO, More than 700 million people with untreated hypertension; https://www.who.int/news/item/25-08-2021-more-than-700-million-people-with-untreated-hypertension

[669] CDC: High Blood Pressure Symptoms and Causes; https://www.cdc.gov/bloodpressure/about.htm?CDC_AA_refVal=https%3A%2F%2Fwww.cdc.gov%2Fbloodpressure%2Ffaqs.htm

Notes

670 Poulter NR, Prabhakaran D, Caulfield M. Hypertension. Lancet. 2015 Aug 22;386(9995):801-12. https://www.thelancet.com/journals/lancet/article/PIIS0140-6736(14)61468-9/fulltext
671 Kearney PM, Whelton M, Reynolds K, Muntner P, Whelton PK, He J. Global burden of hypertension: analysis of worldwide data. Lancet. 2005;365(9455):217–223 Jan. 15, 2005 https://www.thelancet.com/journals/lancet/article/PIIS0140-6736(05)17741-1/fulltext
672 Smith KM, Barraj LM, Kantor M, et al. Relationship between fish intake, n-3 fatty acids, mercury and risk of CHD (National Health and Nutrition Examination Survey 1999–2002). Public Health Nutr. 2009;12:1261–1269. https://pubmed.ncbi.nlm.nih.gov/18986590/
673 Valera B, Dewailly E, Poirier P. 2009: Environmental mercury exposure and blood pressure among Nunavik Inuit adults. Hypertension. 2009 Nov;54 https://pubmed.ncbi.nlm.nih.gov/19805642/
674 Houston MC. 2007: The role of mercury and cadmium heavy metals in vascular disease, hypertension, coronary heart disease, and myocardial infarction. Altern Ther Health Med. 2007 Mar-Apr;13(2):S128-33. https://pubmed.ncbi.nlm.nih.gov/17405690/
675 Mizuno, Y., Shimizu-Furusawa, H., Konishi, S. et al. Associations between urinary heavy metal concentrations and blood pressure in residents of Asian countries. Environ Health Prev Med 26, 101 (2021). https://doi.org/10.1186/s12199-021-01027-y;
676 Xu J, White AJ, Niehoff NM, O'Brien KM, Sandler DP. Airborne metals exposure and risk of hypertension in the Sister Study. Environ Res. 2020 Dec;191:110144.. https://www.ncbi.nlm.nih.gov/pmc/articles/PMC7658027/
677 Zhong, Qi; Wu, Hua-bing, et al 2021: Exposure to multiple metals and the risk of hypertension in adults: A prospective cohort study in a local area on the Yangtze River, China, Environment International, Volume 153, 2021, (https://www.sciencedirect.com/science/article/pii/S016041202100163X)
678 Wang, Xin;. Karvonen-Gutierrez, Carrie A.; et al 2021: Urinary Heavy Metals and Longitudinal Changes in Blood Pressure in Midlife Women: The Study of Women's Health Across the Nation; Hypert. 2021 https://doi.org/10.1161/HYPERTENSIONAHA.121.17295
679 Kim, K., Park, H. Co-exposure to Heavy Metals and Hypertension Among Adults in South Korea. Expo Health 14, 139–147 (2022). https://doi.org/10.1007/s12403-021-00423-7 https://link.springer.com/article/10.1007/s12403-021-00423-7
680 Shih YH, Howe CG, 2021, Argos M. Exposure to metal mixtures in relation to blood pressure among children 5-7 years old: An observational study in Bangladesh. Environ Epidemiol. 2021 Feb 11;5(2): https://www.ncbi.nlm.nih.gov/pmc/articles/PMC7939402/
681 WHO, More than 700 million people with untreated hypertension; https://www.who.int/news/item/25-08-2021-more-than-700-million-people-with-untreated-hypertension
682 Hypertension - the Preventable and Treatable Silent Killer; center for Heart protection; 1 March 2013; https://www.chp.gov.hk/en/features/28272.html
683 Trieme.de Risikofaktor Bluthochdruck; https://www.thieme.de/de/gesundheit/bluthochdruck-21375.htm
684 Ekerdt DJ, Sparrow D, Glynn RJ, Bossé R. Change in blood pressure and total cholesterol with retirement. Am J Epidemiol. 1984 Jul;120(1):64-71. https://pubmed.ncbi.nlm.nih.gov/6741924/
685 McGregor AJ, Mason HJ. Occupational mercury vapour exposure and testicular, pituitary and thyroid endocrine function. Hum Exp Toxicol. 1991;10(3):199–203. https://pubmed.ncbi.nlm.nih.gov/1678950/
686 Lemos NB, Angeli JK, , et al. (2012) Low Mercury Concentration Produces Vasoconstriction, Decreases Nitric Oxide Bioavailability and Increases Oxidative Stress in Rat Conductance Artery. PLoS ONE 7(11): https://doi.org/10.1371/journal.pone.0049005
687 Player, M. S., & Peterson, L. E. (2011). Anxiety Disorders, Hypertension, and Cardiovascular Risk: A Review. The International Journal of Psychiatry in Medicine, 41(4), 365–377. https://doi.org/10.2190/PM.41.4.f;
688 Dr. John Young; All About Chelation Therapy; Young Foundational Health Center; https://youngfoundationalhealth.com/chelation-therapy
689 Chappell LT. EDTA chelation therapy should be more commonly used in the treatment of vascular disease. Altern Ther Hea. Med. 1995 https://pubmed.ncbi.nlm.nih.gov/9359786/
690 CLARKE CN, CLARKE NE, MOSHER RE. Treatment of angina pectoris with disodium ethylene diamine tetraacetic acid. Am J Med Sci. 1956 Dec;232(6):654-66. http://doi.org/10.1097/00000441-195612000-00006.
691 Levine WC, ed. The chelation of heavy metals. In: International Encyclopedia of Pharmacology and Therapeutics. Sec. 70. New York: Pergamon Press; 1979.
692 The Free Library. S.v.: Chelation and cardiovascular disease." Retrieved Feb 09 2023 from https://www.thefreelibrary.com/Chelation+and+cardiovascular+disease.-a0225946869

[693] Schaar, P. , Pahlplatz, R. and Blaurock-Busch, E. (2014) The Effects of Magnesium-EDTA Chelation Therapy on Arterial Stiffness. Health, 6, 2848-2853. https://www.scirp.org/journal/paperinformation.aspx?paperid=52501

[694] Alfonso D. Torres, Ashok N. Rai, Melissa L. Hardiek; Mercury Intoxication and Arterial Hypertension: Report of Two Patients and Review of the Literature. Pediatrics March 2000; 105 (3): e34. 10.1542/peds.105.3.e34 https://publications.aap.org/pediatrics/article-abstract/105/3/e34/62717/Mercury-Intoxication-and-Arterial-Hypertension

[695] bethaniyaclinic : Alternative treatment for varicose veins - bulging veins in legs treatment; https://www.bethaniyaclinic.com/services/alternative-treatment-for-varicose-veins-bulging-v/

[696] totalhealthmagazine.com ; heavy metals 2022; https://totalhealthmagazine.com/tag/heavy-metals.html

[697] Healthline; What's the Difference Between Hemorrhoids and Rectal Varices?; Medically reviewed by Saurabh Sethi, M.D., MPH; September 19, 2022 https://www.healthline.com/health/rectal-varices-vs-hemorrhoids#:~:text=No.,pressure%20in%20the%20lower%20rectum.

[698] Bowdler NC, Beasley DS. Behavioral effects of aluminum ingestion. Pharmacol Biochem Behav 1979; 10: 505-512; & Trapp GA, Miner GD. Aluminum levels in brain in Alzheimer's Disease. Biol Psychiatry 1978; 13: 709-718.

[699] Islam Fahadul, Shohag Sheikh, et al 2022: Exposure of metal toxicity in Alzheimer's disease: An extensive review; Frontiers in Pharmacology; 13 , 2022;; https://www.frontiersin.org/articles/10.3389/fphar.2022.903099/full

[700] Paduraru E, et al 2022: Comprehensive Review Regarding Mercury Poisoning and Its Complex Involvement in Alzheimer's Disease. Int J Mol Sci. 2022 Feb 11;23(4):1992. https://www.ncbi.nlm.nih.gov/pmc/articles/PMC8879904/

[701] Bakulski KM, Seo YA, Hickman RC, Brandt D, Vadari HS, Hu H, Park SK. Heavy Metals Exposure and Alzheimer's Disease and Related Dementias. J Alzheimers Dis. 2020;76(4) https://www.ncbi.nlm.nih.gov/pmc/articles/PMC7454042/#:~:text=In%20cell%20and%20animal%20model,cognitive%20function%20and%20cognitive%20decline.

[702] Xu L, Zhang W, Liu X, et al. Circulatory Levels of Toxic Metals (Aluminum, Cadmium, Mercury, Lead) in Patients with Alzheimer's Disease: A Quantitative Meta-Analysis and Systematic Review. Journal of Alzheimer's Disease : JAD. 2018 ;62(1):361-372. https://europepmc.org/article/med/29439342#:~:text=Meta%2Danalyses%20showed%20significantly%20elevated,AD%20patients%20than%20in%20controls.

[703] Hellstrom HO, Mjoberg B, Mallmin H, et al. The aluminum content of bone increases with age, but is not higher in hip fracture cases with and without dementia compared to controls, Osteoporos Int, 2005, vol. 16 https://europepmc.org/article/MED/16047227

[704] Aoun Sebaiti, M., Abrivard, et al. (2018). Macrophagic myofasciitis-associated dysfunctioning: An update of neuropsychological and neuroimaging features. Best. Pract. Res. Clin. Rheumatol. 32, https://hal.science/hal-03484456v1/preview/S1521694219300579.pdf

[705] Bondy SC 2015. Low levels of aluminum can lead to behavioral and morphological changes associated with Alzheimer's disease and age-related neurodegeneration. Neurotoxicology. 2016 Jan;52:222-9. https://pubmed.ncbi.nlm.nih.gov/26687397/

[706] Hans-Olov Hellström, Karl Michaëlsson, Hans Mallmin, Bengt Mjöberg, 2008: The aluminium content of bone, and mortality risk, Age and Ageing, Volume 37, Issue 2, March 2008, Pages 217–220, https://doi.org/10.1093/ageing/afm152

[707] Pritchard C, Rosenorn-Lanng E. 2015: Neurological deaths of American adults (55-74) and the over 75's by sex compared with 20 Western countries 1989-2010: Cause for concern. Surg Neurol Int. 2015 Jul 23;6:123: https://pubmed.ncbi.nlm.nih.gov/26290774/

[708] Tomaskova H, Kuhnova J, Cimler R, Dolezal O, Kuca K. Prediction of population with Alzheimer's disease in the European Union using a system dynamics model. Neuropsychiatr Dis Treat. 2016 Jun 30;12:1589-98. http://doi.org/10.2147/NDT.S107969..

[709] Chen P, Miah MR, Aschner M. 2016: Metals and Neurodegeneration. F1000 Res. 2016 Mar 17;5:F1000 Faculty Rev-366.; https://pubmed.ncbi.nlm.nih.gov/27006759/

[710] Fulgenzi A, Vietti D, Ferrero ME. 2020: EDTA Chelation Therapy in the Treatment of Neurodegenerative Diseases: An Update. Biomedicines. 2020 Aug 3;8(8):269. https://pubmed.ncbi.nlm.nih.gov/32756375/

[711] Fulgenzi A, Vietti D, Ferrero ME. 2014: Aluminium involvement in neurotoxicity. Biomed Res Int. 2014;2014 https://www.ncbi.nlm.nih.gov/pmc/articles/PMC4160616/

[712] Hameed, O., & Al-Helaly, L. (2020). Levels for some Toxic and Essential Metals in Patients with Neurological Diseases. Rafidain Journal of Science, 29(3), 27-37. https://rsci.mosuljournals.com/article_166316.html

Notes

[713] Chen, S., Huang, W., Xu, Q. et al. The impact of serum copper on the risk of epilepsy: a mendelian randomization study. Acta Epileptologica 5, 15 (2023). https://doi.org/10.1186/s42494-023-00126-3

[714] Patncio F. Reyes et al 1986: Intracranial Calcification in Adults with Chronic Lead Exposure; AJR 146:267-270, https://www.ajronline.org/doi/pdf/10.2214/ajr.146.2.267

[715] Thomson, R.M. and Parry, G.J. (2006), Neuropathies associated with excessive exposure to lead†. Muscle Nerve, 33: 732-741. https://doi.org/10.1002/mus.20510

[716] Shobha N, Taly AB, Sinha S, Venkatesh T. Radial neuropathy due to occupational lead exposure: Phenotypic and electrophysiological characteristics of five patients. Ann Indian Acad Neurol. 2009 Apr;12(2):111-5. http://doi.org10.4103/0972-2327.53080.

[717] Jarup, Lars 2013: Hazards of heavy metal contamination; British Medical Bulletin, Volume 68, Issue 1, December 2003, Pages 167–182, https://doi.org/10.1093/bmb/ldg032

[718] Staff NP, Windebank AJ. Peripheral neuropathy due to vitamin deficiency, toxins, and medications. Continuum (Minneap Minn). 2014 Oct;20(5 Peripheral Nervous System Disorders):1293-306. https://pubmed.ncbi.nlm.nih.gov/25299283/

[719] Jang DH, Hoffman RS. Heavy metal chelation in neurotoxic exposures. Neurol Clin. 2011 Aug;29(3):607-22.. https://pubmed.ncbi.nlm.nih.gov/21803213/

[720] University of Chicago: Types of Peripheral Neuropathy - Toxic/Secondary to Drugs; last modified on 04.16.10 http://peripheralneuropathycenter.uchicago.edu/learnaboutpn/typesofpn/toxic/toxins.shtml

[721] Koszewicz, M.,. et al. 2021: The impact of chronic co-exposure to different heavy metals on small fibers of peripheral nerves. A study of metal industry workers. J Occup Med Toxicol 16, 12 (2021). https://doi.org/10.1186/s12995-021-00302-6

[722] Guo G, Ma H, Wang X. [Psychological and neurobehavioral effects of aluminum on exposed workers]. Zhonghua Yu Fang Yi Xue Za Zhi. 1998 Sep;32(5):292-4. Chinese. https://pubmed.ncbi.nlm.nih.gov/10322775/

[723] Sarihi, S., Niknam, M.,et al (2021). Toxic heavy metal concentrations in multiple sclerosis patients: A systematic review and meta-analysis. EXCLI Journal, 20, 1571–1584. https://doi.org/10.17179/excli2021-3484

[724] Bates MN, Fawcett J, Garrett N, Cutress T, Kjellstrom T. Health effects of dental amalgam exposure: a retrospective cohort study. Int J Epidemiol. 2004 Aug;33(4): https://pubmed.ncbi.nlm.nih.gov/15155698/

[725] Pamphlett R, Kum Jew S. Age-Related Uptake of Heavy Metals in Human Spinal Interneurons. PLoS One. 2016 Sep 9;11(9) https://pubmed.ncbi.nlm.nih.gov/27611334/

[726] Pamphlett, R., et al 2023 Potentially toxic elements in the brains of people with multiple sclerosis. Sci Rep 13, 655 (2023). https://www.nature.com/articles/s41598-022-27169-9

[727] Jirau-Colón H, González-Parrilla L, Martinez-Jiménez J, Adam W, Jiménez-Velez B. Rethinking the Dental Amalgam Dilemma: An Integrated Toxicological Approach. Int J Environ Res Public Health. 2019 Mar 22;16(6) https://pubmed.ncbi.nlm.nih.gov/30909378/

[728] Pyatha S, Kim H, Lee D, Kim K. 2022: Association between Heavy Metal Exposure and Parkinson's Disease: A Review of the Mechanisms Related to Oxidative Stress. Antioxidants (Basel). 2022 Dec 15;11(12):2467. https://www.ncbi.nlm.nih.gov/pmc/articles/PMC9774122/#:~:text=Heavy%20metals%2C%20such%20as%20iron,may%20result%20in%20synergistic%20toxicity.

[729] Kulshreshtha D, Ganguly J, Jog M. Manganese and Movement Disorders: A Review. J Mov Disord. 2021 May;14(2) https://www.ncbi.nlm.nih.gov/pmc/articles/PMC8175808/

[730] Johns Hopkins medicine: Can Environmental Toxins Cause Parkinson's Disease? https://www.hopkinsmedicine.org/health/conditions-and-diseases/parkinsons-disease/can-environmental-toxins-cause-parkinson-disease#:~:text=High%2Ddose%20manganese%20exposure%20—%20%20linked,a%20greater%20risk%20of%20Parkinson%27s.

[731] Bjorklund G, Stejskal V, Urbina MA, Dadar M, Chirumbolo S, Mutter J. Metals and Parkinson's Disease: Mechanisms and Biochemical Processes. Curr Med Chem. 2018;25(19):2198-2214. https://pubmed.ncbi.nlm.nih.gov/29189118/

[732] Ward RJ, Dexter DT, Martin-Bastida A, Crichton RR. Is Chelation Therapy a Potential Treatment for Parkinson's Disease? Int J Mol Sci. 2021 Mar 24;22(7):3338. https://www.ncbi.nlm.nih.gov/pmc/articles/PMC8036775/

[733] Ward RJ, Dexter DT, Martin-Bastida A, Crichton RR. Is Chelation Therapy a Potential Treatment for Parkinson's Disease? Int J Mol Sci. 2021 Mar 24;22(7):3338. https://www.ncbi.nlm.nih.gov/pmc/articles/PMC8036775/#:~:text=In%20recent%20clinical%20trials%2C%20iron,potentially%20slows%20the%20disease%20progression.

[734] Oggiano R, Pisano A, Sabalic A, Farace C,2020: An overview on amyotrophic lateral sclerosis and cadmium. Neurol Sci. 2021 Feb;42(2):531-537. Epub 2020 Dec 5..
https://www.ncbi.nlm.nih.gov/pmc/articles/PMC7843544/
[735] Peters S, Broberg K, Gallo V, Levi M,et al. 2021: Blood Metal Levels and Amyotrophic Lateral Sclerosis Risk: A Prospective Cohort. Ann Neurol. 2021 Jan;89(1):125-133. Epub 2020 Nov 6.
https://www.ncbi.nlm.nih.gov/pmc/articles/PMC7756568/
[736] Peter E A Ash, Uma Dhawan, Samantha Boudeau, Shuwen Lei, Yari Carlomagno, Mark Knobel, et al 2019: , Heavy Metal Neurotoxicants Induce ALS-Linked TDP-43 Pathology, Toxicological Sciences, Volume 167, Issue 1, January 2019, Pages 105–115,
https://doi.org/10.1093/toxsci/kfy267
[737] Figueroa-Romero, C., Mikhail, K.A., Gennings, C., Curtin, P., Bello, G.A., Botero, T.M., Goutman, S.A., Feldman, E.L., Arora, M. and Austin, C. (2020), Early life metal dysregulation in amyotrophic lateral sclerosis. Ann Clin Transl Neurol, 7: 872-882.
https://doi.org/10.1002/acn3.51006
[738] Mangelsdorf I, Walach H, Mutter J: Healing of Amyotrophic Lateral Sclerosis: A Case Report. Complement Med Res 2017; https://www.karger.com/Article/Fulltext/477397#
[739] Shlomo Bar-Sela, Stephen Reingold & Elihu D. Richter (2001) Amyotrophic Lateral Sclerosis in a Battery-factory Worker Exposed to Cadmium, International Journal of Occupational and Environmental Health, 7:2, 109-112,
https://www.tandfonline.com/doi/abs/10.1179/107735201800339470
[740] Rita A. Roelofs-Iverson, Donald W. Mulder, et al 1984: ALS and heavy metals; A pilot case-control study; Neurology Mar 1984, 34 (3) https://n.neurology.org/content/34/3/393
[741] Pamphlett R, Kum Jew S (2016) Age-Related Uptake of Heavy Metals in Human Spinal Interneurons. https://doi.org/10.1371/journal.pone.0162260
[742] Genchi, Giuseppe, Alessia Carocci, Graziantonio Lauria, Maria Stefania Sinicropi, and Alessia Catalano. 2021. "Thallium Use, Toxicity, and Detoxification Therapy: An Overview" Applied Sciences 11, no. 18: 8322. https://doi.org/10.3390/app11188322
[743] Yawei C, Jing S, Wenju S, Yupeng L, Ping Z, Liping H. Mercury as a cause of membranous nephropathy and Guillain–Barre syndrome: case report and literature review. Journal of International Medical Res.. 2021 https://doi.org/10.1177/0300060521999756
[744] Jalal MJ, Fernandez SJ, Menon MK. Acute toxic neuropathy mimicking guillain barre syndrome. J Family Med Prim Care. 2015 Jan-Mar;4(1):137-8.
https://www.ncbi.nlm.nih.gov/pmc/articles/PMC4366988/
[745] Yawei C, Jing S, Wenju S, Yupeng L, Ping Z, Liping H. Mercury as a cause of membranous nephropathy and Guillain–Barre syndrome: case report and literature review. J.of Internat. Medical Research. 2021;49(3). https://doi.org/10.1177/0300060521999756
[746] HORD; Heavy Metal Poisoning; Print; Last updated: March 28, 2008 ; Years published: 1989, 1991, 1998, 2006; https://rarediseases.org/rare-diseases/heavy-metal-poisoning/#:~:text=Neurological%20symptoms%20associated%20with%20lead,%2C%20and%2For%20impaired%20consciousness.
[747] The Raw Truth Teller; Apr 13, 2021; Seizures/Epilepsy & Heavy Metals;
https://www.therawtruthteller.com/post/seizures-epilepsy-heavy-metals
[748]elglaw: Heavy metals and seizures in children with Kanner's syndrome; Michael Bartlett July 04th, 2022; https://www.elglaw.com/blog/heavy-metals-seizures-autism-kanners-syndrome/#:~:text=Lead%20and%20mercury%20are%20the,are%20very%20harmful%20and%20powerful.
[749] Lee, Kuen Su,et al 2023. "The Effect of Maternal Exposure to Air Pollutants and Heavy Metals during Pregnancy on the Risk of Neurological Disorders Using the National Health Insurance Claims Data of South Korea" Medicina 59, no. 5: 951.
https://doi.org/10.3390/medicina59050951
[750] Ran E, Wang M, Yi Y, Feng M, Liu Y. 2021: Mercury poisoning complicated by acquired neuromyotonia syndrome: A case report. Medicine (Baltimore). 2021.
http://doi.org/10.1097/MD.0000000000026910.
[751] M. Szklarek, T. Kostka, 2013: The impact of the use of amalgams in the dentition on the appearance of the symptoms of restless legs syndrome developed by older people, Sleep Medicine, Volume 14, Supplement 1, 2013,
(https://www.sciencedirect.com/science/article/pii/S1389945713018984)
[752] Jiménez-Jiménez FJ, Ayuso P, et al 2017: Serum Trace Elements Concentrations in Patients with Restless Legs Syndrome. Antioxidants (Basel). 2022 Jan 29;11(2):272..
https://www.ncbi.nlm.nih.gov/pmc/articles/PMC8868060/

Notes

[753] Chen P, Totten M, Zhang Z, et al 2019: Iron and manganese-related CNS toxicity: mechanisms, diagnosis and treatment. Expert Rev Neurother. 2019 Mar;19(3): https://www.ncbi.nlm.nih.gov/pmc/articles/PMC6422746/

[754] Chawla S, Gulyani S, Allen RP, Earley CJ, Li X, Van Zijl P, Kapogiannis D. Extracellular vesicles reveal abnormalities in neuronal iron metabolism in restless legs syndrome. Sleep. 2019 Jul 8;42(7):zsz079. https://pubmed.ncbi.nlm.nih.gov/30895312/

[755] Hou YC, Fan YM, et al 2020: Tc-99m TRODAT-1 SPECT is a Potential Biomarker for Restless Leg Syndrome in Patients with End-Stage. J Clin Med. 2020 Mar 24;9(3):889.; https://www.ncbi.nlm.nih.gov/pmc/articles/PMC7141514/

[756] Fulgenzi A, Ferrero ME 2019: EDTA Chelation Therapy for the Treatment of Neurotoxicity. Int J Mol Sci. 2019 https://www.ncbi.nlm.nih.gov/pmc/articles/PMC6429616/

[757] Fulgenzi A, Vietti D, Ferrero ME. 2020: EDTA Chelation Therapy in the Treatment of Neurodegenerative Diseases: An Update. Biomedicines. 2020 Aug 3;8(8):269. https://pubmed.ncbi.nlm.nih.gov/32756375/

[758] Healthstar Clinic: A Toxic Shock: Are Environmental Factors the Source of Your Migraines? by HealthStar Clinic | May 26, 2017 https://www.healthstarclinic.com/toxic-environmental-factors-source-migraines/#:~:text=According%20to%20Dr.,pesticides%20on%20foods%2C%20and%20contraceptives.

[759] Donma, O., Donma, M.M. Association of headaches and the metals. Biol Trace Elem Res 90, 1–14 (2002). https://doi.org/10.1385/BTER:90:1-3:1

[760] Gonullu H, Gonullu E, Karadas S, Arslan M, Kalemci O, Aycan A, Sayin R, Demir H. The levels of trace elements and heavy metals in patients with acute migraine headache. J Pak Med Assoc. 2015, https://pubmed.ncbi.nlm.nih.gov/26160074/

[761] Hameed, O., & Al-Helaly, L. (2020). Levels for some Toxic and Essential Metals in Patients with Neurological Diseases. Rafidain Journal of Science, 29(3), 27-37. http://doi.org/10.33899/rjs.2020.166316

[762] Nesbitt AD, Goadsby PJ. Cluster headache. BMJ 2012;344:e2407. https://doi.org/10.1136/bmj.e2407

[763] Grant ECG. The pill, hormone replacement therapy, vascular and mood over-reactivity, and mineral imbalance. J Nutr Environ Med 1998;8:105-116.

[764] Kundan Singh Dhillon, Jasmer Singh, Jarnail Singh Lyall, A new horizon into the pathobiology, etiology and treatment of migraine, Medical Hypotheses, Volume 77, Issue 1, 2011, https://doi.org/10.1016/j.mehy.2011.03.050.

[765] Ringenberg QS, Doll DC, Patterson WP, Perry MC, Yarbro JW. Hematologic effects of heavy metal poisoning. South Med J. 1988 Sep;81(9):1132-9.

[766] Mount Sinai ; Hemolytic anemia caused by chemicals and toxins; https://www.mountsinai.org/health-library/diseases-conditions/hemolytic-anemia-caused-by-chemicals-and-toxins

[767] Hegazy, A.A., Zaher, M.M., Abd el-hafez, M.A. et al. Relation between anemia and blood levels of lead, copper, zinc and iron among children. BMC Res Notes 3, 133 (2010). https://doi.org/10.1186/1756-0500-3-133

[768] Turgut S. et al, (2009). Relations between Iron Deficiency Anemia and Serum Levels of Copper, Zinc, Cadmium and Lea. Polish Journal of Environmental Studies, 18(2), 273-277. http://www.pjoes.com/Relations-between-Iron-Deficiency-Anemia-r-nand-Serum-Levels-of-Copper-Zinc-r-nCadmium,88231,0,2.html

[769] Hyogo Horiguchi, Etsuko Oguma, Fujio Kayama, 2011: Cadmium Induces Anemia through Interdependent Progress of Hemolysis, Body Iron Accumulation, and Insufficient Erythropoietin Production in Rats, Toxicological Sciences, Volume 122, Issue 1, July 2011, https://doi.org/10.1093/toxsci/kfr100 ;

[770] Huang Chao-Hsin et al: Gender Difference in the Associations among Heavy Metals with Red Blood Cell Hemogram; Int J Environ Res Public Health. 2022 Jan; 19(1): 189. https://www.ncbi.nlm.nih.gov/pmc/articles/PMC8750598/

[771] Nemery B. Metal toxicity and the respiratory tract. Eur Respir J. 1990 Feb;3(2):202-19. https://pubmed.ncbi.nlm.nih.gov/2178966/#:~:text=Exposure%20to%20cadmium%20may%20lead,the%20basis%20of%20allergic%20sensitization.

[772] Wen J, Giri M, Xu L, Guo S. Association between Exposure to Selected Heavy Metals and Blood Eosinophil Counts in Asthmatic Adults: Results from NHANES 2011-2018. J Clin Med. 2023 Feb 15;12(4):1543. http://doi.org/10.3390/jcm12041543..

[773] Giancarlo Pesce et al 2020: Foetal exposure to heavy metals and risk of asthma and allergic diseases in early childhood: a population-based birth-cohort study, EDEN consortium European Resp. J. 2020 http://doi.org/10.1183/13993003.congress-2020.3847

[774] Chia-Yun Hsieh, MSc et al 2021: Combined exposure to heavy metals in PM2.5 and pediatric asthma; ASTHMA AND LOWER AIRWAY DISEASE| VOLUME 147, ISSUE 6, P2171-2180.E13, JUNE 2021; https://doi.org/10.1016/j.jaci.2020.12.634

[775] Jessica M. Madrigal, et al, 2018: Association of heavy metals with measures of pulmonary function in children and youth: Results from the National Health and Nutrition Examination Survey (NHANES), Environment International, Volume 121, Part 1, (https://www.sciencedirect.com/science/article/pii/S0160412018310134)

[776] Nemery B. Metal toxicity and the respiratory tract. Eur Respir J. 1990 Feb;3(2) https://pubmed.ncbi.nlm.nih.gov/2178966/#:~:text=The%20fumes%20or%20gaseous%20forms,o edema%20or%20to%20acute%20tracheobronchitis.

[777] Luoqi Weng, Zhixiao Xu, Chengshui Chen, 2024: Associations of blood cadmium and lead concentrations with all-cause mortality in US adults with chronic obstructive pulmonary disease, Journal of Trace Elements in Medicine and Biology, Volume 81, 2024, (https://www.sciencedirect.com/science/article/pii/S0946672X23002067)

[778] Fei Q, Weng X, et al: The Relationship between Metal Exposure and Chronic Obstructive Pulmonary Disease in the General US Population: NHANES 2015-2016. Int J Environ Res Public Health. 2022 https://pubmed.ncbi.nlm.nih.gov/35206273/

[779] Heo, J., Park, H.S., Hong, Y. et al. Serum heavy metals and lung function in a chronic obstructive pulmonary disease cohort. Toxicol. Environ. Health Sci. 9, 30–35 (2017). https://doi.org/10.1007/s13530-017-0300-x

[780] Wiggers GA, Peçanha FM, et al 2008: Low mercury concentrations cause oxidative stress and endothelial dysfunction in conductance and resistance arteries. Am J Physiol Heart Circ Physiol. 2008 Sep;295(3): https://pubmed.ncbi.nlm.nih.gov/18599595/

[781] Kim, Hyun Soo, et al 2015: An Overview of Carcinogenic Heavy Metal: Molecular Toxicity Mechanism and Prevention; J Cancer Prev. 2015 Dec; 20(4): . https://www.ncbi.nlm.nih.gov/pmc/articles/PMC4699750/

[782] Tinkov AA, Gritsenko VA, Skalnaya MG, Cherkasov SV, Aaseth J, Skalny AV. Gut as a target for cadmium toxicity. Environ Pollut. 2018 Apr;235:429-434. https://pubmed.ncbi.nlm.nih.gov/29310086/

[783] Liu Y, et al (2014) Exposing to Cadmium Stress Cause Profound Toxic Effect on Microbiota of the Mice Intestinal Tract. PLoS https://doi.org/10.1371/journal.pone.0085323

[784] Xue Tian, et al 2023: Gut as the target tissue of mercury and the extraintestinal effects, Toxicology, Volume 484, 2023, https://doi.org/10.1016/j.tox.2022.153396.

[785] Bolan, S. et al. Bioavailability of arsenic, cadmium, lead and mercury as measured by intestinal permeability. Sci Rep 11, https://doi.org/10.1038/s41598-021-94174-9

[786] Choiniere J, Wang L (2016) Exposure to inorganic arsenic can lead to gut microbe perturbations and hepatocellular carcinoma. Acta Pharm Sin B 6(5):426–429 https://doi.org/10.1016/j.apsb.2016.07.011

[787] Kim, Hyun Soo, et al 2015: An Overview of Carcinogenic Heavy Metal: Molecular Toxicity Mechanism and Prevention; J Cancer Prev. 2015 Dec; 20(4): 232–240. Published online 2015 Dec 30. https://www.ncbi.nlm.nih.gov/pmc/articles/PMC4699750/

[788] Carver, A., & Gallicchio, V. S. (2017). Heavy Metals and Cancer. In (Ed.), Cancer Causing Substances. IntechOpen. https://www.intechopen.com/chapters/56652

[789] Society for Risk Analysis. "Heavy metals in our food are most dangerous for kids." ScienceDaily. 12 Dec. 2023. www.sciencedaily.com/releases/2023/12/231212112342.htm

[790] Basal cell carcinoma - Symptoms & causes; Mayo Clinic; https://www.mayoclinic.org/diseases-conditions/basal-cell-carcinoma/symptoms-causes/syc-20354187

[791] Mohammadnezhad K, Sahebi MR, Alatab S, Sajadi A. Investigating heavy-metal soil contamination state on the rate of stomach cancer using remote sensing spectral features. Environ Monit Assess. 2023. https://link.springer.com/article/10.1007/s10661-023-11234-5

[792] Pamphlett, Roger, Andrew J. Colebatch, Philip A. Doble, and David P. Bishop. 2020. "Mercury in Pancreatic Cells of People with and without Pancreatic Cancer" International Journal of Environmental Research and P. Health https://doi.org/10.3390/ijerph17238990

[793] Carrigan PE, Hentz JG, Gordon G, Morgan JL, Raimondo M, Anbar AD, Miller LJ. Distinctive heavy metal composition of pancreatic juice in patients with pancreatic carcinoma. Canc Epidem. Biom. Prev. 2007 https://pubmed.ncbi.nlm.nih.gov/18086771/

[794] Carver, A., & Gallicchio, V. S. (2017). Heavy Metals and Cancer. In (Ed.), Cancer Causing Substances. IntechOpen. https://www.intechopen.com/chapters/56652

[795] Rita Bonfiglio, et al 2024: The impact of toxic metal bioaccumulation on colorectal cancer: Unravelling the unexplored connection, Science of The Total Environment, Volume 906, 2024, https://doi.org/10.1016/j.scitotenv.2023.167667.

Notes

[796] Ge XY, Xie SH, et al : Associations between serum trace elements and the risk of nasopharyngeal carcinoma: a multi-center case-control study in Guangdong Province, southern China. Front Nutr. 2023 http://doi.org/10.3389/fnut.2023.1142861.

[797] Qayyum MA, Shah MH. Disparities in the Concentrations of Essential/Toxic Elements in the Blood and Scalp Hair of Lymphoma Patients and Healthy Subjects. Sci Rep. 2019 Oct 25;9(1):15363 https://www.ncbi.nlm.nih.gov/pmc/articles/PMC6814775/

[798] Deubler EL, Gapstur SM,et al. 2020: Erythrocyte levels of cadmium and lead and risk of B-cell non-Hodgkin lymphoma and multiple myeloma. Int J Cancer. 2020 Dec 1;147(11):3110-3118. https://pubmed.ncbi.nlm.nih.gov/32506449/

[799] Cheah CY, Zucca E, et al Marginal zone lymphoma: present status and future perspectives. Haematologica 2022;107(1) https://doi.org/10.3324/haematol.2021.278755.

[800] Tommaso Iannitti,; et al 2010: Intracellular heavy metal nanoparticle storage: progressive accumulation within lymph nodes with transformation from chronic inflammation to malignancy; Int J Nanomedicine. 2010; 5: 955–960.; 2010 Nov 15. https://www.ncbi.nlm.nih.gov/pmc/articles/PMC3010157/

[801] Caffo M, et al 2014 Heavy metals and epigenetic alterations in brain tumors. Curr Genomics. 2014 Dec;15(6) https://www.ncbi.nlm.nih.gov/pmc/articles/PMC4311389/

[802] Arslan, M., Demir, H., Arslan, H., Gokalp, A. S. & Demir, C. Trace Elements, Heavy Metals and Other Biochemical Parameters in Malignant Glioma Patients. Asian Pacific J. Cancer Prev. 12, 447–451 (2011). https://pubmed.ncbi.nlm.nih.gov/21545211/

[803] Rashidi M, Alavipanah S. Relation between kidney cancer and soil leads in Isfahan Province, Iran between 2007 and 2009. Journal of Cancer Research and Therapeutics. 2016;12(2):716-720. https://pubmed.ncbi.nlm.nih.gov/27461639/

[804] El-Yazigl, A., Al-Saleh, I. & Al-Mefty, O. Concentrations of Ag, Al, Au, Bi, Cd, Cu, Pb, Sb, and Se in Cerebrospinal Fluid of Patients with Cerebral Neoplasms. Clin. Chem. 30, https://citeseerx.ist.psu.edu/document?repid=rep1&type=pdf&doi=871d5d2683a35e81c07b6dcb2ccb93bcdeb0ce75

[805] Stojsavljević, A., Vujotić, L., Rovčanin, B. et al. Assessment of trace metal alterations in the blood, cerebrospinal fluid and tissue samples of patients with malignant brain tumors. Sci Rep 10, 3816 (2020). https://doi.org/10.1038/s41598-020-60774-0

[806] Gaman, Laura; et al (2021) Concentration of heavy metals and rare earth elements in patients with brain tumours: Analysis in tumour tissue, non-tumour tissue, and blood, International Journal of Environmental Health Research, 31:7, 741-754, https://www.tandfonline.com/doi/full/10.1080/09603123.2019.1685079?scroll=top&needAccess=true&role=tab&aria-labelledby=full-article

[807] Nemery B. Metal toxicity and the respiratory tract. Eur Respir J. 1990 Feb;3(2):202-19. https://pubmed.ncbi.nlm.nih.gov/2178966/#:~:text=Exposure%20to%20cadmium%20may%20lead,the%20basis%20of%20allergic%20sensitization.

[808] Mannello F, Tonti GA, et al: Analysis of aluminium content and iron homeostasis in nipple aspirate fluids from healthy women and breast cancer-affected patients. J Appl Toxicol. 2011 Apr;31(3):262-9. https://pubmed.ncbi.nlm.nih.gov/21337589/

[809] Ionescu, John et al (2007). Increased levels of transition metals in breast cancer tissue. Neuro endocrinology letters. 27 Suppl 1. 36-9 https://www.researchgate.net/publication/6979212_Increased_levels_of_transition_metals_in_breast_cancer_tissue

[810] Men Y, Li L, Zhang F, et al: 2019: Evaluation of heavy metals and metabolites in the urine of patients with breast cancer. Oncol Lett. 2020 Feb;19(2): https://www.researchgate.net/publication/337900100_Evaluation_of_heavy_metals_and_metabolites_in_the_urine_of_patients_with_breast_cancer

[811] Darbre PD. Aluminium, antiperspirants and breast cancer. J Inorg Biochem. 2005 Sep;99(9):1912-9. https://pubmed.ncbi.nlm.nih.gov/16045991/

[812] Mannello F, Tonti GA, et al 2011: Analysis of aluminium content and iron homeostasis in nipple aspirate fluids from healthy women and breast cancer-affected patients. J Appl Toxicol. 2011 Apr;31(3):262-9.. https://pubmed.ncbi.nlm.nih.gov/21337589/

[813] Carver, A., & Gallicchio, V. S. (2017). Heavy Metals and Cancer. In (Ed.), Cancer Causing Substances. IntechOpen. https://www.intechopen.com/chapters/56652

[814] Mandriota SJ, Tenan M, et al 2016. Aluminium chloride promotes tumorigenesis and metastasis in normal murine mammary gland epithelial cells. International Journal of Cancer. 2016;139(12):2781-2790. https://www.ncbi.nlm.nih.gov/pmc/articles/PMC5095782/

[815] Darbre PD 2016: Aluminium and the human breast. Morphologie. 2016;100(329):65-74. https://pubmed.ncbi.nlm.nih.gov/26997127/

[816] Jeremiah Morrissey, Marcos Rothstein, et al 1983: Suppression of parathyroid hormone secretion by aluminum, Kidney International, Volume 23, Issue 5, 1983,

(https://www.sciencedirect.com/science/article/pii/S0085253815329513)
[817] Orisakwe OE, Dagur EA, Mbagwu HO, Udowelle NA. Lead levels in vegetables from artisanal mining sites of Dilimi River, Bukuru and Barkin Ladi North Central Nigeria: Cancer and non-cancer risk assessment. Asian Pacific Journal of Cancer Prevention. 2017;18(3) https://www.ncbi.nlm.nih.gov/pmc/articles/PMC5464475/
[818] Chen K, Liao QL, 2014: Association of soil arsenic and nickel exposure with cancer mortality rates, a town-scale ecological study in Suzhou, China. Environ Sci Pollut Res Int. 2015 Apr;22(7):5395-404. https://pubmed.ncbi.nlm.nih.gov/25410308/
[819] Panalyadiyan, S. et al Association of heavy metals and trace elements in carcinoma urinary bladder: A case-controlled study; http://doi.org/10.4103/jju.jju_143_23 yser123AS

[820] Kiani, B., Hashemi Amin, F., Bagheri, N. et al. Association between heavy metals and colon cancer: an ecological study based on geographical information systems in North-Eastern Iran. BMC Cancer 21, 414 (2021). https://doi.org/10.1186/s12885-021-08148-1
[821] Fatfat, M., Merhi, R.A., Rahal, O. et al. 2014: Copper chelation selectively kills colon cancer cells through redox cycling and generation of reactive oxygen species. BMC Cancer 14, 527 (2014). https://doi.org/10.1186/1471-2407-14-527
[822] Mayo Clinic: Kindy cross section: Mayo Foundation for Medical Education and Research https://www.mayoclinic.org/kidney-cross-section/img-20005978
[823] Lentini, P., Zanoli, L., Granata, A., Signorelli, S.S., Castellino, P., & Dell'Aquila, R. (2017). Kidney and heavy metals - The role of environmental exposure (Review). Molecular Medicine Reports, 15, 3413-3419. https://doi.org/10.3892/mmr.2017.6389
[824] Johri, N., Jacquillet, G. & Unwin, R. Heavy metal poisoning: the effects of cadmium on the kidney. Biometals 23, https://link.springer.com/article/10.1007/s10534-010-9328-y

[825] Ting-ting Zhou, Bing Hu, et al 2021: , The associations between urinary metals and metal mixtures and kidney function in Chinese community-dwelling older adults with diabetes mellitus, Ecotoxicology and Environmental Safety, Volume 226, 2021, https://doi.org/10.1016/j.ecoenv.2021.112829.
(https://www.sciencedirect.com/science/article/pii/S0147651321009416)
[826] Chowdhury, Tasrina Rabia; et al 2021: Status of metals in serum and urine samples of chronic kidney disease patients in a rural area of Bangladesh: An observational study
Heliyon : V. 7, 11, E08382, Nov 11, 2021; https://doi.org/10.1016/j.heliyon.2021.e08382
[827] Jayasumana, C., Gunatilake, S. & Siribaddana, S. Simultaneous exposure to multiple heavy metals and glyphosate may contribute to Sri Lankan agricultural nephropathy. BMC Nephrol 16, 103 (2015). https://doi.org/10.1186/s12882-015-0109-2
[828] Satarug S, Vesey DA, Gobe GC. Kidney Cadmium Toxicity, Diabetes and High Blood Pressure: The Perfect Storm. Tohoku J Exp Med. 2017 Jan;241(1):65-87. https://pubmed.ncbi.nlm.nih.gov/28132967/
[829] Lentini, P., Zanoli, L., Granata, A., Signorelli, S.S., Castellino, P., & Dell'Aquila, R. (2017). Kidney and heavy metals - The role of environmental exposure (Review). Molecular Medicine Reports, 15, 3413-3419. https://doi.org/10.3892/mmr.2017.6389
[830] D R Lewis, J W Southwick, R Ouellet-Hellstrom, J Rench, and R L Calderon; 1999, Drinking water arsenic in Utah: A cohort mortality study. Environmental Health Perspectives 107:5 CID: https://doi.org/10.1289/ehp.99107359
[831] Kim NH, Hyun YY,et al 2015: Environmental heavy metal exposure and chronic kidney disease in the general population. J Korean Med Sci. 2015 Mar;30(3):272-7. 2015 Feb 16. https://www.ncbi.nlm.nih.gov/pmc/articles/PMC4330481/
[832] National Institute of Diabetes and Digestive and Kidney Diseases (NIDDK); High Blood Pressure & Kidney Disease; https://www.niddk.nih.gov/health-information/kidney-disease/high-blood-pressure
[833] Salem MM. 2002: Pathophysiology of hypertension in renal failure. Semin Nephrol. 2002 Jan;22(1):17-26. https://pubmed.ncbi.nlm.nih.gov/11785065/
[834] Cleveland Clinic: Renal Hypertension; https://my.clevelandclinic.org/health/diseases/16459-renal-hypertension
[835] Jing Xu et al 2022: Associations of metal exposure with hyperuricemia and gout in general adults; Front. Endocrinol., 02 December 2022; Sec. Systems Endocrinology; Volume 13 - 2022 | https://doi.org/10.3389/fendo.2022.1052784
[836] Lin, Ja-Liang; Yu, et al 2001: Lead chelation therapy and urate excretion in patients with chronic renal diseases and gout, Kidney International, Volume 60, Issue 1, 2001, (https://www.sciencedirect.com/science/article/pii/S0085253815478433)

Notes

[837] Geier D, Carmody T, Kern J, King P, Geier M. A significant dose-dependent relationship between mercury exposure from dental amalgams and kidney integrity biomarkers: A further assessment of the Casa Pia children's dental amalgam trial. Human & Exper, Toxicology. 2013 https://journals.sagepub.com/doi/10.1177/0960327112455671

[838] Krishnan E, Lingala B, 2012 Low-level lead exposure and the prevalence of gout: an observational study. Ann Intern Med. 2012 https://www.researchgate.net/publication/230714399_Low-Level_Lead_Exposure_and_the_Prevalence_of_Gout

[839] Reuters: Even low blood lead levels linked to gout risk ; healthcare & pharma; august 21, 2012 By Amy Norton, Reuters Health; https://www.reuters.com/article/us-blood-lead-gout-idUSBRE87J0X320120820

[840] Jing Xu et al 2022: Associations of metal exposure with hyperuricemia and gout in general adults; Front. Endocrinol., 02 December 2022; Sec. Systems Endocrinology; Volume 13 - 2022 | https://doi.org/10.3389/fendo.2022.1052784

[841] Shi, Z. Cadmium Intake, Dietary Patterns and Hyperuricemia Among Adults in China. Expo Health 13, 219–227 (2021). https://doi.org/10.1007/s 12403-020-00375-4

[842] Jung W, Kim Y, Lihm H, Kang J. 2019 Associations between blood lead, cadmium, and mercury levels with hyperuricemia in the Korean general population: A retrospective analysis of population-based nationally representative data. Int J Rheum Dis. 2019 Aug;22(8). https://pubmed.ncbi.nlm.nih.gov/31215160/

[843] Lin, Ja-Liang; Yu, Chun-Chen; Dan-Tzu Lin-Tan, Huei-Hong Ho, 2001: Lead chelation therapy and urate excretion in patients with chronic renal diseases and gout, Kidney Intern. V. 60, I. 1, 2001, (https://www.sciencedirect.com/science/article/pii/S0085253815478433)

[844] Geier DA, Pretorius HT, Richards NM, Geier MR. A quantitative evaluation of brain dysfunction and body-burden of toxic metals. Med Sci Monit. 2012 Jul;18(7):CR425-31.. https://www.ncbi.nlm.nih.gov/pmc/articles/PMC3560777/

[845] Porphyria, Wikipedia; https://en.wikipedia.org/wiki/Porphyria; 2. 19. 2023

[846] Bralley, Alexander PhD, Richard S. Lord, BS, PhD; Urinary Porphyrins for the Detection of Heavy Metal and Toxic Chemical Exposure; https://clinicalgate.com/urinary-porphyrins-for-the-detection-of-heavy-metal-and-toxic-chemical-exposure/#bib4

[847] Doctor's Data, Science and Insights. Inc; Urine Porphyrins; https://www.doctorsdata.com/urine-porphyrins/

[848] Tsai MT, Huang SY, Cheng SY. Lead Poisoning Can Be Easily Misdiagnosed as Acute Porphyria and Nonspecific Abdominal Pain. Case Rep Emerg Med. 2017;2017:9050713. https://www.ncbi.nlm.nih.gov/pmc/articles/PMC5467293/

[849] AACC.com; Laura M. Parnas Date: DEC.18.2012; Porphyrias; Source Trainee Council in English https://www.aacc.org/science-and-research/clinical-chemistry-trainee-council/trainee-council-in-english/pearls-of-laboratory-medicine/2012/porphyrias

[850] Akshatha L N,, et al 2014:. Lead poisoning mimicking acute porphyria! J Clin Diagn Res. 2014 Dec;8(12):CD01-2. https://pubmed.ncbi.nlm.nih.gov/25653942/

[851] Fujita H, Nishitani C, Ogawa K. Lead, chemical porphyria, and heme as a biological mediator. Tohoku J Exp Med. 2002 Feb;196(2) https://pubmed.ncbi.nlm.nih.gov/12498316/

[852] Fatima, T., McKinney, C., Major, T.J. et al. The relationship between ferritin and urate levels and risk of gout. Arthritis Res Ther 20, 179 (2018). https://doi.org/10.1186/s13075-018-1668-y

[853] James S. Woods, et al Urinary porphyrin profiles as biomarkers of trace metal exposure and toxicity: Studies on urinary porphyrin excretion patterns in rats during prolonged exposure to methyl mercury, Toxicology and Applied Pharmacology, Volume 110, 3, 1991, (https://www.sciencedirect.com/science/article/pii/0041008X91900471)

[854] Sears, M.E. et al 2013: Chelation: Harnessing and Enhancing Heavy Metal Detoxification—A Review; The Scientific World Journal; Hindawi.com https://www.hindawi.com/journals/tswj/2013/219840/tab1/

[855] Osterloh J, Becker CE. Pharmacokinetics of CaNa2EDTA and chelation of lead in renal failure. Clin Pharmacol Ther. 1986 Dec; . https://pubmed.ncbi.nlm.nih.gov/3096624/

[856] Sehnert KW, Clague AF, Cheraskin E. The improvement in renal function following EDTA chelation and multi-vitamin-trace mineral therapy: a study in creatinine clearance. Med Hypotheses. 1984 Nov;15(3):301-4. https://pubmed.ncbi.nlm.nih.gov/6441110/

[857] Tutunji MF, al-Mahasneh QM. Disappearance of heme metabolites following chelation therapy with meso 2,3-dimercaptosuccinic acid (DMSA). J Toxicol Clin Toxicol. 1994;32(3):267-76. https://pubmed.ncbi.nlm.nih.gov/8007034/

[858] Brenner BM, Meyer TW, Hostetter TH. Dietary protein intake and the progressive nature of kidney disease: the role of hemodynamically mediated glomerular injury in the pathogenesis of progressive glomerular sclerosis in aging, renal ablation, and intrinsic renal disease. N Engl J Med. 1982 Sep 9;3 https://pubmed.ncbi.nlm.nih.gov/7050706/

859 Yang SK, Xiao L, Song PA, Xu XX, Liu FY, Sun L. Is lead chelation therapy effective for chronic kidney disease? A meta-analysis. Nephrology (Carlton). 2014 Jan;19(1):56-9.. https://pubmed.ncbi.nlm.nih.gov/24341661/

860 Virginia M. Weaver, MD, MPH et al 2012: Does Calcium Disodium EDTA Slow CKD Progression? Anmerican Journal of Kidney disease: EDITORIAL| VOLUME 60, ISSUE 4, P503-506, OCTOBER 2012; https://www.ajkd.org/article/S0272-6386(12)00958-4/fulltext

861 Foglieni, C., Fulgenzi, A., Ticozzi, P. et al. Protective effect of EDTA preadministration on renal ischemia. BMC Nephrol 7, 5 (2006). https://doi.org/10.1186/1471-2369-7-5 https://bmcnephrol.biomedcentral.com/articles/10.1186/1471-2369-7-5

862 Khalil-Manesh F, et al: Experimental model of lead nephropathy. II. Effect of removal from lead exposure and chelation treatment with dimercaptosuccinic acid (DMSA). Environ Res. 1992 https://pubmed.ncbi.nlm.nih.gov/1317791/

863 Johns Hopkins Medicine 2013: Elevated Cadmium Levels Linked to Liver Disease Men especially affected; Release Date: May 9, 2013; https://www.hopkinsmedicine.org/news/media/releases/elevated_cadmium_levels_linked_to_liver_disease

864 Kiarash Riazi, MD et al. 2022: The prevalence and incidence of NAFLD worldwide: a systematic review and meta-analysis; Lancet; ARTICLES| VOLUME 7, ISSUE 9, P851-861, SEP 2022;: https://doi.org/10.1016/S2468-1253(22)00165-0

865 Jingxuan, Quek et al 2023: Global prevalence of non-alcoholic fatty liver disease and non-alcoholic steatohepatitis in the overweight and obese population: a systematic review and meta-analysis; Lancet: VOLUME 8, ISSUE 1, P20-30, JANUARY 2023; https://www.thelancet.com/journals/langas/article/PIIS2468-1253(22)00317-X/fulltext

866 Kim, Do-Won, Jeongwon Ock, Kyong-Whan Moon, and Choong-Hee Park. 2021. "Association between Pb, Cd, and Hg Exposure and Liver Injury among Korean Adults" International Journal of Environmental Research and Public Health 18, no. 13: 6783. https://doi.org/10.3390/ijerph18136783

867 Zhai, H., Chen, C., Wang, N. et al. Blood lead level is associated with non-alcoholic fatty liver disease in the Yangtze River Delta region of China in the context of rapid urbanization. Environ Health 16, 93 (2017). https://doi.org/10.1186/s12940-017-0304-7

868 Hai Duc Nguyen, Min-Sun Kim, 2022: Cadmium, lead, and mercury mixtures interact with non-alcoholic fatty liver diseases, Environmental Pollution, Volume 309, 2022, 119780, (https://www.sciencedirect.com/science/article/pii/S0269749122009940)

869 Seung Min Chung, Jun Sung Moon, et al 2020: The sex-specific effects of blood lead, mercury, and cadmium levels on hepatic steatosis and fibrosis: Korean nationwide cross-sectional study, Journal of Trace Elements in Medicine and Biology, Volume 62, 2020, , (https://www.sciencedirect.com/science/article/pii/S0946672X20301668)

870 Lin YC, Lian IB, 2017: Association between soil heavy metals and fatty liver disease in men in Taiwan: a cross sectional study. BMJ Open. 2017 Jan 23;7(1):e014215. https://pubmed.ncbi.nlm.nih.gov/28115335/

871 Teerasarntipan, T., Chaiteerakij, R., Prueksapanich, P. et al. Changes in inflammatory cytokines, antioxidants and liver stiffness after chelation therapy in individuals with chronic lead poisoning. BMC Gastro. 20, 263 (2020). https://doi.org/10.1186/s12876-020-01386-w

872 Frediani, J.K., Naioti, E.A., Vos, M.B. et al. 2018: Arsenic exposure and risk of nonalcoholic fatty liver disease (NAFLD) among U.S. adolescents and adults: an association modified by race/ethnicity, NHANES 2005–2014. Environ Health 17, 6 (2018). https://doi.org/10.1186/s12940-017-0350-1

873 Carver, A., & Gallicchio, V. S. (2017). Heavy Metals and Cancer. In (Ed.), Cancer Causing Substances. IntechOpen. https://www.intechopen.com/chapters/56652

874 Jue Tao Lim, et al 2018: Association between serum heavy metals and prostate cancer risk – A multiple metal analysis, Environment International, Volume 132, 2019, https://doi.org/10.1016/j.envint.2019.105109.

875 Pizent A, Anđelković M, et al 2022: Environmental Exposure to Metals, Parameters of Oxidative Stress in Blood and Prostate Cancer: Results from Two Cohorts. Antioxidants. 2022; 11. https://doi.org/10.3390/antiox11102044

876 Stella Bicalho Silva, et al 2023: Impacts of heavy metal exposure on the prostate of murine models: Mechanisms of toxicity, Reproductive Toxicology, Volume 120, 2023, (https://www.sciencedirect.com/science/article/pii/S0890623823001223)

877 E. García-Esquinas, 2020: Cadmium exposure is associated with reduced grip strength in US adults, Environmental Research, Volume 180, 2020,

Notes

(https://www.sciencedirect.com/science/article/pii/S0013935119306164)
878 Ling CH, Taekema D, et al 2010: Handgrip strength and mortality in the oldest old population: the Leiden 85-plus study. CMAJ. 2010 Mar http://doi.org/10.1503/cmaj.091278.
879 Yoo JI, Ha YC, Lee YK, Koo KH. High Levels of Heavy Metals Increase the Prevalence of Sarcopenia in the Elderly Population. J Bone Metab. 2016 May;23(2):101-9. https://www.ncbi.nlm.nih.gov/pmc/articles/PMC4900959/#:~:text=Conclusions,both%20genders %20of%20elderly%20populations.
880 Kyoung-Nam Kim, et al: Associations of Blood Cadmium Levels With Depression and Lower Handgrip Strength in a Community-Dwelling Elderly Population: A Repeated-Measures Panel Study, The Journals of Gerontology: Series A, Volume 71, Issue 11, November 2016, https://doi.org/10.1093/gerona/glw119
881 Wu M, Shu Y, Wang Y. Exposure to mixture of heavy metals and muscle strength in children and adolescents: a population-based study. Environ Sci Pollut Res Int. 2022 Aug https://pubmed.ncbi.nlm.nih.gov/35419687/
882 E. García-Esquinas, 2020: Cadmium exposure is associated with reduced grip strength in US adults, Environmental Research, Volume 180, 2020, 108819 (https://www.sciencedirect.com/science/article/pii/S0013935119306164)
883 Beatrice Battistini, et al 2024: Metals accumulation affects bone and muscle in osteoporotic patients: A pilot study, Enviro Res, V 250, 2024, https://doi.org/10.1016/j.envres.2024.118514. (https://www.sciencedirect.com/science/article/pii/S0013935124004183)
884 Dayer SR, Mears SC, et al 2021: Superior Bone Health Promote a Longer Lifespan? Geriatr Orthop Surg Rehabil. 2021 Aug. https://www.ncbi.nlm.nih.gov/pmc/articles/PMC8358490/
885 creakyjoints.org; Osteoporosis and Mental Health: What You Need to Know; PUBLISHED 11/02/22 BY KERRY WEISS; https://creakyjoints.org/about-arthritis/osteoporosis-and-mental-health-what-you-need-to-know/#1665225653089-68b82cd2-11e7
886 Edward Puzas, Brendan F. Boyce,; Chapter 22 - Metal ion toxicity in the skeleton: lead and aluminum, Editor(s): John P. Bilezikian, T. John Martin, Thomas L. Clemens, Clifford J. Rosen, Principles of Bone Biology (Fourth Edition), Academic Press, 2020 (https://www.sciencedirect.com/science/article/pii/B9780128148419000221)
887 Rodríguez J, et al 2018 A Review of Metal Exposure and Its Effects on Bone Health. J Toxicol. 2018 https://www.ncbi.nlm.nih.gov/pmc/articles/PMC6323513/
888 Akesson A, Bjellerup P, et al 2006: Cadmium-induced effects on bone in a population-based study of women. Environ Health Perspect. 2006 Jun;114(6):830-4. https://www.ncbi.nlm.nih.gov/pmc/articles/PMC1480481/
889 Nowakowski A., Kubaszewski L., Frankowski M., Wilk-Frańczuk M., Ziola-Frankowska A., Czabak-Garbacz R., Kaczmarczyk J., Gasik R., Ann. Agric. Environ. Med. 2015, 22, 362 https://pubmed.ncbi.nlm.nih.gov/26094540/
890 Zhang S, Sun L, Zhang J, Liu S, Han J, Liu Y. 2020: Adverse Impact of Heavy Metals on Bone Cells and Bone Metabolism Dependently and Independently through Anemia. Adv Sci (Weinh). 2020 Aug https://www.ncbi.nlm.nih.gov/pmc/articles/PMC7539179/#:~:text=Mounting%20evidence%20is% 20revealing%20that,degenerative%20disk%20disease%2C%20and%20osteomalacia.
891 Georgetown University; Chronic Back Pain; https://hpi.georgetown.edu/backpain/#:~:text=Some%2016%20million%20adults%20—%208,limited%20in%20certain%20everyday%20activities.
892 Li, Min, 2020: Chronic mercury poisoning causing back pain in spondyloarthritis: a case report, Rheumatology, Volume 59, Issue 11, November 2020, https://doi.org/10.1093/rheumatology/keaa256
893 Hashmi, G. M.et al 2022: Comparative Assessment of Essential and Toxic Metals in the Blood of Spondyloarthropathy Patients and Healthy Subjects; biointerface research; Volume 12, Issue 2, 2022, https://doi.org/10.33263/BRIAC122.19351950
894 Päivi Leino, Guido Magni, 1993: Depressive and distress symptoms as predictors of low back pain, neck-shoulder pain, and other musculoskeletal morbidity: a 10-year follow-up of metal industry employees, Pain, Volume 53, Issue 1, 1993, Pages 89-94,. (https://www.sciencedirect.com/science/article/pii/0304395993900603)
895 Chang, L., Shen, S., Zhang, Z., Song, X., & Jiang, Q. (2018). Study on the relationship between age and the concentrations of heavy metal elements in human bone. Annals Of Translational Medicine, 6(16), 320. https://atm.amegroups.com/article/view/20948/html
896 Md. Shakil Ahmed, et al 2020: Risk assessment and evaluation of heavy metals concentrations in blood samples of plastic industry workers in Dhaka, Bangladesh, Toxicology Reports, Volume 7, 2020, https://doi.org/10.1016/j.toxrep.2020.10.003.

[897] Jarup L, Berglund M, Elinder CG, Nordberg G, Vahter M. 1998: Health effects of cadmium exposure—a review of the literature and a risk estimate. Scand J Work Environ Health1998; 24 (Suppl 1): 1–51 https://pubmed.ncbi.nlm.nih.gov/9569444/

[898] Jakoniuk, Marta, et al 2022: "Concentration of Selected Macronutrients and Toxic Elements in the Blood in Relation to Pain Severity and Hydrogen Magnetic Resonance Spectroscopy in People with Osteoarthritis of the Spine" International Journal of Environmental Research and Public Health 19, https://doi.org/10.3390/ijerph191811377

[899] Irfan S, Rani A, Riaz N, Arshad M, Kashif Nawaz S. Comparative Evaluation of Heavy Metals in Patients with Rheumatoid Arthritis and Healthy Control in Pakistani Population. Iran J Public Health. 2017 May; https://www.ncbi.nlm.nih.gov/pmc/articles/PMC5442275/

[900] Zamudio-Cuevas Yessica Eduviges et al 2022: Impact of cadmium toxicity on cartilage loss in a 3D in vitro model, Environmental Toxicology and Pharmacology, Volume 74, 2020, (https://www.sciencedirect.com/science/article/pii/S1382668919301826)

[901] Xia F, Li Q, Luo X, Wu J. Identification for heavy metals exposure on osteoarthritis among aging people and Machine learning for prediction: A study based on NHANES 2011-2020. Front Public Health. https://www.ncbi.nlm.nih.gov/pmc/articles/PMC9376265/

[902] Chen, L., Zhao, Y., Liu, F. et al. Biological aging mediates the associations between urinary metals and osteoarthritis among U.S. adults. BMC Med 20, 207 (2022). https://doi.org/10.1186/s12916-022-02403-3

[903] Prieto-Alhambra D, Judge A,et al 2014. Incidence and risk factors for clinically diagnosed knee, hip and hand osteoarthritis: influences of age, gender and osteoarthritis affecting other joints. Ann Rheum Dis. 2014 Se https://pubmed.ncbi.nlm.nih.gov/23744977/

[904] Doumouchtsis KK, Doumouchtsis SK, Doumouchtsis EK, Perrea DN. The effect of lead intoxication on endocrine functions. J Endocrinol Invest. 2009 Feb;32(2):175-83. http://doi.org/10.1007/BF03345710.

[905] Markiewicz-Górka I, et al 2022: Cadmium Body Burden and Inflammatory Arthritis: A Pilot Study in Patients from Lower Silesia, Poland. Int J Environ Res Public Health. 2022 Mar 6;19(5):3099. https://www.ncbi.nlm.nih.gov/pmc/articles/PMC8910441/

[906] Jakoniuk, M et al 2022. "Concentration of Selected Macronutrients and Toxic Elements in the Blood in Relation to Pain Severity and Hydrogen Magnetic Resonance Spectroscopy in People with Osteoarthritis of the Spine" International Journal of Environmental Research and Public Health 19, no. 18: 11377. https://doi.org/10.3390/ijerph191811377

[907] Lim HS, Lee HH, Kim TH, Lee BR. 2016: Relationship between Heavy Metal Exposure and Bone Mineral Density in Korean Adult. J Bone Metab. 2016 Nov;23(4):223-231. http://doi.org/10.11005/jbm.2016.23.4.223.

[908] Jalili, C., Kazemi, M., Taheri, E. et al. Exposure to heavy metals and the risk of osteopenia or osteoporosis: a systematic review and meta-analysis. Osteoporos Int 31, 1671–1682 (2020). https://doi.org/10.1007/s00198-020-05429-6

[909] Zengfa Huang et al 2023: Relationship of blood heavy metals and osteoporosis among the middle-aged and elderly adults: A secondary analysis from NHANES 2013 to 2014 and 2017 to 2018; Front. Public Health, 14 March 2023; Sec. Aging and Public Health; Volume 11 - 2023 https://doi.org/10.3389/fpubh.2023.1045020

[910] Brzóska M. M., Moniuszko-Jakoniuk J. Low-level exposure to cadmium during the lifetime increases the risk of osteoporosis and fractures of the lumbar spine in the elderly: Studies on a rat model of human environmental exposure. Toxicological Sciences. 2004;82(2):468–477. http://doi.org/10.1093/toxsci/kfh275.

[911] Moshtaghie, Ali Asghar; Malekpouri, Pedram; et a (2014) "Cobalt induces alterations in serum parameters associated with bone metabolism in male adult rat," Turkish Journal of Biology: Vol. 38: No. 5, Article 1. https://doi.org/10.3906/biy-1312-89

[912] Khalil, Naila, et al 2008: Relationship of Blood Lead Levels to Incident Nonspine Fractures and Falls in Older Women: The Study of Osteoporotic Fractures; JOURNAL OF BONE AND MINERAL RESEARCH; Volume 23, Number 9, 2008 on April 14, 2008; https://asbmr.onlinelibrary.wiley.com/doi/pdf/10.1359/jbmr.080404

[913] Wei-Jie Wang, Chang-Chin Wu, 2013: The associations among lead exposure, bone mineral density, and FRAX score: NHANES, 2013 to 2014, Bone, Volume 128, 2019, https://doi.org/10.1016/j.bone.2019.115045.

[914] Carmouche JJ, Puzas JE, 2005:. Lead exposure inhibits fracture healing and is associated with increased chondrogenesis, delay in cartilage mineralization, and a decrease in osteoprogenitor frequency. Environ Health Perspect. 2005 Jun;113(6) https://www.ncbi.nlm.nih.gov/pmc/articles/PMC1257601/

Notes

915 Campbell JR, et al: The association between blood lead levels and osteoporosis among adults--results from the third national health and nutrition examination survey Envir Health Perspect. 2007 https://www.ncbi.nlm.nih.gov/pmc/articles/PMC1913605/

916 Ezema C. et al 2018: Influence of serum lead level on prevalence of musculoskeletal pain, quality of life and cardiopulmonary function among welders in Enugu metropolis, Southeast, Nigeria; bioRxiv preprint https://doi.org/10.1101/482919.

917 Lim HS, Lee HH, Kim TH, Lee BR. 2016: Relationship between Heavy Metal Exposure and Bone Mineral Density in Korean Adult. Journal of Bone Metabolism. 2016 Nov;23(4):223-231. https://www.ncbi.nlm.nih.gov/pmc/articles/PMC5153379/

918 Blickman JG, Wilkinson RH, Graef JW. The radiologic "lead band" revisited. AJR Am J Roentgenol. 1986 Feb;146(2):245 https://www.ajronline.org/doi/pdf/10.2214/ajr.146.2.245

919 Zhang YF, Xu JW, Yang Y, Huang X, Yu XQ. 2019: The association between body lead levels and childhood rickets: A meta-analysis based on Chinese cohort. Medicine (Baltimore). 2019 Feb;98(8) https://www.ncbi.nlm.nih.gov/pmc/articles/PMC6407931/

920 Järup, L., Alfvén, T. 2004: Low level cadmium exposure, renal and bone effects - the OSCAR stud. Biometals 17, (2004). https://doi.org/10.1023/B:BIOM.0000045729.68774.a1

921 Medscape: Rickets; Updated: Sep 09, 2022; https://emedicine.medscape.com/article/985510-overview

922 smithsonianmag.com: Many Roman Children Suffered From Vitamin D Deficiency New research suggests rickets was common long before the Industrial Revolution, when pollution blocked out sunlight; By Brigit Katz; August 20, 2018; https://www.smithsonianmag.com/smart-news/many-roman-children-suffered-rickets-new-study-has-found-180970074/

923 N. Zoeger,et al 2006: Lead accumulation in tidemark of articular cartilage; Generative AI: New policies, opportunities, and risks; VOLUME 14, ISSUE 9, P906-913, SEPT, 2006 https://doi.org/10.1016/j.joca.2006.03.001

924 Lansdown, A.B.G. (2011). Cartilage and Bone as Target Tissues for Toxic Materials. In General, Applied and Systems Toxicology (eds B. Ballantyne, T.C. Marrs, T. Syversen, D.A. Casciano and S.C. Sahu). https://doi.org/10.1002/9780470744307.gat071

925 Pamphlett Roger, Kum Jew Stephen; 2016: Mercury Is Taken Up Selectively by Cells Involved in Joint, Bone, and Connective Tissue Disorders; Frontiers in Medicine; VOLUME: 6 ;2019 https://www.frontiersin.org/articles/10.3389/fmed.2019.00168/full

926 Baki AE, Yıldızgören MT,2015: Ultrasonographic Measurement of the Achilles and Supraspinatus Tendon Thicknesses in Patients with Chronic Lead Exposure. West Indian Med J. 2015 Sep; https://www.ncbi.nlm.nih.gov/pmc/articles/PMC4909072/

927 Dye BAHR, Brody DJ (2002) The relationship between blood lead levels and periodontal bone loss in the United States, 1988–1994. Envir H. P. 110 https://doi.org/10.1289/ehp.02110997

928 Alhaasmi, A et al 2013: Investigation of periodontal parameters and toxic elements in teeth due to smoking using laser induced breakdown spectroscopy. http://doi.org/10.1109/HONET.2013.6729764

929 Dai, Z., Fu, Y., Tan, Y. et al. Association between metal exposures and periodontitis among U.S. adults: the potential mediating role of biological aging. Environ Sci Eur 36, 123 (2024). https://doi.org/10.1186/s12302-024-00949-y

930 Han DH, Lim SY, Sun BC, et al 2009: Mercury exposure and periodontitis among a Korean population: the Shiwha-Banwol environmental health study. J Periodontol. 2009 Dec;80(12) http://doi.org/10.1902/jop.2009.090293.

931 Ubios AMGM, et al 1991 Uranium inhibits bone formation in physiologic alveolar bone modeling and remodeling. Environ Res; https://doi.org/10.1016/S0013-9351(05)80191-4

932 Malara P, Fischer A, Malara B. Selected toxic and essential heavy metals in impacted teeth and the surrounding mandibular bones of people exposed to heavy metals in the environment. J Occup Med Toxic; https://www.ncbi.nlm.nih.gov/pmc/articles/PMC5154102/

933 Herman M, Golasik M, Piekoszewski W, et al, 2016: Essential and Toxic Metals in Oral Fluid-a Potential Role in the Diagnosis of Periodontal Diseases. Biol Trace Elem Res. 2016 Oct;173(2):275-82. https://www.ncbi.nlm.nih.gov/pmc/articles/PMC5018033/

934 Nycpediatricdentist; Lead Poisoning and Tooth Decay; Increased Risk of Tooth Decay Associated with Lead Poisoning; Nov 28, 2020 by Dr. Sara Babich, DDS (Pediatric Dentist) https://www.nycpediatricdentist.com/lead-poisoning-and-tooth-decay/#:~:text=Lead%20poisoning%20increases%20the%20risk,and%20enhancing%20tooth%20demineralization%20Enamel

935 Asaduzzaman K, et al 2017: Heavy metals in human teeth dentine: A bio-indicator of metals exposure and environmental pollution. Chemosphere. 2017 https://doi.org/10.1016/j.chemosphere.2017.02.114

[936] Asaduzzaman K, Khandaker MU, et al 2017: Heavy metals in human teeth dentine: A bio-indicator of metals exposure and environmental pollution. Chemosphere. 2017 Jun;. http://doi.org/10.1016/j.chemosphere.2017.02.114.

[937] Arora Manish et al 2015: Cumulative Lead Exposure and Tooth Loss in Men: The Normative Aging Study; Environ Health Perspective. 2009 Oct; 117(10): https://www.ncbi.nlm.nih.gov/pmc/articles/PMC2790506/

[938] Cojocaru M, Chicoş B. The role of heavy metals in autoimmunity. Rom J Intern Med. 2014;52(3):189-91. https://pubmed.ncbi.nlm.nih.gov/25509564/

[939] Mishra K. P. et al 2020: Heavy Metals Exposure and Risk of Autoimmune Diseases: A Review; Archives of Immunology and Allergy ISSN: 2639-1848; Volume 3, Issue 2, 2020, PP: 22-26; w https://www.sryahwapublications.com/archives-of-immunology-and-allergy/pdf/v3-i2/4.pdf

[940] Jie Liu; Robert A. Goyer 2023: Toxic Effects of Metals; Casarett & Doull's Essentials of Toxicology, 2e Chapter 23.; https://courseware.cutm.ac.in/wp-content/uploads/2020/07/Chapter-23.-Toxic-Effects-of-Metals.pdf

[941] Vas J, Monesteir M (2008). Immunology of mercury. Annals of the New York Academy of Sciences 1143: 240–267. https://pubmed.ncbi.nlm.nih.gov/19076354/

[942] Cruz-Tapias P, Agmon-Levin N, Israeli E, Anaya JM, Shoenfeld Y. Autoimmune (auto-inflammatory) syndrome induced by adjuvants (ASIA)--animal models as a proof of concept. Curr Med Chem. https://pubmed.ncbi.nlm.nih.gov/23992328/

[943] Bártová J, Procházková J, Krátká Z, Benetková K, Venclíková Z, Sterzl I. Dental amalgam as one of the risk factors in autoimmune diseases. Neuro Endocrinol Lett. 2003 Feb-Apr;24(1-2):65-7. https://pubmed.ncbi.nlm.nih.gov/12743535/

[944] Eggleston DW. Effect of dental amalgam and nickel alloys on T-lymphocytes: preliminary report. J Prosthet Dent. 1984 https://pubmed.ncbi.nlm.nih.gov/6610046/

[945] Anka AU, Usman AB, Kaoje AN, et al. Potential mechanisms of some selected heavy metals in the induction of inflammation and autoimmunity. European Journal of Inflammation. 2022;20. https://www.researchgate.net/publication/364847616_Potential_mechanisms_of_some_selected_heavy_metals_in_the_induction_of_inflammation_and_autoimmunity

[946] Haiyan Xing, Qiang et al 2022: Cadmium mediates pyroptosis of human dermal lymphatic endothelial cells in a NLRP3 inflammasome-dependent manner; https://doi.org/10.2131/jts.47.237

[947] Lu Yiming, Han Yanfei, Yin Hang, Cong Yimei, Shi Guangliang, Li Shu, 2001: Cadmium induces apoptosis of pig lymph nodes by regulating the PI3K/AKT/HIF-1α pathway, Toxicology, Volume 451, 2021, (https://www.sciencedirect.com/science/article/pii/S0300483X21000172)

[948] Offit K, Macris NT. Arsenic-associated angioimmunoblastic lymphadenopathy. Lancet. 1985 Jan 26;1(8422):220. http://doi.org/10.1016/s0140-6736(85)92055-0.

[949] Medical news today; What are lymph nodes? Medically reviewed by Meredith Goodwin, MD, FAAFP - Lauren Martin 2021 https://www.medicalnewstoday.com/articles/lymph-nodes

[950] Grundler F, Séralini G-E, et al (2021) Excretion of Heavy Metals and Glyphosate in Urine and Hair Before and After Long-Term Fasting in Humans. Front. Nutr. https://www.frontiersin.org/articles/10.3389/fnut.2021.708069/full

[951] Vallascas E, De Micco A, Deiana F, Banni S, Sanna E. 2013: Adipose tissue: another target organ for lead accumulation? A study on Sardinian children (Italy). Am J Hum Biol. (2013) 25:789–94. https://pubmed.ncbi.nlm.nih.gov/24022917/

[952] Mymed.com; Bronwen Watson; Handling the psychological and emotional effects of dramatic weight loss; https://www.mymed.com/diseases-conditions/obesity/handling-the-psychological-and-emotional-effects-of-dramatic-weight-loss

[953] Jackson SE, Steptoe A, Beeken RJ, Kivimaki M, Wardle J (2014) Psychological Changes following Weight Loss in Overweight and Obese Adults: A Prospective Cohort Study. PLoS ONE 9(8): e104552. https://doi.org/10.1371/journal.pone.0104552

[954] University College London. (2014, August 7). Losing weight won't necessarily make you happy, researchers say. ScienceDaily. Retrieved March 17, 2023 from www.sciencedaily.com/releases/2014/08/140807105430.htm

[955] Li, Tiezheng, et al 2022. "Associations of Diet Quality and Heavy Metals with Obesity in Adults: A Cross-Sectional Study from National Health and Nutrition Examination Survey (NHANES)" Nutrients 14, no. 19: 4038. https://doi.org/10.3390/nu14194038

[956] Brenda Gamboa-Loira, et al, 2021: Physical activity, body mass index and arsenic metabolism among Mexican women, Environmental Research, Volume 195, 2021, (https://www.sciencedirect.com/science/article/pii/S0013935121001638)

Notes

[957] Kranjac AW, Kranjac D. Explaining adult obesity, severe obesity, and BMI: Five decades of change. Heliyon. 2023 May https://doi.org/10.1016/j.heliyon.2023.e16210

[958] Psychologytoday; Charles Harper Webb; TESTOSTERONE; How Testosterone Is the Jekyll and Hyde of Hormones; December 20, 2022; https://www.psychologytoday.com/us/blog/drawing-the-curtains-back/202211/how-testosterone-is-the-jekyll-and-hyde-of-hormones#:~:text=Testosterone%20increases%20muscle%20mass%20and,i.e.%2C%20adventurousness)%20and%20competition.

[959] Pontzer H, Raichlen DA, Wood BM, Mabulla AZP, Racette SB, Marlowe FW (2012) Hunter-Gatherer Energetics and Human Obesity. PLoS ONE 7(7): e40503. https://doi.org/10.1371/journal.pone.0040503

[960] HERMAN PONTZER: The Exercise Paradox" in Scientific American Magazine Vol. 316 No. 2 (February 2017), p. 26 http://doi.org/10.1038/scientificamerican0217-26

[961] Britannica. ProCon.org : obesity 2016: https://obesity.procon.org/global-obesity-levels/

[962] Wikipedia: List of sovereign states by body mass; index https://en.wikipedia.org/wiki/List_of_sovereign_states_by_body_mass_index

[963] Wikipedia List of countries by food energy intake; 1.2. 2023; https://en.wikipedia.org/wiki/List_of_countries_by_food_energy_intake

[964] Khan MI, Ahmad MF, et al 2022: Arsenic Exposure through Dietary Intake and Associated Health Hazards in the Middle East. Nutrients. 2022 May 20;14(10):2136. https://www.mdpi.com/2072-6643/14/10/2136

[965] Israa M. Shatwan, Noha M. Almoraie, Correlation between dietary intake and obesity risk factors among healthy adults, Clinical Nutrition Open Science, Volume 45, 2022, Pages 32-41, https://doi.org/10.1016/j.nutos.2022.08.007.

[966] Li, Tiezheng, et al 2022. "Associations of Diet Quality and Heavy Metals with Obesity in Adults: A Cross-Sectional Study from National Health and Nutrition Examination Survey (NHANES)" Nutrients 14, no. 19: 4038. https://doi.org/10.3390/nu14194038

[967] Wang X, Mukherjee B, Park SK. 2018: Associations of cumulative exposure to heavy metal mixtures with obesity and its comorbidities among U.S. adults in NHANES 2003-2014. Env. Int 2018 https://www.sciencedirect.com/science/article/pii/S0160412018312650

[968] Huang, W., Igusa, T., Wang, G. et al. In-utero co-exposure to toxic metals and micronutrients on childhood risk of overweight or obesity: new insight on micronutrients counteracting toxic metals. Int J Obes 46, https://doi.org/10.1038/s41366-022-01127-x

[969] Stahr, S., Chiang, Tc., Bauer, M.A. et al. Low-Level Environmental Heavy Metals are Associated with Obesity Among Postmenopausal Women in a Southern State. Expo Health 13, 269–280 (2021). https://doi.org/10.1007/s12403-020-00381-6

[970] Tinkov AA, Aschner M, et al. 2021: Adipotropic effects of heavy metals and their potential role in obesity. Fac Rev. 2021 Mar 26;10:32. https://www.ncbi.nlm.nih.gov/pmc/articles/PMC8103910/

[971] Trasande L, Blumberg B: Endocrine disruptors as obesogens. In Pediatric Obesity. Contemporary Endocrinology. Edited by Freemark MS. Humana Press, Cham. 2018; 243–253. https://link.springer.com/chapter/10.1007/978-3-319-68192-4_14

[972] EPA; Health & Environmental Research Online; Freire, C et al 2020; Adipose tissue concentrations of arsenic, nickel, lead, tin, and titanium in adults from GraMo cohort in Southern Spain: An exploratory study; Science of the Total Environment; 719; 137458; https://hero.epa.gov/hero/index.cfm/reference/details/reference_id/6746555

[973] Tinkov AA, Aschner M, et al. 2021: Adipotropic effects of heavy metals and their potential role in obesity. Fac Rev. 2021 Mar 26;10:32. https://www.ncbi.nlm.nih.gov/pmc/articles/PMC8103910/

[974] Duc, H.N., Oh, H. & Kim, M. 2022: The Effect of Mixture of Heavy Metals on Obesity in Individuals ≥50 Years of Age. Biol Trace Elem Res 200, 3554–3571 (2022). https://doi.org/10.1007/s12011-021-02972-z;

[975] Min Kyong Moon, Inae Lee, et al 2022: Lead, mercury, and cadmium exposures are associated with obesity but not with diabetes mellitus: Korean National Environmental Health Survey (KoNEHS) 2015–2017, Environmental Research, Volume 204, Part A, 2022, (https://www.sciencedirect.com/science/article/pii/S001393512101183X)

[976] Zhong, Q.; et al 2021: Multiple metal exposure and obesity: A prospective cohort study of adults living along the Yangtze River, China, Environmental Pollution, Volume 285, 2021, 117150, (https://www.sciencedirect.com/science/article/pii/S0269749121007326)

[977] Wen WL, Wang CW, Wu DW, Chen SC, Hung CH, Kuo CH. Associations of Heavy Metals with Metabolic Syndrome and Anthropometric Indices. Nutrients. 2020 Sep 1;12(9):2666. https://www.ncbi.nlm.nih.gov/pmc/articles/PMC7551496/

[978] Stahr; S; Su, J. . Positive association between salivary arsenic concentration and obesity in a pilot study of women living in rural communities in the United States. Environmental Epidemiology   3():p   381,   October   2019

https://journals.lww.com/environepidem/Fulltext/2019/10001/Positive_association_between _salivary_arsenic.1163.aspx

[979] Pardo-Manuel De Villena, Fernando National Institute of health; Grantone; Project 2: Arsenic-Obesity- Diabetes Interactions University of North Carolina Chapel Hill, Chapel Hill, NC, United States; https://grantome.com/grant/NIH/P42-ES031007-02-5713

[980] Tseng GH. The potential biological mechanisms of arsenic – induced diabetes mellitus. Toxicol Appl Pharmacol 2004; 197:67–83. https://pubmed.ncbi.nlm.nih.gov/15163543/

[981] Eick SM, Steinmaus C. Arsenic and Obesity: a Review of Causation and Interaction. Curr Envir Health Rep. 2020 Sep; https://www.ncbi.nlm.nih.gov/pmc/articles/PMC7891850/

[982] Arcidiacono B, Iiritano S, Nocera A, Possidente K, Nevolo MT, Ventura V, Foti D, Chiefari E, Brunetti A. Insulin resistance and cancer risk: an overview of the pathogenetic mechanisms. Exp Diabetes Res. https://www.ncbi.nlm.nih.gov/pmc/articles/PMC3372318/

[983] Farkhondeh T, Samarghandian S, Azimi-Nezhad M. The role of arsenic in obesity and diabetes. J Cell Physiol. 2019 Aug;234(8):. https://pubmed.ncbi.nlm.nih.gov/30667058/

[984] Steinmaus, C. et al. 2015:/ Obesity and excess weight in early adulthood and high risks of arsenic-related cancer in later life Environmental Research 142 (2015) 594–601 https://www.ncbi.nlm.nih.gov/pmc/articles/PMC4664040/

[985] Skalnaya MG, Tinkov AA, Demidov VA, Serebryansky EP, Nikonorov AA, Skalny AV. Hair toxic element content in adult men and women in relation to body mass index. Biol Trace Elem Res. 2014 Oct;161(1):13-9. https://pubmed.ncbi.nlm.nih.gov/25048403/

[986] Attia, S.M., Varadharajan, K., Shanmugakonar, M. et al. Cadmium: An Emerging Role in Adipose Tissue Dysfunction. Expo Health 14, (2022). https://doi.org/10.1007/s12403-021-00427-3

[987] Skolarczyk, Justyna & Pekar, Joanna & Skórzyńska-Dziduszko, Katarzyna & Łabądź, Dawid. (2018). Role of heavy metals in the development of obesity: A review of research. Journal of Elementology. 23. https://www.researchgate.net/publication/326629907_Role_of_heavy_metals_in_the_developme nt_of_obesity_A_review_of_research

[988] Park JS, Ha KH, He K, et al 2017.: Association between Blood Mercury Level and Visceral Adiposity in Adults. Diabetes Metab J. 2017; 41(2): 113–20. https://www.researchgate.net/publication/311964019_Association_between_Blood_Mercury_Lev el_and_Visceral_Adiposity_in_Adults

[989] Freire C, Vrhovnik P, Fiket Ž, et al 2020.: Adipose tissue concentrations of arsenic, nickel, lead, tin, and titanium in adults from GraMo cohort in Southern Spain: An exploratory study. Sci Total Environ. 2020; 719: https://www.sciencedirect.com/science/article/abs/pii/S0048969720309682?via%3Dihub

[990] Wang, N. et al 2015: Blood lead level and its association with body mass index and obesity in China - Results from SPECT-China study; December 2015; Sc. Rep 5(1) https://www.researchgate.net/publication/286977704_Blood_lead_level_and_its_association_wit h_body_mass_index_and_obesity_in_China_-_Results_from_SPECT-China_study

[991] Thomas Reinehr, Obesity and thyroid function, Molecular and Cellular Endocrinology, V. 316, 2, 2010 (https://www.sciencedirect.com/science/article/pii/S0303720709003499)

[992] Darbre PD. 2017: Endocrine Disruptors and Obesity. Current Obesity Reports. 2017;6(1):18-27. https://www.ncbi.nlm.nih.gov/pmc/articles/PMC5359373/

[993] Skolarczyk, Justyna & Pekar, Joanna & Skórzyńska-Dziduszko, Katarzyna & Łabądź, Dawid. (2018). Role of heavy metals in the development of obesity: A review of research. J. of Ele. https://hero.epa.gov/hero/index.cfm/reference/details/reference_id/5073901

[994] Holtcamp W.2012: Obesogens: an environmental link to obesity. Environ Health Perspect. 2012 Feb;120(2):a62-8. https://www.ncbi.nlm.nih.gov/pmc/articles/PMC3279464/

[995] Gupta, R. et al 2020: Endocrine disruption and obesity: A current review on environmental obesogens, Current Research in Green and Sustainable Chemistry, Volume 3, 2020, (https://www.sciencedirect.com/science/article/pii/S2666086520300126)

[996] Alexey A. Tinkov, et al 2017; The role of cadmium in obesity and diabetes,; Science of The Total Environment,; Volumes; 601–602,; 2017,; Pages 741-755,; (https://www.sciencedirect.com/science/article/pii/S0048969717313323)

[997] Jia, Xiaoqian; Zhang, Le; et al 2021: Associations between endocrine-disrupting heavy metals in maternal hair and gestational diabetes mellitus: A nested case-control study in China, Environment International, Volume 157, 2021 (https://www.sciencedirect.com/science/article/pii/S0160412021003950)

[998] Wang, R., He, P., Duan, S. et al. Correlation and interaction between urinary metals level and diabetes: A cross sectional study of community-dwelling elderly. Expo Health (2023). https://doi.org/10.1007/s12403-023-00577-6

Notes

[999] Castriota F, Acevedo J, Ferreccio C, Smith AH, Liaw J, Smith MT, Steinmaus C. 2018: Obesity and increased susceptibility to arsenic-related type 2 diabetes in Northern Chile. Environ Res. 2018 Nov;167:248-254. https://doi.org/10.1016/j.envres.2018.07.022.

[1000] Prasanta Kumar Bhattacharyya, et al. (2019). RELATIONSHIP OF HEAVY METAL IN DIABETES AND NON-DIABETIC FOOT ULCER PATIENTS. ISSN: 2320-5407 Int. J. Adv. Res. 7(3), 126-133 https://doi.org/10.5281/zenodo.2644778

[1001] Kimberlie A. Graeme, Charles V. Pollack, 1998: Heavy metal toxicity, part ii: lead and metal fume fever, The Journal of Emergency Medicine, Volume 16, Issue 2, 1998, Pages 171-177, (https://www.sciencedirect.com/science/article/pii/S0736467997002837)

[1002] NORD, Rare Disease Database; Heavy Metal Poisoning; https://rarediseases.org/rare-diseases/heavy-metal-poisoning/

[1003] Pigatto PD, et al. Oral lichen planus due to allergy to mercury dental amalgam. Allergy and Asthma Proceedings. 2013 https://air.unimi.it/handle/2434/616790

[1004] Medical Medium Healing Essential: Addictions Part 2; Anorexia & Bulimia; https://www.medicalmedium.com/blog/addictions-part-2

[1005] Padilla MA, Elobeid M, Ruden DM, Allison DB. An examination of the association of selected toxic metals with total and central obesity indices: NHANES 99-02. Int J Environ Res Public Health. 2010 Sep: https://www.ncbi.nlm.nih.gov/pmc/articles/PMC2954548/

[1006] NORD, Rare Disease Database; Heavy Metal Poisoning; https://rarediseases.org/rare-diseases/heavy-metal-poisoning/

[1007] Su JC, Birmingham CL. Zinc supplementation in the treatment of anorexia nervosa. Eat Weight Disord. 2002 https://www.researchgate.net/publication/286080231_Zinc_supplementation_in_the_treatment_of_anorexia_nervosa

[1008] Casper, Regina & Kirschner Md, Barbara & Jacob, Robert. (1978). Zinc and copper status in anorexia nervosa. Psychopharmacology bulletin. 14. https://www.researchgate.net/publication/22466845_Zinc_and_copper_status_in_anorexia_nervosa

[1009] Abd Elnabi MK, et al Toxicity of Heavy Metals and Recent Advances in Their Removal: A Review. Toxics. 2023 Jul 3;11(7):580. http://doi.org/10.3390/toxics11070580..

[1010] Sheehan MC, Burke TA, Breysse PN, Navas-Acien A, McGready J, Fox MA. Association of markers of chronic viral hepatitis and blood mercury levels in US reproductive-age women from NHANES 2001-2008: a cross-sectional study. Environ Health. 2012; https://ehjournal.biomedcentral.com/articles/10.1186/1476-069X-11-62

[1011] Hu H, Scheidell J et al Associations between blood lead level and substance use and sexually transmitted infection risk among adults in the United States. Environ Res. 2014; https://www.sciencedirect.com/science/article/abs/pii/S0013935114002886?via%3Dihub

[1012] Krueger WS, Wade TJ. Elevated blood lead and cadmium levels associated with chronic infections among non-smokers in a cross-sectional analysis of NHANES data. Environ Health. 2016 http://doi.org/10.1186/s12940-016-0113-4.

[1013] Healing partnership: Dr.Bryan Stern Heavy Metals and Chronic Disease; https://www.healingpartnership.com/articles/heavy-metals-and-chronic-disease/

[1014] Nature: Parasites suck toxins from sharks; Intestinal worms collect heavy metals from the sea. Matt Kaplan; 25 June 2007 | Nature https://www.nature.com/news/2007/070625/full/news070625-1.html

[1015] Brožová A, Jankovská I,et al: Heavy metal concentrations in the small intestine of red fox (Vulpes vulpes) with and without Echinococcus multilocularis infection. Environ Sci Pollut Res Int. 2015 Feb;22(4):3175-9. https://pubmed.ncbi.nlm.nih.gov/25335764/

[1016] Mageed, S. N. et al 2018: Heavy Metal Concentrations in Parasitized Cows and Sheep with Echinococcus as Environmental Bioindicators; International Conference on Pure and Applied Sciences (ICPAS 2018) 41 http://dx.doi.org/10.14500/icpas2018

[1017] Marija Stojkovic, Bruno Gottstein, Thomas Junghanss, 56 - Echinococcosis, Editor(s): Jeremy Farrar, Peter J. Hotez, Thomas Junghanss, Gagandeep Kang, David Lalloo, Nicholas J. White, Manson's Tropical Infectious Diseases (Twenty-third Edition), W.B. Saunders, 2014, https://doi.org/10.1016/B978-0-7020-5101-2.00057-1.

[1018] Schmidberger J, Uhlenbruck J, Schlingeloff P, Maksimov P, Conraths FJ, Mayer B, Kratzer W. Dog Ownership and Risk for Alveolar Echinococcosis, Germany. Emerg Infect Dis. 2022 Aug;28(8):1597-1605. https://www.ncbi.nlm.nih.gov/pmc/articles/PMC9328925/ .

[1019] Sures B, Knopf K, Würtz J, Hirt J. 1999. Richness and diversity of parasite communities in European eels Anguilla anguilla of the River Rhine, Germany, with special reference to helminth parasites. Parasitology. https://pubmed.ncbi.nlm.nih.gov/10503258/

[1020] Graci, Stefania;, et al (2017) Mercury accumulation in Mediterranean Fish and Cephalopods Species of Sicilian coasts: correlation between pollution and the presence of Anisakis parasites, Nat. Product Res, https://doi.org/10.1080/14786419.2016.1230119

[1021] Pascual S, Abollo e. 2003. Accumulation of heavy metals in the whaleworm Anisakis simplex s.l (Nematoda: Anisakidae). J Mar Biol Assoc UK. 83: http://doi.org/10.1017/S0025315403008038h

[1022] Evans DW, Irwin SWB, Fitzpatrick S. 2001. The effect of digenean (Platyhelminthes) infections on heavy metal concentrations in Littorina littorea. J Mar Biol Assoc UK. 81:349–350. https://www.cambridge.org/core/journals/journal-of-the-marine-biological-association-of-the-united-kingdom/article/abs/effect-of-digenean-platyhelminthes-infections-on-heavy-metal-concentrations-in-littorina-littorea/09C4D828E9BAF37D2E562A8CEAF44351

[1023] Thielen, Frankie et al (2004). The intestinal parasite Pomphorhynchus laevis (Acanthocephala) from barbel as a bioindicator for metal pollution in the Danube River near Budapest, Hungary. Environmental pollution (Barking, Essex : 1987). https://www.researchgate.net/publication/5391416_The_intestinal_parasite_Pomphorhynchus_la evis_Acanthocephala_from_barbel_as_a_bioindicator_for_metal_pollution_in_the_Danube_Rive r_near_Budapest_Hungary

[1024] Hassan A., Moharram S., El Helaly H. Role of parasitic helminths in bioremediating some heavy metal accumulation in the tissues of Lethrinus mahsena. Turk. J. Fish. Aquat. Sci. 2018;18:435–443 https://www.trjfas.org/uploads/pdf_1183.pdf

[1025] EL-Hak, H.N.G., Ghobashy, M.A., Mansour, F.A. et al. 2022: Heavy metals and parasitological infection associated with oxidative stress and histopathological alteration in the Clarias gariepinus. Ecotoxicology 31, https://doi.org/10.1007/s10646-022-02569-9

[1026] Teimoori S, Sabour Yaraghi A, Makki MS, Shahbazi F, Nazmara S, Rokni MB, Mesdaghinia A, Salahi Moghaddam A, Hosseini M, Rakhshanpour A, Mowlavi G. Heavy metal bioabsorption capacity of intestinal helminths in urban rats. Iran J Public Health. 2014 Mar;43(3):310-5. https://www.ncbi.nlm.nih.gov/pmc/articles/PMC4419168/

[1027] Mauël, J., Ransijn, A. et al (1989), Lead Inhibits Intracellular Killing of Leishmania Parasites and Extracellular Cytolysis of Target Cells by Macrophages Exposed to Macrophage Activating Facto. J Leukoc Biol, 45: https://doi.org/10.1002/jlb.45.5.401

[1028] TONGO, I; 2018: Tissue and Parasite Accumulation of Heavy Metals in the Giant Rat (Cricetomys gambianus) as Bioindicators of Heavy Metal Pollution; J. Appl. Sci. Environ. Manage. Vol. 22 (10) https://www.ajol.info/index.php/jasem/article/view/180271

[1029] Bożek, Urszula et al 2008 CORRELATION BETWEEN BIOLOGICAL AGENTS AND LEVELS OF HEAVY METALS IN MUNICIPAL SEWAGE SLUDGE;; AAEM; Ann Agric Environ Med 2008, 15, 295–299; https://pubmed.ncbi.nlm.nih.gov/19061266/

[1030] Faith Ngwewa et al 2022: Effects of Heavy Metals on Bacterial Growth, Biochemical Properties and Antimicrobial Susceptibility; Journal of Applied & Environmental Microbiology, 2022, Vol. 10, No. 1, 9-16 http://doi.org/10.12691/jaem-10-1-2

[1031] Omura Y, Beckman SL. Role of mercury (Hg) in resistant infections & effective treatment of Chlamydia trachomatis and Herpes family viral infections[…]. Acupunct Electrother Res. 1995 Aug-Dec;20(3-4): https://pubmed.ncbi.nlm.nih.gov/8686573/

[1032] Eggers, S., et al 2018: Heavy metal exposure and nasal Staphylococcus aureus colonization: analysis of the National Health and Nutrition Examination Survey (NHANES). Environ Health 17, 2 (). https://doi.org/10.1186/s12940-017-0349-7

[1033] Claudia Seiler; et al 2003: Heavy metal driven co-selection of antibiotic resistance in soil and water bodies impacted by agriculture and aquaculture; Front. Microbiol., 14 December 2012; Sec. Antimicrobials, Resistance and Chemotherapy; Volume 3 - 2012 https://doi.org/10.3389/fmicb.2012.00399

[1034] Eggers, Shoshannaha et al 2021: Urinary lead level and colonization by antibiotic resistant bacteria: Evidence from a population-based study. Environ Epid. 5(6):p e175, Dec 2021. | http://doi.org/10.1097/EE9.0000000000000175

[1035] Krueger, W.S., Wade, T.J. Elevated blood lead and cadmium levels associated with chronic infections among non-smokers in a cross-sectional analysis of NHANES data. Environ Health 15, 16 (2016). https://doi.org/10.1186/s12940-016-0113-4

[1036] Victor O. Martinez, et al 2020: Interaction of Toxoplasma gondii infection and elevated blood lead levels on children's neurobehavior, Neuro Toxicology, Volume 78, 2020, Pages 177-185, , https://doi.org/10.1016/j.neuro.2020.03.010.

[1037] Nosheen Aslam, Muhammad Sarfaraz Iqbal, et al 2019: Effects of chelating agents on heavy metals in Hepatitis C Virus (HCV) patients[J]. Mathematical Biosciences and Engineering, 2019, https://www.aimspress.com/fileOther/PDF/MBE/mbe-16-03-054.pdf

Notes

[1038] Zeng HL, Yang Q, Yuan P, Wang X, Cheng L. Associations of essential and toxic metals/metalloids in whole blood with both disease severity and mortality in patients with COVID-19. FASEB J. 2021 Mar https://www.ncbi.nlm.nih.gov/pmc/articles/PMC7995111/

[1039] The Heavy Metal – Fungal Infection Connection; ADVANCED NATUROPATHIC medical center, Dr. Melina Roberts; https://advancednaturopathic.com/the-heavy-metal-fungal-infection-connection/

[1040] Benoit, S.L., Schmalstig, A.A., Glushka, J. et al. 2019: Nickel chelation therapy as an approach to combat multi-drug resistant enteric pathogens. Sci Rep 9, 13851 (2019). https://doi.org/10.1038/s41598-019-50027-0

[1041] Giannakopoulou, Erofili et al 2018: Metal-chelating agents against viruses and parasites; Future Medicinal Chemistry; Future Medicinal Chemistry Vol. 10, NO. 11; 3 May 2018 https://doi.org/10.4155/fmc-2018-0100

[1042] European Patent Office; patent EP1879576A1; Publication of application with search report; Inventor Russell Taylor; https://patents.google.com/patent/EP1879576A1/en#patentCitations

[1043] Débora C Coraça-Huber, et l Iron chelation destabilizes bacterial biofilms and potentiates the antimicrobial activity of antibiotics against coagulase-negative Staphylococci, Pathogens and Disease, Volume 76, Issue 5, July 2018, fty052, https://doi.org/10.1093/femspd/fty052

[1044] Gordeuk VR, et al 1992: Iron chelation with desferrioxamine B in adults with asymptomatic Plasmodium falciparum parasitemia. Blood. 1992 Jan 15;79(2):308-12. https://pubmed.ncbi.nlm.nih.gov/1730079/

[1045] everywomanover29.com Parasites, heavy metals and Lyme disease on the Parasite Summit; September 10, 2017 By Trudy Scott; https://www.everywomanover29.com/blog/parasites-heavy-metals-lyme-disease-parasite-summit/

[1046] isolated spirochetes from the blood of 2 of 36 patients in Long Island and Westchester County, New York, who had signs and symptoms suggestive of Lyme disease; https://pubmed.ncbi.nlm.nih.gov/6828119/

[1047] Lyme Bacteria Hides Inside Parasitic Worms, Causing Chronic Brain Diseases Recent discovery confirmed by state-of-the-art Molecular Beacon DNA probes. Patient Centered Care Advocacy Group; 19 May, 2016, https://www.prnewswire.com/news-releases/lyme-bacteria-hides-inside-parasitic-worms-causing-chronic-brain-diseases-300270742.html

[1048] Akinsanya B, Ayanda IO et al 2020: Heavy metals, parasitologic and oxidative stress biomarker investigations in Heterotis niloticus from Lekki Lagoon, Lagos, Nigeria. Toxi. Rep. 2020 Aug 16; https://www.ncbi.nlm.nih.gov/pmc/articles/PMC7476227/

[1049] Arthur, S. (2007). The effectiveness of Samento, Cumanda, Burbur, and Dr. Lee Cowden's protocol in the treatment of chronic Lyme disease. Townsend Letter: The Examiner of Alternative Medicine, (285), https://link.gale.com/apps/doc/A162234800/AONE?u=anon~4f6cd7d5&sid=googleScholar&xid=b92f118c

[1050] huffpost.com : The Truth About Treating Lyme DiseaseBy Maria Rodale, Contributor; CEO and Chairman of Rodale, Inc. and book author Jul 10, 2014, https://www.huffpost.com/entry/the-truth-about-treating_b_5575564

[1051] flexhealth. Eu; Spirochete Borrelia and Lyme Disease; 28 september 2022; https://flexhealth.eu/en/2022/09/28/768/

[1052] Horowitz, Richard I., and Phyllis R. Freeman. 2018. "Precision Medicine: The Role of the MSIDS Model in Defining, Diagnosing, and Treating Chronic Lyme Disease/Post Treatment Lyme Disease Syndrome and Other Chronic Illness: Part 2" Healthcare 6, no. 4: 129. https://doi.org/10.3390/healthcare6040129

[1053] Aguirre JD, Clark HM, et al: A manganese-rich environment supports superoxide dismutase activity in a Lyme disease pathogen, Borrelia burgdorferi. J Biol Chem. 2013 https://www.jbc.org/article/S0021-9258(19)33493-3/fulltext

[1054] rtoddmaderis.com Dr. Todd Maderis; Associated Conditions Heavy Metal Toxicity PUBLISHED ON OCTOBER 11, 2019 UPDATED ON JANUARY 30, 2023; https://drtoddmaderis.com/heavy-metal-toxicity

[1055] Lyme Mexico; ALL ABOUT CHELATION THERAPY FOR LYME DISEASE; by Lyme Mexico | Sep 22, 2021; https://lymemexico.com/chelation-therapy-lyme-disease/

[1056] THE IMPACT OF HEAVY METALS IN LYME DISEASE; SeAY wellness; https://www.seaywellness.com/the-impact-of-heavy-metals-in-lyme-disease/

[1057] Restorative Health Clinic Portland; Lyme Disease and the Heavy Metal Threat https://restorativehealthclinic.com/lyme-disease-and-the-heavy-metal-threat/

[1058] Li, X., Wang, P., Lutton, A., Olesik, J. (2018). Trace Element Analysis of Borrelia burgdorferi by Inductively Coupled Plasma-Sector Field Mass Spectrometry. In: Pal, U., Buyuktanir, O. (eds) Borrelia burgdorferi. Methods in Molecular Biology, vol 1690. Humana Press, New York, NY. https://doi.org/10.1007/978-1-4939-7383-5_7

[1059] Aguirre, J.Dafhne, et al 2013; A Manganese-rich Environment Supports Superoxide Dismutase Activity in a Lyme Disease Pathogen, Borrelia burgdorferi*, Journal of Biological Chemistry, Volume 288, Issue 12, 2013, https://doi.org/10.1074/jbc.M112.433540.

[1060] Platinumenergysystems: Lyme disease linked to toxicity and mercury; https://platinumenergysystems.ca/blog/post/lyme-disease-linked-to-toxicity-and-mercury

[1061] THE IMPACT OF HEAVY METALS IN LYME DISEASE; SeAY wellness; https://www.seaywellness.com/the-impact-of-heavy-metals-in-lyme-disease/

[1062] Liying Guo, Liping Di, Chen Zhang, Li Lin, Yahui Di, 2022: Influence of urban expansion on Lyme disease risk: A case study in the U.S. I-95 Northeastern corridor, Cities, Volume 125, 2022, https://doi.org/10.1016/j.cities.2022.103633.

[1063] CDC: Lyme disease: https://www.cdc.gov/lyme/transmission/index.html

[1064] CDC: Lyme disease: https://www.cdc.gov/lyme/transmission/index.html#:~:text=If%20you%20remove%20a%20tick,from%20spring%20through%20the%20fall.

[1065] Meves Vet.com: Can humans be affected by the transfer of ticks from domestic animals? Advice; July 19, 2018; https://themewesvets.co.uk/blog/post-215-can-humans-be-affected-by-the-transfer-of-ticks-from-domestic-animals/

[1066] openaccessgovernment.org: Lyme disease diagnoses increased 357% in rural areas August 3, 2022; https://www.openaccessgovernment.org/lyme-disease-diagnoses-increased-357-in-rural-areas/140908/

[1067] US news: Ticks and Lyme Disease Are a Threat for Cities, Too.. By Katelyn Newman, May 15, 2019, https://www.usnews.com/news/healthiest-communities/articles/2019-05-15/lyme-disease-ticks-a-threat-for-cities-study-suggests

[1068] THOMPSON, R.H.S. and KING, E.J. 1964: Biochemical Disorders in Human Disease, 2nd Edition, Published by Academic Press, New York, 1964. https://www.science.org/doi/10.1126/science.147.3660.853.a

[1069] hoffmancentre: Kryptopyrroluria (aka Hemopyrrollactamuria) 2017: A Major Piece of the Puzzle in Overcoming Chronic Lyme Disease; August 2, 2017 by Dietrich Klinghardt; https://hoffmancentre.com/chronic-lyme-disease/

[1070] Carvalho F, Louro F, Zakout R. Adrenal Insufficiency in Metastatic Lung Cancer. World J Oncol. 2015 Jun;6(3):375-377. https://www.ncbi.nlm.nih.gov/pmc/articles/PMC5624663/

[1071] Chabre, Olivier; et al 2017: Group 1. Epidemiology of primary and secondary adrenal insufficiency: Prevalence and incidence, acute adrenal insufficiency, long-term morbidity and mortality, Annales d'Endocrinologie, Volume 78, Issue 6, 2017, Pages 490-494, (https://www.sciencedirect.com/science/article/pii/S0003426617309198)

[1072] Pamphlett R, Kum Jew S, Doble PA, Bishop DP. Mercury in the human adrenal medulla could contribute to increased plasma noradrenaline in aging. Sci Rep. 2021 Feb 3;11(1):2961. https://www.ncbi.nlm.nih.gov/pmc/articles/PMC7858609/

[1073] absolute-health Regenerative clinic; Medical articles; Dr. Chatchai Sribundit https://absolute-health.org/en/blog/post/article-healthtips-4.html

[1074] Mills KC. 1997: Serotonin syndrome; Med Toxicol. 1997;13:763-783. https://pubmed.ncbi.nlm.nih.gov/9330840/

[1075] Nguyen HD. 2023: Interactions between heavy metals and sleep duration among pre-and postmenopausal women: A current approach to molecular mechanisms involved. Environ Pollut. 2023 Jan 1;316(Pt 1) https://pubmed.ncbi.nlm.nih.gov/36347409/

[1076] Kobal AB, Grum DK. 2010: Scopoli's work in the field of mercurialism in light of today's knowledge: past and present perspectives. Am J Ind Med. 2010 May;53(5):535-47. https://pubmed.ncbi.nlm.nih.gov/20112258/

[1077] Spiegel K, Leproult R, Van Cauter E. Impact of sleep debt on metabolic and endocrine function. Lancet. 1999 Oct 23;354(9188):1435-9. http://doi.org/10.1016/S0140-6736(99)01376-8.

[1078] Bhargava P, Gupta N, Vats S and Goel R. 2017: Health Issues and Heavy Metals. Austin J Environ Toxicol. 2017; 3(1): 1018. https://www.researchgate.net/publication/325260555_Health_Issues_and_Heavy_Metals

[1079] Scientific American; Early Lead Exposure Linked to Sleep Problems Long-term study of children ties exposure to sleep disorders later in life; By Rebecca Trager, Chemistry World on November 23, 2015 https://www.scientificamerican.com/article/early-lead-exposure-linked-to-sleep-problems/

[1080] Somsiri Decharat;2018: Urinary Mercury Levels Among Workers in E-waste Shops in Nakhon Si Thammarat Province, Thailand; J Prev Med Public Health 2018; 51(4): 196-204. Published online: June 19, 2018 DOI: https://doi.org/10.3961/jpmph.18.049;

[1081] NIH: Manganese; Fact Sheet for Consumers; March 22, 2021https://ods.od.nih.gov/factsheets/Manganese-Consumer/

Notes

[1082] Videnovic A, Lazar AS, Barker RA, Overeem S. 'The clocks that time us'--circadian rhythms in neurodegenerative disorders. Nat Rev Neurol. 2014 Dec;10(12):683-93. https://www.ncbi.nlm.nih.gov/pmc/articles/PMC4344830/

[1083] Parmalee NL, Aschner M. 2017: Metals and Circadian Rhythms. Adv Neurotoxicol. 2017;1:119-130. https://www.ncbi.nlm.nih.gov/pmc/articles/PMC6361389/

[1084] SUELI REGINA G. ROSSINI et al 2000: Chronic insomnia in workers poisoned by inorganic mercury: psychological and adaptive aspects; Arq. Neuro-Psiquiatr. 58 (1) • Mar 2000, https://doi.org/10.1590/S0004-282X2000000100005

[1085] Rossini SR, Reimão R, Lefèvre BH, Medrado-Faria MA. Chronic insomnia in workers poisoned by inorganic mercury: psychological and adaptive aspects. Arq Neuropsiquiatr. 2000 Mar;58(1):32-8. https://pubmed.ncbi.nlm.nih.gov/10770863/

[1086] Lilis, R, Valciukas, J A, Malkin, J, and Weber, J P. Effects of low-level lead and arsenic exposure on copper smelter workers. U. S. N. p. https://www.osti.gov/biblio/5299978

[1087] Shiue I. Urinary arsenic, pesticides, heavy metals, phthalates, polyaromatic hydrocarbons, and polyfluoroalkyl compounds are associated with sleep troubles in adults: USA NHANES, 2005-2006. Environ Sci Pollut Res Int. 2017 Jan;24(3): https://www.ncbi.nlm.nih.gov/pmc/articles/PMC5340848/

[1088] Shiue I. Low vitamin D levels in adults with longer time to fall asleep: US NHANES, 2005-2006. Int J Cardiol. 2013 Oct 12;168(5) https://pubmed.ncbi.nlm.nih.gov/23938219/

[1089] Song CH, Kim YH, Jung KI. Associations of zinc and copper levels in serum and hair with sleep duration in adult women. Biol Trace Elem Res. 2012 Oct;149(1):16-21. https://pubmed.ncbi.nlm.nih.gov/22476977/

[1090] Zhang HQ, Li N, Zhang Z, Gao S, Yin HY, Guo DM, Gao X. Serum zinc, copper, and zinc/copper in healthy residents of Jinan. Biol Trace Elem Res. 2009 Oct;131(1):25-32. https://pubmed.ncbi.nlm.nih.gov/19340402/

[1091] Environmental Factors in Neurodegenerative Diseases; Metals and Circadian aryphms; Academic Press, 19 Sept 2017; https://www.elsevier.com/books/environmental-factors-in-neurodegenerative-diseases/aschner/978-0-12-812764-3

[1092] Braun JM, Wright RJ,et al. 2014: Relationships between lead biomarkers and diurnal salivary cortisol indices in pregnant women from Mexico City: a cross-sectional study. Environ Health. 2014 Jun 10;13(1):50 https://pubmed.ncbi.nlm.nih.gov/24916609/

[1093] Kosta L, Byrne AR, Zelenko V. Correlation between selenium and mercury in man following exposure to inorganic mercury. Nature. 1975 Mar 20;254(5497):238-9. https://pubmed.ncbi.nlm.nih.gov/1113885/

[1094] Shah, N., Malhotra, A., & Kaltsakas, G. (2020). Sleep disorder in patients with chronic liver disease: a narrative review. Journal Of Thoracic Disease, 12(Suppl 2), S248-S260. https://www.ncbi.nlm.nih.gov/pmc/articles/PMC7642630/

[1095] Endocrine society: People with poor sleep behaviors may be at risk for fatty liver disease; Washington, DC July 28, 2022 https://www.endocrine.org/news-and-advocacy/news-room/2022/people-with-poor-sleep-behaviors-may-be-at-risk-for-fatty-liver-disease

[1096] Wijarnpreecha K, et al 2017: Insomnia and risk of nonalcoholic fatty liver disease: A systematic review and meta-analysis. J Postgrad Med. 2017 Oct-Dec;63(4):226-231.. https://www.ncbi.nlm.nih.gov/pmc/articles/PMC5664866/

[1097] TIMESOFINDIA.COM: Non-alcoholic fatty liver disease: Waking up between 1 am and 4 am could signal liver risk; | Last updated on -Dec 14, 2022; https://timesofindia.indiatimes.com/life-style/health-fitness/health-news/non-alcoholic-fatty-liver-disease-waking-up-between-1-am-and-4-am-could-signal-liver-risk/photostory/96082976.cms

[1098] healthyhabitsliving : Chlorella: All You Need to Know About the Mighty Algae by Carly Neubert, BA, NC on January 16, 2019 https://www.healthyhabitsliving.com/blogs/be-healthy/chlorella-all-you-need-to-know-about-the-mighty-algae

[1099] Benzodiazepine Withdrawal and Heavy Metal Toxicity; Benzodiazepine September 6, 2022 by Carol Gillette; Alternative to Meds Editorial Team; Medically Reviewed by Dr. Samuel Lee MD: https://www.alternativetomeds.com/blog/benzodiazepine-withdrawal-and-heavy-metal-toxicity/

[1100] N. Hu, C. Wang, Y. Liao, Q. Dai, S. Cao, 2021: Smoking and incidence of insomnia: a systematic review and meta-analysis of cohort studies, Public Health, Volume 198, 2021, https://doi.org/10.1016/j.puhe.2021.07.012.

[1101] Kern, Janet & Geier, David & Bjorklund, Geir & King, Paul & Homme, Kristin & Haley, Boyd & Sykes, Lisa & Geier, Mark. (2014). Evidence supporting a link between dental amalgams and chronic illness, fatigue, depression, anxiety, and suicide. Neuro endocrinology letters. 35. https://www.researchgate.net/publication/271536688_Evidence_supporting_a_link_between_dental_amalgams_and_chronic_illness_fatigue_depression_anxiety_and_suicide

[1102] Regland B, Zachrisson O, Stejskal V, Gottfries C (2001). Nickel allergy is found in a majority of women with chronic fatigue syndrome and muscle pain. Journal of Chronic Fatigue Syndrome 8: https://www.melisa.org/pdf/cfs_nickel.pdf

[1103] Sunderman FW Jr. Nasal toxicity, carcinogenicity, and olfactory uptake of metals. Ann Clin Lab Sci. 2001 Jan;31(1):3-24. https://pubmed.ncbi.nlm.nih.gov/11314863/

[1104] Chelation Medical Center; Ray Psonak, D.O. Toxic Heavy Metals; https://www.chelationmedicalcenter.com/toxic-heavy-metals.html

[1105] Block E, Batista VS, Matsunami H, Zhuang H, Ahmed L. The role of metals in mammalian olfaction of low molecular weight organosulfur compounds. Nat Prod Rep. 2017 May 10;34(5):529-557. https://www.ncbi.nlm.nih.gov/pmc/articles/PMC5542778/

[1106] Zheng Y, Shen Y, Zhu Z, Hu H. Associations between Cadmium Exposure and Taste and Smell Dysfunction: Results from the National Health and Nutrition Examination Survey (NHANES), 2011-2014. Int J Environ Res Public Health. 2020 Feb 3;17 https://www.ncbi.nlm.nih.gov/pmc/articles/PMC7037909/

[1107] Sunderman FW Jr. Nasal toxicity, carcinogenicity, and olfactory uptake of metals. Ann Clin Lab Sci. 2001 Jan;31(1):3-24. https://pubmed.ncbi.nlm.nih.gov/11314863/

[1108] Jothimani, Dinesh; Kailasam, Ezhilarasan; 2020: COVID-19: Poor outcomes in patients with zinc deficiency,; International Journal of Infectious Diseases,; Volume 100,; 2020,; Pages 343-349,; https://doi.org/10.1016/j.ijid.2020.09.014.

[1109] Al-Awfi JS (2020) Zinc may have a potential role in taste malfunctions treatment for COVID-19 patients. Integr Food Nutr Metab 7: https://www.researchgate.net/publication/350467107_Zinc_may_have_a_potential_role_in_taste_malfunctions_treatment_for_COVID-19_patients

[1110] Liu, C., Mao, W., You, Z. et al. 2022: Associations between exposure to different heavy metals and self-reported erectile dysfunction: a population-based study using data from the 2001-2004 National Health and Nutrition Examination Survey. Environ Sci Pollut Res 29, https://doi.org/10.1007/s11356-022-20910-x

[1111] Wang W, Xiang LY et al 2023: The association between heavy metal exposure and erectile dysfunction in the United States. Asian J Androl. 2023 Mar-Apr;25(2):271-276. https://pubmed.ncbi.nlm.nih.gov/35708358/

[1112] Liu, Rui-Ji et al 2022: Dietary metal intake and the prevalence of erectile dysfunction in US men: Results from National Health and Nutrition Examination Survey 2001–2004; Front. Nutr., 03 November 2022; Sec. Nutritional Epidemiology Volume 9 - 2022 https://doi.org/10.3389/fnut.2022.974443

[1113] Sun C, Ren Y, Zhang W. Association between skin disease and anxiety: a logistic analysis and prediction. Ann Transl Med 2023. http://doi.org/10.21037/atm-22-6511

[1114] American Psychological Society: The link between skin and psychology: By Rebecca A. Clay; February 2015, Vol 46, No. 2 https://www.apa.org/monitor/2015/02/cover-skin

[1115] MSD Manual: Skin Manifestations of Internal Disease; By Julia Benedetti , MD, Harvard Medical School; Reviewed/Revised Jan 2024; https://www.msdmanuals.com/professional/dermatologic-disorders/approach-to-the-dermatologic-patient/skin-manifestations-of-internal-disease

[1116] Hu Z and Wang T (2023) Beyond skin white spots: Vitiligo and associated comorbidities. Front. Med. 10:1072837. http://doi.org/10.3389/fmed.2023.1072837

[1117] Silverwood RJ, Mansfield KE, Mulick A, et al. Atopic eczema in adulthood and mortality: UK population–based cohort study, 1998-2016. J Allergy Clin Immunol. 2021;147(5) https://jamanetwork.com/journals/jamanetworkopen/fullarticle/2785534

[1118] Oaten M, Stevenson RJ, Case TI. Disease avoidance as a functional basis for stigmatization. Philos Trans R Soc Lond B Biol Sci. 2011 Dec 12;366(1583):3433-52. http://doi.org/10.1098/rstb.2011.0095.

[1119] Stephen Ryan, Megan Oaten et al 2012: Facial disfigurement is treated like an infectious disease, Evolution and Human Behavior, Volume 33, Issue 6, 2012, https://doi.org/10.1016/j.evolhumbehav.2012.04.001.

[1120] Houston, V. and Bull, R. (1994), Do people avoid sitting next to someone who is facially disfigured?. Eur. J. Soc. Psychol., 24: https://doi.org/10.1002/ejsp.2420240205

[1121] Skin Disease and Stigmatization Associated With Decreased Quality of Life dermatologytimes.com October 23, 2023; Rosanna Sutherby, PharmD; https://www.dermatologytimes.com/view/skin-disease-and-stigmatization-associated-with-decreased-quality-of-life

[1122] Borsky, P. et al. Aging in psoriasis vulgaris: female patients are epigenetically older than healthy controls. Immun Ageing 18, 10 (2021). https://doi.org/10.1186/s12979-021-00220-5

Notes

[1123] Rerknimitr P, Kantikosum K, 2019: Chronic occupational exposure to lead leads to significant mucocutaneous changes in lead factory workers. J Eur Acad Dermatol Venereol. 2019 Oct;33(10):1993-2000. https://pubmed.ncbi.nlm.nih.gov/599390/

[1124] Matthews NH, Fitch K, et al. Exposure to Trace Elements and Risk of Skin Cancer: A Systematic Review of Epidemiologic Studies. Cancer Epidemiol Biomarkers Prev. 2019 https://www.ncbi.nlm.nih.gov/pmc/articles/PMC6324965/

[1125] NORD Rare Disease Database; Heavy Metal Poisoning; Last updated: March 28, 2008; https://rarediseases.org/rare-diseases/heavy-metal-poisoning/

[1126] Robert Zaldívar, 1974: Arsenic Contamination of Drinking Water and Foodstuffs Causing Endemic Chronic Poisoning, Beiträge zur Pathologie, Volume 151, Issue 4, 1974, (https://www.sciencedirect.com/science/article/pii/S0005816574800478)

[1127] Rauf AU, Mallongi A, Astuti RDP. Heavy Metal Contributions on Human Skin Disease near Cement Plant: A Systematic Review. Open Access Maced J Med Sci [Internet]. 2020 Jul. 25 [cited 2023 Feb. 22];8(F):117-22. Available from: https://oamjms.eu/index.php/mjms/article/view/4396

[1128] Seulbi Lee, Sung Kyun Park, 2021: Prenatal heavy metal exposures and atopic dermatitis with gender difference in 6-month-old infants using multipollutant analysis, Environmental Research, Volume 195, 2021, (https://www.sciencedirect.com/science/article/pii/S0013935121001596)

[1129] Choi HS, Suh MJ, Hong SC, Kang JW. The Association between the Concentration of Heavy Metals in the Indoor Atmosphere and Atopic Dermatitis Symptoms in Children Aged between 4 and 13 Years: A Pilot Study. Children (Basel). 2021 Nov 3;8(11):1004. https://www.ncbi.nlm.nih.gov/pmc/articles/PMC8625560/

[1130] Tsai T, Wang S, Hsieh C, et al. Association Between Prenatal Exposure to Metals and Atopic Dermatitis Among Children Aged 4 Years in Taiwan. JAMA Netw Open. 2021 https://jamanetwork.com/journals/jamanetworkopen/fullarticle/2785534

[1131] Hon KL, Wang SS, Hung EC, Lam HS, Lui HH, Chow CM, Ching GK, Fok TF, Ng PC, Leung TF. Serum levels of heavy metals in childhood eczema and skin diseases: friends or foes. Pediatr Allergy Immunol. 2010 Aug;21(5) https://pubmed.ncbi.nlm.nih.gov/20337961/

[1132] Giancarlo Pesce et al 2020: Foetal exposure to heavy metals and risk of asthma and allergic diseases in early childhood: a population-based birth-cohort study, EDEN consortium Europ. Respirat J. 2020 http://doi.org/10.1183/13993003.congress-2020.3847

[1133] Granstein RD, Sober AJ. Drug- and heavy metal--induced hyperpigmentation. J Am Acad Dermatol. 1981 Jul;5(1):1-18. https://pubmed.ncbi.nlm.nih.gov/6268671/

[1134] Marta Wacewicz-Muczyńska, et al 2020: Cadmium, lead and mercury in the blood of psoriatic and vitiligo patients and their possible associations with dietary habits; Science of The Total Environment, Volume 757, 2021 https://doi.org/10.1016/j.scitotenv.2020.143967.

[1135] Tsiskarishvili NI,et al. [ELEMENTAL STATUS OF PATIENTS WITH VARIOUS FORMS OF VITILIGO]. Georgian Med News. 2017 Dec;(273): https://pubmed.ncbi.nlm.nih.gov/29328033/

[1136] Mohammed, Mehad & Ahmed, Suhair & Hamid, Suad & Modawe, Gadallah. (2019). - Assessment of Serum Zinc Levels among Sudanese Patients with Vitiligo 12-17; Jouf University Medical Journal (JUMJ), 2019 March 1; 6(1): https://www.researchgate.net/publication/339484365_Modawe_et_al_-_Assessment_of_Serum_Zinc_Levels_among_Sudanese_Patients_with_Vitiligo_Original_Article_Assessment_of_Serum_Zinc_Levels_among_Sudanese_Patients_with_Vitiligo

[1137] Afridi, H.I., Kazi, T.G., Kazi, N. et al. Evaluation of Cadmium, Chromium, Nickel, and Zinc in Biological Samples of Psoriasis Patients Living in Pakistani Cement Factory Area. Biol Trace Elem Res 142, 284–301 (2011). https://doi.org/10.1007/s12011-010-8778-y https://link.springer.com/article/10.1007/s12011-010-8778-y#citeas

[1138] Liaw, FY., Chen, WL., Kao, TW. et al. Exploring the link between cadmium and psoriasis in a nationally representative sample. Sci Rep 7, 1723 (2017). https://doi.org/10.1038/s41598-017-01827-9

[1139] Christophers E. 2007: Comorbidities in psoriasis. Clin Dermatol. 2007 Nov-Dec;25(6):529-34. https://pubmed.ncbi.nlm.nih.gov/18021889/

[1140] Gelfand JM, Yeung H. Metabolic syndrome in patients with psoriatic disease. J Rheumatol Suppl. 2012 Jul; https://pubmed.ncbi.nlm.nih.gov/22751586/

[1141] Ikaraoha CI, Mbadiwe NC, Anyanwu CJ, Odekhian J, Nwadike CN, Amah HC. The Role of Blood Lead, Cadmium, Zinc and Copper in Development and Severity of Acne Vulgaris in a Nigerian Population. Biol Trace Elem Res. 2017 Apr;176(2):251-257. https://pubmed.ncbi.nlm.nih.gov/27600928/

[1142] NYT: Dangerous When Wet; By Charlotte Druckman; Feb. 5, 2006; https://www.nytimes.com/2006/02/05/magazine/dangerous-when-wet.html

[1143] Dermatology Advisor; Heavy Metal Dermatoses: Mercury (Mercury dermatosis: Hydrargyria, mercurialism, acrodynia, "pink disease," Mad Hatter's disease, Hatter's disease, Minamata disease) Ellis Hon Kam Lun | March 13, 2019; https://www.dermatologyadvisor.com/home/decision-support-in-medicine/dermatology/heavy-metal-dermatoses-mercurymercury-dermatosis-hydrargyria-mercurialism-acrodynia-pink-disease-mad-hatters-disease-hatters-disease-minamata-disease/

[1144] Elena, N., Pilnik., V., L., Reinyuk.,et al (2023). The role of anthropogenic dermatotoxicants in the formation of acne in adolescents. Ėkologiâ čeloveka, http://doi.org/10.17816/humeco112524

[1145] Riedel F,et al 2021: Immunological Mechanisms of Metal Allergies and the Nickel-Specific TCR-pMHC Interface. Int J Environ Res Public Health. 2021 Oct 15; http://doi.org/10.3390/ijerph182010867.

[1146] Fowler JF. Allergic Contact Dermatitis to Gold. Arch Dermatol. 1988;124(2):181–182. http://doi.org/10.1001/archderm.1988.01670020013006

[1147] Pigatto PD, Ferrucci SM, Brambilla L, Guzzi G. Alopecia Areata and Toxic Metals. Skin Appendage Disord. 2020 Jun;6(3):177-179. https://www.ncbi.nlm.nih.gov/pmc/articles/PMC7325209/#:~:text=Toxic%20metals%20are%20not%20so,Vicky%20Yu%20and%20colleagues%27%20found.

[1148] Campbell C, et al 2016: Anagen Effluvium Caused by Thallium Poisoning. JAMA Dermatol. https://jamanetwork.com/journals/jamadermatology/fullarticle/2500034

[1149] Toxicology and Iatrogenic ; Disorders; Professional Articles Dr Hayley Willacy Thallium Poisoning; Symptoms, Treatment, Prognosis; 27 Oct 2021 https://patient.info/doctor/thallium-poisoning#:~:text=Thallium%20poisoning%20prognosis,-Of%20those%20who&text=Reports%20of%20persistent%20findings%20most,to%20dementia%2C%20depression%20and%20psychosis.

[1150] Paolo Daniele Pigatto, Silvia Mariel Ferrucci, Lucia Brambilla, Gianpaolo Guzzi; Alopecia Areata and Toxic Metals. Skin Appendage Disord 15 June 2020; 6 (3): 177–179. https://doi.org/10.1159/000507296

[1151] Ozaydin-Yavuz G, Yavuz IH, Demir H, Demir C, Bilgili SG. Alopecia areata different view; Heavy metals. Indian J Dermatol [serial online] 2019 [cited 2023 Apr 21];64:7-11. https://www.e-ijd.org/text.asp?2019/64/1/7/249529

[1152] Yu V, Juhász M,et al: Alopecia and Associated Toxic Agents: A Systematic Review. Skin Appendage Disord 2018; https://www.karger.com/Article/Fulltext/485749#

[1153] TMC: Could Baldness Predict Other Health Risks? By Christine Hall June 6, 2018; https://www.tmc.edu/news/2018/06/could-baldness-predict-other-health-risks/

[1154] Shoenfeld Y, Agmon-Levin N. 'ASIA' - autoimmune/inflammatory syndrome induced by adjuvants. J Autoimmun. 2011 https://pubmed.ncbi.nlm.nih.gov/20708902/

[1155] Koh HY, Kim TH, et al 2019: Serum heavy metal levels are associated with asthma, allergic rhinitis, atopic dermatitis, allergic multimorbidity, and airflow obstruction. J Allergy Clin Immunol Pract. 2019 Nov-Dec;7 https://www.atopona.cz/wp-content/uploads/2020/06/ATO-097-Serum-heavymetal-levels-are-associated-with-asthma-allergic-rhinitis-atopic-dermatitis-allergic-multimorbidity-and-airflow-obstruction.pdf

[1156] Stejska,l Vera 2015: Allergy and Autoimmunity Caused by Metals: A Unifying Concept Vaccines and Autoimmunity, First Edition. Edited by Yehuda Shoenfeld, Nancy Agmon-Levin, and Lucija Tomljenovic. 2015 https://www.melisa.org/wp-content/uploads/2015/11/Allergy-and-autoimmunity-caused-by-metals-2.pdf

[1157] technologynetworks.com Allergic Response May Be Caused by Heavy Metal Food Pollutant;News; 2021; https://www.technologynetworks.com/applied-sciences/news/allergic-response-may-be-caused-by-heavy-metal-food-pollutant-355154

[1158] Gasana J, Dillikar D,et al . Motor vehicle air pollution and asthma in children: a meta-analysis. Environ Res. 2012 https://pubmed.ncbi.nlm.nih.gov/22683007/

[1159] University of Illinois at Chicago. (2017, February 13). Gluten-free diet may increase risk of arsenic, mercury exposure. ScienceDaily. Retrieved August 4, 2023 from www.sciencedaily.com/releases/2017/02/170213131150.htm

[1160] Hideki Kinoshita, et al 2013: Biosorption of heavy metals by lactic acid bacteria and identification of mercury binding protein, Research in Microbiology, Volume 164, Issue 7, https://doi.org/10.1016/j.resmic.2013.04.004.

[1161] Masoumi SJ, Mehrabani D, et al 2021: The effect of yogurt fortified with Lactobacillus acidophilus and Bifidobacterium sp. probiotic in patients with lactose intolerance. Food Sci Nutr. 2021 http://doi.org//10.1002/fsn3.2145.

[1162] AL- Khalifa, Ihab I. 2016: Determination of Some Essential & Non-Essential Metals in Patients with Fibromyalgia Syndrome (FMS); International Journal of Toxicological and Pharmacol. Res. 2016 http://impactfactor.org/PDF/IJTPR/8/IJTPR,Vol8,Issue5,Article1.pdf

Notes

[1163] Stejskal V, et al 2013: Metal-induced inflammation triggers fibromyalgia in metal-allergic patients. Neuro Endocrinol Lett. 2013; https://pubmed.ncbi.nlm.nih.gov/24378456/

[1164] Myroslava Protsiv Catherine Ley Joanna Lankester Trevor Hastie Julie Parsonnet (2020) Decreasing human body temperature in the United States since the Industrial Revolution eLife 9:e49555. https://elifesciences.org/articles/49555

[1165] Wilson's Temperature Syndrome. Check your body temperature https://www.wilsonssyndrome.com/identify/how-are-body-temperatures-measured/

[1166] Smithonian: Even in the Bolivian Amazon, Average Human Body Temperature Is Getting Cooler;; Alex Fox November 19, 2020; https://www.smithsonianmag.com/smart-news/another-study-finds-average-human-body-temperature-dropping-180976335/

[1167] Cleveland Clinic: Heavy Metal Poisoning (Toxicity); https://my.clevelandclinic.org/health/diseases/23424-heavy-metal-poisoning-toxicity

[1168] Martínez F, Vicente I, García F, Peñafiel R, Cremades A. Effects of different factors in lead- and cadmium-induced hypothermia in mice. Eur J Pharmacol. 1993 Aug 2;248(2):199-204. https://pubmed.ncbi.nlm.nih.gov/8223966/

[1169] Christopher J. Gordon , Lela Fogelson & Jerry W. Highfill (1990) Hypothermia and hypometabolism: Sensitive indices of whole-body toxicity following exposure to metallic salts in the mouse, Journal of Toxicology and Environmental Health, 29:2, 185-200, http://doi.org/10.1080/15287399009531382

[1170] Gordon CJ, Stead AG. Effect of nickel and cadmium chloride on autonomic and behavioral thermoregulation in mice. Neurotoxicology. 1986 https://pubmed.ncbi.nlm.nih.gov/3822265/

[1171] Francisco Martínez, et al 1999: Effects of central administration of lead, cadmium and other divalent cations on body temperature in mice, Journal of Thermal Biology, Volume 24, 5–6, 1999, https://doi.org/10.1016/S0306-4565(99)00070-4.

[1172] Vennam S, Georgoulas S,et al Heavy metal toxicity and the aetiology of glaucoma. Eye (Lond). 2020 Jan;34 https://pubmed.ncbi.nlm.nih.gov/31745328/

[1173] Erie, Jay C. 2004: Heavy Metal Concentrations in Human Eyes; American Journal of Ophthalmolog; VOLUME 139, , MAY 01, 2005 https://doi.org/10.1016/j.ajo.2004.12.007;

[1174] Jung SJ, Lee SH. Association between Three Heavy Metals and Dry Eye Disease in Korean Adults: Results of the Korean National Health and Nutrition Examination Survey. Korean J Ophthalmol. 2019 Feb https://www.ncbi.nlm.nih.gov/pmc/articles/PMC6372379/

[1175] Apostoli P, Catalani S, Zaghini A, Mariotti A, Poliani PL, Vielmi V, et al. High doses of cobalt induce optic and auditory neuropathy. Exp Toxicol Pathol. 2013;65:719–27. https://pubmed.ncbi.nlm.nih.gov/23069009/

[1176] Lansdown AB. Metal ions affecting the skin and eyes. Met Ions Life Sci. 2011;8:187-246. https://pubmed.ncbi.nlm.nih.gov/21473382/

[1177] Pastor-Idoate, S., Coco-Martin, R.M., Zabalza, I. et al. Long-term visual pathway alterations after elemental mercury poisoning: report of a series of 29 cases. J Occup Med Toxicol 16, 49 (2021). https://doi.org/10.1186/s12995-021-00341-z

[1178] Khansa, Ibrahim MD*,†; Silver in Wound Care—Friend or Foe?: A Comprehensive Review: Plastic and Reconstructive Surgery - Global Open 7(8):p e2390, August 2019. http://doi.org/10.1097/GOX.0000000000002390

[1179] Wang W, Schaumberg DA, Park SK. Cadmium and lead exposure and risk of cataract surgery in U.S. adults. Int J Hyg Environ Health. 2016 Nov;219(8):850-856. https://www.ncbi.nlm.nih.gov/pmc/articles/PMC5086441/

[1180] Katarzyna Rektor 2020: The influence of heavy metals on cataracts; World News of Natural Science; WNOFNS 33 (2020) 26-37 EISSN 2543-5426; https://www.semanticscholar.org/paper/The-influence-of-heavy-metals-on-cataracts-Rektor-Kamiński/7494e1e602399df552d02cb60edae9edf4da48fe

[1181] S.SABELAISHa et al Ocular manifestations of mercury poisoning https://apps.who.int/iris/bitstream/handle/10665/260865/PMC2366408.pdf?sequence=1&isAllowed=y

[1182] Pamphlett R, Cherepanoff S, (2020) The distribution of toxic metals in the human retina and optic nerve head: Implications for age-related macular degeneration. PLoS ONE 15 https://journals.plos.org/plosone/article?id=10.1371/journal.pone.0241054

[1183] Castellanos MJ, et al : The Adverse Effects of Heavy Metals with and without Noise Exposure on the Human Peripheral and Central Auditory System: A Literature Review. Int J Environ Res Public Health. 2016 https://www.ncbi.nlm.nih.gov/pmc/articles/PMC5201364/

[1184] Shargorodsky J, Curhan SG, Henderson E, Eavey R, Curhan GC. 2011 Heavy Metals Exposure and Hearing Loss in US Adolescents. Arch Otolaryngol Head Neck Surg. 2011;137(12) https://jamanetwork.com/journals/jamaotolaryngology/fullarticle/1106935

[1185] Gabrielli, Paolo et al 2020: Early atmospheric contamination on the top of the Himalayas since the onset of the European Industrial Revolution; PNAS; February 10, 2020; 117 (8) 3967-3973; https://doi.org/10.1073/pnas.1910485117

[1186] Considine R, Tynan R, James C, Wiggers J, Lewin T, Inder K, et al. (2017) The Contribution of Individual, Social and Work Characteristics to Employee Mental Health in a Coal Mining Industry Population. PLoS 12(https://doi.org/10.1371/journal.pone.0168445

[1187] Ana He, Xiaoping Li, Yuwei Ai, Xiaolong Li, Xiaoyun Li, Yuchao Zhang, Yu Gao, Bin Liu, Xu Zhang et al 2020: Potentially toxic metals and the risk to children's health in a coal mining city: An investigation of soil and dust levels, bioaccessibility and blood lead levels, Environ. International, Volume 141, 2020, https://doi.org/10.1016/j.envint.2020.105788.

[1188] Sierra club Toxic Waste and Mining; https://coal.sierraclub.org/the-problem/toxic-waste-and-mining

[1189] Yale.edu: A Troubling Look at the Human Toll of Mountaintop Removal Mining BY RICHARD SCHIFFMAN • NOVEMBER 21, 2017 https://e360.yale.edu/features/a-troubling-look-at-the-human-toll-of-mountaintop-removal-mining

[1190] EPA: Basic Information about Mercury; https://www.epa.gov/mercury/basic-information-about-mercury

[1191] Johan C. Varekamp, Peter R. Buseck, Global mercury flux from volcanic and geothermal sources, Applied Geochemistry, Volume 1, Issue 1, 1986, Pages 65-73, (https://www.sciencedirect.com/science/article/pii/0883292786900387)

[1192] Patrick, Lyn. 2002: "Mercury toxicity and antioxidants: part I: role of glutathione and alpha-lipoic acid in the treatment of mercury toxicity. (Mercury Toxicity)." Alternative Medicine Review, vol. 7, no. 6, Dec. 2002, https://go.gale.com/ps/i.do?p=AONE&u=anon~a695ad01&id=GALE%7CA96416600&v=2.1&it=r&sid=googleScholar&asid=3e698cf0

[1193] Ohle, A. et al 2021: Emission of Mercury and Particulate Matter from Crematory: A Review. https://doi.org/10.1002/cite.202000122

[1194] Rosangela M et al 2010: blood and in calcified tissues from lead-exposed rats, Toxic., V. 271,1–2, 2010, https://www.sciencedirect.com/science/article/pii/S0300483X10000351

[1195] wecologist.com: Drinking Water: Fluoride increases Harm from Lead and Neurotoxins. 2016; https://wecologist.com/2016/02/18/drinking-water-fluoride-increases-harm-from-lead-and-neurotoxins/

[1196] Jarup, Lars 2013: Hazards of heavy metal contamination; British Medical Bulletin, Volume 68, Issue 1, December 2003, Pages 167–182, https://doi.org/10.1093/bmb/ldg032

[1197] Rai, P.K.; Lee, S.S.; Zhang, M.; Tsang, Y.F.; Kim, K.H. Heavy metals in food crops: Health risks, fate, mechanisms, and management. Environ. Int. 2019, 125, 365–385. https://www.sciencedirect.com/science/article/pii/S0160412018327971

[1198] FDA. Arsenic in Rice: Full Analytical Results from Rice/Rice Product Sampling -September 2012. U.S. Food and Drug Administration; 2012. http://www.fda.gov/Food/FoodborneIllnessContaminants/Metals/ucm319916.htm.

[1199] Gutiérrez-Ravelo A, Gutiérrez ÁJ, Paz S, Carrascosa-Iruzubieta C, González-Weller D, Caballero JM, Revert C, Rubio C, Hardisson A. Toxic Metals (Al, Cd, Pb) and Trace Element (B, Ba, Co, Cu, Cr, Fe, Li, Mn, Mo, Ni, Sr, V, Zn) Levels in Sarpa Salpa from the North-Eastern Atlantic Ocean Region. International Journal of Environmental Research and Public Health. 2020; 17(19):7212. https://doi.org/10.3390/ijerph17197212

[1200] Craftsmanship; Issue: Spring 2022: The Vegetable Detective; by todd oppenheimer https://craftsmanship.net/the-vegetable-detective/

[1201] Cher LaCoste, et al 2010: uptake of thallium by vegetables: its significance for human health, phytoremediation, and phytomining; ournal of plant nutrition, 24(8), 1205±1215 (2001); https://kiwiscience.com/JournalArticles/JPlantNutrition2001.pdf

[1202] A. Tremel, et al 1997: Thallium in French agrosystems—II. Concentration of thallium in field-grown rape and some other plant species, Environmental Pollution, Volume 97, Issues 1–2, 1997, https://doi.org/10.1016/S0269-7491(97)00060-2.

[1203] Chemisches und Veterinäruntersuchungsamt Karlsruhe; https://www.ua-bw.de/pub/beitrag.asp?subid=2&Thema_ID=1&ID=2048&lang=DE&Pdf=No#:~:text=Die%20Gesamtaufnahme%20an%20Thallium%20sollte,aus%20übrigen%20Lebensmitteln%20zugrunde%20gelegt.

[1204] Consumer reports: A Third Of Chocolate Products Are High In Heavy Metals, CR's Tests Find; October 25, 2023; By Kevin Loria https://www.consumerreports.org/health/food-safety/a-third-of-chocolate-products-are-high-in-heavy-metals-a4844566398/

[1205] N. Defarge, 2018: Toxicity of formulants and heavy metals in glyphosate-based herbicides and other pesticides, Toxicology Reports, Volume 5, 2018, Pages 156-163, (https://www.sciencedirect.com/science/article/pii/S221475001730149X)

Notes

[1206] Khaled S. Balkhair, Muhammad Aqeel Ashraf, 2018: Field accumulation risks of heavy metals in soil and vegetable crop irrigated with sewage water in western region of Saudi Arabia, Saudi Journal of Biological Sciences, Volume 23, Issue 1, Supplement, 2016, (https://www.sciencedirect.com/science/article/pii/S1319562X15002181)

[1207] Ebrahimi, Mansour et al (2009). Concentration of four heavy metals (cadmium, lead, mercury, and arsenic) in organs of two cyprinid fish (Cyprinus carpio and Capoeta sp.) from the Kor River (Iran). Environmental monitoring and assessment. https://www.researchgate.net/publication/26771131_Concentration_of_four_heavy_metals_cadmium_lead_mercury_and_arsenic_in_organs_of_two_cyprinid_fish_Cyprinus_carpio_and_Capoeta_sp_from_the_Kor_River_Iran

[1208] Aendo, P.; De Garine-Wichatitsky, et al 2022: Potential Health Effects of Heavy Metals and Carcinogenic Health Risk Estimation of Pb and Cd Contaminated Eggs from a Closed Gold Mine Area in Northern Thailand. Foods 2022, 11, 2791. https://www.mdpi.com/2304-8158/11/18/2791

[1209] Second Report Shows Dangerous Levels of Heavy Metals in More Baby Foods 9, 2021; By Baum Hedlund Aristei & Goldman PC; https://www.baumhedlundlaw.com/blog/2021/september/second-report-shows-dangerous-levels-of-heavy-me/

[1210] Healthy Baby Bright Future: Report: What's in my Baby's Food? BabyFoodReport_ENGLISH_R6.pdf https://hbbf.org/report/whats-in-my-babys-food

[1211] Washington post: New report finds toxic heavy metals in popular baby foods. FDA failed to warn consumers of risk; By Laura Reiley; February 4, 2021; https://www.washingtonpost.com/business/2021/02/04/toxic-metals-baby-food/

[1212] consumerreports.org: Heavy Metals in Baby Food: What You Need to Know; By Jesse Hirsch; Published August 16, 2018; https://www.consumerreports.org/food-safety/heavy-metals-in-baby-food-a6772370847/

[1213] Latini, G. et al 2005: Multiple chemical sensitivity as a result of exposure to heterogeneous air pollutants Environmental; Exposure and Health 65; WIT Transactions on Ecology and the Environment, Vol 85, 2005 https://www.witpress.com/Secure/elibrary/papers/EEH05/EEH05007FU.pdf

[1214] Falahi-Ardakani A. Contamination of environment with heavy metals emitted from automotives. Ecotoxicol Environ Saf. 1984 . https://pubmed.ncbi.nlm.nih.gov/6201332/

[1215] Li GJ, Zhang LL, Lu L, Wu P, Zheng W. Occupational exposure to welding fume among welders: alterations of manganese, iron, zinc, copper, and lead in body fluids and the oxidative stress status. J Occup Environ Med. 2004 Mar;46(3):241-8. https://www.ncbi.nlm.nih.gov/pmc/articles/PMC4126160/

[1216] Nessa F, Khan SA,et al. Lead, Cadmium and Nickel Contents of Some Medicinal Agents. Ind J. Pharm. Sci. 2016 https://www.ncbi.nlm.nih.gov/pmc/articles/PMC4852560/

[1217] Contractpharma.com: Heavy Metals in Drug Products Nikki Schopp, Team Leader in charge of ICP-MS, ICP-OES and AA testing, SGS01.29.15; https://www.contractpharma.com/issues/2015-01-01/view_features/heavy-metals-in-drug-products/

[1218] John Kanayochukwu Nduka, et al, 2020: Hazards and risk assessment of heavy metals from consumption of locally manufactured painkiller drugs in Nigeria, Toxicology Reports, V 7, 2020, https://www.sciencedirect.com/science/article/pii/S2214750020303711

[1219] Ada. COVID-19 Symptom Metallic Taste; Written by Ada's Medical Knowledge Team; Updated on September 29, 2022; https://ada.com/covid/covid-19-symptom-metallic-taste/

[1220] Krysiak R,et al. Potentiation of Endocrine Adverse Effects of Lithium by Enalapril and Verapamil. West Ind Med J. 2014 https://www.ncbi.nlm.nih.gov/pmc/articles/PMC4668978/

[1221] Bongiorno, Peter, ND, Lac; Toxicity and Depression; March 23, 2012; In Anxiety/Depression/Mental Health, Detoxification Medicine, Mind/Body; https://ndnr.com/mindbody/toxicity-and-depression/

[1222] CIR Expert Panel Members and Liaisons; Priya Cherian, Scientific Analyst/Writer; May 10, 2019; Re-Review of the Safety Assessment of EDTA and Salts. https://www.cir-safety.org/sites/default/files/EDTA.pdf

[1223] COCAM 3, 16-18 October 2012; SIDS INITIAL ASSESSMENT PROFILE; US/ICCA; https://hpvchemicals.oecd.org/UI/handler.axd?id=73b56220-3a8b-479b-b03c-99c7353bf4d6

[1224] Shearston J.A., et al, 2024: Tampons as a source of exposure to metal(loid)s, Envir Inter. V. 190, 2024, https://www.sciencedirect.com/science/article/pii/S0160412024004355

[1225] Merola M, Affatato S. Materials for Hip Prostheses: A Review of Wear and Loading Considerations. Materials (Basel). 2019 Feb 5;12(3):495. https://www.ncbi.nlm.nih.gov/pmc/articles/PMC6384837/

[1226] David Quig,PhD 2023: Iatrogenic Metal Burdens; The Examiner of Alternative Medicine, Thursday, March 2, 2023; https://www.townsendletter.com/article/iatrogenic-metal-burdens/

[1227] totalmouthfitness.com: BE AWARE OF THE POTENTIALLY HARMFUL METAL COMPONENTS IN YOUR; DENTAL WORK; By Dr. Paul Wilke, DDS, January 9, 2014; https://www.totalmouthfitness.com/dental-education/toxic-metals/

[1228] Benzodiazepine Withdrawal and Heavy Metal Toxicity; Benzodiazepine September 6, 2022 by Carol Gillette; Alternative to Meds Editorial Team; Medically Reviewed by Dr. Samuel Lee MD: https://www.alternativetomeds.com/blog/benzodiazepine-withdrawal-and-heavy-metal-toxicity/

[1229] Anke M, Groppel B, Kronemann H, Grün M. Nickel--an essential element. IARC Sci Publ. 1984;(53):339-65. https://pubmed.ncbi.nlm.nih.gov/6398286/

[1230] Harland BF, Harden-Williams BA. Is vanadium of human nutritional importance yet? J Am Diet Assoc. 1994 Aug;94(8):891-4. https://pubmed.ncbi.nlm.nih.gov/8046184/

[1231] Techtarget: By Katie Terrell Hanna42 (h2g2, meaning of life, The Hitchhiker's Guide to the Galaxy); https://www.techtarget.com/whatis/definition/42-h2g2-meaning-of-life-The-Hitchhikers-Guide-to-the-Galaxy

[1232] Thoughtco.com List is Radioactive Elements and their most stable isotopes.

[1233] Zoroddu MA, Aaseth J,et al.2019 The essential metals for humans: a brief overview. J Inorg Biochem. 2019 https://pubmed.ncbi.nlm.nih.gov/30939379/

[1234] ATSDR's Substance Priority List; What is the Substance Priority List (SPL)? https://www.atsdr.cdc.gov/spl/index.html

[1235] New Jersey department of health, hazardous substances fact sheet; Antimony; https://nj.gov/health/eoh/rtkweb/documents/fs/0141.pdf

[1236] Sax L. Polyethylene terephthalate may yield endocrine disruptors. Environ Health Perspect. 2010 Apr;118(4):445-8. http://doi.org/10.1289/ehp.0901253.

[1237] Shotyk W, Krachler M (2007) Contamination of bottled waters with antimony leaching from polyethylene terephthalate (PET) increases upon storage. Environ Sci Technol 41: https://pubmed.ncbi.nlm.nih.gov/17396641/

[1238] Sax, Leonard , 2010: Polyethylene Terephthalate May Yield Endocrine Disruptors Environmental Health Perspectives 118:4 CID: https://doi.org/10.1289/ehp.0901253; https://ehp.niehs.nih.gov/10.1289/ehp.0901253

[1239] Geetha, T. Endocrine disruptors in boiled drinking water carried in plastic containers: a pilot study in Thrissur, Kerala, India. Appl Water Sci 11, 188 (2021). https://doi.org/10.1007/s13201-021-01524-z

[1240] Antimony: The Most Important Mineral You Never Heard Of; Forbes: David Blackmon: https://www.forbes.com/sites/davidblackmon/2021/05/06/antimony-the-most-important-mineral-you-never-heard-of/?sh=22eaf7962b23

[1241] Baldwin D. E. 1999: Heavy metal poisoning and its laboratory investigation; Ann Clin Bioc. 1999; http://www.vshp.fi/medserv/klkemi/fi/ohjekirja/liitteet/Raskasmetallimyrkytys.pdf

[1242] Basinger MA, Jones MM. Structural requirements for chelate antidotal efficacy in acute antimony(III) intoxication. Res Commun Chem Pathol Pharmacol. 1981 May;32(2). https://pubmed.ncbi.nlm.nih.gov/6264554/

[1243] Adams JB, Baral M, et al 2009: Safety and efficacy of oral DMSA therapy for children with autism spectrum disorders: Part A--medical results. BMC Clin Pharmacol. 2009 Oct https://bmcclinpharma.biomedcentral.com/articles/10.1186/1472-6904-9-17

[1244] Stahl, T., Taschan, H. & Brunn, H. 2011: Aluminium content of selected foods and food products. Environ Sci Eur 23, 37 (2011). https://doi.org/10.1186/2190-4715-23-37

[1245] Reinke CM, Breitkreutz J, Leuenberger H. Aluminium in over-the-counter drugs: risks outweigh benefits? Drug Saf. 2003 ;https://go.gale.com/ps/i.do?p=AONE&u=googlescholar&id=GALE%7CA200344272&v=2.1&it=r&sid=AONE&asid=b8a2fc6c

[1246] CDC: Thimerosal and Vaccines; https://www.cdc.gov/vaccinesafety/concerns/thimerosal/index.html

[1247] Klotz K, Weistenhöfer W, Neff F, Hartwig A, van Thriel C, Drexler H. The Health Effects of Aluminum Exposure. Dtsch Arztebl Int. 2017 Sep 29;114(39) https://www.ncbi.nlm.nih.gov/pmc/articles/PMC5651828/

[1248] Dr. med. Dirk Wiechert; Aluminium - Östrogen, Zusammenhang mit Krebs und neurodegenerativen Erkrankungen?; playtime 1:35; https://www.youtube.com/watch?v=iUPst4vMvHI

[1249] Islam Fahadul, Shohag Sheikh, et al 2022: Exposure of metal toxicity in Alzheimer's disease: An extensive review; Frontiers in Pharmacology; 13 , 2022; https://www.frontiersin.org/articles/10.3389/fphar.2022.903099/full

[1250] Sun H, Hu C, Jia L, Zhu Y, Zhao H, Shao B, Wang N, Zhang Z, Li Y. Effects of aluminum exposure on serum sex hormones and androgen receptor expression in male rats. Biol Trace Elem Res. 2011 Dec;144(1-3) http://doi.org10.1007/s12011-011-9098-6.

Notes

[1251] Yousef, Mokhtar Ibrahim et al 2016: Aluminium oxide nanoparticles-induced spermatotoxicity, oxidative stress and changes in reproductive hormones and testes histopathology in male rats: Possible protective effect of glutathione; Endocrine Abstracts (2016) https://www.endocrine-abstracts.org/ea/0041/ea0041EP719

[1252] Carver, A., & Gallicchio, V. S. (2017). Heavy Metals and Cancer. In (Ed.), Cancer Causing Substances. IntechOpen. https://doi.org/10.5772/intechopen.70348 https://www.intechopen.com/chapters/56652

[1253] Fulgenzi A, De Giuseppe R, et al 2015: Efficacy of chelation therapy to remove aluminium intoxication. J Inorg Biochem. 2015 https://pubmed.ncbi.nlm.nih.gov/26404567/

[1254] Fulgenzi A, Vietti D, Ferrero ME. 2014: Aluminium involvement in neurotoxicity. Biomed Res Int. 2014;2014: https://www.ncbi.nlm.nih.gov/pmc/articles/PMC4160616/

[1255] Fulgenzi A, De Giuseppe R, Bamonti F, Vietti D, Ferrero ME. Efficacy of chelation therapy to remove aluminium intoxication. J Inorg Biochem. 2015 Nov;152:214-8. http://doi.org/10.1016/j.jinorgbio.2015.09.007.

[1256] Ordog, Gary. (2005). 325 ALUMINUM TOXICITY IN ALUMINUM FACTORY WORKERS, TREATED WITH DMSA CHELATION. Journal of Investigative Medicine. 53.. https://www.researchgate.net/publication/304512467_325_ALUMINUM_TOXICITY_IN_ALUMIN UM_FACTORY_WORKERS_TREATED_WITH_DMSA_CHELATION

[1257] Ordog, Gary. (2005). 325 ALUMINUM TOXICITY IN ALUMINUM FACTORY WORKERS, TREATED WITH DMSA CHELATION. Journal of Investigative Medicine. 53. S135.2-S135. http://dx.doi.org/10.2310/6650.2005.00005.324

[1258] Jiayu Gao et al 2019; Role of Gallic Acid in Oxidative Damage Diseases: A Comprehensive Review; https://journals.sagepub.com/doi/10.1177/1934578X19874174

[1259] Castriota F, Acevedo J, Ferreccio C, Smith AH, Liaw J, Smith MT, Steinmaus C. 2018: Obesity and increased susceptibility to arsenic-related type 2 diabetes in Northern Chile. Environ Res. 2018 Nov;167 https://doi.org/10.1016/j.envres.2018.07.022.

[1260][1260] Lansdown AB. 2011: Metal ions affecting the skin and eyes. Met Ions Life Sci. 2011;8:187-246. https://pubmed.ncbi.nlm.nih.gov/21473382/

[1261] Carver, A., & Gallicchio, V. S. (2017). Heavy Metals and Cancer. In (Ed.), Cancer Causing Substances. IntechOpen. https://www.intechopen.com/chapters/56652

[1262] Zartarian VG, Xue J, Ozkaynak H, Dang W, Glen G, Smith L, Stallings C. A probabilistic arsenic exposure assessment for children who contact CCA-treated playsets and decks, Part 1: Model methodology, variability results, and model evaluation. Risk Anal. 2006 Apr;26(2):515-31. https://pubmed.ncbi.nlm.nih.gov/16573637/

[1263] WHO; Arsenic; Dec 7, 2022; https://www.who.int/news-room/fact-sheets/detail/arsenic#:~:text=The%20greatest%20threat%20to%20public%20health%20from%20arsenic%20originates%20from,of%20America%20and%20Viet%20Nam.

[1264] Dyer, C. A., 2007; Heavy Metals as Endocrine-Disrupting Chemicals; 2007/01/01; 111; 133; 978-1-58829-830-0;; 10.1007/1-59745-107-X_5; Endocrine-Disrupting Chemicals: From Basic Science to Clinical Practice; http://eknygos.lsmuni.lt/springer/631/111-133.pdf

[1265] Smith, AH; Arroyo, AP; Mazumdar, DN. Arsenic-induced skin lesions among Atacameno people in northern Chile despite good nutrition and centuries of exposure. Environ. Hea. Perspect 2000, 108, 617–620. https://pubmed.ncbi.nlm.nih.gov/10903614/

[1266] Sharma B, Singh S, Siddiqi NJ. Biomedical implications of heavy metals induced imbalances in redox systems. Biomed Res Int. 2014;2014:640754. https://www.ncbi.nlm.nih.gov/pmc/articles/PMC4145541/

[1267] Md. Shiblur Rahaman, Nathan Mise, Sahoko Ichihara, 2022: Arsenic contamination in food chain in Bangladesh: A review on health hazards, socioeconomic impacts and implications, Hygiene and Environmental Health Advances, Volume 2, 2022, (https://www.sciencedirect.com/science/article/pii/S2773049222000046)

[1268] Islam M S, EuroAquae (2005-2007), Arsenic Contamination In Groundwater In Bangladesh: An Environmental And Social Disaster; Hydro Informatics and Water Management Program, University of Newcastle upon Tyne, Department Of Civil Engineering and Geosciences; IWApublishing; https://www.iwapublishing.com/news/arsenic-contamination-groundwater-bangladesh-environmental-and-social-disaster

[1269] Stanton BA, et al 2015: MDI biological laboratory arsenic summit: Approaches to limiting human exposure to arsenic. Current Environmental Health Reports. 2015;2(3) https://www.researchgate.net/publication/280602751_MDI_Biological_Laboratory_Arsenic_Sum mit_Approaches_to_Limiting_Human_Exposure_to_Arsenic

[1270] Kim, Hyun Soo, et al 2015: An Overview of Carcinogenic Heavy Metal: Molecular Toxicity Mechanism and Prevention; J Cancer Prev. 2015 Dec; 20(4): 232–240. Published online 2015 Dec 30. http://doi.org10.15430/JCP.2015.20.4.232

[1271] CDC, Atsdr: Arsenic Toxicity; How Should Patients Overexposed to Arsenic Be Treated and Managed?; https://www.atsdr.cdc.gov/csem/arsenic/patient_exposed.html

[1272] Kosnett MJ. The role of chelation in the treatment of arsenic and mercury poisoning. J Med Toxicol. 2013 Dec;9(4):347-54. https://pubmed.ncbi.nlm.nih.gov/24178900/

[1273] Kosnett MJ. The role of chelation in the treatment of arsenic and mercury poisoning. J Med Toxicol. 2013 Dec;9(4):347-54. https://pubmed.ncbi.nlm.nih.gov/24178900/

[1274] Flora, S.J.S. et al: Arsenic induced oxidative stress and the role of antioxidant supplementation during chelation: A review; Journal of Environmental Biology April 2007, 28(2) 333-347 (2007); http://jeb.co.in/journal_issues/200704_apr07_supp/paper_01.pdf

[1275] Archna Panghal et al 2020: Gallic acid and MiADMSA reversed arsenic induced oxidative/nitrosative damage in rat red blood cells; VOLUME 6, ISSUE 2, E03431, FEBRUARY 2020; https://doi.org/10.1016/j.heliyon.2020.e03431

[1276] Bhoelan BS, Stevering CH, van der Boog AT, van der Heyden MA. Barium toxicity and the role of the potassium inward rectifier current. Clin Toxicol (Phila). 2014 https://pubmed.ncbi.nlm.nih.gov/24905573/

[1277] Shen Gang, et al 2020: Barium Appendicitis 6 Weeks After Upper Gastrointestinal Imaging; Frontiers in Pediatrics; 8: 2020; https://www.frontiersin.org/articles/10.3389/fped.2020.00535

[1278] Lentini, P., Zanoli, L., Granata, A., Signorelli, S.S., Castellino, P., & Dell'Aquila, R. (2017). Kidney and heavy metals - The role of environmental exposure (Review). Molecular Medicine Reports, 15, 3413-3419. https://doi.org/10.3892/mmr.2017.6389

[1279] Comprehensive Health Center; WHAT YOU NEED TO KNOW ABOUT CHELATION; https://www.comp-health.com/what-you-need-to-know-about-chelation/

[1280] AlMomen, Abdulkareem; and Blaurock-Busch, Eleonore; 2022: Alpha-Lipoic Acid (ALA), fatty acid and promising chelating agent for neurological ailments; World J. of Biolo.l and Pharmac. Research, 2022, 03(01), https://doi.org/10.53346/wjbpr.2022.3.1.0038;

[1281] Su JF, Le DP, Liu CH, Lin JD, Xiao XJ. Critical care management of patients with barium poisoning: a case series. Chin Med J (Engl). 2020 Mar 20;133(6):724-725. https://www.ncbi.nlm.nih.gov/pmc/articles/PMC7190221/

[1282] Perera, Lekamage, 2017: The good without the bad: Selective chelators for beryllium encapsulation; PhD Thesis - University of Auckland; https://researchspace.auckland.ac.nz/handle/2292/35626

[1283] Lenntech WATER TREATMENT SOLUTIONS; Beryllium – Be; https://www.lenntech.com/periodic/elements/be.htm

[1284] Metzger Law group: Beryllium; https://www.toxictorts.com/beryllium/

[1285] CDC: Agency for Toxic Substances and Disease Registry (ATSDR), Beryllium Toxicity Who Is at Risk of Exposure to Beryllium? https://www.atsdr.cdc.gov/csem/beryllium/who_risk.html

[1286] Bazemore AW, Smucker DR. 2002: Lymphadenopathy and malignancy. Am Fam Physician. 2002 Dec 1;66 https://www.aafp.org/pubs/afp/issues/2002/1201/p2103.html

[1287] Drug.com Medications for Berylliosis https://www.drugs.com/condition/berylliosis.html

[1288] Hollins DM, McKinley MA, et al 2009: Beryllium and lung cancer: A weight of evidence evaluation of the toxicological and epidemiological literature. Critical Reviews in Toxicology. 2009;39(1):1-32. http://doi.org/10.1080/10408440902837967

[1289] Figgs LW, Holsinger H, Freitas SJ, Brion GM, Hornung RW, Rice CH, Tollerud D. 2011: Increased suicide risk among workers following toxic metal exposure at the Paducah gaseous diffusion plant from 1952 to 2003: a cohort study. Int J Occup Environ Med. 2011 https://pubmed.ncbi.nlm.nih.gov/23022839/

[1290] Tyson N. Dais; Towards more effective beryllium chelation: an investigation of second-sphere hydrogen bonding; RSC Adv., 2020, 10, 40142; The Royal Society of Chemistry 2020; https://pubs.rsc.org/en/content/articlepdf/2020/ra/d0ra08706h

[1291] Sharma P, Johri S, et al Beryllium-induced toxicity and its prevention by treatment with chelating agents. J Appl Toxicol. 2000 https://pubmed.ncbi.nlm.nih.gov/12557911/

[1292] Pugliese M, Biondi V, Gugliandolo E, Licata P, Peritore AF, Crupi R, Passantino A. D-Penicillamine: The State of the Art in Humans and in Dogs from a Pharmacological and Regulatory Perspective. Antibiotics (Basel). 2021 May 28;10(6):648. https://www.ncbi.nlm.nih.gov/pmc/articles/PMC8229433/

[1293] Johri S, Shukla S, Sharma P. Role of chelating agents and antioxidants in beryllium induced toxicity. Indian J Exp Biol. 2002 May; https://pubmed.ncbi.nlm.nih.gov/12622205/

[1294] Thermo Fisher Scientific; INFOGRAPHIC: Bismuth – The Heaviest Among Heavy Metals; Chris Calam03.01.2016; http://www.thermoscientific.com/content/dam/tfs/ATG/CAD/CAD%20Documents/Application%20&%20Technical%20Notes/Portable%20Analyzers%20for%20Material%20ID/Handheld%20XRF/quality-control-and-assurance-for-lead-free-brass.pdf

Notes

[1295] Fu, Jj., Guo, Jj., Qin, Ap. et al. Bismuth chelate as a contrast agent for X-ray computed tomography. J Nanobiotechnol 18, 110 (2020). https://doi.org/10.1186/s12951-020-00669-4

[1296] Chelation Medical Center; Ray Psonak, D.O. Toxic Heavy Metals; https://www.chelationmedicalcenter.com/toxic-heavy-metals.html

[1297] Adams JB, Baral M, et al 2009: Safety and efficacy of oral DMSA therapy for children with autism spectrum disorders: Part A--medical results. BMC Clin Pharmacol. 2009 Oct 23;9:16.. https://pubmed.ncbi.nlm.nih.gov/19852790/

[1298] Slikkerveer A, Jong HB, Helmich RB, de Wolff FA. Development of a therapeutic procedure for bismuth intoxication with chelating agents. J Lab Clin Med. 1992 1583409. https://pubmed.ncbi.nlm.nih.gov/1583409/

[1299] Ohio State University: Bismuth: Heavy Metal Toxicity What is Bismuth and Where is it Found?; June10 2019; https://u.osu.edu/helmig-mason.1/2019/06/10/bismuth-heavy-metal-toxicity

[1300] Slikkerveer A, Noach LA, Tytgat GN et al.: Comparison of enhanced elimination of bismuth in humans after treatment with meso-2,3 dimercaptosuccinic acid and d,l-2,3-dimercaptopropane-1-sulfonic acid. Analyst. 1998;123:91–92.

[1301] Ohio State University; Bismuth: Heavy Metal Toxicity; June102019; What is Bismuth and Where is it Found? https://u.osu.edu/helmig-mason.1/2019/06/10/bismuth-heavy-metal-toxicity/

[1302] Guidance; Bromine: toxicological overview; 10 June 2022; https://www.gov.uk/government/publications/bromine-properties-incident-management-and-toxicology/bromine-toxicological-overview#:~:text=Health%20effects%20of%20chronic%20exposure,conditioned%20reflexes%20and%20blood%20indexes.

[1303] CDC Facts About Bromine - CDC https://emergency.cdc.gov/agent/bromine/basics/facts.asp#:~:text=Survivors%20of%20serious%20poisoning%20caused,damage%20from%20low%20blood%20pressure

[1304] Cadmium Factsheet UNEP, December 2022; https://www.unep.org/topics/chemicals-and-pollution-action/pollution-and-health/heavy-metals/cadmium

[1305] Nasiadek, M., Danilewicz, M., Sitarek, K. et al.2018: The effect of repeated cadmium oral exposure on the level of sex hormones, estrous cyclicity, and endometrium morphometry in female rats. Environ Sci Pollut Res 25, https://doi.org/10.1007/s11356-018-2821-5

[1306] Hopkinsmedicine; Elevated Cadmium Levels Linked to Liver Disease; Men especially affected: Release Date: May 9, 2013; https://www.hopkinsmedicine.org/news/media/releases/elevated_cadmium_levels_linked_to_liver_disease

[1307] J.P Buchet, R Lauwerys, et al 1990: Renal effects of cadmium body burden of the general population, The Lancet, Volume 336, Issue 8717, 1990, https://doi.org/10.1016/0140-6736(90)92201-R.

[1308] Satarug S. Dietary Cadmium Intake and Its Effects on Kidneys. Toxics. 2018 Mar 10;6(1):15. https://pubmed.ncbi.nlm.nih.gov/29534455/

[1309] Fransson, M.N.; et al 2014: Physiologically-based toxicokinetic model for cadmium using markov-chain monte carlo analysis of concentrations in blood, urine, and kidney cortex from living kidney donors. Toxicol. Sci. https://pubmed.ncbi.nlm.nih.gov/25015660/

[1310] Flora SJ, Pachauri V. Chelation in metal intoxication. Int J Environ Res Public Health. 2010 Jul;7(7):2745-88. http://doi.org/10.3390/ijerph7072745.

[1311] Flora, Swaran J.S., and Vidhu Pachauri. 2010. "Chelation in Metal Intoxication" International Journal of Environmental Research and Public Health 7, no. 7: 2745-2788. https://doi.org/10.3390/ijerph7072745;

[1312] Romero, A. et al 2014: A review of metal-catalyzed molecular damage: protection by melatonin; Journal of Pineal Research: V 56: Is 4;: https://doi.org/10.1111/jpi.12132

[1313] Shlomo Bar-Sela, Stephen Reingold & Elihu D. Richter (2001) Amyotrophic Lateral Sclerosis in a Battery-factory Worker Exposed to Cadmium, International Journal of Occupational and Environmental Health, 7:2, https://pubmed.ncbi.nlm.nih.gov/11373040/

[1314] Dyer, C. A., 2007; Heavy Metals as Endocrine-Disrupting Chemicals; 2007/01/01; 111; 133; 978-1-58829-830-0; Endocrine-Disrupting Chemicals: From Basic Sc. to Clin. Pr. http://eknygos.lsmuni.lt/springer/631/111-133.pdf

[1315] Gay, Flaminia; Laforgia, Vincenza; et al Chronic Exposure to Cadmium Disrupts the Adrenal Gland Activity of the Newt Triturus carnifex (Amphibia, Urodela) https://www.hindawi.com/journals/bmri/2013/424358/

[1316] Nasiadek M, Danilewicz M, Klimczak M, Stragierowicz J, Kilanowicz A.2019: Subchronic Exposure to Cadmium Causes Persistent Changes in the Reproductive System in Female Wistar Rats. Oxid Med Cell Longev. 2019 Dec https://www.hindawi.com/journals/omcl/2019/6490820/

[1317] Lahouaoui, H.; et al 2019: Depression and Anxiety Emerging From Heavy Metals: What Relationship? Source Title: Handbook of Research on Global; Environmental Changes and Human Health; https://www.researchgate.net/publication/330635466_Depression_and_Anxiety_Emerging_From_Heavy_Metals_What_Relationship

[1318] Bernhoft, Robin A.; 2013: Cadmium Toxicity and Treatment; Clinical Detoxification: Elimination of Persistent Toxicants from the Human Body; The Scientific World Journal Volume 2013 https://doi.org/10.1155/2013/394652

[1319] Rafati Rahimzadeh M, Rafati Rahimzadeh M, Kazemi S, Moghadamnia AA. Cadmium toxicity and treatment: An update. Caspian J Intern Med. 2017 Summer;8(3):135-145. doi: 10.22088/cjim.8.3.135. https://www.ncbi.nlm.nih.gov/pmc/articles/PMC5596182/#B82

[1320] Mikirova, Nina et al 2011: Efficacy of oral DMSA and intravenous EDTA in chelation of toxic metals and improvement of the number of stem/ progenitor cells in circulation; TRANSLATIONAL BIOMEDICINE; 2011 Vol. 2 No. 2:2 https://www.transbiomedicine.com/translational-biomedicine/efficacy-of-oral-dmsa-and intravenous-edta-in-chelation-of-toxic-metals-and-improvement-of-the-number-of-stem-progenitor-cells-in-circulation.pdf

[1321] Sarić, M.M., Blanuša, M., Jureša, D., Šarić, M., Varnai, V.M. and Kostial, K. (2004), Combined Early Treatment with Chelating Agents DMSA and CaDTPA in Acute Oral Cadmium Exposure. Basic & Clinical Pharmacology & Toxicology, 94: 119-123. https://doi.org/10.1111/j.1742-7843.2004.pto940304.x

[1322] Tandon SK, et al Chelation in metal intoxication: influence of cysteine or N-acetyl cysteine on the efficacy of 2,3-dimercaptopropane-1-sulphonate in the treatment of cadmium toxicity. J Appl Toxicol. 2002 Jan-Feb https://pubmed.ncbi.nlm.nih.gov/11807931/

[1323] Olivier Barbier, Grégory Jacquillet, Michel Tauc, Marc Cougnon, Philippe Poujeol; Effect of Heavy Metals on, and Handling by, the Kidney. Nephron Physiology 1 April 2005; 99 (4): p105–p110. https://doi.org/10.1159/000083981

[1324] W. Smith, 2013: The Role of Chelation in the Treatment of Other Metal Poisonings Silas J Med Toxicol. 2013 Dec; 9 .https://www.ncbi.nlm.nih.gov/pmc/articles/PMC3846962/

[1325] Kargacin B, Kostial K. Age-related efficiency of Ca-DTPA to reduce 141Ce retention in rats. Toxicol Lett. 1986 Sep;32(3):243-7.. https://pubmed.ncbi.nlm.nih.gov/3775807/

[1326] Wikipedia Cobalt poisoning; 12-20- 2022 https://en.wikipedia.org/wiki/Cobalt_poisoning

[1327] NORD, Rare Disease Database; Heavy Metal Poisoning; https://rarediseases.org/rare-diseases/heavy-metal-poisoning/

[1328] Noboru Yamagata, Sadao Murata, Tetsuya Torii, The Cobalt Content of Human Body, Journal of Radiation Research, Volume 3, Issue 1, March 1962, Pages 4–8, https://doi.org/10.1269/jrr.3.4

[1329] Steens, W., Loehr, J.F., von Foerster, G. et al. Chronische Kobaltvergiftung in der Endoprothetik. Orthopäde 35, 860–864 (2006). https://link.springer.com/article/10.1007/s00132-006-0973-3

[1330] David Quig, PhD 2023: Iatrogenic Metal Burdens; The Examiner of Alternative Medicine, Thursday, March 2, 2023; https://www.townsendletter.com/article/iatrogenic-metal-burdens/

[1331] nutritionalbalancing.org Copper Excess: Low Energy and Chronic Fatigue; https://nutritionalbalancing.org/center/htma/science/articles/copper-excess

[1332] Richard Malter : Copper Excess (Toxicity): Psychological Implications for Children, Adolescents, and Adults; April, 1984 June, 2001 https://rickmalter.com/articles/f/copper-excess-psychological-implications

[1333] mountsinai; Copper poisoning; 2023 Icahn School of Medicine at Mount Sinai https://www.mountsinai.org/health-library/poison/copper-poisoning#:~:text=Sudden%20(acute)%20copper%20poisoning%20is,is%20to%20the%20body%27s%20organs.

[1334] GREENBLATT, JAMES, MD; The Role Of Heavy Metals And Environmental Toxins In Psychiatric Disorders; July 10, 2017 https://www.immh.org/article-source/2017/7/10/the-role-of-heavy-metals-and-environmental-toxins-in-psychiatric

[1335] Baldwin D. E. 1999: Heavy metal poisoning and its laboratory investigation; Ann Clin Bioc. 1999; http://www.vshp.fi/medserv/klkemi/fi/ohjekirja/liitteet/Raskasmetallimyrkytys.pdf

[1336] LiverTox: Clinical and Research Information on Drug-Induced Liver Injury [Internet]. Bethesda (MD): National Institute of Diabetes and Digestive and Kidney Diseases; 2012-. Wilson Disease Agents. [Updated 2020]. https://www.ncbi.nlm.nih.gov/books/NBK548883/

[1337] Cao Y, Skaug MA, et al 2014: Chelation therapy in intoxications with mercury, lead and copper. J Trace Elem Med Biol. https://pubmed.ncbi.nlm.nih.gov/24894443/

Notes

[1338] LiverTox: Clinical and Research Information on Drug-Induced Liver Injury [Internet]. Bethesda (MD): National Institute of Diabetes and Digestive and Kidney Diseases; 2012-. Trientine. [Updated 2020 Jul 25]. https://www.ncbi.nlm.nih.gov/books/NBK548119/

[1339] Dayan AD, Paine AJ. Mechanisms of chromium toxicity, carcinogenicity and allergenicity: review of the literature from 1985 to 2000. Hum Exp Toxicol. 2001;20:439–51. https://www.researchgate.net/publication/11582421_Mechanisms_of_Chromium_Toxicity_Carcinogenicity_and_Allergenicity_Review_of_the_Literature_from_1985_to_2000

[1340] ATSDR: hromium Toxicity, What Are the Physiologic Effects of Chromium Exposure? https://www.atsdr.cdc.gov/csem/chromium/physiologic_effects_of_chromium_exposure.html

[1341] David Quig,PhD 2023: Iatrogenic Metal Burdens; The Examiner of Alternative Medicine, March 2, 2023; https://www.townsendletter.com/article/iatrogenic-metal-burdens/

[1342] Kotaś J, et al: Chromium occurrence in the environment and methods of its speciation. Environ Pollut. 2000; https://www.sciencedirect.com/science/article/abs/pii/S0269749199001682

[1343] Kim HS, Kim YJ, Seo YR. An Overview of Carcinogenic Heavy Metal: Molecular Toxicity Mechanism and Prevention. J Cancer Prev. 2015 Dec;20(4):232-40. https://www.ncbi.nlm.nih.gov/pmc/articles/PMC4699750/

[1344] Kim, Hyun Soo, et al 2015: An Overview of Carcinogenic Heavy Metal: Molecular Toxicity Mechanism and Prevention; J Cancer Prev. 2015 Dec; 20(4): 232–240. Published online 2015 Dec 30. https://www.ncbi.nlm.nih.gov/pmc/articles/PMC4699750/

[1345] Iranmanesh M, Fatemi SJ, Ebrahimpour R, Dahooee Balooch F. Chelation of chromium(VI) by combining deferasirox and deferiprone in rats. Biometals. 2013 Jun;26(3):465-71. https://doi.org/10.1007/s10534-013-9631-5

[1346] W. Banner, et al 1986: Experimental chelation therapy in chromium, lead, and boron intoxication with N-acetylcysteine and other compounds, Toxicology and Applied Pharmacology, Volume 83, Issue 1, 1986, Pages 142-147, (https://www.sciencedirect.com/science/article/pii/0041008X86903315)

[1347] Poonam, Neema Tufchi et al 2018: Detoxification of Arsenic and Chromium through Chelators and enzymes: an In-silico approach; International Journal of Applied Engineering Research ISSN 0973-4562 Volume 13, Number 10 (2018) pp. 8249-8271 © Research India Publications. http://www.ripublication.com

[1348] Gallium Oxide Toxicology; CAS # :12024-21-4 https://digitalfire.com/hazard/gallium+oxide+toxicology#:~:text=Chronic%20Toxicity%20Studies,of%20the%20bone%20marrow%20function.

[1349] Zahra Mirhoseiny, Asghar Amiri, et al (2015) Chelation therapy improves spatial learning and memory impairment in gallium arsenide intoxicated rats, Toxin Reviews, 34:4, 177-183, https://doi.org/10.3109/15569543.2015.1127259

[1350] Domingo, J.L., Llobet, J.M. & Corbella, J. Relative efficacy of chelating agents as antidotes for acute gallium nitrate intoxication. Arch Toxicol 59, 382–383 (1987). https://doi.org/10.1007/BF00295095

[1351] Rees, J.A., Deblonde, G.JP., An, D.D. et al. 2018: Evaluating the potential of chelation therapy to prevent and treat gadolinium deposition from MRI contrast agents. Sci Rep 8, 4419 (2018). https://doi.org/10.1038/s41598-018-22511-6

[1352] Contrast caution: Dr. Chris Ramirez: HSC Newsroom 2022 Contrast Caution By Michael Haederle | February 24, 2022; https://hsc.unm.edu/news/2022/02/doctor-researches-toxic-side-effects-rare-earth-metals-mri.html

[1353] Working Group for COVID Vaccine Analysis; SUMMARY OF PRELIMINARY FINDINGS; 06.07.2022; https://www.documentcloud.org/documents/22140176-report-from-working-group-of-vaccine-analysis-in-germany

[1354] Boyken J, et al 2019: Impact of Treatment With Chelating Agents Depends on the Stability of Administered GBCAs: A Comparative Study in Rats. Invest Radiol. 2019 Feb;54(2):76-82. https://pubmed.ncbi.nlm.nih.gov/30358694/

[1355] Rydahl, Casper MD. Et al 2008: High Prevalence of Nephrogenic Systemic Fibrosis in Chronic Renal Failure Patients Exposed to Gadodiamide, a Gadolinium-Containing Magnetic Resonance Contrast Agent. Investigative Radiology 43(2):p 141-144, February 2008. https://www.frontiersin.org/articles/10.3389/fenvs.2022.948041/full#B102

[1356] Boyken J, Frenzel T,et al 2019: Impact of Treatment With Chelating Agents Depends on the Stability of Administered GBCAs: A Comparative Study in Rats. Invest Radiol. 2019 Feb;54(2): https://www.ncbi.nlm.nih.gov/pmc/articles/PMC6310454/

[1357] CLINICAL RESEARCH PROTOCOL 2016: Effects of IV-Administered Ca-DTPA and Zn-DTPA To Treat Patients With Gadolinium Deposition Disease, https://classic.clinicaltrials.gov/ProvidedDocs/22/NCT02947022/Prot_SAP_000.pdf

[1358] Weinreb JC et al :Use of intravenous gadolinium-based contrast media in patients with kidney disease: Consensus statements from the American College of Radiology and the Nat Kidney Found. Radiology 2021 Jan; (https://doi.org/10.1148/radiol.2020202903.

[1359] Martino F, Amici G, Rosner M, Ronco C, Novara G. Gadolinium-Based Contrast Media Nephrotoxicity in Kidney Impairment: The Physio-Pathological Conditions for the Perfect Murder. J Clin Med. 2021 Jan 13;10(2):271. http://doi.org/10.3390/jcm10020271.

[1360] Dean Sherry; et al 2009: Primer on gadolinium chemistry; 24 November 2009; MRI; Volume 30, Issue 6; December 2009; https://doi.org/10.1002/jmri.21966

[1361] Wikipedia. 11.23. 2022; https://en.wikipedia.org/wiki/Gadolinium

[1362] Chen, F., et al. Controllable Fabrication and Optical Properties of Uniform Gadolinium Oxysulfate Hollow Spheres. Sci Rep 5, (2016). https://doi.org/10.1038/srep17934

[1363] Dean Sherry; et al 2009: Primer on gadolinium chemistry; 24 November 2009; MRI; Volume 30, Issue 6; December 2009; https://doi.org/10.1002/jmri.21966

[1364] Wikipedia, Gadolinium; 8-15-2023; https://en.wikipedia.org/wiki/Gadolinium

[1365] Marlei Veiga, et al 2020: Presence of other rare earth metals in gadolinium-based contrast agents, Talanta, V. 216, 2020, https://doi.org/10.1016/j.talanta.2020.120940

[1366] Yale Radiology and Biomedical Imaging: https://medicine.yale.edu/diagnosticradiology/patientcare/policies/faq%20gadolinium%20retentio n_339594_284_11023_v1.pdf

[1367] Iyad, Nebal et al: Gadolinium contrast agents- challenges and opportunities of a multidisciplinary approach: Literature review; https://doi.org/10.10161/j.ejro.2023.100503

[1368] Semelka RC, et al 2018: Intravenous Calcium-/Zinc-Diethylene Triamine Penta-Acetic Acid in Patients With Presumed Gadolinium Deposition Disease: A Preliminary Report on 25 Patients. Invest Radiol. 2018 Jun http://doi.org/10.1097/RLI.0000000000000453.

[1369] NIH: Clinical trial.gov: DTPA (Diethylenetriaminepenta-acetate) Chelation for Symptoms After Gadolinium-assisted MRI Exposure; First Posted: May 4, 2022; ClinicalTrials.gov Identifier: https://clinicaltrials.gov/ct2/show/NCT05359835;

[1370] Rees, J.A., Deblonde, G.JP., An, D.D. et al. 2018: Evaluating the potential of chelation therapy to prevent and treat gadolinium deposition from MRI contrast agents. Sci Rep 8, 4419 (2018). https://doi.org/10.1038/s41598-018-22511-6

[1371] Broschova, M. et al 2002: Structure and magnetic properties of gadolinium hexacyanoferrate Prussian blue analogue *) Czechoslovak Journal of Physics, Vol. 52 (2002), https://home.saske.sk/~mihalik/Hrabcak/Prussian/2002-Brosch-CzJPhy325.pdf

[1372] Web MD: Germanium - Uses, Side Effects, and More; https://www.webmd.com/vitamins/ai/ingredientmono-459/germanium#:~:text=Spirogermanium%20and%20propagermanium%20are%20examples.ele mental)%20germanium%20is%20LIKELY%20UNSAFE.

[1373] Havarinasab S, Johansson U, Pollard KM, Hultman P. Gold causes genetically determined autoimmune and immunostimulatory responses in mice. Clin Exp Immunol. 2007 Oct;150(1):179-88. http://doi.org/10.1111/j.1365-2249.2007.03469.x.

[1374] Zohdi, H., Emami, M., & Reza, H. (2012). Galvanic Corrosion Behavior of Dental Alloys. InTech. http://doi.org/10.5772/52319

[1375] AETNA Chelation Therapy; Number: 0234 https://www.aetna.com/cpb/medical/data/200_299/0234.html

[1376] Yoshihiro Takahashi, et al 1995: The utility of chelating agents as antidotes for nephrotoxicity of gold sodium thiomalate in adjuvant-arthritic rats, Toxicology, Volume 97, Issues 1–3, 1995, https://doi.org/10.1016/0300-483X(94)02944-P.

[1377] Kojima S, Takahashi Y, Kiyozumi M, Funakoshi T, Shimada H. Characterization of gold in urine and bile following administration of gold sodium thiomalate with chelating agents to rats. Toxicology. 1992 Aug;74 https://doi.org/10.1016/0300-483X(92)90038-G

[1378] Flora, Swaran J.S., and Vidhu Pachauri. 2010. "Chelation in Metal Intoxication" International Journal of Environmental Research and Public Health 7, no. 7: 2745-2788. https://doi.org/10.3390/ijerph7072745;

[1379] Sripetchwandee J, Pipatpiboon N, Chattipakorn N, Chattipakorn S (2014) Combined Therapy of Iron Chelator and Antioxidant Completely Restores Brain Dysfunction Induced by Iron Toxicity.. https://doi.org/10.1371/journal.pone.0085115

[1380] Dr. Milton Tenenbein (2001) Hepatotoxicity in Acute Iron Poisoning, Journal of Toxicology: Clinical Toxicology, 39:7, https://www.tandfonline.com/doi/abs/10.1081/CLT-100108513

[1381] Ferrero, Maria Elena. 2022. "Neuron Protection by EDTA May Explain the Successful Outcomes of Toxic Metal Chelation Therapy in Neurodegenerative Diseases" Biomedicines 10, no. 10: 2476. https://doi.org/10.3390/biomedicines10102476

[1382] Correia S, Hubbard E, et al 2010: Basal ganglia MR relaxometry in obsessive-compulsive disorder: T2 depends upon age of symptom onset. Brain Imaging Behav. 2010 Mar;4(1):35-45. https://www.ncbi.nlm.nih.gov/pmc/articles/PMC3018344/

[1383] Moore C Jr, Ormseth M, Fuchs H. Causes and significance of markedly elevated serum ferritin levels in an academic medical center. J Clin Rheumatol. 2013 Sep;19(6):324-8. https://europepmc.org/article/med/23965472

[1384] Iron Disorders Institute, Iron Reduction: Chelation Therapy https://irondisorders.org/chelation-therapy/

[1385] Corsello, Serafinaet al. (2009). The usefulness of chelation therapy for the remission of symptoms caused by previous treatment with mercury-containing pharmaceuticals: A case report. Cases journal. 2. 199. https://www.researchgate.net/publication/40039582_The_usefulness_of_chelation_therapy_for_t he_remission_of_symptoms_caused_by_previous_treatment_with_mercury-containing_pharmaceuticals_A_case_report

[1386] Rudolph CJ, 1991; Effect of EDTA Chelation on Serum Iron; Journal of Advancement in Medicine; Volumen 4, Number 1, Spring 1991; https://mcdonaghmed.com/wp-content/uploads/2019/07/paper26.pdf

[1387] Ferrero, Maria Elena 2016: Rationale for the Successful Management of EDTA Chelation Therapy in Human Burden by Toxic Metals; Hindawi; V. 2016 https://doi.org/10.1155/2016/8274504https://www.hindawi.com/journals/bmri/2016/8274504/

[1388] Saleh, S. et al 2014: Chelation of Thallium (III) in Rats Using Combined Deferasirox and Deferiprone Therapy; https://koreascience.kr/article/JAKO201731242008041.pdf

[1389] Bloodbank: ; Chelating Agents; Accession Number DBCAT000624 https://go.drugbank.com/drugs/DB01609

[1390] Scarano, A. et al 2023: The Chelation ability of Plant Polyphenols Can affect Iron Homeostasis and Gut Microbiota; J. Antioxidants; http://doi.org/10.3390/antiox12030630

[1391] Jennrich, Peter, 2009: die medizinische bedeutung chronischer metallbelastungen – ein Überblick umwelt·medizin·gesellschaft | 22 | 3/2009; http://tierversuchsfreie-medizin.de/download/chronische_Metallbelastungen_Ueberblick.pdf

[1392] Lanphear BP, Rauch S, Auinger P, Allen RW, Hornung RW. Low-level lead exposure and mortality in US adults: a population-baseno d cohort study. Lancet Public Health.; 2018;3(4):E177-E184. https://www.researchgate.net/publication/323742199_Low-level_lead_exposure_and_mortality_in_US_adults_A_population-based_cohort_study

[1393] Fewtrell LJ, et al 2004: Estimating the global burden of disease of mild mental retardation and cardiovascular diseases from environmental lead exposure. Environ Res. 2004 Feb;94(2):120-33.. https://pubmed.ncbi.nlm.nih.gov/14757375/

[1394] Reuters: Even low blood lead levels linked to gout risk; healthcare & pharma; august 21, 2012 By Amy Norton, Reuters Health; https://www.reuters.com/article/us-blood-lead-gout-idUSBRE87J0X320120820

[1395] Dyer, C.A.2007; Heavy Metals as Endocrine-Disrupting Chemicals; 2007/01/01; 111; 133; 978-1-58829-830-0;; 10.1007/1-59745-107-X_5; Endocrine-Disrupting Chemicals: From Basic Science to Clinical Practice; http://eknygos.lsmuni.lt/springer/631/111-133.pdf

[1396] Shoshan, Michal S 2022:; Will Short Peptides Revolutionize Chelation Therapy? Zurich Open Repository and Archive; Univ. of Zurich; https://www.zora.uzh.ch/id/eprint/230581/1/ZORA_5418.pdf

[1397] CHE-WA (Collaborative on Health and the Environment, Washington State chapter; by Steven G. Gilbert.; https://www.healthandenvironment.org/environmental-health/social-context/history/thomas-midgley-jr.-developed-tetraethyl-lead-for-gasoline

[1398] Smithsonian: Leaded Gas Was a Known Poison the Day It Was Invented; Kat Eschner; December 9, 2016; https://www.smithsonianmag.com/smart-news/leaded-gas-poison-invented-180961368 /

[1399] Wikipedia Timeline of alcohol Fuel; 3.4. 2023 https://en.wikipedia.org/wiki/Timeline_of_alcohol_fuel

[1400] Jarup, Lars 2013: Hazards of heavy metal contamination; British Medical Bulletin, Volume 68, Issue 1, December 2003, Pages 167–182, https://doi.org/10.1093/bmb/ldg032

[1401] EPA Requires Phase-Out of Lead in All Grades of Gasoline; [EPA press release - November 28, 1973] https://www.epa.gov/archive/epa/aboutepa/epa-requires-phase-out-lead-all-grades-gasoline.html

[1402] Grist: Leaded gasoline is finally gone – but its toxic legacy lingers; Yvette Cabrera; Aug 31, 2021; https://grist.org/regulation/leaded-gasoline-lead-poisoning-united-nations/

[1403] Kelly T.D. & Matos G.R. 2005 Historical statistics for mineral and material commodities in the United States. In: U.S. Geological Survey, 140,, Lead: 20.08.2011, at http://pubs.usgs.gov/ds/2005/140/.

[1404] McFarland M. J. et al 2022: Half of US population exposed to adverse lead levels in early childhood; PROCEEDINGS OF THE NATIONAL ACADEMY OF SCIENCES; Vol. 119 | No. 11; March 15, 2022; https://doi.org/10.1073/pnas.2118631119

[1405] EWG's Tap Water Database — 2021; https://www.ewg.org/tapwater/reviewed-lead.php

[1406] Pulitzercenter.: 50 Years of Research Shows there is No Safe Level of Childhood Lead Exposure; JUNE 16, 2022 Michael Coren GRANTEE; https://pulitzercenter.org/stories/50-years-research-shows-there-no-safe-level-childhood-lead-exposure

[1407] Adriyan Pramono et al 2017: Low zinc serum levels and high blood lead levels among school-age children in coastal area, IOP Conf. Ser.: Earth Environ. Sci. 55 012058 https://iopscience.iop.org/article/10.1088/1755-1315/55/1/012058

[1408] Rhodes, Daniel MD, MPH; Spiro, Avron III PhD; Aro, Antonio PhD; Hu, Howard MD, MPH, ScD. Relationship of Bone and Blood Lead Levels to Psychiatric Symptoms: The Normative Aging Study. Journal of Occupational and Environmental Medicine: November 2003 - Volume 45 - Issue 11 https://www.jstor.org/stable/44996906

[1409] Papanikolaou, N.C.; Hatzidaki, E.G.; Belivanis, S.; Tzanakakis, G.N.; Tsatsakis, A.M. Lead toxicity update. A brief review. Med. Sci. Monit. 2005, 11, 329–336.

[1410] Lahouaoui, H.; et al 2019: Depression and Anxiety Emerging From Heavy Metals: What Relationship? Source Title: Handbook of Research on Global; Environmental Changes and Human Health; 2019 http://doi.org/10.4018/978-1-5225-7775-1.ch015

[1411] Patient: Lead Poisoning; Causes, Symptoms, and Treatment; Authored by Dr Colin Tidy, Reviewed by Dr Laurence Knott | 24 Nov 2021; https://patient.info/doctor/lead-poisoning-pro

[1412] Gardella, C. (2001). Lead exposure in pregnancy: A review of the literature and argument for routine prenatal screening. Obstetrical & Gynecological Survey, 56(4), https://pubmed.ncbi.nlm.nih.gov/11285436/

[1413] Levander, O. (1979). Lead Toxicity and Nutritional Deficiencies. Environmental Health Perspectives, 29, 115-125. https://ehp.niehs.nih.gov/doi/abs/10.1289/ehp.7929115

[1414] Mense, S., Zhang, L. Heme: a versatile signaling molecule controlling the activities of diverse regulators ranging from transcription factors to MAP kinases. Cell Res 16, 681–692 (2006). https://doi.org/10.1038/sj.cr.7310086

[1415] Qiao, W., Pan, D., Zheng, Y. et al. 2022: Divalent metal cations stimulate skeleton interoception for new bone formation in mouse injury models. Nat Commun 13, 535 (2022). https://doi.org/10.1038/s41467-022-28203-0 https://www.nature.com/articles/s41467-022-28203-0

[1416] Weiss G, Carver PL. Role of divalent metals in infectious disease susceptibility and outcome. Clin Microbiol Infect. 2018 Jan;24(1) https://pubmed.ncbi.nlm.nih.gov/28143784/

[1417] Hegazy AA, Zaher MM, Abd El-Hafez MA, Morsy AA, Saleh RA. 2010: Relation between anemia and blood levels of lead, copper, zinc and iron among children. BMC Res Notes. 2010 May 12 https://bmcresnotes.biomedcentral.com/articles/10.1186/1756-0500-3-133

[1418] Katarzyna Kordas, 2017; The "Lead Diet": Can Dietary Approaches Prevent or Treat Lead Exposure? Journal of paediatrics; VOLUME 185, P224-231.E1, JUNE 01, 2017

[1419] Carraccio CL, Bergman GE, Daley BP. 1987: Combined iron deficiency and lead poisoning in children. Effect on FEP levels. Clin Pediatr (Phila). 1987 Dec;26(12):644-7.. https://pubmed.ncbi.nlm.nih.gov/3677534/

[1420] Washingtonpost: Study Concludes Beethoven Died From Lead Poisoning; By Rick Weiss; December 6, 2005; https://www.washingtonpost.com/archive/politics/2005/12/06/study-concludes-beethoven-died-from-lead-poisoning/042021b3-d515-4d9b-aadd-e42310e1f466/

[1421] Reiter C, Prohaska T. Beethoven's death-the result of medical malpractice? Wien Med Wochenschr. 2021 Nov;171(15-16) https://www.ncbi.nlm.nih.gov/pmc/articles/PMC8553724/#:~:text=The%20results%20revealed%20the%20presence,100%20times%20the%20normal%20value.

[1422] Brigitte M. Gensthaler: Beethoven und Blei - Tödliches Zusammenspiel. In: Pharmazeutische Zeitung, 30, 2001, abgerufen am 12. Mai 2018.

[1423] Smithsonian: Sugar of Lead: A Deadly Sweetener: Did ancient Romans, Pope Clement II or Ludwig van Beethoven overdose on a sweet salt of lead? J. Rhodes; 2012; https://www.smithsonianmag.com/arts-culture/sugar-of-lead-a-deadly-sweetener-89984487/

[1424] Kasperczyk, Aleksandra et al 2012: The Effect of Occupational Lead Exposure on Blood Levels of Zinc, Iron, Copper, Selenium and Related Proteins; Biol Trace Elem Res. 2012 Dec; 150(https://www.ncbi.nlm.nih.gov/pmc/articles/PMC3510413/?report=classic

[1425] Muran PJ., DMSA, vitamin C, and glutathione: an observational clinical review. Altern Ther Health Med. 2006 May-Jun;12(3):70-5. https://pubmed.ncbi.nlm.nih.gov/16708769/

[1426] Clarkson TW, Magos L, Myers GJ. The toxicology of mercury –

current exposures and clinical manifestations. N Engl J Med. 2003; 3https://pubmed.ncbi.nlm.nih.gov/16973445/

[1427] Houston, M.C. (2011), Role of Mercury Toxicity in Hypertension, Cardiovascular Disease, and Stroke. The Journal of Clinical Hypertension, 13: https://doi.org/10.1111/j.1751-7176.2011.00489.x

[1428] Salonen JT, Seppanen K, Nyyssonen K, et al. Intake of mercury from fish, lipid peroxidation, and the risk of myocardial infarction and coronary, cardiovascular, and any death in eastern Finnish men. Circulation. 1995 https://pubmed.ncbi.nlm.nih.gov/7828289/

[1429] EDF: Mercury pollution from coal plants is still a dang. Mercury pollution from coal plants is still a danger to Americans. We need stronger standards to protect us. Ashley Maiolatesi / Published: Feb. 22, 2022; https://blogs.edf.org/climate411/2022/02/22/mercury-pollution-from-coal-plants-is-still-a-danger-to-americans-we-need-stronger-standards-to-protect-us/

[1430] Public Health Benefits Associated with Mercury Emissions Reductions from U.S. Power Plants; 04/11/2022 | Harvard Chan C-CHANGE; https://www.hsph.harvard.edu/c-change/news/mercury-emissions-reductions/

[1431] Selin, N.E. Global Biogeochemical Cycling of Mercury: A Review Noelle Eckley Selin. Annu. Rev. Environ. Resour. 2009, 34, 43–63.

[1432] Mondino BJ, Salamon SM, Zaidman GW. Allergic and toxic reactions of soft contact lens wearers. Surv Ophthalmol. 1982 May-Jun;26(6):337-44. http://doi.org10.1016/0039-6257(82)90126-6.

[1433] CDC: Thimerosal and Vaccines; https://www.cdc.gov/vaccinesafety/concerns/thimerosal/index.html

[1434] shimadzu-: Mercury in your eye; https://www.shimadzu-webapp.eu/magazine/issue-2011-1_en/mercury-in-your-eye/

[1435] Swiss Medical detox: PUBLICATIONS; 18 January 2019; Environmental diseases The chelation, an indispensable therapy with a future; http://www.swissmedicaldetox.ch/en/publications-2/

[1436] Justin McCurry 2006: Japan remembers Minamata Lancet: WORLD REPORT| VOLUME 367, ISSUE 9505, P99-100, JANUARY 14, 2006 https://doi.org/10.1016/S0140-6736(06)67944-0

[1437] Houston MC. The role of mercury and cadmium heavy metals in vascular disease, hypertension, coronary heart disease, and myocardial infarction. Altern Ther Health Med. 2007 Mar-Apr;13(2):S128-33. https://pubmed.ncbi.nlm.nih.gov/17405690/

[1438] World Health Organization. Mercury in Health Care: Policy Paper. Geneva, Switzerland; August 2005. Available from WHO Web site: Accessed December 22, 2015. http://www.who.int/water_sanitation_health/medicalwaste/mercurypolpaper.pdf.

[1439] Houston MC. The role of mercury and cadmium heavy metals in vascular disease, hypertension, coronary heart disease, and myocardial infarction. Altern Ther Health Med. 2007 Mar-Apr;13(2):S128-33. https://pubmed.ncbi.nlm.nih.gov/17405690/

[1440] Houston MC. 2007: The role of mercury and cadmium heavy metals in vascular disease, hypertension, coronary heart disease, and myocardial infarction. Altern Ther Health Med. 2007 Mar-Apr;13(2):S128-33. https://pubmed.ncbi.nlm.nih.gov/17405690/

[1441] Kern, J. K..et al 2014: Evidence supporting a link between dental amalgams and chronic illness, fatigue, depression, anxiety, and suicide: Neuroendocrinology Letters Volume 35 No. https://pubmed.ncbi.nlm.nih.gov/25617876/

[1442] Rowland IR, Robinson RD, Doherty RA. Effect of diet on mercury metabolism and excretion in mice given methylmercury: role of gut flora. Arch Env Health. 1984;39:401–408. https://pubmed.ncbi.nlm.nih.gov/6524959/

[1443] Marina Robas, et al 2021:Mercury and Antibiotic Resistance Co-Selection in Bacillus sp. Isolates from the Almadén Mining District; Int J Environ Res Public Health. 2021 Aug; 18(16): 8304. . http://doi.org/10.3390/ijerph18168304

[1444] Ask, K.; Åkesson, A.; Berglund, M.; Vahter, M. Inorganic mercury and methylmercury in placentas of Swedish women. Environ. Health Perspect. 2002, 110, https://www.jstor.org/stable/3455340

[1445] Kern, Janet & Geier, David & Bjorklund, et al (2014). Evidence supporting a link between dental amalgams and chronic illness, fatigue, depression, anxiety, and suicide. Neuro endocrinology letters. 35.https://www.researchgate.net/publication/271536688_Evidence_supporting_a_link_between_dental_amalgams_and_chronic_illness_fatigue_depression_anxiety_and_suicide

[1446] Jarup, Lars 2013: Hazards of heavy metal contamination; British Medical Bulletin, Volume 68, Issue 1, December 2003, Pages 167–182, https://doi.org/10.1093/bmb/ldg032

[1447] Houston, M.C. (2011), Role of Mercury Toxicity in Hypertension, Cardiovascular Disease, and Stroke. The Journal of Clinical Hypertension, 13: https://doi.org/10.1111/j.1751-7176.2011.00489.x

[1448] Swiss Medical detox: Publications; 18 January 2019; Environmental diseases The chelation, an indispensable therapy with a future; http://www.swissmedicaldetox.ch/en/publications-2/

[1449] Graham N. George Mercury Binding to the Chelation Therapy Agents DMSA and DMPS, and the Rational Design of Custom Chelators for Mercury.; https://www-ssrl.slac.stanford.edu/~george/pickup/hg-chelator.pdf

[1450] EPA; Technical Report ; The Use Of 2,3 Dimercaptopropane Sodium Sulfonate (DMPS) In Mercury Chelation Therapy ; Battistone, GC; Miller, RA; Rubin, M ; 1977 https://hero.epa.gov/hero/index.cfm/reference/details/reference_id/1784943

[1451] Koh AS, Simmons-Willis TA, Pritchard JB, Grassl SM, Ballatori N. Identification of a mechanism by which the methylmercury antidotes N-acetylcysteine and dimercaptopropanesulfonate enhance urinary metal excretion: transport by the renal organic anion transporter-1. Mol Pharm. 2002; https://pubmed.ncbi.nlm.nih.gov/12237339/

[1452] Lindh U, Hudecek R, Danersund A, Eriksson S, Lindvall A (2002). Removal of dental amalgam and other metal alloys supported by antioxidant therapy alleviates symptoms and improves qual- ity of life in patients with amalgam-associated ill health. Neuro Endocrinology Letters 23: https://www.researchgate.net/publication/10975536_Removal_of_dental_amalgam_and_other_metal_alloys_supported_by_antioxidant_therapy_alleviates_symptoms_and_improves_quality_of_life_in_patients_with_amalgam-associated_ill_health

[1453] Parmalee NL, Aschner M. 2017: Metals and Circadian Rhythms. Adv Neurotoxicol. 2017; https://www.ncbi.nlm.nih.gov/pmc/articles/PMC6361389/

[1454] Zheng W, Jiang YM, Zhang Y, Jiang W, Wang X, Cowan DM. Chelation therapy of manganese intoxication with para-aminosalicylic acid (PAS) in Sprague-Dawley rats. Neurotoxicology. 2009 Mar;30(2):240-8 https://doi.org/10.1016/j.neuro.2008.12.007

[1455] RODIER J. Manganese poisoning in Moroccan miners. Br J Ind Med. 1955 Jan;12(1):21-35. https://pubmed.ncbi.nlm.nih.gov/14351643/

[1456] NIH: Manganese; Fact Sheet for Consumers; March 22, 2021https://ods.od.nih.gov/factsheets/Manganese-Consumer/

[1457] ATSDR: Toxicological Profile for Manganese; https://www.atsdr.cdc.gov/toxprofiles/tp151-c2.pdf

[1458] Klos KJ, Chandler M, Kumar N, Ahlskog JE, Josephs KA. Neuropsychological profiles of manganese neurotoxicity. European Journal of Neurology. 2006;13:1139-1141

[1459] Aaseth, Jan O., and Valeria M. Nurchi. 2022. "Chelation Combination—A Strategy to Mitigate the Neurotoxicity of Manganese, Iron, and Copper?" Biomolecules 12, no. 11: 1713. https://doi.org/10.3390/biom12111713

[1460] Aaseth JO, Nurchi VM. Chelation Combination-A Strategy to Mitigate the Neurotoxicity of Manganese, Iron, and Copper? Biomolecules. 2022 Nov 18;12(11):1713. https://pubmed.ncbi.nlm.nih.gov/36421727/

[1461] Zheng W, Jiang YM, Zhang Y, Jiang W, Wang X, Cowan DM. Chelation therapy of manganese intoxication with para-aminosalicylic acid (PAS) in Sprague-Dawley rats. Neurotoxicology. 2009 Mar https://www.ncbi.nlm.nih.gov/pmc/articles/PMC2677987/

[1462] NIH National Institutes of Health: Molybdenum, Fact Sheet for Consumers; https://ods.od.nih.gov/factsheets/Molybdenum-Consumer/

[1463] Ellithorpe, Rita & Jimenez,et al (2009). Calcium disodium EDTA chelation suppositories: A novel approach for removing heavy metal toxins in clinical practice. January 2009; In book: Anti-Aging Therapeutics (pp.107-118) Chapter: 14; American Academy of Anti-Aging Medicine; Editors: R. Klatz, R. Goldma https://www.researchgate.net/publication/235923312_Calcium_disodium_EDTA_chelation_suppositories_A_novel_approach_for_removing_heavy_metal_toxins_in_clinical_practice

[1464] Jurgita Šulinskien: Effect of Zinc on the Oxidative Stress Biomarkers in the Brain of Nickel-Treated Mice. Volume 2019 | Article ID 8549727 | Oxidative Medicine and Cellular Longevity/.2019 https://doi.org/10.1155/2019/8549727

[1465] Nickel. IN: Dietary Reference Intakes for Vitamin A, Vitamin K, Arsenic, Boron, Chromium, Copper, Iodine, Iron, Manganese, Molybdenum, Nickel, Silicon, Vanadium, and Copper Archived September 22, 2017, at the Wayback Machine. National Academy Press. 2001, PP. 521–529. https://pubmed.ncbi.nlm.nih.gov/25057538/

[1466] Anke M, Groppel B, Kronemann H, Grün M. Nickel--an essential element. IARC Sci Publ. 1984;(53):339-65. PMID: 6398286. https://pubmed.ncbi.nlm.nih.gov/6398286/

[1467] totalmouthfitness.com: BE AWARE OF THE POTENTIALLY HARMFUL METAL COMPONENTS IN YOUR; DENTAL WORK; By Dr. Paul Wilke, DDS, January 9, 2014; https://www.totalmouthfitness.com/dental-education/toxic-metals/

Notes

[1468] Eggleston DW. Effect of dental amalgam and nickel alloys on T-lymphocytes: preliminary report. J Prosthet Dent. 1984 May; https://pubmed.ncbi.nlm.nih.gov/6610046/

[1469] Nielsen NH, Menné T, Kristiansen J, Christensen JM, Borg L, Poulsen LK. Effects of repeated skin exposure to low nickel concentrations: a model for allergic contact dermatitis to nickel on the hands. Br J Dermatol. 1999; https://pubmed.ncbi.nlm.nih.gov/10583115/

[1470] Grimsrud TK, Berge SR, Martinsen JI, Andersen A. 2003: Lung cancer incidence among Norwegian nickel-refinery workers 1953–2000. J Environ Monit. 2003;5:190–7. https://www.researchgate.net/publication/10776490_Lung_cancer_incidence_among_Norwegian_nickel-refinery_workers_1953-2000

[1471] Kim, Hyun Soo, et al 2015: An Overview of Carcinogenic Heavy Metal: Molecular Toxicity Mechanism and Prevention; J Cancer Prev. 2015 Dec; 20(4): 232–240. Published online 2015 Dec 30. https://www.ncbi.nlm.nih.gov/pmc/articles/PMC4699750/

[1472] Public Health England: Nickel Toxicological Overview https://assets.publishing.service.gov.uk/government/uploads/system/uploads/attachment_dMice treated with Niata/file/337433/Nickel_Toxicological_Overview_phe_v1.pdf

[1473] Jurgita Šulinskien: Effect of Zinc on the Oxidative Stress Biomarkers in the Brain of Nickel-Treated Mice. Volume 2019 | Article ID 8549727 | Oxidative Medicine and Cellular Longevity/.2019 https://doi.org/10.1155/2019/8549727

[1474] Benoit, S.L., Schmalstig, A.A., Glushka, J. et al. Nickel chelation therapy as an approach to combat multi-drug resistant enteric pathogens. Sci Rep 9, 13851 (2019). https://doi.org/10.1038/s41598-019-50027-0

[1475] Sunderman FW Sr. Chelation therapy in nickel poisoning. Ann Clin Lab Sci. 1981 Jan-Feb;11(1):1-8.. https://pubmed.ncbi.nlm.nih.gov/6260008/

[1476] AlMomen, Abdulkareem; and Blaurock-Busch, E.; 2022: Alpha-Lipoic Acid (ALA), fatty acid and promising chelating agent for neurological ailments; World Journal of Biological and Pharmaceutical Research, 2022, 03(01), https://doi.org/10.53346/wjbpr.2022.3.1.0038;

[1477] Dr. rer. nat. Eleonore Blaurock-Busch: DMSA – die sanfte und effektive orale Entgiftung; OM & Ernährung 2011 | Nr. 134; DMSA-Artikel-Entgiftung.pdf

[1478] Rengaswamy Gopal, S.2009: Chelating efficacy of CaNa2 EDTA on nickel-induced toxicity in Cirrhinus mrigala (Ham.) through its effects on glutathione peroxidase, reduced glutathione and lipid peroxidation, Comptes Rendus Biologies, Volume 332, Issue 8, 2009, Pp 685-696, https://www.sciencedirect.com/science/article/pii/S1631069109000870

[1479] Petr Dusek, Jan Aaseth, Chapter 3 - Diagnosis and Evaluation of Metal Poisonings and Chelation Therapy, Editor(s): Jan Aaseth, Guido Crisponi, Ole Andersen, Chelation Therapy in the Treatment of Metal Intoxication, Academic Press, 2016, Pages 63-83, (https://www.sciencedirect.com/science/article/pii/B9780128030721000031)

[1480] Rundle, Chandler; Jacob, Sharon E..2017: Chelation Therapy for Nickel Allergy. Journal of the Dermatology Nurses' Association 9(1):p 46-49, 1/2 2017 https://journals.lww.com/jdnaonline/Abstract/2017/01000/Chelation_Therapy_for_Nickel_Allergy.13.aspx https://www.medscape.com/viewarticle/753985_7

[1481] Topical and Systemic Therapies for Nickel Allergy; Antonella Tammaro; Alessandra Narcisi; Severino Persechino; Cristiano Caperchi; Anthony Gaspari; Dermatitis. 2011;22(05):251-255. https://www.medscape.com/viewarticle/753985_7

[1482] Michigan Department of Community Health: Osmium Tetroxide; Information for the Public https://www.michigan.gov/-/media/Project/Websites/mdhhs/Folder1/Folder29/mdch-osmium_tetroxide_fs.pdf?rev=8716ae8a59fe4652aa8ef95e4c8ebe5b#:~:text=Acute%2Fshort%2Dterm%3A%20Osmium,ultimately%2C%20death%20at%20high%20concentrations.

[1483] Platinum - Biomonitoring Summary | CDC Centers for Disease Control and Prevention Platinum; CAS No. 7440-06-4: https://www.cdc.gov/biomonitoring/Platinum_BiomonitoringSummary.html

[1484] Staff NP, Cavaletti G, Islam B, Lustberg M, Psimaras D, Tamburin S. Platinum-induced peripheral neurotoxicity: From pathogenesis to treatment. J Peripher Nerv Syst. 2019 Oct;24 Suppl 2(Suppl 2):S26-S39. http://doi.org/10.1111/jns.12335.

[1485] Graziano, Joseph & Jones, Brian & Pisciotto, Patricia. (1981). The effect of heavy metal chelators on the renal accumulation of platinum after cis-dichlorodiammineplatinum(II) administration to the rat. British journal of pharmacology. 73. 649-54. http://doi.org/10.1111/j.1476-5381.1981.tb16800.x.

[1486] Science (directory) Dutch Anti Amalgam Foundation Stichting Amalgaamvrij Nederland IAOMT-protocol for removal of amalgam fillings https://stgvisie.home.xs4all.nl/AMALGAM/EN/SCIENCE/paladium.html

[1487] Wikipedia: Dimethylglyoxime; https://en.wikipedia.org/wiki/Dimethylglyoxime

[1488] Brmi; Therapeutics - Metal Detoxification – Palladium
https://www.biologicalmedicineinstitute.com/palladium
[1489] CDC. cdc.gov/radiation-health/data-research/facts-stats/cigarette- Facts about Cigarette Smoking and Radiation
[1490] Aaseth J, Nurchi VM, Andersen O. Clinical Therapy of Patients Contaminated with Polonium or Plutonium. Curr Med Chem. 2021;28(35):7238-7246.
https://pubmed.ncbi.nlm.nih.gov/33081668/
[1491] AcciDental Blow Up in Medicine: Battle Plan for Your Life (2019);
https://preventionandhealing.com/books/
[1492] Mass.gov: Health effects of Radium radiation exposure; https://www.mass.gov/info-details/health-effects-of-radium-radiation-exposure#:~:text=Exposure%20to%20Radium%20over%20a,bones%20(reduced%20bone%20growth).
[1493] Marcus, Carol S, PhD, MD: Administration Of Decorporation Drugs To Treat Internal Radionuclide Contamination; Medical Emergency Response To Radiologic Incidents;
http://rdcms-snmmi.s3.amazonaws.com/files/production/public/docs/DMAT-Adm%20Decorp%20Drugs%20Int%20Rad%20Contam%2012-01-0311.pdf
[1494] lenntech.com Rhodium – Rh; Chemical properties of rhodium - Health effects of rhodium - Environmental effects of rhodium:
https://www.lenntech.com/periodic/elements/rh.htm#:~:text=Health%20effects%20of%20rhodium&text=All%20rhodium%20compounds%20should%20be,granular%20form%2C%20mixed%20with%20air.
[1495] R Razavi DFT Study and Investigation of Desferrioxamine and Deferiprone in Removal of Rhodium and Iron from Biological System: https://www.sid.ir/FileServer/SE/247E20131896.pdf
[1496] Lenntech; Ruthenium – Ru Chemical properties of ruthenium - Health effects of ruthenium - Environmental effects of ruthenium
https://www.lenntech.com/periodic/elements/ru.htm#:~:text=Health%20effects%20of%20rutheniu m,-Ruthenium%20compounds%20are&text=All%20ruthenium%20compounds%20should%20be,vol atile%2C%20and%20to%20be%20avoided.
[1497] Catsch, A 1963: Rare earths and ruthenium: metabolism and removal from the mammalian body; nternational Atomic Energy Agency (IAEA)
https://inis.iaea.org/search/search.aspx?orig_q=RN:44058815
[1498] Healthmatters; Rubidium; https://healthmatters.io/understand-blood-test-results/rubidium#:~:text=Rubidium%20has%20been%20used%20in,enzymes%2C%20and%20h epatic%20lipid%20composition.
[1499] Hardeep Singh Bambra, Mod Mazhar, 2019: Prussian Blue- An Radioactive De-Corporation Agent; International Journal of Trend in Scientific Research and Development (ITSRD) Volume: 3 | Issue: 4 | May-lun 2019 Available Online: www.ijtsrd.com e-ISSN:
https://www.slideshare.net/ijtsrd/prussian-blue-an-radioactive-de-corporation-agent
[1500] Baldwin D. E. 1999: Heavy metal poisoning and its laboratory investigation; Ann Clin Bioc. 1999; http://www.vshp.fi/medserv/klkemi/fi/ohjekirja/liitteet/Raskasmetallimyrkytys.pdf
[1501] Schwermetalle und ihre Wirkung auf die Gesundheit - Dr. Klinghardt 1998; 10:45 min;
https://www.youtube.com/watch?v=N0RgeRq2h2g&t=667s
[1502] Hultman P, Johansson U, Turley SJ, Lindh U, Eneström S, Pollard KM. Adverse immunological effects and autoimmunity induced by dental amalgam and alloy in mice. FASEB J. 1994 Nov;8(14):1183-90.. https://pubmed.ncbi.nlm.nih.gov/7958626/
[1503] Havarinasab S, Pollard KM, Hultman P. Gold- and silver-induced murine autoimmunity--requirement for cytokines and CD28 in murine heavy metal-induced autoimmunity. Clin Exp Immunol. 2009 Mar;155(3):567-76.. https://doi.org/10.1111/j.1365-2249.2008.03831.x
[1504] Korani, Mitra, Ghazizadeh, Elham, Korani, Shahla, Hami, Zahra and Mohammadi-Bardbori, Afshin. "Effects of silver nanoparticles on human health" European Journal of Nanomedicine, vol. 7, no. 1, 2015, pp. 51-62. https://doi.org/10.1515/ejnm-2014-0032
[1505] Gonzalez-Carter, D., Leo, B., Ruenraroengsak, P. et al. 2017: Silver nanoparticles reduce brain inflammation and related neurotoxicity through induction of H2S-synthesizing enzymes. Sci Rep 7, 42871 (2017). https://doi.org/10.1038/srep42871
[1506] Korani, Mitra, Ghazizadeh, Elham, Korani, Shahla, Hami, Zahra and Mohammadi-Bardbori, Afshin. "Effects of silver nanoparticles on human health" European Journal of Nanomedicine, vol. 7, no. 1, 2015, pp. 51-62. https://doi.org/10.1515/ejnm-2014-0032
[1507] William J. Trickler, et al 2010: Silver Nanoparticle Induced Blood-Brain Barrier Inflammation and Increased Permeability in Primary Rat Brain Microvessel Endothelial Cells, Toxicological Sciences, Volume 118, Issue 1, November 2010, Pages 160–170,
https://doi.org/10.1093/toxsci/kfq244

Notes

[1508] Havarinasab S, Johansson U, Pollard KM, Hultman P. Gold causes genetically determined autoimmune and immunostimulatory responses in mice. Clin Exp Immunol. 2007 Oct;150(1). https://pubmed.ncbi.nlm.nih.gov/17680821/

[1509] Korani, Mitra, Ghazizadeh, Elham, Korani, Shahla, Hami, Zahra and Mohammadi-Bardbori, Afshin. "Effects of silver nanoparticles on human health" European Journal of Nanomedicine, vol. 7, no. 1, 2015, pp. 51-62. https://doi.org/10.1515/ejnm-2014-0032

[1510] PAMELA L. DRAKE, KYLE J. HAZELWOOD, Exposure-Related Health Effects of Silver and Silver Compounds: A Review, The Annals of Occupational Hygiene, Volume 49, Issue 7, October 2005, Pages 575–585, https://doi.org/10.1093/annhyg/mei019

[1511] Aaseth, J., Halse, J. and Falch, J. (1986), CHELATION OF SILVER IN ARGYRIA. Acta Pharmacologica et Toxicologica, Volume 59, Issues 7 December 1986; https://onlinelibrary.wiley.com/doi/abs/10.1111/j.1600-0773.1986.tb02805.x

[1512] Heavy Metal Poisoning; Last updated: March 28, 2008; https://rarediseases.org/rare-diseases/heavy-metal-poisoning/

[1513] Sears, M.E. et al 2013: Chelation: Harnessing and Enhancing Heavy Metal Detoxification—A Review; The Scientific World Journal; Hindawi.com https://www.hindawi.com/journals/tswj/2013/219840/tab1/

[1514] Chelat-Substanzen und Ihre Bindungen ; Seegarten Klinik AG Kilchberg ZH Switzerland - Copyright 2023 https://sgk.swiss/chelat-substanzen.html

[1515] Grzelak A,et al: Crucial role of chelatable iron in silver nanoparticles induced DNA damage and cytotoxicity. Redox Biol. 2018 http://doi.org/10.1016/j.redox.2018.01.006.

[1516] Ku, HH., Lin, P. & Ling, MP. Assessment of potential human health risks in aquatic products based on the heavy metal hazard decision tree. BMC Bioinformatics 22 (Suppl 5), 620 (2021). https://doi.org/10.1186/s12859-022-04603-3

[1517] Ortega A, Gómez M, Domingo JL, Corbella J. The removal of strontium from the mouse by chelating agents. Arch Environ Contam Toxicol. 1989 Jul-Aug;18(4) http://doi.org/10.1007/BF01055029.

[1518] Fukuda S. et al Removal of strontium by the chelating agent acetylamino propylidene diphosphonic acid in rats. H. Phys. 1999 http://doi.org/10.1097/00004032-199905000-00004.

[1519] Hardeep Singh Bambra, Mod Mazhar, 2019: Prussian Blue- An Radioactive De-Corporation Agent; International Journal of Trend in Scientific Research and Development (ITSRD) Volume: 3 | Issue: 4 | May-Iun 2019 Available Online: www.ijtsrd.com e-ISSN: https://www.slideshare.net/ijtsrd/prussian-blue-an-radioactive-de-corporation-agent

[1520] Aik Doulgeridou et al 2020: Review of Potentially Toxic Rare Earth Elements, Thallium and Tellurium in Plant-based Foods; efsa Journal; 26 November 2020; Volume 18, Issue S1; https://doi.org/10.2903/j.efsa.2020.e181101

[1521] Mark C. Yarema, Steven C. Curry; Acute Tellurium Toxicity From Ingestion of Metal-Oxidizing Solutions. Pediatrics August 2005; 116 (2): e319–e321. 10.1542/peds.2005-0172 https://publications.aap.org/pediatrics/article-abstract/116/2/e319/62918/Acute-Tellurium-Toxicity-From-Ingestion-of-Metal?redirectedFrom=fulltext

[1522] Ferrero, Maria Elena 2016: Rationale for the Successful Management of EDTA Chelation Therapy in Human Burden by Toxic Metals; Hindawi; V. 2016 https://doi.org/10.1155/2016/8274504https://www.hindawi.com/journals/bmri/2016/8274504/

[1523] How Linus Pauling almost gave Matt Meselson tellurium breath; By Wavefunction on Thursday, June 11, 2015; http://wavefunction.fieldofscience.com/2015/06/how-linus-pauling-almost-gave-matt.html

[1524] Mark C. Yarema, Steven C. Curry; Acute Tellurium Toxicity From Ingestion of Metal-Oxidizing Solutions. Pediatrics August 2005; 116 (2): https://publications.aap.org/pediatrics/article-abstract/116/2/e319/62918/Acute-Tellurium-Toxicity-From-Ingestion-of-Metal?redirectedFrom=fulltext

[1525] Genchi, Giuseppe, Alessia Carocci, et al. 2021. "Thallium Use, Toxicity, and Detoxification Therapy: An Overview" Applied Sciences 11, no. 18: 8322. https://doi.org/10.3390/app11188322

[1526] CHEMNOTE: THALLIUM POISONING https://www.chemsee.com/commercial/food-poisons/resources/chemnotes-food-poison-detection/thallium-poisoning-chemnote/

[1527] Metametrix 2011; ELEMENTS; INTERPRETIVE GUIDE BLOOD, HAIR & URINE; https://www.gdx.net/uk/core-uk/interpretive-guides-uk/Elements-IG.pdf

[1528] Medscape; Dec 12, 2021 ;Author: David Vearrier, MD https://emedicine.medscape.com/article/821465-overview

[1529] Y. Luo, Z. Weng, Y. Lin, B. Han, X. Ou, Y. Zhou and J. Jiang, 2022: Coordination/cation exchangeable dual sites intercalated multilayered T3C2Tx MXene for selective and ultrafast removal of thallium(I) from water Environ. Sci.: Nano, 2022, 9, https://pubs.rsc.org/en/content/articlelanding/2022/en/d2en00392a

[1530] CDC; National Biomonitoring Program; Thallium; CAS No. 7440-28-0;
https://www.cdc.gov/biomonitoring/Thallium_BiomonitoringSummary.html
[1531] Safe work Australia: Health monitoring; Guide for thallium;
https://www.safeworkaustralia.gov.au/system/files/documents/2002/health_monitoring_guidance_-_thallium.pdf
[1532] Francesco Esposito, et al 2018: A systematic risk characterization related to the dietary exposure of the population to potentially toxic elements through the ingestion of fruit and vegetables from a potentially contaminated area. A case study: The issue of the "Land of Fires" area in Campania region, Italy, Environmental Pollution, V. 243, Part B, 2018,
https://www.sciencedirect.com/science/article/abs/pii/S0269749118322668
[1533] Campanella B, et al 2019: Toxicity of Thallium at Low Doses: A Review. Int J Environ Res Public Health. 2019 Nov 27; https://www.ncbi.nlm.nih.gov/pmc/articles/PMC6926957/
[1534] Mitochondria as a Key Intracellular Target of Thallium Toxicity; Sergey Korotkov Academic Press, 1 Jun 2022 https://shop.elsevier.com/books/mitochondria-as-a-key-intracellular-target-of-thallium-toxicity/korotkov/978-0-323-95531-7
[1535] MedScaoe Thallium Toxicity, 2021; Author: David Vearrier,
https://emedicine.medscape.com/article/821465-overview?form=fpf
[1536] Toxicology and Iatrogenic Disorders; Thallium Poisoning; Symptoms, Treatment, Prognosis; by Dr Hayley Willacy; 27 Oct 2021; https://patient.info/doctor/thallium-poisoning#:~:text=Thallium%20poisoning%20prognosis,-Of%20those%20who&text=Delay%20in%20receiving%20treatment%20is,the%20feet%20and%20lower%20extremities.
[1537] Liu H, Liao G. Long-term misdiagnosis and neurologic outcomes of thallium poisoning: A case report and literature review. Brain Behav. 2021 Mar;11(3):e02032. doi: 10.1002/brb3.2032.
https://www.ncbi.nlm.nih.gov/pmc/articles/PMC7994691/
[1538] de Carvalho Machado C, Dinis-Oliveira RJ. Clinical and Forensic Signs Resulting from Exposure to Heavy Metals and Other Chemical Elements of the Periodic Table. J Clin Med. 2023 Mar 29;12(7):2591. https://www.ncbi.nlm.nih.gov/pmc/articles/PMC10095087/
[1539] Daniel E. Rusyniak, CHAPTER 24 - Thallium, Editor(s): MICHAEL R. DOBBS, Clinical Neurotoxicology, W.B. Saunders, 2009
https://www.sciencedirect.com/science/article/pii/B9780323052603500307
[1540] Staff NP, Windebank AJ. Peripheral neuropathy due to vitamin deficiency, toxins, and medications. Continuum (Minneap Minn). 2014 Oct;20(5 Peripheral Nervous System Disorders):1293-306. http://doi/org10.1212/01.CON.0000455880.06675.5a.
[1541] Ku, HH., Lin, P. & Ling, MP. Assessment of potential human health risks in aquatic products based on the heavy metal hazard decision tree. BMC Bioinformatics 22 (Suppl 5), 620 (2021).
https://doi.org/10.1186/s12859-022-04603-3
[1542] Guifang Yang, et al 2018: Hair Loss: Evidence to Thallium Poisoning; Case Reports in Emergency Medicine; Volume 2018 (2018), Article ID 1313096, 3 pages
https://doi.org/10.1155/2018/1313096
[1543] Hanzel CE, Verstraeten SV. 2006 Thallium induces hydrogen peroxide generation by impairing mitochondrial function. Toxicol Appl Pharmacol. 2006 Nov 1;216(3).
https://pubmed.ncbi.nlm.nih.gov/16934846/
[1544] Lansdown AB. Metal ions affecting the skin and eyes. Met Ions Life Sci. 2011;..
https://pubmed.ncbi.nlm.nih.gov/16934846/
[1545] Tjälve, H., Nilsson, M. and Larsson, B. (1982), Thallium-201: Autoradiography in Pigmented Mice and Melanin-binding in Vitro. Acta Pharmacologica et Toxicologica, 51: 147-153.
https://doi.org/10.1111/j.1600-0773.1982.tb01006.x
[1546] Yumoto T, et al. A Successfully Treated Case of Criminal Thallium Poisoning. J Clin Diagn Res. 2017 Apr;11 https://www.ncbi.nlm.nih.gov/pmc/articles/PMC5449837/
[1547] Toxicology and Iatrogenic ; Disorders; Professional Articles Dr Hayley Willacy Thallium Poisoning; Symptoms, Treatment, Prognosis; 27 Oct 2021, https://patient.info/doctor/thallium-poisoning#:~:text=Thallium%20poisoning%20prognosis,-Of%20those%20who&text=Reports%20of%20persistent%20findings%20most,to%20dementia%2C%20depression%20and%20psychosis.
[1548] Mingyang Wu, Lulin Wang, 2020: The association between prenatal exposure to thallium and shortened telomere length of newborns, Chemosphere, V. 265, 2021.
https://www.sciencedirect.com/science/article/pii/S0045653520332227
[1549] Genchi, Giuseppe, Alessia Carocci, Graziantonio Lauria, Maria Stefania Sinicropi, and Alessia Catalano. 2021. "Thallium Use, Toxicity, and Detoxification Therapy: An Overview" Applied Sciences 11, no. 18: 8322. https://doi.org/10.3390/app11188322

Notes

[1550] Genchi, Giuseppe, Alessia Carocci, Graziantonio Lauria, Maria Stefania Sinicropi, and Alessia Catalano. 2021. "Thallium Use, Toxicity, and Detoxification Therapy: An Overview" Applied Sciences 11, no. 18: 8322. https://doi.org/10.3390/app11188322

[1551] Saljooghi AS, et al2016: Chelation of thallium by combining deferasirox and desferrioxamine in rats. Toxicol Ind H. 2016 https://pubmed.ncbi.nlm.nih.gov/24021432/

[1552] Kamerbeek, H.H., et al (1971), Dangerous Redistribution Of Thallium By Treatment With Sodium Diethyldithiocarbamate. Acta Medica Scandinavica, 189: https://doi.org/10.1111/j.0954-6820.1971.tb04356.x

[1553] World Health Organization (2009). Stuart MC, Kouimtzi M, Hill SR (eds.). WHO Model Formulary 2008. World Health Org. p. 65. https://apps.who.int/iris/handle/10665/44053

[1554] Gupta, Ramesh C. 2016: Chapter 47 - Non-Anticoagulant Rodenticides, Editor(s): Ramesh C. Gupta, Veterinary Toxicology (Third Edition), Academic Press, 2018, https://doi.org/10.1016/B978-0-12-811410-0.00047-7.

[1555] EPA Provisional Peer Reviewed Toxicity Values for Prussian Blue (Ferric Ferrocyanide) (CASRN 14038-43-8) EPA/690/R-05/020F Final 11-22-2005 https://cfpub.epa.gov/ncea/pprtv/documents/PrussianBlueFerricFerrocyanide.pdf

[1556] Giacomo Dacarro et al 2018: Prussian Blue Nanoparticles as a Versatile Photothermal Tool; Molecules 2018, 23(6), https://doi.org/10.3390/molecules23061414

[1557] L Doveri, 2023: Prussian Blue nanoparticles: An FDA-approved substance ... ScienceDirect; https://www.sciencedirect.com/science/article/abs/pii/S0927776523002515

[1558] United States patent US8092783B2; Gadolinium containing Prussian blue nanoparticles as nontoxic MRI contrast agents having high relativity. 2009-04-03; Application filed by Kent State Univ.. https://patents.google.com/patent/US8092783B2/en

[1559] Hodorowicz M, Szklarzewicz J, Jurowska A. The Role of Prussian Blue-Thallium and Potassium Similarities and Differences in Crystal Structures of Selected Cyanido Complexes of W, Fe and Mo. Materials (Basel). 2022 Jun 29;15(13):. https://www.ncbi.nlm.nih.gov/pmc/articles/PMC9267926/

[1560] Ole Andersen: A review of pitfalls and progress in chelation treatment of metal poisonings; Journal of Trace Elements in Medicine and Biology Volume 38, December 2016, Pages 74-80 https://doi.org/10.1016/j.jtemb.2016.03.013

[1561] Guido Crisponi, Valeria Marina Nurchi, Chapter 2 - Chelating Agents as Therapeutic Compounds—Basic Principles, Editor(s): Jan Aaseth, Guido Crisponi, Ole Andersen, Chelation Therapy in the Treatment of Metal Intoxication, Academic Press, 2016, https://doi.org/10.1016/B978-0-12-803072-1.00002-X.

[1562] Estelrich J, Busquets MA. Prussian Blue: A Safe Pigment with Zeolitic-Like Activity. Int J Mol Sci. 2021 Jan 15;22(2):780. https://pubmed.ncbi.nlm.nih.gov/33467391/

[1563] Phys.org OCT 2, 2019; A blue pigment found to be a high-performance ammonia adsorbent; https://phys.org/news/2019-10-blue-pigment-high-performance-ammonia-adsorbent.html#google_vignette

[1564] Mohammad, Adil & Yang, Y & Khan, Mansoor & Faustino, Patrick. (2015). Long-term stability study of Prussian blue—A quality assessment of water content and cyanide release. Clinical toxicology (Philadelphia, Pa.). 53. 1-6. https://www.tandfonline.com/doi/full/10.3109/15563650.2014.998337

[1565] Rusyniak, Daniel & Kao,et al (2003). Dimercaptosuccinic Acid and Prussian Blue in the Treatment of Acute Thallium Poisoning in Rats. Journal of toxicology. Clinical toxicology. 41. https://www.researchgate.net/publication/10771493_Dimercaptosuccinic_Acid_and_Prussian_Blue_in_the_Treatment_of_Acute_Thallium_Poisoning_in_Rats

[1566] Genchi, Giuseppe, Alessia Carocci, Graziantonio Lauria, Maria Stefania Sinicropi, and Alessia Catalano. 2021. "Thallium Use, Toxicity, and Detoxification Therapy: An Overview" Applied Sciences 11, no. 18: 8322. https://doi.org/10.3390/app11188322

[1567] Ríos C, Monroy-Noyola A. D-penicillamine and prussian blue as antidotes against thallium intoxication in rats. Toxicology. 1992 https://pubmed.ncbi.nlm.nih.gov/1514189/

[1568] Salehi S, et al 2017: Chelation of Thallium (III) in Rats Using Combined Deferasirox and Deferiprone Therapy. Toxicol Res. 2017 https://www.ncbi.nlm.nih.gov/pmc/articles/PMC5654193/

[1569] Malbrain ML, Lambrecht GL, et al: Treatment of severe thallium intoxication. J Toxicol Clin Toxicol. 1997;35(1):97-100. https://pubmed.ncbi.nlm.nih.gov/9022660/

[1570] Bank WJ, Pleasure DE, Suzuki K, Nigro M, Katz R. Thallium Poisoning. Arch Neurol. 1972; https://jamanetwork.com/journals/jamaneurology/article-abstract/571343

[1571] Feng J. He, et al 2005: Randomized trials have shown that increasing potassium intake lowers blood pressure.; 21 Feb 2005 Hypertension. 2005; https://www.ahajournals.org/doi/10.1161/01.hyp.0000158264.36590.19

[1572] Wikipeedia Natriuresis
https://en.wikipedia.org/wiki/Natriuresis#:~:text=Natriuresis%20is%20the%20process%20of,by%20chemicals%20such%20as%20aldosterone.

[1573] Neal, Bruce; et al 2021: Effect of Salt Substitution on Cardiovascular Events and Death; September 16, 2021 N Engl J Med 2021
https://www.nejm.org/doi/full/10.1056/nejmoa2105675#article_Abstract

[1574] Chaouali N, Gana I,et al 2013: Potential Toxic Levels of Cyanide in Almonds (Prunus amygdalus), Apricot Kernels (Prunus armeniaca), and Almond Syrup. ISRN Toxicol. 2013
https://www.ncbi.nlm.nih.gov/pmc/articles/PMC3793392/

[1575] Mohammad, Adil; et al 2015:   Long-term stability study of Prussian blue—A quality assessment of water content and cyanide release; Clinical Toxicology (2015), 53, 102–107
https://www.researchgate.net/publication/271222354

[1576] https://www.kremer-pigmente.com/elements/resources/products/files/45202.pdf

[1577] National Caner; Institute; Thorium: December 8, 2022 https://www.cancer.gov/about-cancer/causes-prevention/risk/substances/thorium#:~:text=And%20there%20is%20research%20evidence,may%20be%20stored%20in%20bone.

[1578] J. Rencová, V. Volf, R. Burgada, Chelation Therapy of Thorium Deposited in Rat Lung, Radiation Protection Dosimetry, Volume 79, Issue 1-4, 1 October 1998, Pages 459–462,
https://doi.org/10.1093/oxfordjournals.rpd.a032449

[1579] Nord rarediseases.org: Heavy Metal Poisoning;: March 28, 2008;
https://rarediseases.org/rare-diseases/heavy-metal-poisoning/

[1580] Chelation Medical Center; Ray Psonak, D.O. Toxic Heavy Metals;
https://www.chelationmedicalcenter.com/toxic-heavy-metals.html

[1581] Winship KA. Toxicity of tin and its compounds. Adverse Drug React Acute Poisoning Rev. 1988 Spring;7(1):19-38.. https://pubmed.ncbi.nlm.nih.gov/3291572/

[1582] Ksenia S. Egorova et al 2017: Toxicity of Metal Compounds: Knowledge and Myths; Organometallics 2017 https://doi.org/10.1021/acs.organomet.7b00605

[1583] Ashok Kumar Jaiswal, et al. 2019: TIN Toxicity with Analytical Aspects and its Management. International Journal of Forensic Science. 2019;
https://www.rfppl.co.in/subscription/upload_pdf/Ashok%20Kumar%20Jaiswal%207_10171.pdf

[1584] Stephen A. Lawrence 2018 : Toxicity from Metal Hip Implants; January 17,
https://www.wellnessdentalcare.com/1935/toxicity-metal-hip-implants/

[1585] Kim KT, Eo MY, Nguyen TTH, Kim SM. General review of titanium toxicity. Int J Implant Dent. 2019 Mar 11 https://www.ncbi.nlm.nih.gov/pmc/articles/PMC6409289/ .

[1586] Sandip P. Tarpada, Jeremy Loloi, Evan M. Schwechter, A Case of Titanium Pseudotumor and Systemic Toxicity After Total Hip Arthroplasty Polyethylene Failure, Arthroplasty Today, Volume 6, Issue 4, 2020, https://doi.org/10.1016/j.artd.2020.07.033.

[1587] American Heart Association News: Low-level toxic metal exposure may raise the risk for clogged arteries; Published: December 9, 2021; https://www.heart.org/en/news/2021/12/09/low-level-toxic-metal-exposure-may-raise-the-risk-for-clogged-arteries

[1588] Stephen A. Lawrence 2018 : Toxicity from Metal Hip Implants; January 17,
https://www.wellnessdentalcare.com/1935/toxicity-metal-hip-implants/

[1589] Toxicology: investigating environmental drivers of disease.; NMPhA Annual Convention; June 12th, 2022; Dr. Alicia Bolt; University of New Mexico Col. of Pharmacy;
https://www.nmpharmacy.org/resources/Convention%202022/Bolt_Toxicology_NMPhA_Presentation_June2022.pdf

[1590] Ferrero, Maria Elena 2016: Rationale for the Successful Management of EDTA Chelation Therapy in Human Burden by Toxic Metals; Hindawi; Volume 2016
https://doi.org/10.1155/2016/8274504https://www.hindawi.com/journals/bmri/2016/8274504/

[1591] VanderSchee, C.R., Kuter, D., Bolt, A.M. et al. Accumulation of persistent tungsten in bone as in situ generated polytungstate. Commun Chem 1, 8 (2018). https://doi.org/10.1038/s42004-017-0007-6

[1592] Alicia M. Bolt, Chapter Five - Tungsten toxicity and carcinogenesis, Editor(s): Max Costa, Advances in Pharmacology, Academic Press, Volume 96, 2023, Pages 119-150,
https://doi.org/10.1016/bs.apha.2022.10.004.

[1593] Shah Idil, Ahmad & Donaldson, Nick. (2018). The use of tungsten as a chronically implanted material. J. of Neural Engin. 15. http://doi.org/10.1088/1741-2552/aaa502.

[1594] Chelation Medical Center; Ray Psonak, D.O. Toxic Heavy Metals;
https://www.chelationmedicalcenter.com/toxic-heavy-metals.html

[1595] Avila, Maria D.; Escolar, Esteban; Lamas, Gervasio A.. Chelation therapy after the Trial to Assess Chelation Therapy: results of a unique trial. Current Opinion in Cardiology 29(5):p 481-

Notes

488, September 2014. https://journals.lww.com/co-cardiology/fulltext/2014/09000/chelation_therapy_after_the_trial_to_assess.13.aspx

[1596] Fulgenzi A, Vietti D, Ferrero ME. 2020: EDTA Chelation Therapy in the Treatment of Neurodegenerative Diseases: An Update. Biomedicines. 2020 https://pubmed.ncbi.nlm.nih.gov/32756375/

[1597] Whish SR, Mayer LP, et al Uranium is an estrogen mimic and causes changes in female mouse reproductive tissues. The Endocrine Society 87th Annual Meeting 2005; Abstract P2-261.

[1598] Dyer, C. A., 2007; Heavy Metals as Endocrine-Disrupting Chemicals; 2007/01/01; 111; Endocrine-Disrupting Chemicals: From Basic Science to Clinical Practice http://eknygos.lsmuni.lt/springer/631/111-133.pdf

[1599] Anees A. Al-Hamzawi et al 2020 In vitro detection of urinary uranium of healthy subjects in Babylon governorate, Iraq; J. Phys.: Conf. Ser. 1591 https://iopscience.iop.org/article/10.1088/1742-6596/1591/1/012011/pdf

[1600] Paquet F, et al 2006: Accumulation and distribution of uranium in rats after chronic exposure by ingestion. H. Phys. 2006 http://doi.crg/10.1097/01.hp.0000174527.66111.83

[1601] Lawrence, G., Patel, K. & Nusbaum, A. (2014). Uranium toxicity and chelation therapy. Pure and Applied Chemistry, 86(7), https://doi.org/10.1515/pac-2014-0109

[1602] Lawrence, G., Patel, K. & Nusbaum, A. (2014). Uranium toxicity and chelation therapy. Pure and Applied Chemistry, 86(7). https://doi.org/10.1515/pac-2014-0109

[1603] Hardeep Singh Bambra, Mod Mazhar, 2019: Prussian Blue- An Radioactive De-Corporation Agent; International Journal of Trend in Scientific Research and Development (ITSRD) Volume: 3 | Issue: 4 | May-Jun 2019 Available Online: www.ijtsrd.com e-ISSN: https://www.slideshare.net/ijtsrd/prussian-blue-an-radioactive-de-corporation-agent

[1604] Ohmachi Y, Imamura T, et al: Sodium bicarbonate protects uranium-induced acute nephrotoxicity through uranium-decorporation by urinary alkalinization in rats. J Toxicol Pathol. 2015 http://doi.org/10.1293/tox.2014-0041.

[1605] Beatriz Martínez, A., Bettina Bozal, C., Soledad Orona, N., Ruth Tasat, D., & Matilde Ubios, A. (2020). Bisphosphonates as Chelating Agents in Uranium Poisoning. IntechOpen. http://doi.org/10.5772/intechopen.92220

[1606] Beatriz Martínez, A., Bettina Bozal, C., et al: (2020). Bisphosphonates as Chelating Agents in Uranium Poisoning. Intech Open. http://doi.org/10.5772/intechopen.92220

[1607] Uehara A, Matsumura D,et al: Uranium chelating ability of decorporation agents in serum evaluated by X-ray absorption spectroscopy. Anal Methods. 2022 Jun 23;14(24). https://pubmed.ncbi.nlm.nih.gov/35694955/

[1608] Lawrence, Glen D., Patel, Kamalkumar S. and Nusbaum, Aviva. "Uranium toxicity and chelation therapy" Pure and Applied Chemistry, vol. 86, no. 7, 2014, pp. 1105-1110. https://doi.org/10.1515/pac-2014-0109

[1609] Elmileegy IMH, et al: Gallic acid rescues uranyl acetate induced-hepatic dysfunction in rats by its antioxidant and cytoprotective potentials. BMC Complement Med Ther. 2023 http://doi.org/10.1186/s12906-023-04250-y.

[1610] Bhuia, Md.Shimul et al 2023Neurobiological Effects of gallic acid: current perspectives. Chinese Medicine 18; https:/doi.org/10.1186/s13020-023-00735-7

[1611] Kim JS, Cho EW, Chung HW, Kim IG. Effects of Tiron, 4,5-dihydroxy-1,3-benzene disulfonic acid, on human promyelotic HL-60 leukemia cell differentiation and death. Toxicology. 2006 Jun 1;223(1-2):36-45. http://doi.org/10.1016/j.tox.2006.03.004.

[1612] Wilk A, Szypulska-Koziarska D: The toxicity of vanadium on gastrointestinal, urinary and reproductive system, and its influence on fertility and fetuses malformations. Postepy Hig Med Dosw (Online). 2017 Sep 25;71(0) https://pubmed.ncbi.nlm.nih.gov/29039350/

[1613] Fredrick, Randi, Ph.D; Chelation Therapy and Mental HealthMentalhelp.net; https://www.mentalhelp.net/blogs/chelation-therapy-and-mental-health/

[1614] Wilk A, Szypulska-Koziarska et al 2017: The toxicity of vanadium on gastrointestinal, urinary and reproductive system, and its influence on fertility and fetuses malformations. Postepy Hig Med Dosw (Online). 2017 Sep 25 https://pubmed.ncbi.nlm.nih.gov/29039350/

[1615] Shrivastava S, Jadon A, et al Chelation therapy and vanadium: effect on reproductive organs in rats. Indian J Exp Biol. 2007 Jun; https://pubmed.ncbi.nlm.nih.gov/17585685/

[1616] Shrivastava S, Jadon A, Shukla S, Mathur R. Chelation therapy and vanadium: effect on reproductive organs in rats. Indian J Exp Biol. 2007 Jun;45(6):515-23.

[1617] Fredrick, Randi, Ph.D; Chelation Therapy and Mental HealthMentalhelp.net; https://www.mentalhelp.net/blogs/chelation-therapy-and-mental-health/

[1618] Fosmire GJ. Zinc toxicity. Am J Clin Nutr. 1990. https://pubmed.ncbi.nlm.nih.gov/2407097/

[1619] Ku, HH., Lin, P. & Ling, MP. Assessment of potential human health risks in aquatic products based on the heavy metal hazard decision tree. BMC Bioinformatics 22 (Suppl 5), 620 (2021). https://doi.org/10.1186/s12859-022-04603-3

[1620] Radford RJ, Lippard SJ. Chelators for investigating zinc metalloneurochemistry. Curr Opin Chem Biol. 2013 Apr;17(2) https://www.ncbi.nlm.nih.gov/pmc/articles/PMC3634875/#:~:text=The%20most%20common%20intracellular%20zinc,TPEN)%20(Figure%202).

[1621] Mehri A. Trace Elements in Human Nutrition (II) - An Update. Int J Prev Med. 2020 Jan 3;11:2. https://www.ncbi.nlm.nih.gov/pmc/articles/PMC6993532/

[1622] Pizzorno L. Nothing Boring About Boron. Integr Med (Encinitas). 2015 Aug;14(4):35-48. https://www.ncbi.nlm.nih.gov/pmc/articles/PMC4712861/ .

[1623] Healthline: Can Boron Boost Testosterone Levels or Treat ED? By Tim Jewell on October 11, 2019 https://www.healthline.com/health/boron-testosterone

[1624] Turkez H, Geyikoglu F, Tatar A, Keles MS, Kaplan I. The effects of some boron compounds against heavy metal toxicity in human blood. Exp Toxicol Pathol. 2012 Jan;64 (1-2):93-101. https://pubmed.ncbi.nlm.nih.gov/20663653/

[1625] NIH: Boron; Fact Sheet for Health Professionals; June 9, 2022 https://ods.od.nih.gov/factsheets/Boron-HealthProfessional/

[1626] W. Banner, et al 1986: Experimental chelation therapy in chromium, lead, and boron intoxication with N acetylcysteine and other compounds, Toxicology and Applied Pharmacology, Volume 83, Issue 1, 1986 https://doi.org/10.1016/0041-008X(86)90331-5.

[1627] Nonaka S, Hough CJ, Chuang DM. Chronic lithium treatment robustly protects neurons in the central nervous system against excitotoxicity by inhibiting N-methyl-D-aspartate receptor-mediated calcium influx. Proc Natl Acad Sci U S A. 1998 Mar 3;95(5):2642-7. https://www.ncbi.nlm.nih.gov/pmc/articles/PMC19446/

[1628] Institute Of Mineral Research; Life Sciences - Health & Wellness; Lithium as a Nutrient; Timothy M. Marshall, Ph.D.; https://instituteofmineralresearch.org/lithium-as-a-nutrient-2/

[1629] psychcentral.com Can Lithium Help Treat Schizophrenia? https://psychcentral.com/schizophrenia/lithium-for-schizophrenia

[1630] Schrauzer GN, Shrestha KP, Flores-Arce MF. Lithium in scalp hair of adults, students, and violent criminals. Effects of supplementation and evidence for interactions of lithium with vitamin B12 and with other trace elements. Biol Trace Elem Res 1992; Aug;34(2):161-76.

[1631] Schrauzer GN, de Vroey E.1994: Effects of nutritional lithium supplementation on mood,A. placebo-controlled study with former drug users. Biol Trace Elem Res 1994; 40(1):89- 101.

[1632] Schrauzer GN, Shrestha KP. Lithium in drinking water and the incidences of crimes, suicides, and arrests related to drug addictions. Biol Trace Elem Res 1990 May;25(2):105-13

[1633] Sugawara N, Yasui-Furukori N, Ishii N, Iwata N, Terao T. Lithium in tap water and suicide mortality in Japan. Int J Environ Res Public Health. 2013 Nov 12;10(11):6044-8. https://www.ncbi.nlm.nih.gov/pmc/articles/PMC3863886/#:~:text=After%20adjusting%20for%20confounders%2C%20a,risk%20of%20suicide%20among%20females.

[1634] VICE news: By Max Daly; August 5, 2020: https://www.vice.com/en/article/akzyeb/link-between-lithium-in-drinking-water-study

[1635] Jared Ng, Manne Sjöstrand & Nir Eyal, 2011: Adding Lithium to Drinking Water for Suicide Prevention—The Ethics; Public Health Ethics 12 (3):274-286 (2019); https://gwern.net/doc/psychiatry/lithium/2019-ng.pdf

[1636] Erden A, Karagöz H, et al 2013: intoxication and nephrogenic diabetes insipidus: a case report and review of literature. Int J Gen Med. 2013 Jul 3;6:535-9. doi: 10.2147/IJGM.S46383. https://pubmed.ncbi.nlm.nih.gov/23861592/

[1637] Pingchuan Zhang et al 2022: Lithium-induced nephropathy; One medication with multiple side effects: a case report; BMC Nephrology (2022) 23:309 https://doi.org/10.1186/s12882-022-02934-0 https://bmcnephrol.biomedcentral.com/counter/pdf/10.1186/s12882-022-02934-0.pdf

[1638] Haussmann, R., Bauer, M., von Bonin, S. et al. Treatment of lithium intoxication: facing the need for evidence. Int J Bipolar Disord 3, 23 (2015). https://doi.org/10.1186/s40345-015-0040-2 https://journalbipolardisorders.springeropen.com/articles/10.1186/s40345-015-0040-2

[1639] Haussmann, R., Bauer, M., von Bonin, S. et al. Treatment of lithium intoxication: facing the need for evidence. Int J Bipolar Disord 3, 23 (2015). https://doi.org/10.1186/s40345-015-0040-2

[1640] Korani, Mitra, Ghazizadeh, Elham, Korani, Shahla, Hami, Zahra and Mohammadi-Bardbori, Afshin. "Effects of silver nanoparticles on human health" European Journal of Nanomedicine, vol. 7, no. 1, 2015, pp. 51-62. https://doi.org/10.1515/ejnm-2014-0032

[1641] Abd-Elhakim,Y. et al 2021: Effects of Co-Exposure of Nanoparticles and Metals on Different Organisms: A Rev.Tox https://www.ncbi.nlm.nih.gov/pmc/articles/PMC8623643/

[1642] Zhiyong Liu et al 2023: Anionic nanoplastic contaminants promote Parkinson's disease–associated α-synuclein aggregation SCIENCE ADVANCES; VOL. 9, NO. 46; https://www.science.org/doi/10.1126/sciadv.adi8716

Notes

[1643] Working Group for COVID Vaccine Analysis; SUMMARY OF PRELIMINARY FINDINGS; 06.07.2022; https://www.documentcloud.org/documents/22140176-report-from-working-group-of-vaccine-analysis-in-germany

[1644] Ou, L., Song, B., Liang, H. et al. Toxicity of graphene-family nanoparticles: a general review of the origins and mechanisms. Part Fibre Toxicol 13, 57 (2016). https://doi.org/10.1186/s12989-016-0168-y

[1645] Amrollahi-Sharifabadi, Mohammad et al. "In vivo toxicological evaluation of graphene oxide nanoplatelets for clinical application." International journal of nanomedicine vol. 13 4757-4769. 22 Aug. 2018, http://doi.org/10.2147/IJN.S168731

[1646] Perini, Giordano et al. "Unravelling the Potential of Graphene Quantum Dots in Biomedicine and Neuroscience." International journal of molecular sciences vol. 21,10 3712. 25 May. 2020, http://doi.org/10.3390/ijms21103712.

[1647] Baojin Ma, Shi Guo, et al2021: Reaction between Graphene Oxide and Intracellular Glutathione Affects Cell Viability and Proliferation; ACS Appl. Mater. Interfaces 2021, 13, 3, https://doi.org/10.1021/acsami.0c17523

[1648] Gurunathan S, Arsalan Iqbal M, Qasim M, Park CH, Yoo H, Hwang JH, Uhm SJ, Song H, Park C, Do JT, Choi Y, Kim JH, Hong K. Evaluation of Graphene Oxide Induced Cellular Toxicity and Transcriptome Analysis in Human Embryonic Kidney Cells. Nanomaterials (Basel). 2019 Jul 2;9(7):969. https://pubmed.ncbi.nlm.nih.gov/31269699/

[1649] Shaobin Liu et al 2011: Antibacterial Activity of Graphite, Graphite Oxide, Graphene Oxide, and Reduced Graphene Oxide: Membrane and Oxidative Stress ACS Nano 2011, 5, 9, 6971–6980; https://doi.org/10.1021/nn202451x

[1650] Iczak, Katarzyna, Witold Jakubowski, and Witold Szymański. 2023. "Bactericidal Activity of Graphene Oxide Tests for Selected Microorganisms" Materials 16, no. 11: 4199. https://doi.org/10.3390/ma16114199

[1651] Senthil Kumar Kandasamy, Chapter 8 - Graphene oxide, Editor(s): Yarub Al-Douri, In Woodhead Publishing Series in Electronic and Optical Materials, Graphene, Nanotubes and Quantum Dots-Based Nanotechnology, Woodhead Publishing, 2022, https://doi.org/10.1016/B978-0-323-85457-3.00024-4.

[1652] Shilpent;: How to remove graphene oxide from the body? November 5, 2022 By Shilpent; https://blog.shilpent.com/how-to-remove-graphene-oxide-from-the-body/

[1653] IV Drip Bali; Copyright ©2024 https://ivdripsbali.com/vita-spike/

[1654] Valentina Palmieri et al Biocompatible N-acetyl cysteine reduces graphene oxide and persists at the surface as a green radical scavenger; Chemical communications: ssue 29, 2019; https://doi.org/10.1039/C9CC00429G

[1655] Schwalfenberg Gerry K.2021: N-Acetylcysteine: A Review of Clinical Usefulness (an Old Drug with New Tricks) Journal of Nutrition and Metabolism, Volume 2021; https://doi.org/10.1155/2021/9949453

[1656] Zhang M, Hou C, Halder A, Ulstrup J, Chi Q. Interlocked graphene-Prussian blue hybrid composites enable multifunctional electrochemical applications. Biosens Bioelectron. 2017 Mar 15;89(Pt 1 https://daneshyari.com/article/preview/5031724.pdf

[1657] Xiao-Wang Liu, et al 2010: Graphene oxide sheet–prussian blue nanocomposites: Green synthesis and their extraordinary electrochemical properties, Colloids and Surfaces B: Biointerfaces, Vol 81,2, 2010, https://doi.org/10.1016/j.colsurfb.2010.07.049.

[1658] Yuan X, Peng D, Jing Q, Niu J, Cheng X, Feng Z, Wu X. Green and Effective Removal of Aqueous Graphene Oxide under UV-Light Irradiation. Nanomaterials (Basel). 2018 Aug 24;8(9):654. http://doi.org/10.3390/nano8090654.

[1659] Nanogrfi.com https://nanografi.com/blog/what-is-the-difference-between-graphene-oxide-and-reduced-graphene-oxide/?utm_term=&utm_campaign=Graphene+%7C+Americas-A+(Test)&utm_source=adwords&utm_medium=ppc&hsa_acc=1992861092&hsa_cam=20567115314&hsa_grp=155336864044&hsa_ad=674540790896&hsa_src=g&hsa_tgt=dsa-1657884057109&hsa_kw=&hsa_mt=&hsa_net=adwords&hsa_ver=3&gad_source=1&gclid=Cjw KCAiA7t6sBhAiEiwAsaieYrDk0m_dnQL_doPEeDtybPQa32BSNdMmSdiFM_sBzmUcvIsNQIqHQ xoC7qUQAvD_BwE

[1660] Chao-Zhi Zhang, Ting Li, et al 2016: An efficient and environment-friendly method of removing graphene oxide in wastewater and its degradation mechanisms, Chemosphere, Volume 153, 2016, https://doi.org/10.1016/j.chemosphere.2016.03.094.

[1661] Marina Kryuchkova and Rawil Fakhrullin, 2018: Kaolin Alleviates Graphene Oxide Toxicity; Environmental Science & Technology Letters 2018 5 (5), 295-300 https://doi.org/10.1021/acs.estlett.8b00135

[1662] Rozhina E, Batasheva S, Danilushkina A, Kryuchkova M, Gomzikova M, Cherednichenko Y, Nigamatzyanova L, Akhatova F, Fakhrullin R. Kaolin alleviates the toxicity of graphene oxide for mammalian cells. Medchemcomm. 2019 Jun https://doi.org/10.1039/C8MD00633D

1663 Smith, Peter 2013: How to detoxify Heavy Metals; –Holistic Medicine Practitioner- (updated 2/2013); Better Mental Health with Natural Remedies https://www.balancingbrainchemistry.co.uk/peter-smith/28/Heavy-Metal-Toxicity-Depression-&-Anxiety.html
1664 Smith, Peter 2013: How to detoxify Heavy Metals; –Holistic Medicine Practitioner- (updated 2/2013); Better Mental Health with Natural Remedies https://www.balancingbrainchemistry.co.uk/peter-smith/28/Heavy-Metal-Toxicity-Depression-&-Anxiety.html
1665 Lichtenstein E. et al, 1976: Letter: Diagonal ear-lobe crease and coronary artery sclerosis. Ann Intern Med. 1976 Sep;85(3) http://doi.org/10.7326/0003-4819-85-3-337.
1666 Apollo Hospitals central cyanosis: 2023: https://www.apollohospitals.com/central-cyanosis/
1667 Prozialeck WC, Edwards JR, et al 2008: The vascular system as a target of metal toxicity. Toxicol Sci. 2008 Apr;102(2):207-18. http://doi.org/10.1093/toxsci/kfm263.
1668 Parizanganeh A, Zamani A, Bijnavand V, Taghilou B. Human nail usage as a Bio-indicator in contamination monitoring of heavy metals in Dizajabaad, Zanjan province-Iran. J Environ Health Sci Eng. 2014 Dec 14;12(1):147. 10.1186/s40201-014-0147-x
1669 Wikipedia Mees' lines 5.4. 2023 https://en.wikipedia.org/wiki/Mees%27_lines
1670 Antonella Tosti, Massimiliano Pazzaglia, Chapter 18 - Occupational Nail Disorders, Editor(s): Richard K Scher, Antonella Tosti, Boni E Elewski, C Ralph Daniel, Philip Fleckman, Phoebe Rich, Nails (Third Edition), W.B. Saunders, 2005, Pages 205-214, (https://www.sciencedirect.com/science/article/pii/B9781416023562500244)
1671 MSD Manual; consumer version: https://www.msdmanuals.com/home/multimedia/image/mees-lines-leukonychia-striata
1672 Stanford Medicine Examination of the Hand (The Hand in Diagnosis); The examination of the hand and nails can lead to a number of diagnoses. Some of these include liver disease (Terry's nails), kidney disease (Lindsay's nails), lung disease (nail clubbing), endocarditis and many others. https://stanfordmedicine25.stanford.edu/the25/hand.html
1673 Keya, M. K. (2004). Mental health of arsenic victims in Bangladesh. South Afr Anthropol, 4, 215-23. http://www.romanpub.com/resources/Socio%20v1-1-6-Mahbuba_Kaniz_Keya.pdf
1674 Khan, M. M. H., Aklimunnessa, K., Ahsan, N., Kabir, M., & Mori, M. (2006). Case-control study of arsenicosis in some arsenic contaminated villages of Bangladesh. https://sapmed.repo.nii.ac.jp/?action=pages_view_main&active_action=repository_view_main_item_detail&item_id=14531&item_no=1&page_id=13&block_id=21
1675 American College for Advancement in Medicine: Why All Americans Should Know About Chelation Therapy; Posted By Guest Post by Malissa Stawicki of Natural Medicine & Detox, Friday, September 13, 2019; https://www.acam.org/blogpost/1092863/331320/Why-All-Americans-Should-Know-About-Chelation-Therapy
1676 Muñoz D, Grijota FJ, et al: Serum and urinary concentrations of arsenic, beryllium, cadmium and lead after an aerobic training period of six months in aerobic athletes and sedentary people. J Int Soc Sports Nutr. 2020 Aug 17;17(1):43. http://doi.org/10.1186/s12970-020-00372-7.
1677 Morgan, G. T., & Drew, H. D. K. (1920). CLXII.—Researches on residual affinity and co-ordination. Part II. Acetylacetones of selenium and tellurium. J. of the Chemical Society, Transac, 117 https://pubs.rsc.org/en/content/articlelanding/1920/ct/ct9201701456/unauth
1678 Bjorklund, Geir, Guido Crisponi, et al 2019: "A Review on Coordination Properties of Thiol-Containing Chelating Agents Towards Mercury, Cadmium, and Lead" Molecules 24, no. 18: 3247. https://www.ncbi.nlm.nih.gov/pmc/articles/PMC6767255/
1679 Paolieri Matteo: Ferdinand Münz: EDTA and 40 years of inventions In: ACS Bulletin for the History of Chemistry. 42(2), 2017, S. 133–140. https://www.researchgate.net/publication/321552574_Ferdinand_Munz_EDTA_and_40_years_of_inventions
1680 PETERS, R., STOCKEN, L. & THOMPSON, R. British Anti-Lewisite (BAL). Nature 156, 616–619 (1945). https://doi.org/10.1038/156616a0
1681 Tennessee Poison Center | FREE 24/7 Poison Help Hotline 800.222.1222 Donna Seger, MD; Medical Director; Tennessee Poison Center ; https://www.vumc.org/poison-control/toxicology-question-week/nov-12-2012-what-history-behind-development-bal
1682 Marissa Hauptman, Alan D. Woolf, Chapter 3.4 - British anti-lewisite (dimercaprol), Editor(s): Alan D. Woolf, In History of Toxicology and Environmental Health, History of Modern Clinical Toxicology, Academic Press, 2022, https://doi.org/10.1016/B978-0-12-822218-8.00050-8.
1683 Bjorklund, Geir, Guido Crisponi, et al 2019: "A Review on Coordination Properties of Thiol-Containing Chelating Agents Towards Mercury, Cadmium, and Lead" Molecules 24, no. 18: 3247. https://www.ncbi.nlm.nih.gov/pmc/articles/PMC6767255/

Notes

[1684] Miller AL. Dimercaptosuccinic acid (DMSA), a non-toxic, water-soluble treatment for heavy metal toxicity. Altern Med Rev. 1998 Jun;3(3):199-207. https://wellnesspharmacy.com/wp-content/uploads/2015/01/dmsa-heavymetaltoxicity.pdf

[1685] Bjorklund, Geir, Guido Crisponi, Valeria Marina Nurchi, Rosita Cappai, Aleksandra Buha Djordjevic, and Jan Aaseth. 2019: "A Review on Coordination Properties of Thiol-Containing Chelating Agents Towards Mercury, Cadmium, and Lead" Molecules 24, no. 18: 3247. https://doi.org/10.3390/molecules2418324

[1686] Dr. rer. nat. Eleonore Blaurock-Busch: DMSA – die sanfte und effektive orale Entgiftung; OM & Ernährung 2011 | Nr. 134; DMSA-Artikel-Entgiftung.pdf

[1687] Mikirova, Nina et al 2011: Efficacy of oral DMSA and intravenous EDTA in chelation of toxic metals and improvement of the number of stem/ progenitor cells in circulation; TRANSLATIONAL BIOMEDICINE; 2011 Vol. 2 No. 2:2 https://www.transbiomedicine.com/translational-biomedicine/efficacy-of-oral-dmsa-and-intravenous-edta-in-chelation-of-toxic-metals-and-improvement-of-the-number-of-stem-progenitor-cells-in-circulation.pdf

[1688] Aposhian HV, Maiorino RM, Dart RC, Perry DF. Urinary excretion of meso-2,3-dimercaptosuccinic acid in human subjects. Clin Pharmacol Ther. 1989 May. http://doi.oeg/10.1038/clpt.1989.67.

[1689] Aposhian HV. DMSA and DMPS--water soluble antidotes for heavy metal poisoning. Annu Rev Pharmacol Toxicol. 1983; http://doi.org/10.1146/annurev.pa.23.040183.001205.

[1690] Bradberry S, Vale A. Dimercaptosuccinic acid (succimer; DMSA) in inorganic lead poisoning. Clin Toxicol (Phila). 2009 Aug; https://pubmed.ncbi.nlm.nih.gov/19663612/

[1691] Vander Schaar, P. IBCMT Textbuch der Klinischen Metalltoxikologie. 2008

[1692] Aaseth, J.; Jacobsen, D.; Andersen, O.; Wickstrøm, E. Treatment of mercury and lead poisonings with dimercaptosuccinic acid and sodium dimercaptopropanesulfonate: A review. Analyst 1995 https://pubs.rsc.org/en/content/articlelanding/1995/an/an9952000853

[1693] Adams JB, Baral M, et al 2009: Safety and efficacy of oral DMSA therapy for children with autism spectrum disorders: Part A--medical results. BMC Clin Pharmacol. 2009 Oct 23;9:16.. https://pubmed.ncbi.nlm.nih.gov/19852790/

[1694] Sears, M.E. et al 2013: Chelation: Harnessing and Enhancing Heavy Metal Detoxification—A Review; The Scientific World Journal; Hindawi.com https://www.hindawi.com/journals/tswj/2013/219840/tab1/

[1695] Bjorklund, Geir, Guido Crisponi, et al: 2019: A Review on Coordination Properties of Thiol-Containing Chelating Agents Towards Mercury, Cadmium, and Lead" Molecules 24, no. 18: 3247. https://doi.org/10.3390/molecules2418324

[1696] Jeanne A. Drisko, Chapter 107 - Chelation Therapy, Editor(s): David Rakel, Integrative Medicine (Fourth Edition), Elsevier, 2018, https://doi.org/10.1016/B978-0-323-35868-2.00107-9.

[1697] Blaurock-Busch, Eleonore 2011: DMSA – die sanfte und effektive orale Entgiftung; OM & Ernährung 2011 | Nr. 134; DMSA-Artikel-Entgiftung.pdf https://microtrace.de/fileadmin/uploads/pdf/de/DMSA-Artikel-Entgiftung.pdf

[1698] Blaurock-Busch, Eleonore 2011: DMSA – die sanfte und effektive orale Entgiftung; OM & Ernährung 2011 | Nr. 134; DMSA-Artikel-Entgiftung.pdf https://microtrace.de/fileadmin/uploads/pdf/de/DMSA-Artikel-Entgiftung.pdf

[1699] Blaurock-Busch, E.; Naturheilkunde 06/ 2016; https://microtrace.de/fileadmin/uploads/pdf/de/Die_DMSA-Chelattherapie.pdf

[1700] Sears, M.E. et al 2013: Chelation: Harnessing and Enhancing Heavy Metal Detoxification—A Review; The Scientific World Journal; Hindawi.com https://www.hindawi.com/journals/tswj/2013/219840/tab1/

[1701] Medscape succimer (Rx); Brand and Other Names:Chemet; Occupational and Environmental Medicine: Lead Exposure Occupational and Environmental Medicine: Lead Exposure https://reference.medscape.com/drug/chemet-succimer-343751#5

[1702] Mary Jean Brown, Alan D. Woolf, Chapter 1.8 - Zamfara gold mining lead poisoning disaster—Nigeria, Africa, 2010, Editor(s): Alan D. Woolf, In History of Toxicology and Environmental Health, History of Modern Clinical Toxicology, Academic Press, 2022, https://doi.org/10.1016/B978-0-12-822218-8.00012-0.

[1703] Zetpil™ DMSA Chelation Suppository; https://www.zetpilnutrition.com/product/zetpil-dmsa-chelation-suppository/

[1704] Bjorklund, Geir, Guido Crisponi, et al 2019: "A Review on Coordination Properties of Thiol-Containing Chelating Agents Towards Mercury, Cadmium, and Lead" Molecules 24, no. 18: 3247. https://www.ncbi.nlm.nih.gov/pmc/articles/PMC6767255/

[1705] Flora, Swaran J.S., and Vidhu Pachauri. 2010. "Chelation in Metal Intoxication" International Journal of Environmental Research and Public Health 7, no. 7: https://doi.org/10.3390/ijerph7072745;

[1706] Sears, M.E. et al 2013: Chelation: Harnessing and Enhancing Heavy Metal Detoxification—A Review; The Scientific World Journal; Hindawi.com https://www.hindawi.com/journals/tswj/2013/219840/tab1/

[1707] Muran PJ. 2006 Mercury elimination with oral DMPS, DMSA, vitamin C, and glutathione: an observational clinical review. Altern Ther Health Med. 2006 https://citeseerx.ist.psu.edu/document?repid=rep1&type=pdf&doi=c3561142922c93da4a18bcd6d bbd94f2069f2af2

[1708] Muran PJ. 2006: Mercury elimination with oral DMPS, DMSA, vitamin C, and glutathione: an observational clinical review. Altern Ther Health Med. 2006 https://citeseerx.ist.psu.edu/document?repid=rep1&type=pdf&doi=c3561142922c93da4a18bcd6d bbd94f2069f2af2

[1709]chemie-schule.de Ethylendiamintetraessigsäure https://www.chemie-schule.de/KnowHow/Ethylendiamintetraessigsäure

[1710] Gordon,. Garry, M.D. 1997; EDTA Chelation The Real "Miracle" Therapy for Vascular Disease; life-enhancement: https://life-enhancement.com/pages/edta-chelation-the-real-miracle-therapy-for-vascular-disease;

[1711] Wikipedia; Sodium calcium edetate, 4.3. 2023: https://en.wikipedia.org/wiki/Sodium_calcium_edetate

[1712] Clarke NE, Clarke CN, Mosher RE. Treatment of angina pectoris with disodium ethylene diamine tetraacetic acid. Am J Med Sci.1956; December:654-666.

[1713] Gordon, Garry, M.D. 1997; EDTA Chelation The Real "Miracle" Therapy for Vascular Disease; life-enhancement: https://life-enhancement.com/pages/edta-chelation-the-real-miracle-therapy-for-vascular-disease;

[1714] Calcium disodium edetate and disodium edetate. Federal Register, Volume 35, No. 8, Tuesday, January 13, 1970, 585-587. https://www.federalregister.gov/documents/2000/08/08/00-19990/food-additives-permitted-for-direct-addition-to-food-for-human-consumption-calcium-disodium-edta-and

[1715] Ward Dean, MD. 2021: Chelation with EDTA and the Hidden Causes of Heart Disease; https://warddeanmd.com/chelation-with-edta-and-the-hidden-causes-of-heart-disease/

[1716] Fulgenzi A. 2016: New Insights into EDTA In Vitro Effects on Endothelial Cells and on In Vivo Labeled EDTA Biodistribution; Journal of Heavy Metal Toxicity and Diseases; (2016) Volume 1, Issue 2; March 14, 2016; https://www.primescholars.com/articles/new-insights-into-edta-in-vitro-effects-on-endothelial-cells-and-on-in-vivo-labeled-edta-biodistribution-96476.html

[1717] Ferrero, Maria Elena. 2022. "Neuron Protection by EDTA May Explain the Successful Outcomes of Toxic Metal Chelation Therapy in Neurodegenerative Diseases" Biomedicines 10, no. 10: 2476. https://doi.org/10.3390/biomedicines10102476

[1718] Gordon, Garry, M.D. 1997; EDTA Chelation The Real "Miracle" Therapy for Vascular Disease; life-enhancement: https://life-enhancement.com/pages/edta-chelation-the-real-miracle-therapy-for-vascular-disease;

[1719] Corsello, Serafina et al. (2009). The usefulness of chelation therapy for the remission of symptoms caused by previous treatment with mercury-containing pharmaceuticals: A case report. Cases journal. 2. 199. http://doi.org/10.1186/1757-1626-2-199.

[1720] Evstatiev, R., Cervenka, A., (2021). et al. The food additive EDTA aggravates colitis and colon carcinogenesis in mouse models. Sci Rep 11, https://doi.org/10.1038/s41598-021-84571-5 https://www.nature.com/articles/s41598-021-84571-5

[1721] EU Risk assessment Report, for EDETIC ACID (EDTA) 2004: Institute for Health and Consumer Protection European Chemicals Bureau; Special Publication I.04.279; Germany https://echa.europa.eu/documents/10162/5ed7db13-e932-4999-8514-378ce88ca51f

[1722] Final Report on the Safety Assessment of EDTA, Calcium Disodium EDTA, .. International Journal of Toxicology, 21(Suppl. 2):95–142, 2002 Copyright c 2002 Cosmetic Ingredient Review; https://journals.sagepub.com/doi/pdf/10.1080/10915810290096522

[1723] Final Report on the Safety Assessment of EDTA, Calcium Disodium EDTA, .. International Journal of Toxicology, 21(Suppl. 2):95–142, 2002 Copyright c 2002 Cosmetic Ingredient Review; https://journals.sagepub.com/doi/pdf/10.1080/10915810290096522

[1724] Wikipedia: Salt poisoning; https://en.wikipedia.org/wiki/Salt_poisoning;

[1725] EPA January 28, 2004; MEMORANDUM; Tolerance Reassessment Decisions Completed by the Lower Toxicity Pesticide Chemical Focus Group; https://www.epa.gov/sites/default/files/2015-04/documents/edta.pdf

[1726] accessdata.fda.gov CENTER FOR DRUG EVALUATION AND RESEARCH; 2009; APPLICATION NUMBER: 022560Orig1s000 PHARMACOLOGY REVIEW(S); P.10 https://www.accessdata.fda.gov/drugsatfda_docs/nda/2010/022560Orig1s000PharmR.pdf

Notes

[1727] Wikipedia Liste der Lebensmittelzusatzstoffe EU, 3.21.2021
https://de.wikipedia.org/wiki/Liste_der_Lebensmittelzusatzstoffe
[1728] Wreesmann, C.T.J. (2014), Reasons for raising the maximum ADI of EDTA. Matern Child Nutr, 10: 481-495. https://doi.org/10.1111/mcn.12110
[1729] FDA: CFR - Code of Federal Regulations Title 21;
https://www.accessdata.fda.gov/scripts/cdrh/cfdocs/cfcfr/CFRSearch.cfm?fr=172.135&SearchTerm=disodium%20edta
[1730] The Japan Food chemical Research Foundation; Standards for Use, according to Use Categories; June 3 2018:
https://www.ffcr.or.jp/en/upload/StandardsforUseofFoodAdditivesfeb2018_2.pdf
[1731] Goodseedventures: Worldwide Food Consumption Per Capita; DECEMBER 2, 2021https://goodseedventures.com/worldwide-food-consumption-per-capita-2/
[1732] Ward Dean, M.D. CHELATION UPDATE: EXCERPT FROM NOVEMBER 2001 GORDON RESEARCH INSTITUTE REPORT; https://warddeanmd.com/chelation-update-excerpt-from-november-2001-gordon-research-institute-report/
[1733] Healthline: Is Calcium Disodium EDTA a Safe Additive?; Medically reviewed by Imashi Fernando, MS, RDN; By Kaitlyn Berkheiser; February 8, 2023
https://www.healthline.com/nutrition/calcium-disodium-edta
[1734] Jeanne A. Drisko, 2018: Chapter 107 - Chelation Therapy, Editor(s): David Rakel, Integrative Medicine (Fourth Edition), Elsevier, 2018,
(https://www.sciencedirect.com/science/article/pii/B9780323358682001079)
[1735] sciencedirect.com: Chelation Therapy; Jeanne A. Drisko MD, in Integrative Medicine (Fourth Edition), 2018; EDTA; https://www.sciencedirect.com/topics/immunology-and-microbiology/ethylenediaminetetraacetic-acid
[1736] Drugbank, online; PHARMACOLOGY ; Edetate calcium disodium;
https://go.drugbank.com/drugs/DB14598
[1737] Ellithorpe, Rita & Mazur, et al (2007). Comparison of the Absorption, Brain and Prostate Distribution, and Elimination of CaNa2 EDTA of Rectal Chelation Suppositories to Intravenous Administration. Journal of the American Nutraceutical Association. 10. 38-44.
https://www.researchgate.net/publication/235954753_Comparison_of_the_Absorption_Brain_and_Prostate_Distribution_and_Elimination_of_CaNa2_EDTA_of_Rectal_Chelation_Suppositories_to_Intravenous_Administration
[1738] Ward Dean, M.D. CHELATION UPDATE: EXCERPT FROM NOVEMBER 2001 GORDON RESEARCH INSTITUTE REPORT; https://warddeanmd.com/chelation-update-excerpt-from-november-2001-gordon-research-institute-report/
[1739] Ward Dean, MD. 2021: Chelation with EDTA and the Hidden Causes of Heart Disease;
https://warddeanmd.com/chelation-with-edta-and-the-hidden-causes-of-heart-disease/
[1740] Perry H.M. Schroeder, H.A. 1955: Depression of cholesterol levels in human plasma following ethylenediamine tetracetate and hydralazine, Journal of Chronic Diseases, Volume 2, Issue 5, 1955, https://doi.org/10.1016/0021-9681(55)90151-X.
[1741] Schroeder, Henry A 1956: A practical method for the reduction of plasma cholesterol in man, Journal of Chronic Diseases, Volume 4, Issue 5, 1956,
(https://www.sciencedirect.com/science/article/pii/0021968156900650)
[1742] Spencer Feldman; Effects of Magnesium Di-Potassium EDTA suppositories on blood chemistry values; OAW Health; 2000;
https://oawhealth.com/article/effects-of-magnesium-di-potassium-edta-suppositories-on-blood-chemistry-values/
[1743] Ellithorpe, Rita & Mazur, et al (2007). Comparison of the Absorption, Brain and Prostate Distribution, and Elimination of CaNa2 EDTA of Rectal Chelation Suppositories to Intravenous Administration. Journal of the American Nutraceutical Association. 10. 38-44.
https://www.researchgate.net/publication/235954753_Comparison_of_the_Absorption_Brain_and_Prostate_Distribution_and_Elimination_of_CaNa2_EDTA_of_Rectal_Chelation_Suppositories_to_Intravenous_Administration
[1744] Magnesium di-potassium EDTA complex and method of administration; US20020169211A1; United States; 2002-11-14; Publication of US20020169211A1
https://patents.google.com/patent/US20020169211A1/en
[1745] Ellithorpe, Rita & Jimenez,et al (2009). Calcium disodium EDTA chelation suppositories: A novel approach for removing heavy metal toxins in clinical practice. January 2009; In book: Anti-Aging Therapeutics (pp.107-118) Chapter: 14; American Academy of Anti-Aging Medicine; Editors: R. Klatz, R. Goldma
https://www.researchgate.net/publication/235923312_Calcium_disodium_EDTA_chelation_suppositories_A_novel_approach_for_removing_heavy_metal_toxins_in_clinical_practice

[1746] myhealth.alberta Chelation Therapy; Adam Husney MD - Adam Husney MD; https://myhealth.alberta.ca/Health/Pages/conditions.aspx?hwid=ty3205spec

[1747] Ferrero, Maria Elena. 2022. "Neuron Protection by EDTA May Explain the Successful Outcomes of Toxic Metal Chelation Therapy in Neurodegenerative Diseases" Biomedicines 10, no. 10: 2476. https://doi.org/10.3390/biomedicines10102476

[1748] Holleman, A.F.et al. (2001) Inorganic Chemistry. Academic Press, San Diego, https://www.scirp.org/%28S%28vtj3fa45qm1ean45vvffcz55%29%29/reference/referencespapers.aspx?referenceid=2434024

[1749] Teerasarntipan, T., Chaiteerakij, R., Prueksapanich, P. et al. Changes in inflammatory cytokines, antioxidants and liver stiffness after chelation therapy in individuals with chronic lead poisoning. BMC Gastroenterol. (2020). https://doi.org/10.1186/s12876-020-01386-w

[1750] Mikirova, Nina et al 2011: Efficacy of oral DMSA and intravenous EDTA in chelation of toxic metals and improvement of the number of stem/ progenitor cells in circulation; TRANSLATIONAL BIOMEDICINE; 2011 Vol. 2 No. 2:2 https://www.transbiomedicine.com/translational-biomedicine/efficacy-of-oral-dmsa-and-intravenous-edta-in-chelation-of-toxic-metals-and-improvement-of-the-number-of-stem-progenitor-cells-in-circulation.pdf

[1751] Ghibu S, Richard C,e t al [An endogenous dithiol with antioxidant properties: alpha-lipoic acid, potential uses in cardiovascular diseases]. Ann Cardiol Angeiol (Paris). 2008 Jun;57(3):161-5. French. http://doi.org/10.1016/j.ancard.2008.02.018.

[1752] Cakatay U. Pro-oxidant actions of alpha-lipoic acid and dihydrolipoic acid. Med Hypotheses. 2006;66(1):110-7. https://pubmed.ncbi.nlm.nih.gov/16165311/

[1753] Patrick, L. Mercury toxicity and antioxidants: Part I: Role of glutathione and alpha-lipoic acid in the treatment of mercury toxicity. Altern. Med. Rev. 2002, 7, 456–471. https://pubmed.ncbi.nlm.nih.gov/12495372/

[1754] Sivaprasad R, Nagaraj M, Varalakshmi P. Lipoic acid in combination with a chelator ameliorates lead-induced peroxidative damages in rat kidney. Arch Toxicol. 2002 https://www.researchgate.net/publication/11202878_Lipoic_acid_in_combination_with_a_chelator_ameliorates_lead-induced_peroxidative_damage_in_rat_kidney

[1755] Pande M, Flora SJ. 2002: Lead induced oxidative damage and its response to combined administration of alpha-lipoic acid and succimers in rats. Toxicology. 2002 Aug 15;177(2-3) https://www.sciencedirect.com/science/article/abs/pii/S0300483X02002238

[1756] Nagaraja Haleagrahara, Tan Jackie, Srikumar Chakravarthi and Anupama Bangra Kulur, 2011. Protective Effect of Alpha-lipoic Acid Against Lead Acetate-Induced Oxidative Stress in the Bone Marrow of Rats. International Journal of Pharmacology, 7: 217-227.: https://scialert.net/abstract/?doi=ijp.2011.217.22 7

[1757] Gurer H, Ozgunes H, Oztezcan S, Ercal N. 1999: Antioxidant role of alpha-lipoic acid in lead toxicity. Free Radic Biol Med. 1999 July https://pubmed.ncbi.nlm.nih.gov/10443922/

[1758] Samy A. Hussein, et al 2014: Protective effects of alpha-lipoic acid against lead-induced oxidative stress in erythrocytes of rats; BENHA VETERINARY MEDICAL J. VOL. 27, NO. 2:382-395, DEc 2014; https://www.bvmj.bu.edu.eg/issues/27-2/38.pdf

[1759] AlMomen, Abdulkareem; and Blaurock-Busch, Eleonore; 2022: Alpha-Lipoic Acid (ALA), fatty acid and promising chelating agent for neurological ailments; World J. of Biolog. and Pharmaceutical Research, 2022, https://doi.org/10.53346/wjbpr.2022.3.1.0038;

[1760] Bjorklund G, Aaseth J,et al. 2019: Insights on alpha lipoic and dihydrolipoic acids as promising scavengers of oxidative stress and possible chelators in mercury toxicology. J Inorg Biochem. 2019 https://pubmed.ncbi.nlm.nih.gov/30939378/

[1761] AlMomen, Abdulkareem; and Blaurock-Busch, Eleonore; 2022: Alpha-Lipoic Acid (ALA), fatty acid and promising chelating agent for neurological ailments; World J. of Biological and Pharmaceut. Research, 2022, https://doi.org/10.53346/wjbpr.2022.3.1.0038;

[1762] Monica Morini, et al 2004: α-Lipoic acid is effective in prevention and treatment of experimental autoimmune encephalomyelitis, Journal of Neuroimmunology, Volume 148, Issues 1–2, 2004, , https://doi.org/10.1016/j.jneuroim.2003.11.021.

[1763] Deore MS, S K, Naqvi S, Kumar A, Flora SJS. Alpha-Lipoic Acid Protects Co-Exposure to Lead and Zinc Oxide Nanoparticles Induced Neuro, Immuno and Male Reproductive Toxicity in Rats. Front Pharmacol. 2021 Jul https://www.frontiersin.org/articles/10.3389/fphar.2021.626238/full

[1764] WARNER ORTHOPEDICS & WELLNESS; WHY YOU SHOULD BE TAKING ALPHA-LIPOIC ACID; https://warnerorthopedics.com/alpha-lipoic-acid-supplement-benefits/

[1765] Ziegle, D.; Reljanovic, M; Mehnert, H; Gries, F. A. (1999). "α-Lipoic acid in the treatment of diabetic polyneuropathy in Germany". Experimental and Clinical Endocrinology & Diabetes. 107 (7): 421–30. http://doi.org/10.1055/s-0029-1212132

Notes

[1766] Hauptman M, Bruccoleri RAn Update on Childhood Lead Poisoning. Clin Pediatr Emerg Med. 2017 Sep;18(3) https://www.ncbi.nlm.nih.gov/pmc/articles/PMC5645046/

[1767] Flora, Swaran J.S., and Vidhu Pachauri. 2010. "Chelation in Metal Intoxication" International Journal of Environmental Research and Public Health 7, no. 7: 2745-2788. https://doi.org/10.3390/ijerph7072745;

[1768] Bloodbank: ; Chelating Agents; Accession Number DBCAT000624 https://go.drugbank.com/drugs/DB01609

[1769] Lanz J, Biniaz-Harris N, Kuvaldina M, Jain S, Lewis K, Fallon BA. Disulfiram: Mechanisms, Applications, and Challenges. Antibiotics (Basel). 2023 Mar 6;12(3):524. https://www.ncbi.nlm.nih.gov/pmc/articles/PMC10044060/#:~:text=Later%20studies%20identified%20diethyldithiocarbamate%20(DDTC,zinc%20%5B10%2C16%5D. .

[1770] Antonella Tammaro; et al; Topical and Systemic Therapies for Nickel Allergy DISCLOSURES Dermatitis. 2011;22(05) https://www.medscape.com/viewarticle/753985_7

[1771] Takako Tominaga, et al 2021 Effects of the chelating agent DTPA on naturally accumulating metals in the body, Toxicology Letters, Volume 350, 2021, https://doi.org/10.1016/j.toxlet.2021.08.001.

[1772] Benoit, S.L., Schmalstig, A.A., Glushka, J. et al. Nickel chelation therapy as an approach to combat multi-drug resistant enteric pathogens. Sci Rep 9, 13851 (2019). https://doi.org/10.1038/s41598-019-50027-0

[1773] Wikipedia: Dimethylglyoxime; https://en.wikipedia.org/wiki/Dimethylglyoxime

[1774] Dimethylglyoxime; Material Safety Data Sheet; STATEMENT OF HAZARDOUS NATURE https://datasheets.scbt.com/sc-211355.pdf

[1775] Benoit, S.L., Schmalstig, A.A., Glushka, J. et al. Nickel chelation therapy as an approach to combat multi-drug resistant enteric pathogens. Sci Rep 9, 13851 (2019). https://doi.org/10.1038/s41598-019-50027-0

[1776] Weiss KH, Thurik F,et al ; EUROWILSON Consortium. Efficacy and safety of oral chelators in treatment of patients with Wilson disease. Clin Gastroenterol Hepatol. 2013 Aug;11(8): https://pubmed.ncbi.nlm.nih.gov/23542331/

[1777] Pugliese M, Biondi V, Gugliandolo E, Licata P, Peritore AF, Crupi R, Passantino A. D-Penicillamine: The State of the Art in Humans and in Dogs from a Pharmacological and Regulatory Perspective. Antibiotics (Basel). 2021 May https://www.ncbi.nlm.nih.gov/pmc/articles/PMC8229433/

[1778] https://remm.hhs.gov/penicillamine.htm

[1779] N.V. BHAGAVAN, CHAPTER 2 - Amino Acids, Editor(s): N.V. BHAGAVAN, Medical Biochemistry (Fourth Edition), Academic Press, 2002, (https://www.sciencedirect.com/science/article/pii/B9780120954407500044)

[1780] Rxlist; HOW DO COPPER CHELATORS WORK?; Medical Author: Nazneen Memon, BHMS, PGDCR; Medical and Pharmacy Editor: Sarfaroj Khan, BHMS, PGD Health Operations; https://www.rxlist.com/copper_chelators/drug-class.htm

[1781] Fatfat, M., Merhi, R.A., Rahal, O. et al. 2014: Copper chelation selectively kills colon cancer cells through redox cycling and generation of reactive oxygen species. BMC Cancer 14, 527 (2014). https://doi.org/10.1186/1471-2407-14-527

[1782] MedScape: Hypocitraturia Overview of Potassium Citrate and Calcium Citrate Updated: May 18, 2023 ; Author: Gates B Colbert, https://emedicine.medscape.com/article/444968-overview?form=fpf

[1783] Lawrence, Glen D., Patel, Kamalkumar S. and Nusbaum, Aviva. "Uranium toxicity and chelation therapy" Pure and Applied Chemistry, vol. 86, no. 7, 2014, https://doi.org/10.1515/pac-2014-0109

[1784] Bitter, E.E. et al 1992: Citrate as an aluminum chelator and positive effector of the sodium efflux in single barnacle muscle fibers. Biochim. Biophys Acta. http://doi.org/10.1016/0005-2736(92)90027-j.

[1785] Granchi D, et al 2019: Role of Citrate in Pathophysiology and Medical Management of Bone Diseases. Nutrients. 2019 http://doi.org/10.3390/nu11112576.

[1786] Magshoud Nabilpour, et al 2024: Acute effects of sodium citrate supplementation on competitive performance and lactate level of elite fitness challenge athletes: A crossover, placebo-controlled, double-blind study, Journal of Exercise Science & Fitness, Volume 22, I2, 2024, https://doi.org/10.1016/j.jesf.2024.02.001.

[1787] Boudou, F. et al 2019: Assessment of a new approach of metal ions chelation by Gallic acid; https://www.researchgate.net/publication/338778369_Assessment_of_a_new_approach_of_metal_ions_chelation_by_Gallic_acid

[1788] Janaina E. Rocha, et al 2019: Identification of the gallic acid mechanism of action on mercury chloride toxicity reduction using infrared spectroscopy and antioxidant assays, Internat. Biodet. & Biodegrad, Vol. 141, 2019, https://doi.org/10.1016/j.ibiod.2018.07.002.

[1789] Bhuia, M.S., Rahaman, M.M., Islam, T. et al. Neurobiological effects of gallic acid: current perspectives. Chin Med 18, 27 (2023). https://doi.org/10.1186/s13020-023-00735-7

[1790] Elmileegy IMH, et al: Gallic acid rescues uranyl acetate induced-hepatic dysfunction in rats by its antioxidant and cytoprotective potentials. BMC Complement Med Ther. 2023 http://doi.org/10.1186/s12906-023-04250-y.

[1791] Phenol-explorer.eu Showing all foods in which the polyphenol gallic acid is found

[1792] AndyCutler.com; New to chelating? Start here; https://andy-cutler-chelation.com

[1793] Lu SC. 2012: Glutathione synthesis. Biochim Biophys Acta. 2013 May;1830(5):3143-53..bbagen.2012.09.008. https://www.ncbi.nlm.nih.gov/pmc/articles/PMC3549305/#:~:text=Glutathione%20(GSH)%20is%20present%20in,%2C%20immune%20function%2C%20and%20fibrogenesis. .

[1794] Jozefczak M, Remans T, Vangronsveld J, Cuypers A. 2012: Glutathione is a key player in metal-induced oxidative stress defenses. Int J Mol Sci. 2012;13(3):3145-3175. https://pubmed.ncbi.nlm.nih.gov/22489146/

[1795] C. D. Klaassen, J. Liu, and B. A. Diwan, "Metallothionein protection of cadmium toxicity," Toxicology and Applied Pharmacology, vol. 238, no. 3, pp. 215–220, 2009. https://www.ncbi.nlm.nih.gov/pmc/articles/PMC2740813/

[1796] Patent Pharmaceutical preparations of glutathione and methods of administration thereof; 2002; Inventor Harry B. DemopolosMyron L. Seligman Current Assignee Molecular Defenses Holdings LLC; https://patents.google.com/patent/US6896899B2/en

[1797] Ilya E. Zlobin, A, 2017: Different roles of glutathione in copper and zinc chelation in Brassica napus roots, Plant Physiology and Biochemistry, Volume 118, 2017, (https://www.sciencedirect.com/science/article/pii/S0981942817302206)

[1798] Sharma DK, Sharma P. Augmented Glutathione Absorption from Oral Mucosa and its Effect on Skin Pigmentation: A Clinical Review. Clin Cosmet Investig Dermatol. 2022 Sep 10;15:1853-1862. https://www.ncbi.nlm.nih.gov/pmc/articles/PMC9473545/

[1799] Patent Pharmaceutical preparations of glutathione and methods of administration thereof; 2002; Inventor Harry B. DemopolosMyron L. Seligman Current Assignee Molecular Defenses Holdings LLC; https://patents.google.com/patent/US6896899B2/en

[1800] Premranjan Kumar, PhD, et al 2023: Supplementing Glycine and N-Acetylcysteine (GlyNAC) in Older Adults Improves Glutathione Deficiency, Oxidative Stress, Mitochondrial Dysfunction, Inflammation, Physical Function, and Aging Hallmarks: A Randomized Clinical Trial, The J. of Gerontology: Se. A, .78, 1, J. 2023, https://doi.org/10.1093/gerona/glac135

[1801] Richie JP, Nichenametla S, Neidig W, et al. Randomized con- trolled trial of oral glutathione supplementation on body stores of glutathione. Eur J Nutr. 2015;54(2):251-263. https://pubmed.ncbi.nlm.nih.gov/24791752/

[1802] Sharma DK, Sharma P. Augmented Glutathione Absorption from Oral Mucosa and its Effect on Skin Pigmentation: A Clinical Review. Clin Cosmet Investig Dermatol. 2022 Sep 10;15:1853-1862. https://www.ncbi.nlm.nih.gov/pmc/articles/PMC9473545/

[1803] Bjorklund, Geir, Guido Crisponi, et al 2019: "A Review on Coordination Properties of Thiol-Containing Chelating Agents Towards Mercury, Cadmium, and Lead" Molecules 24, no. 18: 3247. https://www.ncbi.nlm.nih.gov/pmc/articles/PMC6767255/

[1804] W. Banner, et al 1986: Experimental chelation therapy in chromium, lead, and boron intoxication with N-acetylcysteine and other compounds, Toxicology and Applied Pharmac, V. 83,1, 1986, https://www.sciencedirect.com/science/article/pii/0041008X86903315)

[1805] Orisakwe OE. 2014: The role of lead and cadmium in psychiatry. N Am J Med Sci. 2014 Aug;6(8):370-6. https://www.ncbi.nlm.nih.gov/pmc/articles/PMC4158644/

[1806] Schwalfenberg Gerry K.2021:,N-Acetylcysteine: A Review of Clinical Usefulness (an Old Drug with New Tricks) Journal of Nutrition and Metabolism, Volume 2021 https://www.hindawi.com/journals/jnme/2021/9949453/

[1807] Kondala R. Atkuri N-acetylcysteine - a safe antidote for cysteine/glutathione deficiency; Curr Opin Pharmacol. 2007 Aug; 7(4): 355–359.; https://www.ncbi.nlm.nih.gov/pmc/articles/PMC4540061/

[1808] Schwalfenberg Gerry K.2021:,N-Acetylcysteine: A Review of Clinical Usefulness (an Old Drug with New Tricks) Journal of Nutrition and Metabolism, Volume 2021 https://www.hindawi.com/journals/jnme/2021/9949453/

[1809] Smith, Peter 2013: How to detoxify Heavy Metals; –Holistic Medicine Practitioner- (updated 2/2013); Better Mental Health with Natural Remedies https://www.balancingbrainchemistry.co.uk/peter-smith/28/Heavy-Metal-Toxicity-Depression-&-Anxiety.html

[1810] Flora, S. et al . (2004). Lead induced oxidative stress and its recovery following co-administration of melatonin or N-acetylcysteine during chelation with succimer in male rats. Cellular and molecular biology, https://pubmed.ncbi.nlm.nih.gov/15555419/

[1811] Olsson, B, et al . et al. Pharmacokinetics and bioavailability of reduced and oxidized N-acetylcysteine. Eur J Clin Pharmacol 34, (1988). https://doi.org/10.1007/BF01061422

[1812] Zetpil CoQ10 450 with N-Acetyl-Cysteine Suppositories https://www.drvitaminsolutions.com/products/zetpil-coq10-450-with-n-acetyl-cysteine-suppositories-30-count/

[1813] Tenório MCdS, Graciliano NG, Moura FA, Oliveira ACMd, Goulart MOF. N-Acetylcysteine (NAC): Impacts on Human Health. Antioxidants. 2021; 10(6):967. https://doi.org/10.3390/antiox10060967

[1814] Kadioglu Simsek G. Arayici S. Buyuktiryaki M. Okur N. Kanmaz Kutman G. Suna Oguz S. Oral N. Acetyl Cysteine for Meconium Ileus of Preterm Infants. Gynecol Obstet Reprod Med. 2019;25(3):169-173 https://pdfs.semanticscholar.org/b189/872685ccae3152c39fac5473c58b14dd9833.pdf

[1815] Izquierdo JL, Soriano JB, et al 2022: Use of N-Acetylcysteine at high doses as an oral treatment for patients hospitalized with COVID-19. Sci Prog. 2022 Jan-Mar;105(1): http://doi.org/10.1177/00368504221074574.

[1816] N-Acetylcysteine (NAC) Supplements; Benefits, uses, side effects of NAC supplements; By Jennifer Lefton, MS, RD/N, CNSC, FAND Updated on June 30, 2023 https://www.verywellhealth.com/the-benefits-of-n-acetylcysteine-89416

[1817] Nutraingredients NAC supplements back on Amazon; By Stephen Daniells 25-Aug-2022 https://www.nutraingredients-usa.com/Article/2022/08/25/NAC-supplements-back-on-Amazon#:~:text=Despite%20being%20used%20as%20in,prior%20approval%20as%20a%20drug.

[1818] McCarty MF, O'Keefe JH, DiNicolantonio JJ. Dietary Glycine Is Rate-Limiting for Glutathione Synthesis and May Have Broad Potential for Health Protection. Ochsner J. 2018 Spring;18(1):81-87. https://pubmed.ncbi.nlm.nih.gov/29559876/

[1819] Michael A. Borowitzka, Chapter 3 - Biology of Microalgae, Editor(s): Ira A. Levine, Joël Fleurence, Microalgae in Health and Disease Prevention, Academic Press, 2018, Pages 23-72, , https://doi.org/10.1016/B978-0-12-811405-6.00003-7.

[1820] Radwan, E. K.,et al (2020). Bioremediation of potentially toxic metal and reactive dye-contaminated water by pristine and modified Chlorella vulgaris. Environmental Science and Pollution Research, 27,. https://link.springer.com/article/10.1007/s11356-020-08550-5

[1821] Kim YJ, Kwon S, Kim MK. Effect of Chlorella vulgaris intake on cadmium detoxification in rats fed cadmium. Nutr Res Pract. 2009 Summer;3(2):89-94. https://www.ncbi.nlm.nih.gov/pmc/articles/PMC2788181/

[1822] Seegarten Klinik, Switzerland https://sgk.swiss/achtung-chorella.html

[1823] Mahendra Yadav et al 2022: ; Quantitative evaluation of Chlorella vulgaris for removal of toxic metals from body; Journal of Applied Phycology volume 34, pages 2743–2754 (2022); https://link.springer.com/article/10.1007/s10811-021-02640-8#:~:text=Most%20of%20the%20metal%20ions,%E2%88%921%20in%20SGF%2C%20respectively.

[1824] Merino JJ, , et al: The Long-Term Algae Extract (Chlorella and Fucus sp) and Aminosulphurate Supplementation Modulate SOD-1 Activity and Decrease Heavy Metals (Hg++, Sn) Levels in Patients with Long-Term Dental Titanium Implants and Amalgam Fillings Restorations. Antioxidants (Basel). 2019 https://www.mdpi.com/2076-3921/8/4/101

[1825] Yunes Panahi, Roghayeh Badeli, Gholam-Reza Karami, Zeinab Badeli, Amirhossein Sahebkar 2015:A randomized controlled trial of 6-week Chlorella vulgaris supplementation in patients with major depressive disorder, Complementary Therapies in Medicine, Volume 23, Issue 4, 2015, Pages 598-602, https://doi.org/10.1016/j.ctim.2015.06.010.

[1826] Mehrangiz Ebrahimi-Mameghani, Zahra Sadeghi, et al, 2017: Glucose homeostasis, insulin resistance and inflammatory biomarkers in patients with non-alcoholic fatty liver disease: Beneficial effects of supplementation with microalgae Chlorella vulgaris: A double-blind placebo-controlled randomized clinical trial, Clinical Nutrition, Volume 36, Issue 4, 2017, (https://www.sciencedirect.com/science/article/pii/S0261561416301704)

[1827] Velaga MK, Yallapragada PR, Williams D, Rajanna S, Bettaiya R. 2014: Hydroalcoholic seed extract of Coriandrum sativum (Coriander) alleviates lead-induced oxidative stress in different regions of rat brain. Biol Trace Elem Res. 2014 Jun;159(1-3):351-63. https://pubmed.ncbi.nlm.nih.gov/24793421/

[1828] cleangreensimple.com, Cilantro vs. Parsley: What's the Difference? by Sara Seitz on October 1, 2020; https://cleangreensimple.com/article/cilantro-vs-parsley/

[1829] Mlay,P.S. et al 2008: Effect of cilantro on plasma lead levels and some hematological parameters in rats; Tanzaniane Vereinarian Journal ; Vol. 25 No. 2 (2008); DOI: 10.4314/tvj.v25i2.42036. ; https://www.ajol.info/index.php/tvj/article/view/42036

[1830] Donia, G.R.. (2020). PROTECTIVE EFFECT OF CORIANDER (CORINDRUM SATIVUM) AGAINST LEAD TOXICITY IN RABBITS. https://www.researchgate.net/publication/340033032_PROTECTIVE_EFFECT_OF_CORIANDE R_CORINDRUM_SATIVUM_AGAINST_LEAD_TOXICITY_IN_RABBITS

[1831] Gordanić SV, Kostić AŽ, et al: A detailed survey of agroecological status of Allium ursinum across the republic of Serbia: Mineral composition and bioaccumulation potential. Heliyon. 2023 Nov 10;9. http://doi.org/10.1016/j.heliyon.2023.e22134.

[1832] Belviso, Claudia. 2020. "Zeolite for Potential Toxic Metal Uptake from Contaminated in tSoil: A Brief Review" Processes 8, no. 7: 820. https://doi.org/10.3390/pr8070820

[1833] Belviso, Claudia. 2020. "Zeolite for Potential Toxic Metal Uptake from Contaminated Soil: A Brief Review" Processes 8, no. 7: 820. https://doi.org/10.3390/pr8070820

[1834] Kraljević Pavelić S, et al 2022: Clinical Evaluation of a Defined Zeolite-Clinoptilolite Supplementation Effect on the Selected Blood Parameters of Patients. Front Med (Lausanne). 2022 May 27;9:851782. http://doi.org/10.3389/fmed.2022.851782.

[1835] Flowers J, Lonky SA, Deitsch EJ. Clinical evidence supporting the use of an activated clinoptilolite suspension as an agent to increase urinary excretion of toxic heavy metals. Nutrition and Dietary Supplements. 2009; https://doi.org/10.2147/NDS.S8043

[1836] Kraljević Pavelić S, et al 2022: Clinical Evaluation of a Defined Zeolite-Clinoptilolite Supplementation Effect on the Selected Blood Parameters of Patients. Front Med (Lausanne). 2022. http://doi.org/10.3389/fmed.2022.851782.

[1837] Eliaz I, Hotchkiss AT, et al: The effect of modified citrus pectin on urinary excretion of toxic elements. Phytother Res. 2006 https://pubmed.ncbi.nlm.nih.gov/16835878/

[1838] Life Extension Magazine: Fighting Cancer Metastasis and Heavy Metal Toxicities With Modified Citrus Pectin https://www.lifeextension.com/magazine/2009/3/modified-citrus-pectin-fighting-cancer-metastasis-heavy-metal-toxicities#:~:text=Modified%20Citrus%20Pectin%20and%20Chelation&text=A%20pilot%20trial%20evaluating%20MCP%27s,urinary%20excretion%20of%20toxic%20metals.

[1839] Zhao ZY, Liang L, et al 2008: The role of modified citrus pectin as an effective chelator of lead in children hospitalized with toxic lead levels. Alt. Ther H. Med. 2008 https://www.researchgate.net/publication/5236772_The_role_of_modified_citrus_pectin_as_an_e ffective_chelator_of_lead_in_children_hospitalized_with_toxic_lead_levels

[1840] Singh NP, Thind IS, et al 1979: Intake of magnesium and toxicity of lead: an experimental model. Arch Environ Health. 1979 https://pubmed.ncbi.nlm.nih.gov/453925/

[1841] S.J.S. Flora, S.K. Tandon, Beneficial effects of zinc supplementation during chelation treatment of lead intoxication in rats, Toxicology, V. 64 2, 1990, https://doi.org/10.1016/0300-483X(90)90130-9.

[1842] Olivier Barbier, et al: Effect of Heavy Metals on, and Handling by, the Kidney. Nephron Physiology 1 April 2005; 99 (4): p105–p110. https://doi.org/10.1159/000083981

[1843] Zhang D, Liu J, Gao J, et al. (2014) Zinc Supplementation Protects against Cadmium Accumulation and Cytotoxicity in Madin-Darby Bovine Kidney Cells. https://doi.org/10.1371/journal.pone.0103427

[1844] Zhai Q, Narbad A, Chen W. Dietary strategies for the treatment of cadmium and lead toxicity. Nutrients. 2015 Jan 14;7(1):552-71. http://doi.org/10.3390/nu7010552.

[1845] Hsu PC, Guo YL. Antioxidant nutrients and lead toxicity. Toxicology. 2002 Oct 30;180(1):33-44. https://pubmed.ncbi.nlm.nih.gov/12324198/

[1846] Patrick, Lyn. 2006: "Lead toxicity Part II: the role of free radical damage and the use of antioxidants in the pathology and treatment of lead toxicity." Alternative Medicine Review, vol. 11, no. 2, 2006, https://go.gale.com/ps/anonymous?id=GALE%7CA148424512&sid=googleScholar&v=2.1&it=r&li nkaccess=abs&issn=10895159&p=AONE&sw=w

[1847] Valko M, Morris H, Cronin MT. Metals, toxicity and oxidative stress. Curr Med Chem. 2005;12(10) http://doi.org/10.2174/0929867053764635.

[1848] Flora SJ, Shrivastava R, Mittal M. Chemistry and pharmacological properties of some natural and synthetic antioxidants for heavy metal toxicity. Curr Med Chem.2013;20(36) http://doi.org/10.2174/09298673113209990146.

[1849] https://www.medivere.de/shop/Alle/Schwermetall-Urintest-Plus.html?listtype=search&searchparam=metall

[1850] Doctor's Data; Urine Toxic & Essential Elements https://www.holisticheal.com/urine-toxic-essential-elements.html

Notes

[1851] Ellithorpe, Rita & Jimenez,et al (2009). Calcium disodium EDTA chelation suppositories: A novel approach for removing heavy metal toxins in clinical practice. January 2009; In book: Anti-Aging Therapeutics (pp.107-118) Chapter: 14; American Academy of Anti-Aging Medicine; Editors: R. Klatz, R. Goldma
https://www.researchgate.net/publication/235923312_Calcium_disodium_EDTA_chelation_supp ositories_A_novel_approach_for_removing_heavy_metal_toxins_in_clinical_practice

[1852] Adams JB, Baral M, et al 2009: Safety and efficacy of oral DMSA therapy for children with autism spectrum disorders: Part A--medical results. BMC Clin Pharmacol. 2009 Oct
https://bmcclinpharma.biomedcentral.com/articles/10.1186/1472-6904-9-17

[1853] Mount Sinai, Ethylenediaminetetraacetic acid; Chelation therapy; EDTA;
https://www.mountsinai.org/health-library/supplement/ethylenediaminetetraacetic-acid

[1854] Dimaval® (DMPS) 100 mg Hartkapseln; Activesubstance: (RS)-2,3-Bis(sulfanyl)propane-1-sulfonicacid, sodium salt 1 H2O; https://www.heyl-berlin.de/img_upload/pdf/PIL_Dimaval-cps_EN_2020-06.pdf

[1855] Kostial, K., et al (2000), Combined treatment with racemic-DMSA and EDTA for lead mobilization in rats. J. Trace Elem. Exp. Med., 13: 277-284. https://doi.org/10.1002/1520-670X(2000)13:3<277::AID-JTRA5>3.0.CO;2-2

[1856] Sears, M.E. et al 2013: Chelation: Harnessing and Enhancing Heavy Metal Detoxification—A Review; The Scientific World Journal; Hindawi.com
https://www.hindawi.com/journals/tswj/2013/219840/tab1/

[1857] Besunder, J., Anderson, R., Pope, J. et al. Randomized Clinical Trial of EDTA Vs EDTA + DMSA in Lead (Pb) Poisoned Children. Pediatr Res 45, 65 (1999).
https://doi.org/10.1203/00006450-199904020-00388

[1858] Treatment Options for Mercury/Metal Toxicity in Autism and Related Developmental Disabilities: Consensus Position Paper; February 2005; AUTISM RESEARCH INSTITUTE; p. 6
https://vce.org/mercury/merctreat.pdf

[1859] visceralsynergy ; Challenge Testing for Heavy Metals
https://visceralsynergy.com/assets/challenge-testing-for-heavy-metals.pdf

[1860] URINE HEAVY METAL TESTING; The Healing Sanctuary
https://healingsanctuary.clinic/wp-content/uploads/handouts/services/Heavy%20Metal%20Testing.pdf

[1861] Zetpil test kit https://www.zetpilnutrition.com/product/dmsa-cana2edta-for-provocation-urine-test/

[1862] Muran PJ. 2006: Mercury elimination with oral DMPS, DMSA, vitamin C, and glutathione: an observational clinical review. Altern Ther Health Med. 2006
https://citeseerx.ist.psu.edu/document?repid=rep1&type=pdf&doi=c3561142922c93da4a18bcd6d bbd94f2069f2af2

[1863] Yuan, X., Chapman, R.L. and Wu, Z. (2011), Analytical methods for heavy metals in herbal medicines. Phytochem. Anal., 22: 189-198. https://doi.org/10.1002/pca.1287

[1864] Alexandre Soares Leal et al 2013: Determination of metals in medicinal plants highly consumed in Brazil; Brazilian Journal of Pharmaceutical Sciences vol. 49, n. 3, jul./sep., 2013;
https://www.scielo.br/j/bjps/a/WPdNC7Kdkjm5y8xCwR9TJRy/?format=pdf&lang=en

[1865] Shailendra K. Dwivedi & Sahadeb Dey (2002) Medicinal Herbs: A Potential Source of Toxic Metal Exposure for Man and Animals in India, Archives of Environmental Health: An International Journal, 57:3, 229-231, http://doi.org/10.1080/00039890209602941

[1866] U.S. Department of Health and Human Services NIH: Ayurvedic Medicine: In Depth;
https://www.nccih.nih.gov/health/ayurvedic-medicine-in-depth

[1867] health.state.mn Minnesota.gov : Metal Toxicity from Ayurvedic Medications;
https://www.health.state.mn.us/communities/environment/lead/fs/ayurvedic.html

[1868] E. Ernst. 2021: Heavy metals in traditional Indian remedies; ; . Eur J Clin Pharmacol 57, 891–896 (2002). https://doi.org/10.1007/s00228-001-0400-y

[1869] Saper RB, Kales SN, Paquin J, et al. Heavy metal content of ayurvedic herbal medicine products. JAMA. 2004;292(23): https://pubmed.ncbi.nlm.nih.gov/15598918/

[1870] Fernöstliche Bleivergiftung; Deutschlandfunk; Susanne Schrammar | 30.01.2009
https://www.deutschlandfunk.de/fernoestliche-bleivergiftung-100.html

[1871] SHU-MEI LI et al 2012: Heavy Metals in Chinese Therapeutic Foods and Herbs; J.Chem.Soc.Pak., Vol. 34, No.5, 2012;., p.1091: https://jcsp.org.pk/PublishedVersion/d2c6b93a-1690-4238-8cd7-ad2002b0568aManuscript%20no%206,%201st%20gally%20proof%20of%208998%20_Shu-Mei%20Li_.pdf

[1872] FDA In Brief: FDA releases test results identifying dangerous levels of heavy metals in certain kratom products. April 3, 2019; Media Inquiries; FDA Office of Media Affairs; 301-796-

4540; https://www.fda.gov/news-events/fda-brief/fda-brief-fda-releases-test-results-identifying-dangerous-levels-heavy-metals-certain-kratom

[1873] Li AM, Chan MHM, Leung TF, et al Mercury intoxication presenting with tics Archives of Disease in Childhood 2000;83:174-175. https://adc.bmj.com/content/83/2/174

[1874] Dinu, Cristina, , et al. 2021. "Toxic Metals (As, Cd, Ni, Pb) Impact in the Most Common Medicinal Plant (Mentha piperita)" International Journal of Environmental Research and Public Health 18, no. 8: https://doi.org/10.3390/ijerph18083904

[1875] Brannan, Elizabeth H. MD*; Su, Sharon MD*†; Alverson, Brian K. MD*†. Elemental Mercury Poisoning Presenting as Hypertension in a Young Child. Pediatric Emergency Care 28(8):p 812-814, August 2012. | https://www.researchgate.net/publication/230618913_Elemental_Mercury_Poisoning_Presenting_as_Hypertension_in_a_Young_Child

[1876] Țincu RC, , et al. 2016: Acute mercury poisoning from occult ritual use. Rom J Anaesth Intensive Care. 2016 https://www.ncbi.nlm.nih.gov/pmc/articles/PMC5505367/

[1877] New York Times: Ritual Use of Mercury Prompts Testing of Children for Illness; Dec. 14, 1997 By Mirta Ojito; https://www.nytimes.com/1997/12/14/nyregion/ritual-use-of-mercury-prompts-testing-of-children-for-illness.html

[1878] TASK FORCE ON RITUALISTIC USES OF MERCURY REPORT; United States Environmental Protection Agency; December 2002; https://clu-in.org/download/contaminantfocus/mercury/Task-Force-on-Ritualistic.pdf

[1879] Țincu RC, Cobilinschi C, Ghiorghiu Z, Macovei RA. Acute mercury poisoning from occult ritual use. Rom J Anaesth Intensive Care. 2016 Apr;23(1):73-76.. https://www.ncbi.nlm.nih.gov/pmc/articles/PMC5505367/ .

[1880] Țincu RC, Cobilinschi C, Acute mercury poisoning from occult ritual use. Rom J Anaesth Intensive Care. 2016 https://www.ncbi.nlm.nih.gov/pmc/articles/PMC5505367/ .

[1881] https://niguanta.wordpress.com/2019/04/15/gypsy-magic/

[1882] Ferrero, Maria Elena 2016: Rationale for the Successful Management of EDTA Chelation Therapy in Human Burden by Toxic Metals; Hindawi; Volume 2016 https://pubmed.ncbi.nlm.nih.gov/27896275/

[1883] Sukheeja, D. et al 2014 Subcutaneous Mercury Injection by a Child: AHistopathologicy Case Report: J. LabPhysicians 2014 Jan. Jun; 6 (1) http://doi.org/10.4103/0974-2727.129095

[1884] Krajcovicová-Kudládková M, Ursínyová M, Masánová V, Béderová A, Valachovicová M. Cadmium blood concentrations in relation to nutrition. Cent Eur J Public Health. 2006 Sep;14(3):126-9.. https://pubmed.ncbi.nlm.nih.gov/17152224/

[1885] Li, H., Fagerberg, B., Sallsten, G. et al. Smoking-induced risk of future cardiovascular disease is partly mediated by cadmium in tobacco: Malmö Diet and Cancer Cohort Study. Environ Health 18, 56 (2019). https://doi.org/10.1186/s12940-019-0495-1

[1886] Veganhealth.org; Cadmium; by Jack Norris, RD https://veganhealth.org/cadmium/

[1887] The Vegan Review: The heavy metals found in vegan protein powders By Tijen Najarian; https://theveganreview.com/the-heavy-metals-found-in-vegan-protein-powders/

[1888] Sean Callan 2018: New Study of Protein Powders from Clean Label Project Finds Elevated Levels of Heavy Metals and BPA in 53 Leading Brands; Denver, CO – February 27, 2018; https://cleanlabelproject.org/blog-post/new-study-of-protein-powders-from-clean-label-project-finds-elevated-levels-of-heavy-metals-and-bpa-in-53-leading-brands/

[1889] skinsalvationsf.com: acne-causing heavy metals in protein powders - how a client's own detective research cleared him up! By kerry Watson; September 03, 2018; https://skinsalvationsf.com/blogs/blog/acne-causing-heavy-metals-in-protein-powders-how-a-clients-own-detective-research-cleared-him-up

[1890] TIMESOFINDIA.COM Created: May 6, 2020, https://timesofindia.indiatimes.com/life-style/health-fitness/diet/vegetarians-and-vegans-are-more-likely-to-be-depressed-than-meat-eaters-claims-study/articleshow/75555301.cms

[1891] Joseph R. Hibbeln, Kate Northstone, Jonathan Evans, Jean Golding, 2018: Vegetarian diets and depressive symptoms among men, Journal of Affective Disorders, Volume 225, 2018, Pages 13-17, https://doi.org/10.1016/j.jad.2017.07.051.

[1892] Raehsler SL, Choung RS, Marietta EV, Murray JA. Accumulation of Heavy Metals in People on a Gluten-Free Diet. Clin Gastroenterol Hepatol. 2018 Feb;16(2):244-251. https://pubmed.ncbi.nlm.nih.gov/28223206/

[1893] https://www.pharmacytimes.com/view/does-ibuprofen-disrupt-testosterone-production#

[1894] Loren Cordain, et al, 2000: Plant-animal subsistence ratios and macronutrient energy estimations in worldwide hunter-gatherer diets, The American Journal of Clinical Nutrition, Volume 71, (https://www.sciencedirect.com/science/article/pii/S0002916523070582)

Notes

[1895] Patisaul, H. (2017). Endocrine disruption by dietary phyto-oestrogens: Impact on dimorphic sexual systems and behaviours. Proceedings of the Nutrition Society, 76(2), 130-144. http://doi:10.1017/S0029665116000677

[1896] Adgent, M. A., Daniels, J. L., Edwards, L. J., Siega-Riz, A. M., & Rogan, W. J. (2011). Early-life soy exposure and gender-role play behavior in children. Environmental health perspectives, 119(12), 1811–1816. https://doi.org/10.1289/ehp.1103579

[1897] Video: K G Vegans Before and After 1; parts 1-3 https://www.youtube.com/watch?v=9Qo9peKk_gQ&t=1160s

[1898] DeMartini, et al 2001: Lead Arthropathy and Systemic Lead Poisoning from an Intra-articular bullet; AJR 176; https://www.ajronline.org/doi/pdfplus/10.2214/ajr.176.5.1761144

[1899] TIME.com: They Survived Mass Shootings. Years Later, The Bullets Are Still Trying to Kill Them; Melissa Chan; May 31, 2019 https://time.com/longform/gun-violence-survivors-lead-poisoning/

[1900] Weiss D, Tomasallo CD, et al 2003: Elevated Blood Lead Levels Associated with Retained Bullet Fragments - United States, 2003-2012. MMWR Morb Mortal Wkly Rep. 2017 Feb 10;66(5):130-133. https://www.cdc.gov/mmwr/volumes/66/wr/mm6605a2.htm

[1901] CNN: Bullet fragments linked to lead poisoning, CDC study says CNN; Susan Scutti, Updated 0855 GMT (1655 HKT) February 13, 2017; https://edition.cnn.com/2017/02/13/health/bullets-blood-lead-study/index.html

[1902] Walker, JT: 1940: Bullet Holes and Chemical Residues in Shooting Cases; Northwestern University; Journal of Criminal Law and Criminology; Volume 31; Issue 4 https://scholarlycommons.law.northwestern.edu/cgi/viewcontent.cgi?article=2991&context=jclc

[1903] Pryor, A. (2021). The development of inductively coupled plasma mass spectrometry for use in the provenance establishment of lead projectiles. [Doctoral Thesis, The University of Western Australia]. https://doi.org/10.26182/an31-va68

[1904] Pogisego Dinake, Onneetse Maphane,et al: (Reviewing editor) (2018) Pollution status of shooting range soils from Cd, Cu, Mn, Ni and Zn found in ammunition, C. Envi Scie, 4:1 http://doi.org/10.1080/23311843.2018.1528701

[1905] Thiboutot, 2001: Evaluation of Heavy Metals Contamination at CFAD Dundurn Resulting from Small-Arms Ammunition Incineration; Defense Technical Information Center; https://apps.dtic.mil/sti/tr/pdf/ADA396586.pdf

[1906] Tindel, Nathaniel L. et al 2001: The Effect of Surgically Implanted Bullet Fragments on the Spinal Cord in a Rabbit Model; The Journal of Bone & Joint Surgery: June 2001 - Volume 83 - Issue 6 - https://pubmed.ncbi.nlm.nih.gov/11407797/

[1907] Ken-ichiro Nakao, Kazuhiko Kibayashi, Takashi Taki, and Hiroyoshi Koyama. Journal of Neurotrauma.Oct 2010. https://www.liebertpub.com/doi/abs/10.1089/neu.2010.1379

[1908] Linden MA, et al 1982: Lead poisoning from retained bullets. Pathogenesis, diagnosis, and management. Ann Surg. 1982 Mar;195(3) http://doi:10.1097/00000658-198203000-00010.

[1909] Bilen, Bukem et al 2018: Examination of metal mobilization from a gunshot by scanning acoustic microscopy, scanning electron microscopy, energy-dispersive X-ray spectroscopy, and inductively coupled plasma optical emission spectroscopy: a case report; Journal of Medical Case Reports volume 12, Article number: 391 (2018) https://link.springer.com/article/10.1186/s13256-018-1905-7

[1910] McQuirter, Joseph L. et al 2001: The Effects of Retained Lead Bullets on Body Lead Burden; June 2001; The Journal of trauma 50(5):892-9; https://www.researchgate.net/publication/11966133_The_Effects_of_Retained_Lead_Bullets_on_Body_Lead_Burden

[1911] Araújo GCSd, Mourão NT, Pinheiro IN, Xavier AR, Gameiro VS, 2015: Lead Toxicity Risks in Gunshot Victims. PLoS ONE 10(10) https://doi.org/10.1371/journal.pone.0140220;

[1912] Nickel WN, Steelman TJ, et al. Extra-Articular Retained Missiles; Is Surveillance of Lead Levels Needed? Mil Med. 2018 https://pubmed.ncbi.nlm.nih.gov/29365163/

[1913] Sclafani SJ, Vuletin JC, Twersky J. Lead arthropathy: arthritis caused by retained intra-articular bullets. Radiology. 1985 Aug; https://pubmed.ncbi.nlm.nih.gov/4011890/

[1914] Chandrasekar, Suraj, et al 2015; Systemic Lead Toxicity; Orthopedics. 2015;38(10):592, 644-647 https://doi.org/10.3928/01477447-20151002-01

[1915] Apte, Anisha MD; et al 2019: Lead toxicity from retained bullet fragments: A systematic review and meta-analysis, Journal of Trauma and Acute Care Surgery: September 2019 - Volume 87 - Issue 3 - https://pubmed.ncbi.nlm.nih.gov/30939573/

[1916] Eline Vandebroek, et al Occupational Exposure to Metals in Shooting Ranges: A Biomonitoring Study, Safety and Health at Work, Volume 10, Issue 1, 2019, https://doi.org/10.1016/j.shaw.2018.05.006.

[1917] Tariba B. Metals in wine--impact on wine quality and health outcomes. Biol Trace Elem Res. 2011 Dec;144(1-3):143-56. https://pubmed.ncbi.nlm.nih.gov/21479541/

[1918] Georgiana-Diana Dumitriu (Gabur), et al 2021: Heavy metals assessment in the major stages of winemaking: Chemometric analysis and impacts on human health and environment, Journal of Food Composition and Analysis, Volume 100, 2021, (https://www.sciencedirect.com/science/article/pii/S0889157521001356

[1919] Violina ANGELOVA, et al 1999: HEAVY METAL (Pb, Cu, Zn and Cd) CONTENT IN WINE PRODUCED FROM GRAPE CULTIVAR MAVRUD, GROWN IN AN INDUSTRIALLY POLLUTED REGION; J. Int. Sci. Vigne Vin, 1999, 33, n°3, 119-131 Vigne et Vin Publications Internationales (Bordeaux, France);

[1920] WebMD: Heavy Metals Found in Wine; Daniel J. DeNoon; Medically Reviewed by Louise Chang, MD on October 29, 2008; https://www.webmd.com/food-recipes/food-poisoning/news/20081029/heavy-metals-found-in-wine

[1921] Brent W. Morgan, et al, 2001: Elevated blood lead levels in urban moonshine drinkers, Annals of Emergency Medicine, Volume 37, Issue 1, 2001, Pages 51-54, https://doi.org/10.1067/mem.2001.111708.

[1922] Gerhardt RE, Crecelius EA, Hudson JB. Moonshine-related arsenic poisoning. Arch Intern Med. 1980 Feb;140(2):211-3. https://pubmed.ncbi.nlm.nih.gov/7352816/

[1923] Rezaie M, Abolhassanzadeh SZ, Haghighinejad H. Comparing serum lead level in drug abuse pregnant women with non-addicted pregnant mothers referring to Shiraz university hospitals in 2017-2018. J Family Med Prim Care. 2019 May;8(5):1653-1657 https://www.ncbi.nlm.nih.gov/pmc/articles/PMC6559079/ .

[1924] Aghababaei R, Javadi I, Nili-Ahmadabadi A, Parsafar S, Ahmadimoghaddam D. Occurrence of bacterial and toxic metals contamination in illegal opioid-like drugs in Iran: a significant health challenge in drug abusers. Daru. 2018 Sep;26(1):77-83. https://www.ncbi.nlm.nih.gov/pmc/articles/PMC6154484/

[1925] Fishbein, Diana H., et al 2008: Relationship between lead exposure, cognitive function, and drug addiction: Pilot study and research agenda,; Environmental Research,; Volume 108, Issue 3,; 2008, (https://www.sciencedirect.com/science/article/pii/S0013935108001576)

[1926] Busse FP, Fiedler GM, Leichtle A, Lead poisoning due to adulterated marijuana in leipzig. Dtsch Arztebl Int. 2008 https://pubmed.ncbi.nlm.nih.gov/19623274/

[1927] McGraw KE, Nigra AE, Klett J, et al. Blood and urinary metal levels among exclusive marijuana users in nhanes (2005–2018). Environ Health Perspect. 2023 https://doi.org/10.1289/EHP12074

[1928] Banafshe HR, Ghaderi A. Thallium Intoxication in Relation to Drug Abuse and Cigarette Smoking in Iran. International Journal of Medical Toxicology and Forensic Medicine. 2018; 8(2):41-44. https://journals.sbmu.ac.ir/ijmtfm/article/view/22090

[1929] Salimi, Majid & Assareh, Mohammad & Khodayar, Mohammad & Mousavi, Zahra. (2017). Investigating the Source of Contamination Opioid into Lead in Forensic Medicine. Journal of Heavy Metal Toxicity and Diseases. https://www.primescholars.com/articles/investigating-the-source-of-contamination-opioid-into-lead-in-forensic-medicine.pdf

[1930] Alinejad, S., Aaseth, J., Abdollahi, M., Hassanian-Moghaddam, H. and Mehrpour, O. (2018), Clinical Aspects of Opium Adulterated with Lead in Iran: A Review. Basic Clin Pharmacol Toxicol, 122: 56-64. https://doi.org/10.1111/bcpt.12855

[1931] Soltaninejad K, Shadnia S. Lead Poisoning in Opium Abuser in Iran: A Systematic Review. Int J Prev Med. 2018 Jan 5;9:3.

[1932] Hayatbakhsh, M.M., Oghabian, Z., Conlon, E. et al. Lead poisoning among opium users in Iran: an emerging health hazard. Subst Abuse Treat Prev Policy 12, 43 (2017). https://doi.org/10.1186/s13011-017-0127-0

[1933] Bernhard, David; et al 2005: Metals in Cigarette Smoke; IUBMB Life, 57(12): 805 – 809, Decr 2005 https://iubmb.onlinelibrary.wiley.com/doi/pdf/10.1080/15216540500459667

[1934] Li, Y, Wu, F, Mu, Q, et al. 2022: Metal ions in cerebrospinal fluid: Associations with anxiety, depression, and insomnia among cigarette smokers. CNS Neurosci Ther. 2022; 28: 2141- 2147. Http://doi:10.1111/cns.13955

[1935] N. Abd El-Aziz, et al 2005: Natural radioactivity contents in tobacco, International Congress Series, Volume 1276, 2005,, https://doi.org/10.1016/j.ics.2004.11.166.

[1936] José Ignacio de Granda-Orivea, et al 2020: E-waste: Rare earth elements, new toxic substances in cigarettes and electronic cigarettes; Archivos de Bronconeumologia Vol. 56. Issue 8. pages 477-478 (August 2020) http://doi.org/10.1016/j.arbr.2019.10.011

[1937] Hammer, D. I.,et al (1973). Cadmium and Lead in Autopsy Tissues. Journal of Occupational Medicine, 15(12), 956–963. http://www.jstor.org/stable/45010941

[1938] Caruso RV, et al: Toxic metal concentrations in cigarettes obtained from U.S. smokers in 2009: results from the International Tobacco Control (ITC) United States survey cohort. Int J Env Res Public Health. 2013 https://www.ncbi.nlm.nih.gov/pmc/articles/PMC3924441/

Notes

[1939] World Health Organization: Chapter 6.3 Cadmium;
https://www.euro.who.int/__data/assets/pdf_file/0016/123073/AQG2ndEd_6_3Cadmium.PDF

[1940] cen.acs.org; 26 Mar 2020 https://cen.acs.org/safety/consumer-safety/Vaping-exposes-users-toxic-metals/98/i12

[1941] Fowles J, Barreau T, Wu N. Cancer and Non-Cancer Risk Concerns from Metals in Electronic Cigarette Liquids and Aerosols. Int J Environ Res Public Health. 2020 Mar 24;17(6):2146. https://www.ncbi.nlm.nih.gov/pmc/articles/PMC7142621/

[1942] Hess, Catherine Ann, Olmedo Pablo, et al, 2017: E-cigarettes as a source of toxic and potentially carcinogenic metals, Environmental Research, Volume 152, 2017, (https://www.sciencedirect.com/science/article/pii/S0013935116306995)

[1943] Zhao D, Aravindakshan A, Hilpert M, Olmedo P, Rule AM, Navas-Acien A, Aherrera A. Metal/Metalloid Levels in Electronic Cigarette Liquids, Aerosols, and Human Biosamples: A Systematic Review. Environ Health Perspect. 2020 Mar;128(3):36001.

[1944] NIH: Environmental Factor; Your Online Source for NIEHS News; FEBRUARY 2022; https://factor.niehs.nih.gov/2022/2/feature/3-feature-e-cigarettes-and-toxic-metals

[1945] Badea, Mihaela, et al 2018: Body burden of toxic metals and rare earth elements in non-smokers, cigarette smokers and electronic cigarette users, Environmental Research, Volume 166, 2018, https://doi.org/10.1016/j.envres.2018.06.007.

[1946] Smokers urged to weigh the 'facts' during the 'Great American Smoke-Out,' Vital Signs, The Daily Progress, Charlottesville, Virginia, Nov. 14, 1993, by June Russell, Smoke-Free Charlottesville https://www.medicalnewstoday.com/releases/9703#1

[1947] UCLA https://www.uclahealth.org/news/no-such-thing-as-harmless-tobacco-products#:~:text=Smokeless%20tobacco%20also%20contains%20heavy,as%20the%20tobacco%20plant%20grows.&text=Smokeless%20products%20may%20spare%20the,developing%20a%20range%20of%20cancers.

[1948] Whashington Post: Ink and infection: 10 percent have skin problems after getting tattoos; Lenny Bernstein; May 28, 2015; https://www.washingtonpost.com/news/to-your-health/wp/2015/05/28/ink-and-infection-10-percent-have-skin-problems-after-getting-tattoos/

[1949] Medermislaserclinic: Tattoo Ink Safety: What Are They Made From ?; https://medermislaserclinic.com/blog/what-are-tattoo-inks-made-from/

[1950] Schreiver, I., Hesse, B., Seim, C. et al. 2017: Synchrotron-based v-XRF mapping and µ-FTIR microscopy enable to look into the fate and effects of tattoo pigments in human skin. Sci Rep 7 https://doi.org/10.1038/s41598-017-11721-z

[1951] AGING MATTERS MAGAZINE ; Think before you ink – tattoos can take a toll on your body; September 5th, 2019; https://aging-matters.com/think-before-you-ink-tattoos-can-take-a-toll-on-your-body/

[1952] Inter Clinic Labratories; TOXINS IN TATTOO INKS AND HEALTH IMPACTS 26 July 2023; https://interclinical.com.au/newsletter/toxins-in-tattoo-inks-and-health-impacts/

[1953] psychcentral.com People With Tattoos More Likely to Also Have Mental Health Issues; https://psychcentral.com/news/2019/01/27/people-with-tattoos-more-likely-to-also-have-mental-health-issues#1

[1954] Raspa RF, Cusack J. Psychiatric implications of tattoos. Am Fam Physician. 1990 May;41(5):1481-6. https://pubmed.ncbi.nlm.nih.gov/2333825/

[1955] Study: Rate of homicidal poisoning is increasing; UGA today. .

[1956] Soltaninejad K. Poison and Drugs Used in Homicidal Poisoning: A Systematic Review http://doi.org(10.23880/ijfsc-16000335

[1957] U.S. Attorney's Office FBI: Kimber Pleads Guilty to Using Mercury as a Chemical Weapon at Albany Medical Center; November 29, 2012; https://archives.fbi.gov/archives/albany/press-releases/2012/kimber-pleads-guilty-to-using-mercury-as-a-chemical-weapon-at-albany-medical-center

[1958] Kern, Janet & Geier, David et al (2014). Evidence supporting a link between dental amalgams and chronic illness, fatigue, depression, anxiety, and suicide. Neuro endocrinology letters. 35. 537-552. https://www.researchgate.net/publication/271536688_Evidence_supporting_a_link_between_dental_amalgams_and_chronic_illness_fatigue_depression_anxiety_and_suicide

[1959] https://en.wikipedia.org/wiki/List_of_sovereign_states_by_body_mass_index

[1960] Jayasumana C, Fonseka S,et al 2015: Phosphate fertilizer is a main source of arsenic in areas affected with chronic kidney disease of unknown etiology in Sri Lanka. Springerplus. 2015 Feb 24;4:90. https://doi.org/10.1186/s40064-015-0868-z

[1961] Environmental distribution of heavy metals on Nauru, Central Pacific, and possible relationships to human health; Nauru Environmental Data Portal; https://nauru-data.sprep.org/resource/environmental-distribution-heavy-metals-nauru-central-pacific-and-possible-relationships

[1962] Tubing Yin 2019; Effects of acid and phosphate on arsenic solidification in a phosphogypsum-based cement backfill process; RSC Adv., 2019, 9, 28095; https://pubs.rsc.org/en/content/articlepdf/2019/ra/c9ra04624k

[1963] Khelifi F, Caporale AG,et al: Bioaccessibility of potentially toxic metals in soil, sediments and tailings from a north Africa phosphate-mining area: Insight into human health risk assessment. J E. M. 2021 https://doi.org/10.1016/j.jenvman.2020.111634

[1964] Sabiha-Javied, T. Mehmood, et al 2008:, Heavy metal pollution from phosphate rock used for the production of fertilizer in Pakistan, Microchemical Journal, V. 91, I. 1 https://doi.org/10.1016/j.microc.2008.08.009.

[1965] Chen, Y.-p et al. 2018: Environmental toxicants impair liver and kidney function and sperm quality of captive pandas; Ecotoxicology and Environmental Safety 162 (2018) 218–224; https://harvardforest.fas.harvard.edu/sites/default/files/ellison-pubs/2018/Chen-etal_2018-EES.pdf

[1966] Chen, Yi-ping, Ying-juan Zheng, Qiang Liu, Yi Song, Zhi-sheng An, Qing-yi Ma, and Aaron M. Ellison. 2017. "Atmospheric Deposition Exposes Qinling Pandas to Toxic Pollutants." Ecological Applications 27 (2) (March): http://doi.org/10.1002/eap.1494.

[1967] Zheng YJ, Chen YP, Maltby L, Jin XL. Highway increases concentrations of toxic metals in giant panda habitat. Environ Sci Pollut Res Int. 2016 Nov;23(21):21262-21272. http://doi.org/10.1007/s11356-016-7221-0.

[1968] Tian, Z., Liu, X., Sun, W. et al. Characteristics of heavy metal concentrations and risk assessment for giant pandas and their habitat in the Qinling Mountains, China. Environ Sci Pollut Res 27, 1569–1584 (2020). https://doi.org/10.1007/s11356-019-06769-5

[1969] Fangyuan Bian, Zheke Zhong, et al: Bamboo – An untapped plant resource for the phytoremediation of heavy metal contaminated soils, Chemosphere, Volume 246, 2020, https://doi.org/10.1016/j.chemosphere.2019.125750.

[1970] M. De Keersmaecker et al. A Short Historical Overview on the Use of Lead; Universiteit Gent; Academic Bibliography; https://biblio.ugent.be/publication/8558334/file/8558350.pdf

[1971] NDNR: METAL AND MINERAL TOXICITY PRESENTING AS NEUROLOGICAL COMPLAINTS; By Editor1 Posted December 28, 2008 https://ndnr.com/neurology/metal-and-mineral-toxicity-presenting-as-neurological-complaints-2/

[1972] ARCHIBALD ANNA; The Disturbingly Long History of Lead Toxicity in Winemaking BY https://www.winemag.com/2020/07/20/lead-toxicity-wine-history/

[1973] M. De Keersmaecker et al. A Short Historical Overview on the Use of Lead; Universiteit Gent; Acad. Biblio; https://biblio.ugent.be/publication/8558334/file/8558350.pdf

[1974] Dr. Herbert L. Needleman; HISTORY OF LEAD POISONING IN THE WORLD; http://103.24.47.157/history_of_lead_poisoning_in_the_world.htm

[1975] Lead poisoning in ancient Rome; Encyclopaedia Romana; http://penelope.uchicago.edu/~grout/encyclopaedia_romana/wine/leadpoisoning.html

[1976] Aneni, Monica. (2018). Lead Poisoning in Ancient Rome. Department of Classics, University of Ibadan; https://www.researchgate.net/publication/325023100_Lead_Poisoning_in_Ancient_Rome

[1977] Aneni, Monica. (2018). Lead Poisoning in Ancient Rome. Department of Classics, University of Ibadan; https://www.researchgate.net/publication/325023100_Lead_Poisoning_in_Ancient_Rome

[1978] Joanna Moore, et al 2021: The Family in Past Perspective; Edition 1st Edition; First Published 2021; Imprint Routledge; P. 22

[1979] Sohn, Emily; Lead: Versatile Metal, Long Legacy; Dartmouth Toxic Metals Superfund Research Program; ; https://sites.dartmouth.edu/toxmetal/more-metals/lead-versatile-metal-long-legacy/

[1980] GVGK Tang ; Of Gods & Emperors: Trans Experiences in Ancient Rome; https://notchesblog.com/2017/11/14/of-gods-emperors-trans-experiences-in-ancient-rome/

[1981] Challenging Gender Boundaries: A Trans Biography Project by Students of Catherine Jacquet; Fall 2012 class at the University of Illinois, Chicago. https://outhistory.org/exhibits/show/tgi-bios/elagabalus#:~:text=Castration%2C%20according%20to%20Dio%20Cassius,would%20toda y%20be%20called%20transsexualism.

[1982] Wikipedia, Elagabalus, Aug 8 2014: https://en.wikipedia.org/wiki/Elagabalus#:~:text=Dio%20says%20that%20Elagabalus%20prostitu ted,mistress%2C%20wife%2C%20and%20queen.

[1983]https://en.wikipedia.org/wiki/Elagabalus#:~:text=The%20Augustan%20History%20claims%20 that,that%20Zoticus%20was%20his%20cubicularius.

[1984] Wikipedia: Homosexuality in ancient Rome; 8.8. 2024 https://en.wikipedia.org/wiki/Homosexuality_in_ancient_Rome

Notes

[1985] Lead poisoning in ancient Rome; Encyclopaedia Romana;
http://penelope.uchicago.edu/~grout/encyclopaedia_romana/wine/leadpoisoning.html
[1986] Healthliine, How Alcohol Affects Testosterone; https://www.healthline.com/health/how-alcohol-affects-testosterone
[1987] Retief, FP; Cilliers, L. 2005: LEAD POISONING IN ANCIENT ROME; Acta Theologica Supplementum 7 Vol. 26 No. 2 https://www.ajol.info/index.php/actat/article/view/52570
[1988] Olalla López-Costas, et al 2020: Human bones tell the story of atmospheric mercury and lead exposure at the edge of Roman World, Science of The Total Environment, Volume 710, 2020, https://doi.org/10.1016/j.scitotenv.2019.136319.
[1989] López-Costas, Olalla, et al 2020: Human bones tell the story of atmospheric mercury and lead exposure at the edge of Roman World,; Science of The Total Environment,; V. 710,; 2020 https://doi.org/10.1016/j.scitotenv.2019.136319.(https://www.sciencedirect.com/science/article/pii/S0048969719363156)
[1990] Siblerud RL, Motl J, Kienholz E. Psychometric evidence that mercury from silver dental fillings may be an etiological factor in depression, excessive anger, and anxiety. Psychol Rep. 1994 Feb;74(1):67-80. http://doi.org/10.2466/pr0.1994.74.1.67.
[1991] Zhu X, Kusaka Y, Sato K, Zhang Q. The endocrine disruptive effects of mercury. Environ Health Prev Med. 2000 Jan;4(4):174-83. http://doi.org/10.1007/BF02931255.
[1992] New York Met:, The Story of Cinnabar and Vermilion (HgS) at The Met February 28, 2018 Ellen Spindler, Volunteer, Department of Objects Conservation https://www.metmuseum.org/blogs/collection-insights/2018/cinnabar-vermilion
[1993] Seeker; John Dyer; Antimony Poisoning — Not Lead — May Have Contributed to the Roman Empire's Fall; Analysis of a 2,000-year-old Roman pipe fragment from Pompeii revealed traces of antimony, a chemical that's even more toxic than lead. 8/17/2017
[1994] Sax L. 2010: Polyethylene terephthalate may yield endocrine disruptors. Environ Health Perspect. 2010 Apr;118(4):445-8. http://doi.org10.1289/ehp.0901253.
[1995] Duncan E. Cook, et al 2022:: Novel Insights into Mercury Sources and Behavior in the Surface Earth Environment; Environmental legacy of pre-Columbian Maya mercury Front. Environ. Sci., 23 September 2022; Sec. Toxicology, Pollution and the Environment Volume 10 - 2022 | https://doi.org/10.3389/fenvs.2022.986119 www.frontiersin.org
[1996] The guardian: Researcher reports 'large quantities' of the substance under ruins of Teotihuacan in discovery that could shed light on city's mysterious leaders. Alan Yuhas in New York; 24 Apr 2015; https://www.theguardian.com/world/2015/apr/24/liquid-mercury-mexican-pyramid-teotihuacan
[1997] Philippe Grandjean & Clair C. Patterson (1988) Ancient Skeletons as Silent Witnesses of Lead Exposures in the Past, CRC Critical Reviews in Toxicology, 19: http://doi.org/10.3109/10408448809040815
[1998] Patterson C, Ericson J, Manea-Krichten M, Shirahata H. Natural skeletal levels of lead in Homo sapiens sapiens uncontaminated by technological lead. Sci Total Environ. 1991 Sep; 107:205-236.
[1999] Zbigniew Jaworowski, et al 1985; Heavy metals in human and animal bones from ancient and contemporary France, Science of The Total Environment, Volume 43, Issues 1–2, 1985, Pages 103-126, https://doi.org/10.1016/0048-9697(85)90034-8. (https://www.sciencedirect.com/science/article/pii/0048969785900348)
[2000] Zbigniew Jaworowski, et al 1985; Heavy metals in human and animal bones from ancient and contemporary France, Science of The Total Environment, Volume 43, Issues 1–2, 1985, Pages 103-126, https://doi.org/10.1016/0048-9697(85)90034-8. (https://www.sciencedirect.com/science/article/pii/0048969785900348)
[2001] González-Reimers, E. et al 2003: Bone cadmium and lead in prehistoric inhabitants and domestic animals from Gran Canaria, Science of The Total Environment, Volume 301, Issues 1–3, 2003, (https://www.sciencedirect.com/science/article/pii/S0048969702002991)
[2002] M. Arnay-de-la-Rosa, et al (2003) Bone Cadmium and Lead in 18th Century Population Groups from the Canary Islands, Journal of Trace and Microprobe Techniques, 21:1, http://doi.org/10.1081/TMA-120017916
[2003] Monge, G., Jimenez-Espejo, F., García-Alix, A. et al. Earliest evidence of pollution by heavy metals in açrchaeological sites. Sci Rep 5, (2015). https://doi.org/10.1038/srep14252